New Insights into Immunology and Microbiology

New Insights into Immunology and Microbiology

Editor: Addison Boyd

AMERICAN
MEDICAL PUBLISHERS
www.americanmedicalpublishers.com

AMERICAN
MEDICAL PUBLISHERS
www.americanmedicalpublishers.com

Cataloging-in-Publication Data

New insights into immunology and microbiology / edited by Addison Boyd.
p. cm.
Includes bibliographical references and index.
ISBN 979-8-88740-332-8
1. Immunology. 2. Microbiology. 3. Clinical immunology. 4. Medical microbiology. I. Boyd, Addison.
QR181 .N49 2023
616.079--dc23

American Medical Publishers,
41 Flatbush Avenue,
1st Floor, New York,
NY 11217, USA

ISBN 979-8-88740-332-8 (Hardback)

Contents

Preface

Over the recent decade, advancements and applications have progressed exponentially. This has led to the increased interest in this field and projects are being conducted to enhance knowledge. The main objective of this book is to present some of the critical challenges and provide insights into possible solutions. This book will answer the varied questions that arise in the field and also provide an increased scope for furthering studies.

Microbiology comprises the study of various microorganisms like bacteria, fungi and viruses. It is focused on gaining knowledge of all the aspects associated with these microorganisms, like physiology, behavior, biochemistry, evolution and ecology. It also assesses the pathology of the disease caused by them. According to the taxonomy, various branches of microbiology include bacteriology, nematology, protozoology, immunology, parasitology, mycology, and phycology. Microbiology includes a range of subsets from immunology, from genetic engineering to microbial genetics. Immunology studies the manner in which the immune system in humans protects them from microbes causing infectious disease. It is concerned with understanding the relationships between the hosts and pathogens like viruses and bacteria. The integrated approach to immunology and microbiology can be utilized in understanding the effect that microbes have on the health of humans. This book unfolds the innovative aspects of immunology and medical microbiology, which will be crucial for the progress of this field in the future. It will provide comprehensive knowledge to the readers.

I hope that this book, with its visionary approach, will be a valuable addition and will promote interest among readers. Each of the authors has provided their extraordinary competence in their specific fields by providing different perspectives as they come from diverse nations and regions. I thank them for their contributions.

Editor

1

Emergence of CD4+ and CD8+ Polyfunctional T Cell Responses Against Immunodominant Lytic and Latent EBV Antigens in Children with Primary EBV Infection

Janice K. P. Lam[1†], K. F. Hui[1†], Raymond J. Ning[1], X. Q. Xu[1], K. H. Chan[2] and Alan K. S. Chiang[1]*

[1] Department of Paediatrics and Adolescent Medicine, Li Ka Shing Faculty of Medicine, Queen Mary Hospital, The University of Hong Kong, Pokfulam, Hong Kong, [2] Department of Microbiology, Li Ka Shing Faculty of Medicine, Queen Mary Hospital, The University of Hong Kong, Pokfulam, Hong Kong

***Correspondence:**
Alan K. S. Chiang
chiangak@hku.hk

† These authors have contributed equally to this work.

Long term carriers were shown to generate robust polyfunctional T cell (PFC) responses against lytic and latent antigens of Epstein-Barr virus (EBV). However, the time of emergence of PFC responses against EBV antigens, pattern of immunodominance and difference between CD4+ and CD8+ T cell responses during various stages of EBV infection are not clearly understood. A longitudinal study was performed to assess the development of antigen-specific PFC responses in children diagnosed to have primary symptomatic (infectious mononucleosis [IM]) and asymptomatic (AS) EBV infection. Evaluation of IFN-γ secreting CD8+ T cell responses upon stimulation by HLA class I-specific peptides of EBV lytic and latent proteins by ELISPOT assay followed by assessment of CD4+ and CD8+ PFC responses upon stimulation by a panel of overlapping EBV peptides for co-expression of IFN-γ, TNF-α, IL-2, perforin and CD107a by flow cytometry were performed. Cytotoxicity of T cells against autologous lymphoblastoid cell lines (LCLs) as well as EBV loads in PBMC and plasma were also determined. Both IM and AS patients had elevated PBMC and plasma viral loads which declined steadily during a 12-month period from the time of diagnosis whilst decrease in the magnitude of CD8+ T cell responses toward EBV lytic peptides in contrast to increase toward latent peptides was shown with no significant difference between those of IM and AS patients. Both lytic and latent antigen-specific CD4+ and CD8+ T cells demonstrated polyfunctionality (defined as greater or equal to three functions) concurrent with enhanced cytotoxicity against autologous LCLs and steady decrease in plasma and PBMC viral loads over time. Immunodominant peptides derived from BZLF1, BRLF1, BMLF1 and EBNA3A-C proteins induced the highest proportion of CD8+ as well as CD4+ PFC responses. Diverse functional subtypes of both CD4+ and CD8+ PFCs were shown to emerge at 6–12 months. In conclusion, EBV antigen-specific CD4+ and CD8+ PFC responses emerge during the first year of primary EBV infection, with greatest responses toward immunodominant epitopes in both lytic and latent proteins, correlating to steady decline in PBMC and plasma viral loads.

Keywords: EBV, polyfunctional T cells, immunodominance, infectious mononucleosis, asymptomatic primary infection

INTRODUCTION

Epstein-Barr virus (EBV) is a human gamma-1 herpes virus which infects more than 95% of the population (Young and Rickinson, 2004). This virus is strongly associated with a range of lymphoid and epithelial malignancies and autoimmune diseases (Longnecker and Neipel, 2007; Posnett, 2008; Salvetti et al., 2009). EBV preferentially infects naïve B cells at oropharyngeal lymphoid tissues and subsequently establishes a persistent infection in the circulating memory B cells (Babcock et al., 1998; Rickinson et al., 2014). Once EBV establishes a latent infection, it downregulates the expression of most of the viral genes thereby evading the host immune responses (Kurth et al., 2000). Primary EBV infection typically occurs during childhood without apparent clinical symptoms and evolves into a non-symptomatic persistent virus carrier state (Hislop et al., 2007). Delayed primary infection in some individuals leads to the development of a self-limiting disease called infectious mononucleosis (IM) (Krabbe et al., 1981; Sumaya and Ench, 1985; Niedobitek et al., 1997; Rickinson et al., 2014). EBV has transforming capability as manifested by the occurrence of uncontrolled malignant B cell proliferation in immunosuppressed individuals such as solid organ or stem cell transplantation recipients (Murukesan and Mukherjee, 2012).

The understanding of the mechanisms by which the human immune system controls EBV infection is incomplete due to the difficulties in identifying specific EBV peptides across a wide range of HLA alleles and the fact that EBV can express a large number of lytic and latent proteins displaying hierarchy of immunodominance in its life cycle (Pudney et al., 2005). IM, which is characterized by large expansions of CD8+ T cells and NK cells, provides an excellent model for the study of immune responses against EBV (Callan et al., 1996; Rickinson et al., 2014). The current knowledge on EBV-specific T-cell immunity is mostly derived from studies of IM peripheral blood mononuclear cell (PBMC) samples using either MHC-specific tetramers to determine the percentages of EBV-specific T cells or Enzyme-linked immunosorbent spot (ELISPOT) assay to detect the production of interferon-gamma (IFN-γ) by EBV-specific CD8+ T cells (McCutcheon et al., 1997; Schmittel et al., 1997; Helms et al., 2000; Jennes et al., 2002). However, the functional roles of CD4+ and CD8+ T cells in the control of EBV infection are not completely understood.

Polyfunctional T cells (PFC) are T cells which have multiple functions, such as degranulation of cytotoxic proteins and production of multiple cytokines such as IFN-γ, tumor necrosis factor-alpha (TNF-α), interleukin-2 (IL-2) simultaneously. Accumulating evidence suggests that PFC are associated with more effective control of chronic microbial infections including human immunodeficiency virus (HIV), hepatitis C virus (HCV), and cytomegalovirus (CMV) (Harari et al., 2005; Casazza et al., 2006; Ciuffreda et al., 2008; Duvall et al., 2008; Qiu et al., 2012). We and other groups have studied EBV-specific PFC in long term carriers and found that they produced more cytokines per cell than the single functional T cells and may be functionally superior (Smith et al., 2009; Ning et al., 2011). Another study found that frequencies of PFC were higher in HIV non-progressors than in progressors (Betts et al., 2006). Interestingly, a recent study demonstrated that polyfunctional and IFN-γ mono-functional CD4+ T cells are molecularly distinct and the polyfunctional gene signatures in response to *Plasmodium falciparum* infection and influenza infection were highly conserved (Burel et al., 2017). These findings support the notion that PFC contribute to more robust T-cell immunity in the control of virus infections. However, how PFC arise during primary EBV infection and evolve over time as well as their role in the long term control of EBV from primary infection stage to long term persistence remain unclear.

Here, we conducted a longitudinal study to assess the development and maturation of T cell responses to EBV from acute infection stage to long term persistence in two primary infection cohorts in children, those presenting as IM and those as asymptomatic primary infection (AS). ELISPOT assay was first performed to detect the IFN-γ secreting CD8+ T cell responses upon stimulation by HLA class I-specific peptides of EBV lytic and latent proteins in 18 longitudinally followed IM cases and 12 AS cases. A 9-color flow cytometric assay which simultaneously delineates five parameters: production of IFN-γ, perforin, TNF-α and IL-2, and surface mobilization of CD107a (degranulation marker), upon stimulation by overlapping peptide pools of 4 EBV lytic and 5 latent cycle proteins was then performed to further evaluate the EBV-specific CD4+ and CD8+ PFC responses in another 11 IM cases. Corresponding PBMC and plasma viral loads were determined as measurement of viral control. T cell lysis against autologous lymphoblastoid cell line (LCL) in three IM patients was measured to assess the cytotoxic function of the EBV-specific T cells.

MATERIALS AND METHODS

Subject Recruitment

Two cohorts of study subjects consisting of 29 children with infectious mononucleosis (IM) and 12 with asymptomatic primary infection (AS) were recruited. Serological screening for EBV was performed to confirm their primary infection state of EBV (Supplementary Table 1). Children with positive viral capsid antigen (VCA)-IgM, VCA-IgG, negative EBNA1 IgG and showed clinical symptoms were identified as IM subjects. For those who showed a serological profile of primary EBV infection with positive or negative VCA-IgM, positive VCA-IgG, negative EBNA1 and low VCA-IgG avidity without symptoms were recruited as AS subjects. As the maturation of VCA-IgG antibody from low to high avidity takes up to 6 months, AS patients were estimated to have been infected by EBV within a period of 6 months. Heparinized peripheral blood samples were collected at the time of first examination and subsequently, at 1, 2–5, and 6–12 months after diagnosis for the longitudinal study. Plasma was isolated and stored in −80°C until use. Peripheral blood mononuclear cells (PBMC) were isolated by standard Ficoll-Hypaque density gradient method. Collected PBMC were cryopreserved in fetal bovine serum (FBS) (Invitrogen, Carlsbad, CA, United States) with 10% DMSO under liquid nitrogen until use. All patient samples were handled as potential biohazardous material following the institutional safety procedures. The study protocol was approved by the Institutional Review Board of the University of Hong Kong. Informed written consent was obtained from each participant prior to the study.

DNA Extraction, HLA Typing and Quantitative PCR (qPCR)

Qiagen DNeasy blood mini kit (Qiagen) and NucliSENS easyMag instrument (BioMerieux) were used to extract DNA from PBMC and plasma, respectively, in accordance to the manufacturer's instruction. Part of the DNA samples were transferred to The University of Birmingham and the HLA laboratory in Queen Mary Hospital, The University of Hong Kong for HLA typing. The HLA types of all subjects recruited in ELISPOT assay were documented (Supplementary Table 3). The rest of the DNA was used to measure the EBV loads by qPCR with ABI PRISM 7900 sequence detector (Applied Biosystems, United States). EBV loads in PBMC were determined by the amplification of viral DNA polymerase (Pol, BALF5) sequence. Human β2 microglobulin sequence was detected as an internal control. Plasma EBV loads were quantified by expression of the BamH1W repeats in the EBV genome.

Synthetic EBV Peptides

Two types of synthetic peptides consisting of 24 HLA class I-restricted peptides and 9 overlapping peptide pools were utilized. All HLA class I-restricted peptides were kindly provided by Professor Alan B. Rickinson (The University of Birmingham, Birmingham, United Kingdom) and their sequences and identities are listed in Supplementary Table 2. The HLA class-I restricted peptides were diluted into 2 μg/mL in CTL-Test Medium (Cellular Technology Limited, United States) and 100 μl was added to each well in 96-well plate. Fifteen-mer peptides overlapped by 11 amino acids spanning each of the EBV latent proteins, EBNA1, EBNA3A, EBNA3B, EBNA3C and LMP2 and the lytic proteins, BZLF1, BRLF1, BMLF1 and GP350 were purchased from JPT Peptide Technologies, Berlin, Germany. The lyophilized peptide pools of each EBV protein were reconstituted according to manufacturer's instruction. Final concentration of overlapping peptides was 10 μg/ml per million cells. The HLA class-I restricted peptides were used in the ELISPOT assay and overlapping peptides were used in the flow cytometric analysis.

ELISPOT Assay

Interferon-gamma (IFN-γ) producing EBV-specific CD8+ T cell responses were quantified in duplicate by ELISPOT assay. Cryopreserved PBMC and HLA class-I restricted peptides were used. The peptide epitopes tested for each individual were listed in Supplementary Table 3. Wells containing phytohemagglutinin (PHA) (1 mg/ml) were used as positive control and wells with only cells were used as a negative control. IFN-γ producing cells were counted by immunospot plate reader (Cellular Technology Limited-ImmunoSpot S5 Macro Analyzer) and expressed in spot-forming cells (SFC)/10^6 PBMC. Spots were defined as positive when the SFC/10^6 PBMC was higher than 20. Only positive results were reported in the present study.

Expansion of T Cells

For better sensitivity of the flow cytometric analysis, the EBV lytic and latent protein-specific T cells were expanded by adding recombinant IL-4 and IL-7 according to a protocol provided by Professor Cliona M Rooney, Baylor College of Medicine, United States (Jones et al., 2010; Gerdemann et al., 2011). In brief, cryopreserved PBMC were thawed and washed with 10% FBS in RPMI 1640. Cells were seeded and incubated with relevant peptide pools, IL-4 and IL-7 at 2 μg/ml, 1000 U/ml and 10 ng/ml (PreproTech) respectively for 5 days at 37°C, 5% CO_2 in 24-well plate (1×10^6 PBMC/ml). PBMC cultured with IL-4 and IL-7 for 5 days were used as negative control.

Re-stimulation of T Cells

After expansion of T cells for 5 days, PBMC were rested overnight at 37°C, 5% CO_2 prior to peptide re-stimulation. PBMC were then re-stimulated with corresponding overlapping peptide pools at 2 μg/ml, together with PE-Cy5-conjugated anti-CD107a monoclonal antibody (BD Biosciences Pharmingen, United States), co-stimulatory reagents containing anti-CD28 monoclonal antibody at 1 μg/ml (BD Pharmingen, United States), anti-CD49d monoclonal antibody at 1 μg/ml (BD Pharmingen, United States) and brefeldin A at 10 μg/ml (BD Biosciences Pharmingen, United States) for 6 h at 37°C, 5% CO_2. Cells stimulated with 1 μg/ml staphylococcal enterotoxin B (SEB) were used as a positive control whereas unstimulated PBMC were used as negative control. Both positive and a negative controls were treated with the same costimulatory reagents.

Flow Cytometric Analysis

After incubation for 6 h, the treated cells were washed in PBS and stained with Aqua Blue Dye (Invitrogen, United States) for 20 min for dead cell exclusion. APC-Cy7-conjugated anti-CD3 (BD Pharmingen, United States), PE-Texas Red-conjugated anti-CD4 (Life Technologies, United States) and Pacific Blue-conjugated anti-CD8 (BD Pharmingen, United States) monoclonal antibody were subsequently added for surface marker staining. The stained cells were washed, fixed and permeabilized by BD FACS fixation/permeabilization kit (BD Bioscience). Subsequently, PBMC were washed and stained intracellularly with FITC-conjugated anti-IFN-γ (BD Pharmingen, United States), PE-conjugated anti-perforin (Abcam, United States BD-48 clone), PE-Cy7-conjugated anti-TNF-α (BD Pharmingen, United States) and allophycocyanin (APC)-conjugated anti-IL-2 monoclonal antibody (BD Pharmingen, United States) for 30 min. Cells were washed and resuspended in 1% paraformaldehyde prior to flow cytometric analysis. Around 10^6 cells were acquired on FACS LSR-II flow cytometer (BD Biosciences, United States). FACS data was analyzed by FlowJo (Tree Star, United States). The data with lymphocytes and live cells below 20% of the total population were excluded. The combinations of T cell functions were analyzed by the Boolean combination gate in FlowJo software.

T cells with more than or equal to 3 functions were defined as PFCs.

Isolation of CD3+ T Cells and Cytolysis Assay

CD3+ T cells, which were used as effector cells in this study, were isolated and purified from PBMC of 3 IM patients by negative selection using Magnetic Beads Sorting Kit (Pan T cell isolation kit, Miltenyi, Germany). The purity of isolated CD3+ T cells was determined by staining with anti-CD3 monoclonal antibody, followed by analysis with BD LSRII flow cytometer. Highly purified CD3+ T cells (>95%) were obtained after sorting. Autologous LCLs (target cells) were stained with 5- and 6-carboxyfluorescein diascetate succinimidyl ester (CFSE) and incubated in 10% FBS/RPMI at 10^6 cells/ml at 37°C, 5% CO_2. The purified and stimulated CD3+ T cells (effector cells) were co-cultured with the target cells at a ratio 10:1 for 4 h at 37°C, 5% CO2 and stained with propidium iodide (PI) (Life Technologies). Cells were analyzed by flow cytometry. Percentage of PI positive cells within the CFSE positive population was obtained. Cultures with either autologous LCLs or isolated CD3+ T cells alone served as negative controls.

Statistical Analysis

Comparisons of EBV loads in PBMC and plasma amongst the longitudinal samples of IM or AS subjects across the study time points were performed using repeated measure ANOVA. Bonferroni's correction was applied. P-value < 0.0001 was regarded as statistically significant. Comparisons between groups of T cell responses across the study time points were performed by Kruskal–Wallis test and Mann–Whitney Test. P-value < 0.05 was regarded as statistically significant. Prism 6 (GraphPad Software, La Jolla, CA, United States) was used for calculations and illustrations.

RESULTS

Magnitude of IFN-γ Secreting CD8+ T Cell Responses Toward EBV Lytic Peptides Decreased but Those Toward Latent Peptides Increased Over Time in Both IM and AS Individuals

We measured the magnitude of EBV-specific CD8+ T cell responses toward EBV lytic and latent peptides in both IM and AS individuals by IFN-γ ELISPOT assay. HLA typing of 18 PBMC samples of IM patients (IM1–18) and 12 AS individuals (AS 1–12) were performed (Supplementary Table 3). HLA-class I specific EBV lytic and latent peptides were used to stimulate the PBMC of HLA-class I matched individuals (Supplementary Tables 2, 3). The number of spot-forming cells (SFC) per million PBMC of the IM and AS individuals is shown in **Table 1**. Trend in changes of the EBV antigen-specific T cell response was deduced by comparing the SFC per million PBMC at the earliest time point to that at the longest time point for each study subject (**Table 1**). Difference in the magnitude of the T cell responses less than or equal to 20 SFC per million PBMC was defined as a stable trend whereas that greater than 20 SFC per million PBMC was defined as an increasing or decreasing trend. As indicated in **Table 1**, the magnitude of IFN-γ secreting CD8+ T cell responses toward EBV lytic peptides tended to decrease over time from day 0 to 12 months whereas those toward latent peptides tended to increase over time in the majority of IM and AS subjects. The ELISPOT data of 2 representative cases, IM16 and IM17, were shown in **Figure 1**. PBMC of IM16 (HLA-type: A2, A26, B46 and cw1) collected at 1, 3, 6, and 12 months post-diagnosis were stimulated by 7 peptide epitopes (TLD, VLK, GLC, YVL, SLR, CLG, VQP). Prominent IFN-γ secreting CD8+ T cell responses against an immediate lytic cycle protein BRLF1-derived peptide (YVL) and a latent cycle protein EBNA3A-derived peptide (VQP) were observed (**Figure 1A**). YVL stimulated 793 SFC at 1 month and decreased to 115 SFC at 12 months. In contrast, VQP stimulated 58 SFC at 1 month and increased to 215 SFC at 12 months. IM17 (HLA-type: A1, A11, B4001, B13, Cw7 and Cw10) showed similar trend of T cell responses (**Figure 1B**). Response against ATI, the A11-restricted BRLF1-derived peptide, was found to decrease from 2193 to 433 SFC whereas the response against SSCS, the LMP2A-derived peptide, was found to increase from 15 to 180 SFC from 1 to 12 months (**Figure 1B**). The decreasing trend of IFN-γ secreting CD8+ T cell responses toward lytic peptides and increasing trend of responses toward latent peptides were observed in the majority of the IM and AS subjects (**Table 1**). No significant difference between the responses in IM and AS individuals was detected.

PBMC and Plasma Viral Loads in Both IM and AS Individuals Decreased Over Time

High PBMC viral loads in IM patients during acute infection and substantial decrease of viral loads over time were observed in previous studies (Kimura et al., 1999; Balfour et al., 2005; Cheng et al., 2007). We also determined the viral loads in both PBMC and plasma of 29 IM patients and 12 AS subjects by qPCR. The median PBMC viral load in IM patients decreased from 21878 EBV copies/million PBMC at diagnosis (D0) to 209 copies/million PBMC at 12 months after diagnosis (**Figure 2A**). The median plasma viral loads also decreased from 37154 to 5 copies/mL plasma from day 0 to 12 months (**Figure 2A**). Decreases in PBMC and plasma viral loads were also observed in AS individuals (**Figure 2B**). In both IM and AS subjects, the PBMC and plasma viral loads peaked at diagnosis and declined substantially afterward. The viral loads were the lowest at the end of the study period, indicating an establishment of effective viral control. Repeated measure ANOVA with Bonferroni's correction was applied for multiple comparisons. Cases which had a complete set of time points (day 0, day 7 and 1, 3, 6, and 12 months) were evaluated by the program. The results showed that the PBMC ($n = 9$) and plasma viral loads ($n = 7$) significantly decreased over time in the IM samples with values [$F(5,40) = 12.76$, $P < 0.0001$] and [$F(5,30) = 13.23$, $P < 0.0001$], respectively. In addition, the PBMC and plasma viral loads at day 7 and 1, 3, 6, and 12 months were significantly lower than those at day 0 (Supplementary Figure 1).

Kinetics of Development of CD4+ and CD8+ T Cell Responses to EBV Lytic and Latent Cycle Antigens After Primary Infection

Next, we carried out a detailed characterization of the development of CD4+ and CD8+ T cell responses to several immunodominant EBV lytic and latent antigens in IM patients from primary infection to long term persistence by multi-color flow cytometric assays. Due to the low frequencies of EBV-specific T cells, an expansion of T cells was necessary for the accurate analysis of the subtle changes of functional T cell subsets in the IM patients during different stages of infection (Jennes et al., 2002; Jones et al., 2010). We adopted a T cell expansion protocol provided by Prof. Cliona M Rooney (Baylor College of Medicine, United States) in order to increase the sensitivity of our flow cytometric assay (Gerdemann et al., 2011). Such expansion protocol using IL4 and IL7 had been used in different T cell studies and found to maintain the survival of most of the cytokine secreting T cells in similar magnitude (Vella et al., 1997, 1998; Gerdemann et al., 2011; Shmarov et al., 2016). To confirm the validity of the flow cytometric assay, we stimulated the PBMC with EBV overlapping peptide pools (EBNA1, EBNA-3A, -3B, -3C and BZLF1) in an IM patient and an EBV-seronegative donor. EBV-specific T cells were clearly detected in the IM patient but not in the seronegative donor except for the pre-loaded perforin in a small proportion of T cells (Supplementary Figure 2). In addition, the increasing trend of latent antigen-specific IFN-γ secreting CD8+ T cell responses and decreasing trend of lytic antigen-specific responses detected by ELISPOT could also be replicated by this flow cytometric assay (Supplementary Figure 3).

We proceeded to analyze the EBV-specific T cell responses of 11 longitudinally followed IM patients (IM19-29) toward 4 lytic and 5 latent overlapping EBV peptides. The magnitude of responses was measured as the frequency of responsive T cells which presented at least one function (either IFN-γ, perforin, TNF-α, IL-2, or CD107a) after stimulation by the overlapping peptide pools. No discernible differences in the magnitude and quality of T cell responses were found among the IM patients of different age groups. The overall magnitude of responses of CD4+ T cells to overlapping peptide pools of lytic and latent cycle proteins was similar to that of CD8+ T cells (**Figure 3**). At diagnosis, all EBV lytic peptide pools could stimulate both CD4+ and CD8+ T cell responses, presenting a broad response spectrum. Remarkably, the frequency of EBNA3A, 3B and 3C-specific CD4+ and CD8+ T cells clearly increased over time and dominated at 1 year after diagnosis. In contrast, responses toward other EBV lytic and latent peptides were relatively stable throughout the period of our study (**Figure 3**).

Diversity of CD4+ and CD8+ Polyfunctional T Cells (PFC) Responses Increased Over Time

Polyfunctional T cells, which execute multiple functions upon stimulation by a specific antigen, were reported to elicit stronger immune responses (Betts et al., 2006; Almeida et al., 2007; Smith et al., 2009). We examined the evolution of the magnitude and functionality of lytic and latent cycle antigen-specific CD4+ and CD8+ T cells. The functional profiles of CD4+ and CD8+ PFC (with three or more functions) of a representative case, IM 25, are shown in **Figure 4.** Low percentages of lytic and latent antigen-specific CD4+ and CD8+ responsive T cells with 2 or more functions appeared at diagnosis. The CD4+ and CD8+ responsive T cells against the latent antigen EBNA3B increased dramatically over time. Particularly, the frequency of EBNA3B-specific CD8+ PFC increased from approximately 1% at diagnosis to 30% of total antigen-reactive CD8+ T cells at 12 months after diagnosis. In contrast, BZLF1-responsive cells decreased over time and EBNA1- responsive cells remained stable across the time points from day 0 to 12 months (**Figures 4A,B**). At day 0, most of the CD4+ and CD8+ PFC only displayed a restricted number of combinations of functions. Very low percentages of 4-functional CD4+ PFC (IFNγ+/IL-2+/perforin+/TNF-α+) and 3-functional CD8+ PFC (CD107a+/IL-2+/TNF-α+) were detected (**Figures 4A,B**). At later time points, these CD4+ and CD8+ PFC became more highly functional as 4- and 5-functional T cells started to emerge. Interestingly, a dramatic increase in the diversity of functional subsets of both CD4+ and CD8+ T cells was observed (**Figures 4C,D**). Such diverse functional subsets were found in 8 out of the 11 IM cases whereas the remaining 3 cases showed a constant level or slightly decreased variety of combination of functions in the later time points (Supplementary Figure 4).

Emergence of CD4+ and CD8+ Polyfunctional T Cell Responses Toward EBV Lytic and Latent Antigens

We summarized the development of EBV-specific CD4+ and CD8+ PFC for all IM patients (**Figure 5**). EBV lytic and latent cycle antigen-specific CD4+ PFC (with three or more functions) existed at diagnosis but the mean frequencies were less than 3% of total responsive CD4+ T cells (**Figure 5A**). The mean frequencies of CD4+ PFC against lytic and latent cycle antigens did not change significantly over time from primary infection to long term persistent stage. The abilities of EBV lytic and latent cycle antigen-specific CD8+ T cells to generate PFC were relatively stronger when compared with CD4+ cells and appeared to change over time (**Figure 5B**). During acute infection, the mean frequencies of EBV-specific CD8+ PFC were less than 3% of the total responsive CD8+ T cells after stimulation. The percentages of CD8+ PFC against early lytic antigen, BMLF1, BRLF1 and BZLF1, increased slightly whereas those of CD8+ PFC against the latent antigens, EBNA3A, 3B and 3C, increased significantly over time. Other subdominant antigens such as EBNA1, LMP2 and GP350 did not stimulate any significant changes in the proportion of PFC. Although the PFC responses were induced by the immunodominant latent antigens derived from EBNA3A-C in most of the IM patients (**Figure 5**), it should be noted that PFC responses could also be induced

TABLE 1 | Table showing the T cell responses against HLA-class I restricted EBV lytic and latent peptides determined by ELISPOT.

Status	Peptide	Protein	Type	D0	D7	1 m	3 m	6 m	12 m	Trend
IM1	SSCS	LMP2A	Latent	–	3	18	35	45	55	Increasing
IM1	ATI	BRLF1	Lytic	–	413	268	65	65	43	Decreasing
IM1	SEN	BZLF1	Lytic	–	50	23	18	35	20	Decreasing
IM2	SSCS	LMP2A	Latent	–	–	–	165	–	–	–
IM3	VSF	EBNA3B	Latent	1610	–	–	2065	–	–	Increasing
IM4	RPP	EBNA3A	Latent	1823	393	603	525	–	298	Decreasing
IM4	RPQG	BMRF1	Lytic	533	138	310	293	–	93	Decreasing
IM5	YVL	BRLF1	Lytic	–	–	813	893	328	–	Decreasing
IM5	SSCS	LMP2A	Latent	–	–	23	30	123	–	Increasing
IM5	ATI	BRLF1	Lytic	–	–	453	370	163	–	Decreasing
IM6	VSF	EBNA3B	Latent	–	–	–	785	1380	1753	Increasing
IM6	SLR	EBNALP	Latent	–	–	–	470	365	470	Stable
IM7	EPL	BZLF1	Lytic	–	505	–	1008	–	805	Increasing
IM8	SEN	BZLF1	Lytic	–	3423	2260	1133	–	1025	Decreasing
IM9	GLC	BMLF1	Lytic	–	333	–	–	–	93	Decreasing
IM9	AVF	EBNA3B	Latent	–	985	–	–	–	8	Decreasing
IM9	VQP	EBNA3A	Latent	–	18	–	–	–	123	Increasing
IM9	SSCS	LMP2A	Latent	–	33	–	90	–	–	Increasing
IM10	IED	LMP2A	Latent	–	63	–	1488	413	223	Increasing
IM10	SEN	BZLF1	Lytic	–	488	–	305	245	28	Decreasing
IM11	SSCS	LMP2A	Latent	–	0	113	–	298	–	Increasing
IM11	VSF	EBNA3B	Latent	–	383	563	–	383	–	Stable
IM11	ATI	BRLF1	Lytic	–	78	80	–	75	–	Stable
IM12	VSF	EBNA3B	Latent	–	775	–	–	393	283	Decreasing
IM13	VLK	EBNA1	Latent	–	30	–	83	–	258	Increasing
IM13	SLR	EBNALP	Latent	–	75	–	78	–	88	Stable
IM14	YVL	BRLF1	Lytic	–	–	133	90	25	28	Decreasing
IM14	AVF	EBNA3B	Latent	–	–	8	548	163	178	Increasing
IM14	IED	LMP2A	Latent	–	–	43	525	385	403	Increasing
IM15	ATI	BRLF1	Lytic	–	–	18	53	60	73	Increasing
IM15	VSF	EBNA3B	Latent	–	–	263	225	103	155	Decreasing
IM15	SSCS	LMP2A	Latent	–	–	13	73	78	93	Increasing
IM16	YVL	BRLF1	Lytic	–	–	793	590	260	115	Decreasing
IM16	VQP	EBNA3A	Latent	–	–	58	150	170	215	Increasing
IM17	SSCS	LMP2A	Latent	–	–	15	310	143	180	Increasing
IM17	ATI	BRLF1	Lytic	–	–	2193	1575	663	433	Decreasing
IM17	SEN	BZLF1	Lytic	–	–	65	90	48	20	Decreasing
IM18	VLK	EBNA1	Latent	–	–	–	375	180	370	Stable
IM18	SSCS	LMP2A	Latent	–	–	–	128	15	150	Increasing
AS6	VSF	EBNA3B	Latent	–	–	305	530	–	–	Increasing
AS7	AVF	EBNA3B	Latent	–	–	0	20	–	98	Increasing
AS7	SSCS	LMP2A	Latent	–	–	90	510	–	223	Increasing
AS7	ATI	BRLF1	Lytic	–	–	213	148	–	28	Deceasing
AS8	SSCS	LMP2A	Latent	–	–	–	45	168	–	Increasing
AS11	AVF	EBNA3B	Latent	–	–	–	185	295	275	Increasing
AS11	SSCS	LMP2A	Latent	–	–	–	23	95	93	Increasing
AS12	VSF	EBNA3B	Latent	–	–	–	185	408	273	Increasing

Results are expressed as numbers of spot-forming cells (SFC). "–" represents sample not available.

by antigens derived from immediately early (BZLF1 and BRLF1) and early (BMLF1) EBV proteins in some individuals (Refer to **Figures 4**, **5** and Supplementary Figure 4). Taken together, our data suggested that the CD4+ and CD8+ T cells specific to the immunodominant EBV proteins, including BZLF1, BRLF1, BMLF1, EBNA-3A, -3B, and -3C, became highly functional during the long term persistent phase.

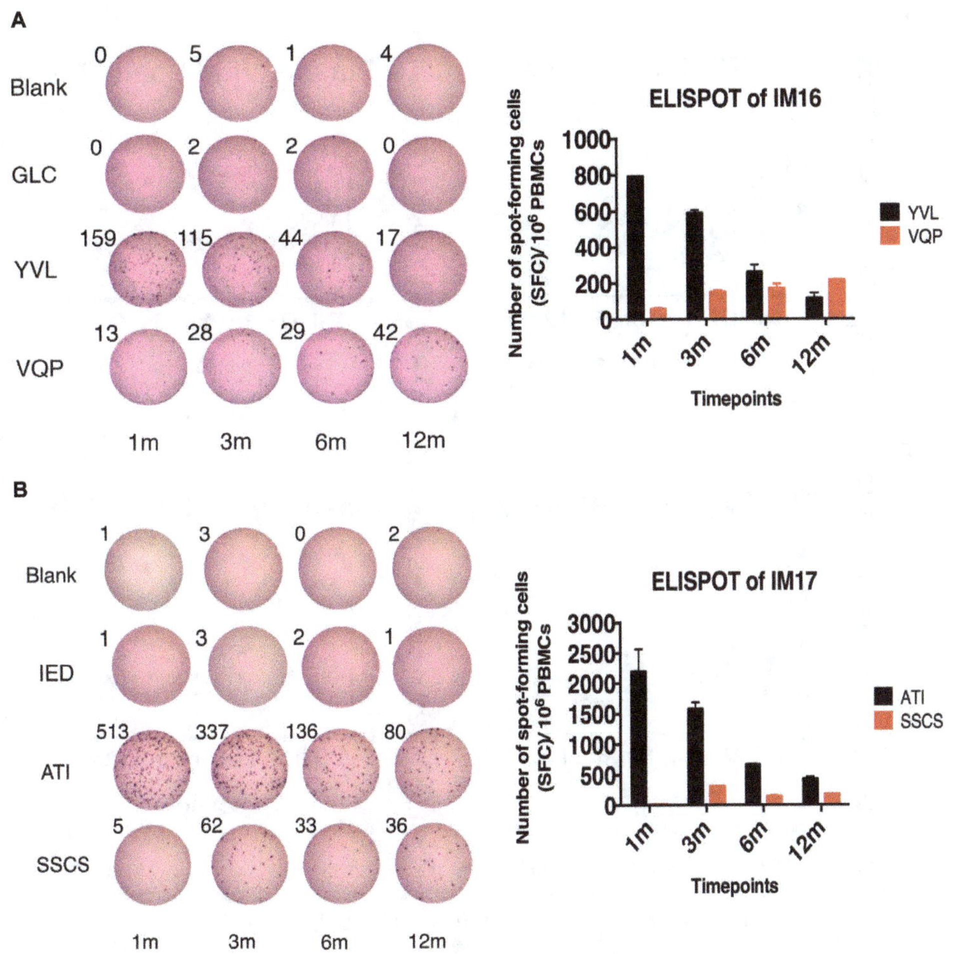

FIGURE 1 | IFN-γ producing EBV-specific CD8+ T cell responses in IM16 and IM 17. **(A)** IM16 cells collected at 0, 1, 3, 6, and 12 months post-diagnosis (0, 1, 3, 6, and 12 m) were stimulated with 7 different peptides (TLD, VLK, GLC, YVL, SLR, CLG, and VQP) in duplicate wells. IM16 reacted to only two of the peptides. GLC was shown as representative negative control. **(B)** IM17 cells collected at 0, 1, 3, 6, and 12 months post-diagnosis (0, 1, 3, 6, and 12 m) were stimulated with 5 different peptides (ATI, SSCS, AVF, IED, and SEN) in duplicate wells. IM17 reacted to only two of the peptides. IED was shown as representative negative control. Wells with cells only (blank) were also shown as negative controls. The numbers of spots were shown above the wells. Positive results in histogram were expressed in the mean ± SEM of numbers of spot-forming cells (SFC) per million PBMC.

Increased Cytotoxicity of T Cells Against Autologous LCL in IM Patients Over Time

Cytotoxicity assay was carried out to examine whether increased polyfunctionality is accompanied by enhanced cytotoxicity of EBV-specific T cells. T cells were stimulated and expanded by overlapping peptide pools from the immunodominant EBNA3A or 3B protein of each donor. The CD3+ T cells were then purified by negative selection using Miltenyl Magnetic Beads Cell Sorting system. The purity of the T cells was on average greater than 95%, and the viability of T cells after sorting did not change significantly.

The cytotoxicity of T cells against autologous LCL, after stimulation with EBNA3 overlapping peptide pools, was assessed longitudinally for three IM patients (**Figure 6A**). The cytotoxicity of T cells against LCL increased over time. These results were consistent with elevated frequencies of perforin- and CD107a-expressing T cells (**Figure 6B**). Cytotoxic potential was further enhanced by stimulating the T cells with EBNA3 overlapping peptide pools for 5 days prior to setting up the lysis assay, concurrent with increasing polyfunctionality, perforin production, and degranulation (**Figure 6B**).

DISCUSSION

Identification of polyfunctional CD8+ T cells in the immune control of viral infection had been reported (Betts et al., 2006; Almeida et al., 2007; Smith et al., 2009). However, most of these studies focused on assessing CD8+ T cell responses to human immunodeficiency virus (HIV) and their mechanisms in killing. Much less is known about the role of PFC responses in the control of stable persistent DNA virus such as EBV. Here, we describe a comprehensive study in which the development of EBV-specific CD4+ and CD8+ T cells, as well as their

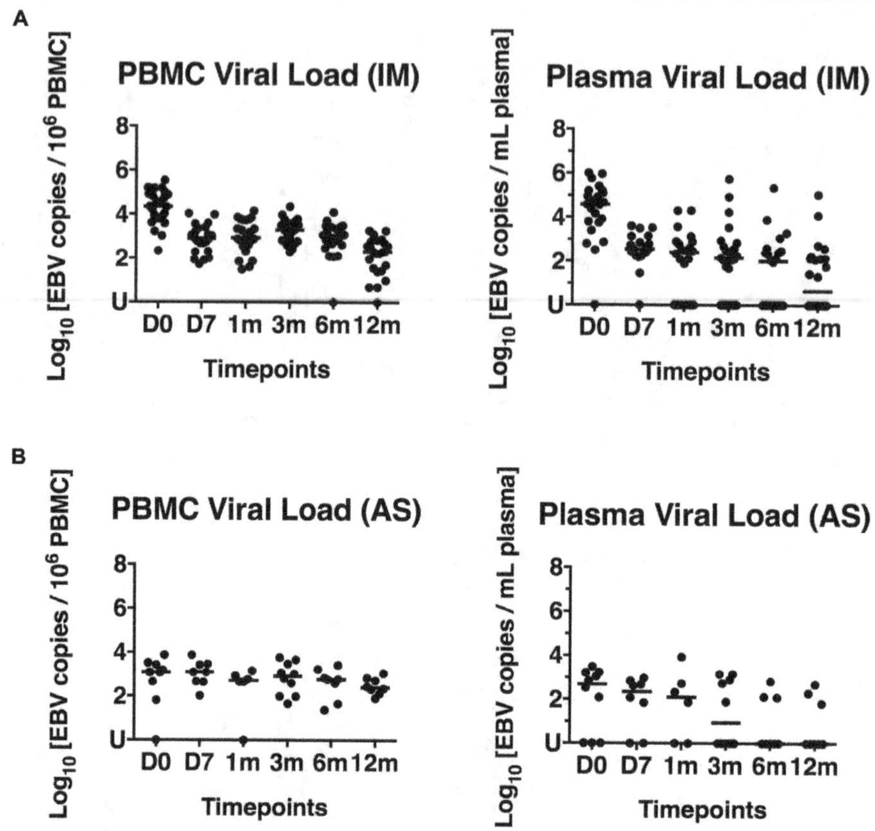

FIGURE 2 | PBMC and plasma viral loads of 29 IM patients and 12 AS individuals. **(A)** EBV loads in PBMC and plasma of IM1-29. **(B)** EBV loads in PBMC and plasma of AS1-12. The spots represent the copy numbers of EBV per million PBMC and copy numbers of EBV per mL plasma in different IM and AS individuals collected at Day 0, 7 and 1, 3, 6, and 12 months post-diagnosis (D0, D7, 1 m, 3 m, 6 m, and 12 m). U, undetectable.

magnitude and polyfunctionality were monitored from primary infection to long-term persistence in two cohorts of children with infectious mononucleosis (IM) and asymptomatic (AS) primary EBV infection, respectively.

The IFN-γ secreting CD8+ T cells were characterized as the major population of T cells participating in viral control (Callan et al., 1996; Shi and Lutz, 2002). IFN-γ ELISPOT assay became a common quantitative detection method of virus-specific CD8+ cells (Larsson et al., 1999; Yang et al., 2000). A previous study had demonstrated the diagnostic potential of IFN-γ and IL-2 ELISPOT assays in distinguishing active and latent tuberculosis in children infected with *Mycobacterium tuberculosis* (Chiappini et al., 2012). In the present study, the kinetics of IFN-γ producing CD8+ T cell responses in IM patients and AS subjects was first assessed by ELISPOT assay. The decreasing pattern of IFN-γ producing CD8+ T cell responses toward EBV lytic peptides and increasing pattern of T cell responses toward EBV latent peptides were identified over time in both IM and AS subjects. There was no discernible difference in the trend of evolution of T cell responses in these two study cohorts. However, this widely accepted IFN-γELISPOT assay using HLA-type restricted epitopes to detect EBV antigen-specific T cells could not simultaneously assess the CD4+ cell responses and determine the expression of other functional cytokines (Casazza et al., 2006; Scherrenburg et al., 2008). The difficulties in choosing the specific EBV peptides across a wide range of HLA alleles also restricted the panel of antigen-specific cells to be tested which could result in missing of potentially important information (Supplementary Tables 2, 3).

Accumulating evidence indicated that the "quality" of T cell responses should be assessed by functionality (Seder et al., 2008). The more functions the T cells possess, the more robust the immune protection they can provide (Makedonas et al., 2010). We have also shown that long term carriers could generate robust PFC responses against lytic and latent EBV antigens with the greatest responses toward the immunodominant epitopes of the EBNA3 proteins (Ning et al., 2011). However, the time of emergence of PFC responses against EBV lytic or latent antigens, differences between CD4+ and CD8+ T cell responses, and concurrent EBV loads in PBMC and plasma from acute to chronic stage of infection are not clearly understood. To address these questions, we performed a longitudinal study to assess the development of PFC responses to EBV in 11 IM patients. We assessed five functional parameters: IFN-γ, TNF-α, IL-2, perforin, and CD107a, all of which are typical functions of T cells that were reported in previous studies (Harari et al., 2006; Pantaleo and Harari, 2006; Precopio et al., 2007; Makedonas et al., 2010). T cells with three or more functions after stimulation are defined

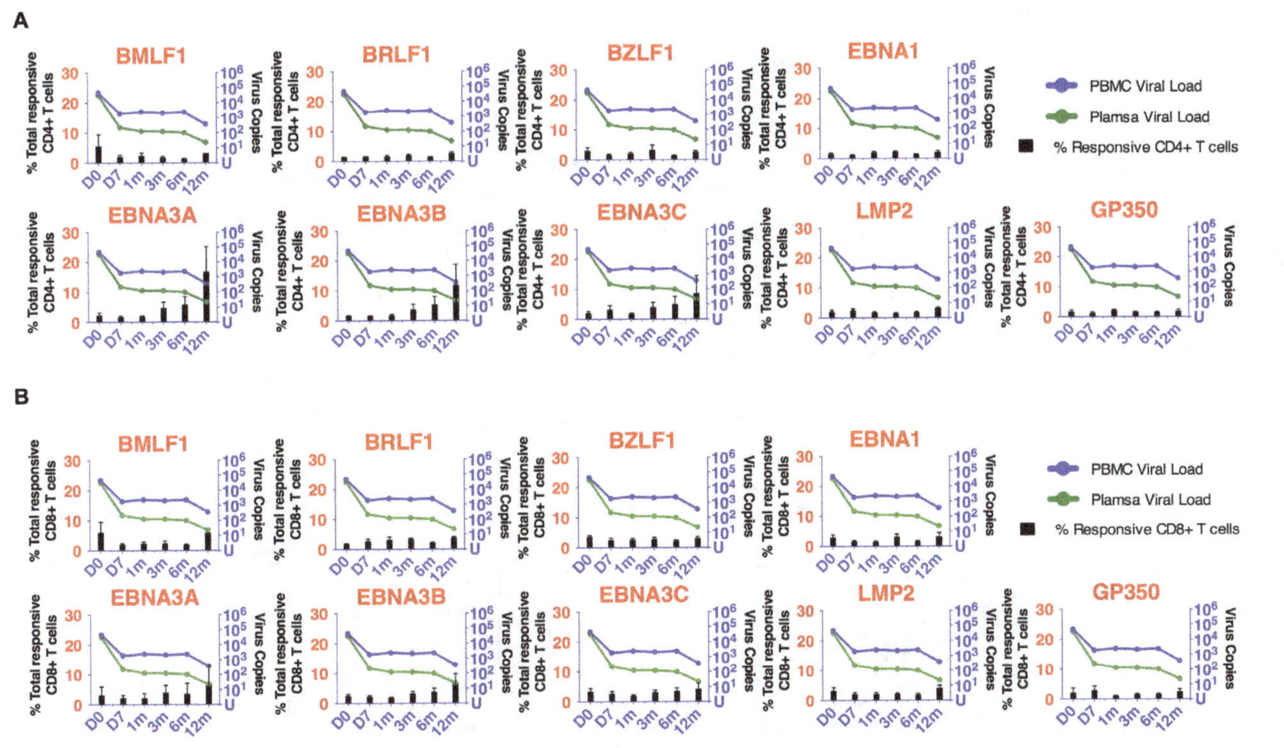

FIGURE 3 | Kinetics of development of CD4+ and CD8+ T cell responses to EBV lytic and latent cycle antigens after primary infection. **(A)** Kinetic changes of the percentages of EBV-specific CD4+ T cells and EBV loads. **(B)** Kinetic changes of the percentages of EBV-specific CD8+ T cells and EBV loads. T cells were expanded by overlapping peptide pools for 5 days and re-stimulated by the corresponding peptide pools for 6 h before flow cytometric assays. Each bar represents the mean percentages of EBV-specific T cells in the 11 IM patients (IM 19–29) at different time points. The corresponding viral loads in PBMC (blue curve) and plasma (green curve) at different time points are shown. Each dot in the line curve represents the mean viral load of the 11 IM patients.

as PFC. EBV-specific lytic and latent antigen-derived overlapping peptides were used to stimulate both CD4+ and CD8+ T cell responses. Similar trend of response of IFN-γ specific CD8+ cells was observed as that detected by ELISPOT assay, validating the reliability of data generated by both methods (Supplementary Figure 3). In the IM patients, EBV-specific CD4+ and CD8+ PFC were detectable at diagnosis toward lytic and latent cycle antigens. These CD4+ and CD8+ PFC only displayed a restricted combination of functions, such as the 4- functional CD4+ PFC (IFNγ+/IL-2+/perforin+/TNF-α+) and the 3-functional CD8+ PFC (CD107a+/IL-2+/TNF-α+) (refer to **Figure 4**). At later time points, these CD4+ and CD8+ PFC became more highly functional as 4- and 5-functional T cells started to emerge. The development of PFC responses toward different specific peptides varied among the individuals. In most of the IM patients, the PFC responses were induced by the immunodominant antigens derived from EBNA3A-C (**Figure 5**). Interestingly, in some of the individuals, antigens derived from immediately early (BZLF1 and BRLF1) and early (BMLF1) EBV proteins induced the highest proportion of CD8+ as well as CD4+ PFCs (refer to **Figures 4, 5** and Supplementary Figure 4). In addition, low frequencies of EBNA1-specific CD4+ T cells were detected at both diagnosis and 6 and 12 months in some IM patients (Supplementary Figure 4), in contrast to the findings of previous studies in which EBNA1-specific CD4+ T cells were not detected until months after the initial diagnosis (Long et al., 2013; Rickinson et al., 2014). Since EBNA1-specific effector T cells might be important in the control of EBV-positive lymphoproliferative diseases (Jones et al., 2010), it is interesting to follow whether the proportion of EBNA1-responsive PFC would increase at longer time points in the future. Diverse combinations of three or more functions of both antigen-specific CD4+ and CD8+ T cells were shown to emerge at 6–12 months, suggesting a potential co-operative relationship between the CD4+ and CD8+ PFC in the long term viral control (**Figures 4C,D** and Supplementary Figure 4). Presence of CD107a+ and perforin-releasing cytotoxic CD4+ PFC was demonstrated in this study (**Figure 4C**). Similarly, a rare population of CD4+ cytotoxic T cells was previously identified in the patients with chronic viral infection of CMV (Casazza et al., 2006). The presence of cytotoxic CD4+ PFC indicates that CD4+ T cells may also play a direct role in the control of persistent EBV infection. The clinical preparation of virus-specific T cells for the control of post-transplant lymphoproliferative disorders was shown to require the presence of CD4+ T cells (Gerdemann et al., 2011; Linnerbauer et al., 2014). In fact, CD4+ PFC was found to be molecularly distinct from IFN-γ mono-functional CD4+ T cells and associate with favorable clinical outcomes in patients with *Plasmodium falciparum* infection (Burel et al., 2017). Taken together, our data clearly demonstrated the development and

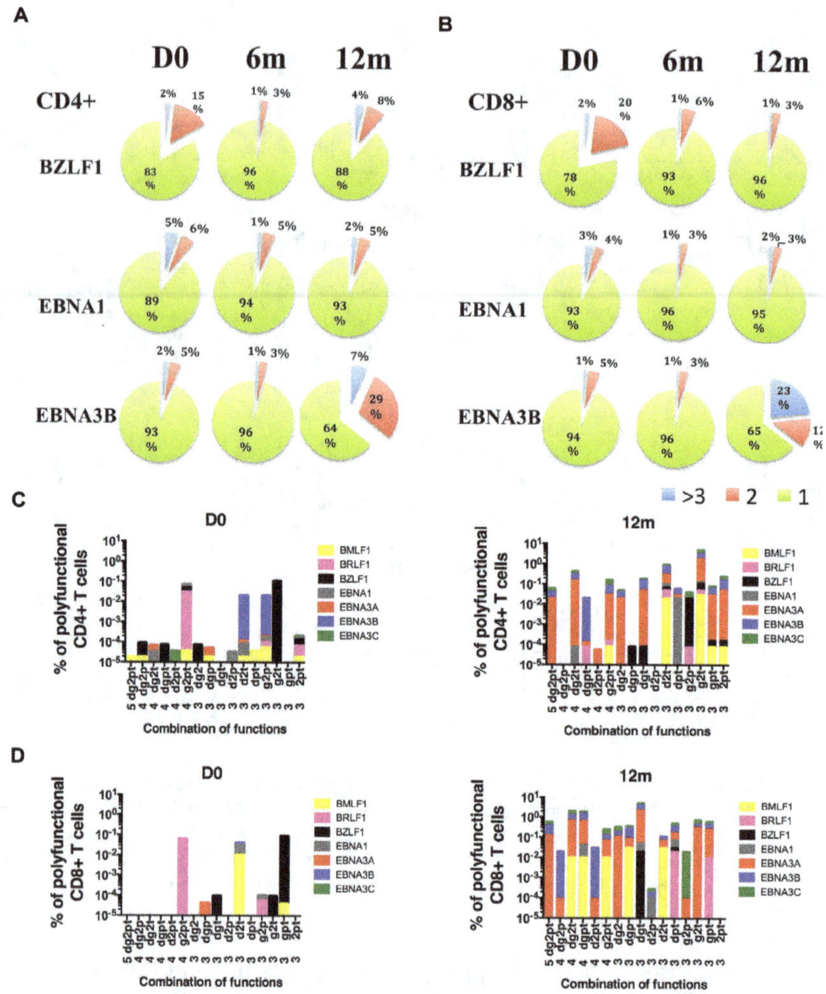

FIGURE 4 | Longitudinal functional profiles of EBV-specific T cells in one representative IM patient (IM25). The pie charts represent the proportions of **(A)** CD4+ T cells and **(B)** CD8+ T cells with single (green), double (red), triple or more (blue) functions upon stimulation with BZLF1, EBNA3B, and EBNA1 overlapping peptide pools. T cells were expanded with 4 lytic and 5 latent antigens overlapping peptides pools for 5 days and re-stimulated by the corresponding peptide pools for 6 h before flow cytometric assays. Flow cytometric assays were performed at an early time point ranged from D0 to 3 m, a middle time point ranged from 3 to 6 m and a late time point ranged from 6 to 12 m. D0, at diagnosis; 6 m, 6 months after diagnosis; 12 m, 1 year after diagnosis. The percentages of responsive **(C)** CD4+ and **(D)** CD8+ T cells with different combinations of functions upon stimulation by BMLF1, BRLF1, BZLF1, EBNA1, EBNA3A, EBNA3B and EBNA3C at diagnosis (D0) and 1 year after diagnosis (12 m). d, CD107a; g, Interferon-gamma; 2, Interleukin-2; p, Perforin; t, Tumor-necrosis factor-alpha.

maturation of both CD4+ and CD8+ PFC from early to long term infection stages in IM patients.

Decreasing patterns of EBV loads in PBMC and plasma were illustrated in both IM and AS subjects (**Figure 2**), indicating that both study subjects were capable of generating sufficient T-cell immunity for viral control. Moreover, the viral loads *per se* could not explain the development of IM symptoms in some individuals, although elevated viral loads were observed in both IM and AS individuals during acute EBV infection (Silins et al., 2001). Manifestation of the self-limiting immunopathological conditions arising in IM patients might be related to the inadequate NK cell cytotoxicity toward infected cells during acute infection (Rickinson et al., 2014). In both IM and AS subjects, plasma loads declined dramatically to low or undetected levels, yet, PBMC viral loads showed a slower decline (**Figure 2**). The sharp decrease in plasma loads was probably due to the initial control by NK cell and the early lytic cycle antigen-specific CD8+ T cell responses. In contrast, the slow decline of PBMC was due to the gradual emergence of both lytic and latent antigen-specific polyfunctional CD4+ and CD8+ T cell responses at about 6 months. Indeed, a natural decay of PBMC viral loads in the early stage of infection independent of EBV-specific T-cell immunity was previously proposed (Hadinoto et al., 2008). The viral control thereafter was probably mediated by the development and strengthening of PFC responses toward the immunodominant antigens derived from BZLF1, BRLF1, BMLF1, EBNA3A, 3B and 3C proteins from about 6 to 12 months post-infection. The sustained decline of EBV loads during this period correlated well with the emergence of T cells capable of presenting multiple functions. To further assess

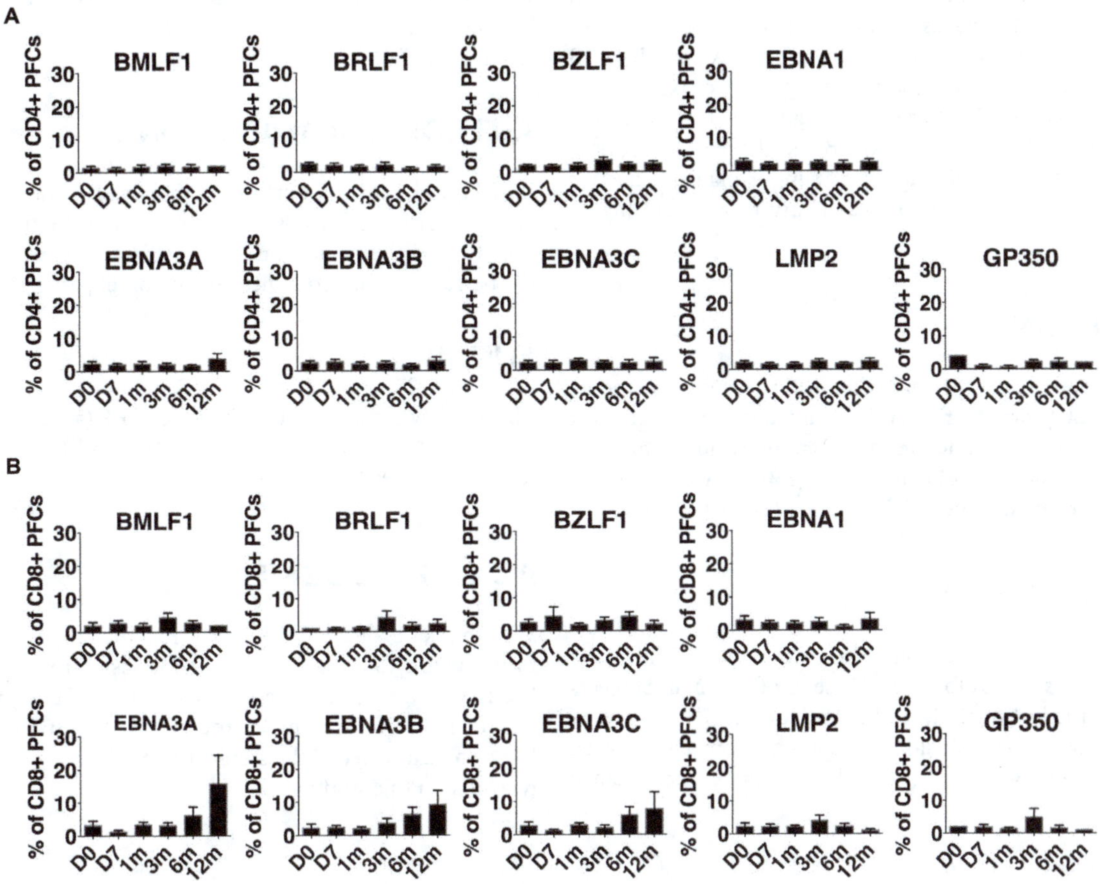

FIGURE 5 | Development of EBV lytic and latent antigen-specific polyfunctional T cells from acute primary infection stage to long-term persistence. **(A)** CD4+ T cells and **(B)** CD8+ T cells in 11 IM patients. T cells were expanded by overlapping peptide pools for 5 days and re-stimulated by the corresponding peptide pools for 6 h before flow cytometric assays. Each bar represents the mean ± SEM percentages of polyfunctional T cells (three or more functions after stimulation) out of total EBV-specific T cells upon stimulation with a specific latent overlapping peptide pool.

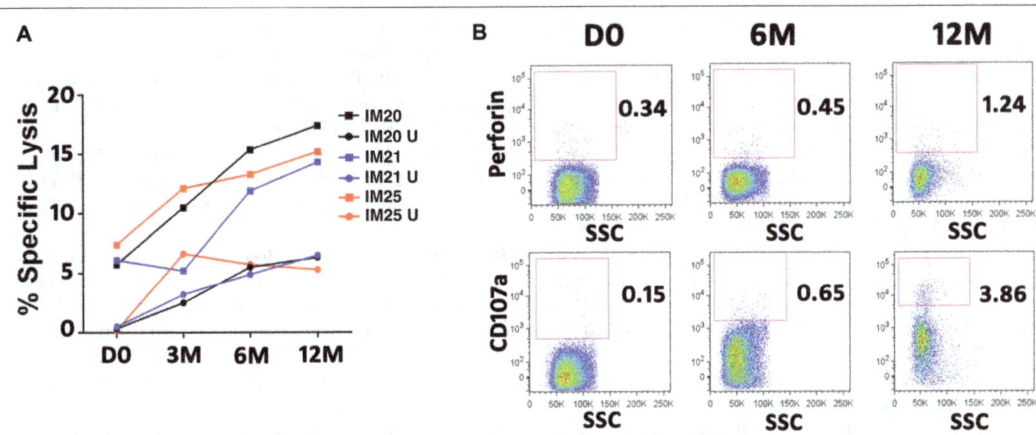

FIGURE 6 | Cytotoxicity of EBNA3-specific T cells against autologous LCLs in three IM patients. T cells were expanded for 5 days in the presence of overlapping peptide pools of EBNA3A or EBNA3B. Autologous B-LCL (target cells) were stained with CFSE and co-cultured with activated purified T cells (effector cells) for 4 h at an Effector/Target ratio of 10:1. Dead cells were discriminated from live cells by propidium iodide (PI). Autologous LCLs were killed by T cells. The percentage of specific lysis is calculated by subtracting the background (LCL co-cultured with unstimulated T cells). **(A)** Cytotoxicity of EBNA3-specific T cells at different time points in 3 IM patients. PBMC of IM20 and IM21 and IM25 patients were stimulated and expanded with overlapping peptide pools of EBNA3A and EBNA3B, respectively. U, LCL co-cultured with unstimulated T cells. **(B)** Development of Perforin producing T cells (upper row) and CD107a positive T cells (lower row) in IM25.

whether increased PFC responses correlated to viral control in the IM patients, a cytotoxic assay was performed. We stimulated the T cells of three IM patients with EBNA3A or EBNA3B peptide pools and found a steady increase in cytotoxicity of T cells against autologous LCL over time (**Figure 6**). The increasing proportions of EBNA3A- or EBNA3B-specific PFC correlated with the enhanced cytotoxic capacities, supporting that effective viral control was achieved by the capability to generate highly functional T cells.

CONCLUSION

EBV antigen-specific CD4+ and CD8+ PFC responses emerge during the first year of primary EBV infection, with greatest responses toward immunodominant epitopes in both lytic (BZLF1, BRLF1 and BMLF1) and latent (EBNA3A-C) proteins, correlating to steady decline in PBMC and plasma viral loads.

ETHICS STATEMENT

This study was carried out in accordance with the recommendations of "Informed Consent of Human Subjects of Research, Institutional Review Board of the University of Hong Kong" with written informed consent from all subjects. All subjects gave written informed consent in accordance with the Declaration of Helsinki. The protocol was approved by the "Institutional Review Board of the University of Hong Kong."

AUTHOR CONTRIBUTIONS

JL, KH, RN, and XX performed the experiments, data analysis, and interpretation. JL, KH, and AC wrote the manuscript. AC coordinated the project and recruited and followed all patients. KC performed the serological assays for all patients.

FUNDING

This work was supported by the RGC-GRF (# HKU739403M and HKU763407M), CRCG (# 104002548), and Epstein-Barr Virus research (# 20004525) grants.

ACKNOWLEDGMENTS

We thank Professor Alan B. Rickinson of University of Birmingham for providing us HLA-class I restricted peptides. We thank Mr. T. F. Chan and Mr. Wilfred H. S. Wong of The University of Hong Kong for their advices on statistical analyses. We also acknowledge the support of all the parents and patients recruited in this study.

REFERENCES

Almeida, J. R., Price, D. A., Papagno, L., Arkoub, Z. A., Sauce, D., Bornstein, E., et al. (2007). Superior control of HIV-1 replication by CD8+ T cells is reflected by their avidity, polyfunctionality, and clonal turnover. *J. Exp. Med.* 204, 2473–2485. doi: 10.1084/jem.20070784

Babcock, G. J., Decker, L. L., Volk, M., and Thorley-Lawson, D. A. (1998). EBV persistence in memory B cells in vivo. *Immunity* 9, 395–404. doi: 10.1016/S1074-7613(00)80622-6

Balfour, H. H. Jr., Holman, C. J., Hokanson, K. M., Lelonek, M. M., Giesbrecht, J. E., White, D. R., et al. (2005). A prospective clinical study of Epstein-Barr virus and host interactions during acute infectious mononucleosis. *J. Infect. Dis.* 192, 1505–1512. doi: 10.1086/491740

Betts, M. R., Nason, M. C., West, S. M., De Rosa, S. C., Migueles, S. A., Abraham, J., et al. (2006). HIV nonprogressors preferentially maintain highly functional HIV-specific CD8+ T cells. *Blood* 107, 4781–4789. doi: 10.1182/blood-2005-12-4818

Burel, J. G., Apte, S. H., Groves, P. L., McCarthy, J. S., and Doolan, D. L. (2017). Polyfunctional and IFN-γamma monofunctional human CD4+ T cell populations are molecularly distinct. *JCI Insight* 2:e87499. doi: 10.1172/jci.insight.87499

Callan, M. F., Steven, N., Krausa, P., Wilson, J. D., Moss, P. A., Gillespie, G. M., et al. (1996). Large clonal expansions of CD8+ T cells in acute infectious mononucleosis. *Nat. Med.* 2, 906–911. doi: 10.1038/nm0896-906

Casazza, J. P., Betts, M. R., Price, D. A., Precopio, M. L., Ruff, L. E., Brenchley, J. M., et al. (2006). Acquisition of direct antiviral effector functions by CMV-specific CD4+ T lymphocytes with cellular maturation. *J. Exp. Med.* 203, 2865–2877. doi: 10.1084/jem.20052246

Cheng, C. C., Chang, L. Y., Shao, P. L., Lee, P. I., Chen, J. M., Lu, C. Y., et al. (2007). Clinical manifestations and quantitative analysis of virus load in Taiwanese children with Epstein-Barr virus-associated infectious mononucleosis. *J. Microbiol. Immunol. Infect.* 40, 216–221.

Chiappini, E., Della Bella, C., Bonsignori, F., Sollai, S., Amedei, A., Galli, L., et al. (2012). Potential role of M. tuberculosis specific IFN-γamma and IL-2 ELISPOT assays in discriminating children with active or latent tuberculosis. *PLOS One* 7:e46041. doi: 10.1371/journal.pone.0046041

Ciuffreda, D., Comte, D., Cavassini, M., Giostra, E., Buhler, L., Perruchoud, M., et al. (2008). Polyfunctional HCV-specific T-cell responses are associated with effective control of HCV replication. *Eur. J. Immunol.* 38, 2665–2677. doi: 10.1002/eji.200838336

Duvall, M. G., Precopio, M. L., Ambrozak, D. A., Jaye, A., McMichael, A. J., Whittle, H. C., et al. (2008). Polyfunctional T cell responses are a hallmark of HIV-2 infection. *Eur. J. Immunol.* 38, 350–363. doi: 10.1002/eji.200737768

Gerdemann, U., Vera, J. F., Rooney, C. M., and Leen, A. M. (2011). Generation of multivirus-specific T cells to prevent/treat viral infections after allogeneic hematopoietic stem cell transplant. *J. Vis. Exp.* 51:2736. doi: 10.3791/2736

Hadinoto, V., Shapiro, M., Greenough, T. C., Sullivan, J. L., Luzuriaga, K., and Thorley-Lawson, D. A. (2008). On the dynamics of acute EBV infection and the pathogenesis of infectious mononucleosis. *Blood* 111, 1420–1427. doi: 10.1182/blood-2007-06-093278

Harari, A., Dutoit, V., Cellerai, C., Bart, P. A., Du Pasquier, R. A., and Pantaleo, G. (2006). Functional signatures of protective antiviral T-cell immunity in human virus infections. *Immunol. Rev.* 211, 236–254. doi: 10.1111/j.0105-2896.2006.00395.x

Harari, A., Vallelian, F., Meylan, P. R., and Pantaleo, G. (2005). Functional heterogeneity of memory CD4 T cell responses in different conditions of antigen exposure and persistence. *J. Immunol.* 174, 1037–1045. doi: 10.4049/jimmunol.174.2.1037

Helms, T., Boehm, B. O., Asaad, R. J., Trezza, R. P., Lehmann, P. V., and Tary-Lehmann, M. (2000). Direct visualization of cytokine-producing recall antigen-specific CD4 memory T cells in healthy individuals and HIV patients. *J. Immunol.* 164, 3723–3732. doi: 10.4049/jimmunol.164.7.3723

Hislop, A. D., Taylor, G. S., Sauce, D., and Rickinson, A. B. (2007). Cellular responses to viral infection in humans: lessons from Epstein-barr virus. *Annu. Rev. Immunol.* 25, 587–617. doi: 10.1146/annurev.immunol.25.022106.141553

Jennes, W., Kestens, L., Nixon, D. F., and Shacklett, B. L. (2002). Enhanced ELISPOT detection of antigen-specific T cell responses from cryopreserved specimens with addition of both IL-7 and IL-15–the Amplispot assay. *J. Immunol. Methods* 270, 99–108. doi: 10.1016/S0022-1759(02)00275-2

Jones, K., Nourse, J. P., Morrison, L., Nguyen-Van, D., Moss, D. J., Burrows, S. R., et al. (2010). Expansion of EBNA1-specific effector T cells in posttransplantation lymphoproliferative disorders. *Blood* 116, 2245–2252. doi: 10.1182/blood-2010-03-274076

Kimura, H., Morita, M., Yabuta, Y., Kuzushima, K., Kato, K., Kojima, S., et al. (1999). Quantitative analysis of Epstein-Barr virus load by using a real-time PCR assay. *J. Clin. Microbiol.* 37, 132–136.

Krabbe, S., Hesse, J., and Uldall, P. (1981). Primary Epstein-Barr virus infection in early childhood. *Arch. Dis. Child.* 56, 49–52. doi: 10.1136/adc.56.1.49

Kurth, J., Spieker, T., Wustrow, J., Strickler, G. J., Hansmann, L. M., Rajewsky, K., et al. (2000). EBV-infected B cells in infectious mononucleosis: viral strategies for spreading in the B cell compartment and establishing latency. *Immunity* 13, 485–495. doi: 10.1016/S1074-7613(00)00048-0

Larsson, M., Jin, X., Ramratnam, B., Ogg, G. S., Engelmayer, J., Demoitie, M. A., et al. (1999). A recombinant vaccinia virus based ELISPOT assay detects high frequencies of Pol-specific CD8 T cells in HIV-1-positive individuals. *AIDS* 13, 767–777. doi: 10.1097/00002030-199905070-00005

Linnerbauer, S., Behrends, U., Adhikary, D., Witter, K., Bornkamm, G. W., and Mautner, J. (2014). Virus and autoantigen-specific CD4+ T cells are key effectors in a SCID mouse model of EBV-associated post-transplant lymphoproliferative disorders. *PLOS Pathog.* 10:e1004068. doi: 10.1371/journal.ppat.1004068

Long, H. M., Chagoury, O. L., Leese, A. M., Ryan, G. B., James, E., Morton, L. T., et al. (2013). MHC II tetramers visualize human CD4+ T cell responses to Epstein–Barr virus infection and demonstrate atypical kinetics of the nuclear antigen EBNA1 response. *J. Exp. Med.* 210, 933–949. doi: 10.1084/jem.20121437

Longnecker, R., and Neipel, F. (2007). "Introduction to the human gamma-herpesviruses," in *Human Herpesviruses: Biology, Therapy, and Immunoprophylaxis*, eds A. Arvin, G. Campadelli-Fiume, E. Mocarski, P. S. Moore, B. Roizman, R. Whitley, et al. (Cambridge: Cambridge University Press).

Makedonas, G., Hutnick, N., Haney, D., Amick, A. C., Gardner, J., Cosma, G., et al. (2010). Perforin and IL-2 upregulation define qualitative differences among highly functional virus-specific human CD8 T cells. *PLOS Pathog.* 6:e1000798. doi: 10.1371/journal.ppat.1000798

McCutcheon, M., Wehner, N., Wensky, A., Kushner, M., Doan, S., Hsiao, L., et al. (1997). A sensitive ELISPOT assay to detect low-frequency human T lymphocytes. *J. Immunol. Methods* 210, 149–166. doi: 10.1016/S0022-1759(97)00182-8

Murukesan, V., and Mukherjee, S. (2012). Managing post-transplant lymphoproliferative disorders in solid-organ transplant recipients. *Drugs* 72, 1631–1643. doi: 10.2165/11635690-000000000-00000

Niedobitek, G., Agathanggelou, A., Herbst, H., Whitehead, L., Wright, D. H., and Young, L. S. (1997). Epstein-Barr virus (EBV) infection in infectious mononucleosis: virus latency, replication and phenotype of EBV-infected cells. *J. Pathol.* 182, 151–159. doi: 10.1002/(SICI)1096-9896(199706)182:2<151::AID-PATH824>3.0.CO;2-3

Ning, R. J., Xu, X. Q., Chan, K. H., and Chiang, A. K. (2011). Long-term carriers generate Epstein-Barr virus (EBV)-specific CD4(+) and CD8(+) polyfunctional T-cell responses which show immunodominance hierarchies of EBV proteins. *Immunology* 134, 161–171. doi: 10.1111/j.1365-2567.2011.03476.x

Pantaleo, G., and Harari, A. (2006). Functional signatures in antiviral T-cell immunity for monitoring virus-associated diseases. *Nat. Rev. Immunol.* 6, 417–423. doi: 10.1038/nri1840

Posnett, D. N. (2008). Herpesviruses and autoimmunity. *Curr. Opin. Investig. Drugs* 9, 505–514.

Precopio, M. L., Betts, M. R., Parrino, J., Price, D. A., Gostick, E., Ambrozak, D. R., et al. (2007). Immunization with vaccinia virus induces polyfunctional and phenotypically distinctive CD8(+) T cell responses. *J. Exp. Med.* 204, 1405–1416. doi: 10.1084/jem.20062363

Pudney, V. A., Leese, A. M., Rickinson, A. B., and Hislop, A. D. (2005). CD8+ immunodominance among Epstein-Barr virus lytic cycle antigens directly reflects the efficiency of antigen presentation in lytically infected cells. *J. Exp. Med.* 201, 349–360. doi: 10.1084/jem.20041542

Qiu, Z., Zhang, M., Zhu, Y., Zheng, F., Lu, P., Liu, H., et al. (2012). Multifunctional CD4 T cell responses in patients with active tuberculosis. *Sci. Rep.* 2:216. doi: 10.1038/srep00216

Rickinson, A. B., Long, H. M., Palendira, U., Munz, C., and Hislop, A. D. (2014). Cellular immune controls over Epstein-Barr virus infection: new lessons from the clinic and the laboratory. *Trends Immunol.* 35, 159–169. doi: 10.1016/j.it.2014.01.003

Salvetti, M., Giovannoni, G., and Aloisi, F. (2009). Epstein-Barr virus and multiple sclerosis. *Curr. Opin. Neurol.* 22, 201–206. doi: 10.1097/WCO.0b013e32832b4c8d

Scherrenburg, J., Piriou, E. R., Nanlohy, N. M., and van Baarle, D. (2008). Detailed analysis of Epstein-Barr virus-specific CD4+ and CD8+ T cell responses during infectious mononucleosis. *Clin. Exp. Immunol.* 153, 231–239. doi: 10.1111/j.1365-2249.2008.03699.x

Schmittel, A., Keilholz, U., and Scheibenbogen, C. (1997). Evaluation of the interferon-gamma ELISPOT-assay for quantification of peptide specific T lymphocytes from peripheral blood. *J. Immunol. Methods* 210, 167–174. doi: 10.1016/S0022-1759(97)00184-1

Seder, R. A., Darrah, P. A., and Roederer, M. (2008). T-cell quality in memory and protection: implications for vaccine design. *Nat. Rev. Immunol.* 8, 247–258. doi: 10.1038/nri2274

Shi, Y., and Lutz, C. T. (2002). Interferon-gamma control of EBV-transformed B cells: a role for CD8+ T cells that poorly kill EBV-infected cells. *Viral Immunol.* 15, 213–225. doi: 10.1089/088282402317340350

Shmarov, V. A., Malashchenko, V. V., Meniailo, M. E., Gazatova, N. D., Todosenko, N. M., Melashchenko, O. B., et al. (2016). Direct effects of interleukin-7 on the function of human T cells *in vitro*. *Eur. Cytokine Netw.* 27, 102–107. doi: 10.1684/ecn.2016.0385

Silins, S. L., Sherritt, M. A., Silleri, J. M., Cross, S. M., Elliott, S. L., Bharadwaj, M., et al. (2001). Asymptomatic primary Epstein-Barr virus infection occurs in the absence of blood T-cell repertoire perturbations despite high levels of systemic viral load. *Blood* 98, 3739–3744. doi: 10.1182/blood.V98.13.3739

Smith, C., Beagley, L., and Khanna, R. (2009). Acquisition of polyfunctionality by Epstein-Barr virus-specific CD8+ T cells correlates with increased resistance to galectin-1-mediated suppression. *J. Virol.* 83, 6192–6198. doi: 10.1128/JVI.00239-09

Sumaya, C. V., and Ench, Y. (1985). Epstein-Barr virus infectious mononucleosis in children. I. Clinical and general laboratory findings. *Pediatrics* 75, 1003–1010.

Vella, A., Teague, T. K., Ihle, J., Kappler, J., and Marrack, P. (1997). Interleukin 4 (IL-4) or IL-7 prevents the death of resting T cells: stat6 is probably not required for the effect of IL-4. *J. Exp. Med.* 186, 325–330. doi: 10.1084/jem.186.2.325

Vella, A. T., Dow, S., Potter, T. A., Kappler, J., and Marrack, P. (1998). Cytokine-induced survival of activated T cells *in vitro* and *in vivo*. *Proc. Natl. Acad. Sci. U.S.A.* 95, 3810–3815. doi: 10.1073/pnas.95.7.3810

Yang, J., Lemas, V. M., Flinn, I. W., Krone, C., and Ambinder, R. F. (2000). Application of the ELISPOT assay to the characterization of CD8(+) responses to Epstein-Barr virus antigens. *Blood* 95, 241–248.

Young, L. S., and Rickinson, A. B. (2004). Epstein-Barr virus: 40 years on. *Nat. Rev. Cancer* 4, 757–768. doi: 10.1038/nrc1452

2

Secretome of Intestinal *Bacilli:* A Natural Guard Against Pathologies

Olga N. Ilinskaya[1], Vera V. Ulyanova[1], Dina R. Yarullina[1] and Ilgiz G. Gataullin[2]*

[1] *Department of Microbiology, Kazan Federal University, Kazan, Russia,* [2] *Department of Surgery and Oncology, Regional Clinical Cancer Center, Kazan, Russia*

***Correspondence:**
Olga N. Ilinskaya
ilinskaya_kfu@mail.ru*

Current studies of human gut microbiome usually do not consider the special functional role of transient microbiota, although some of its members remain in the host for a long time and produce broad spectrum of biologically active substances. Getting into the gastrointestinal tract (GIT) with food, water and probiotic preparations, two representatives of *Bacilli* class, genera *Bacillus* and *Lactobacillus*, colonize epithelium blurring the boundaries between resident and transient microbiota. Despite their minor proportion in the microbiome composition, these bacteria can significantly affect both the intestinal microbiota and the entire body thanks to a wide range of secreted compounds. Recently, insufficiency and limitations of pure genome-based analysis of gut microbiota became known. Thus, the need for intense functional studies is evident. This review aims to characterize the *Bacillus* and *Lactobacillus* in GIT, as well as the functional roles of the components released by these members of microbial intestinal community. Complex of their secreted compounds is referred by us as the "bacillary secretome." The composition of the bacillary secretome, its biological effects in GIT and role in counteraction to infectious diseases and oncological pathologies in human organism is the subject of the review.

Keywords: *Lactobacillus*, *Bacillus*, gastrointestinal tract, metabolites, secretome

INTRODUCTION

The human gut microbiota consists of about 1500 microbial species which constitute 10^{12} bacteria per gram of stool (Browne et al., 2016). The gastrointestinal microbiota of healthy human adults consists primarily of bacteria belonging to phyla *Firmicutes* and *Bacteroidetes*, and to a lesser extent to phyla *Actinobacteria* and *Proteobacteria* (Dethlefsen et al., 2008; Yang and Jobin, 2014). Density and composition of microbiota varies along both the length of the gut and the cross-section (Nava and Stappenbeck, 2011; Tropini et al., 2017). Changes in nutrients, availability of oxygen, and presence of immune effectors in local microenvironment determine species variation and abundance (Donaldson et al., 2016). The most dominant taxa have the highest stability in the gut (Martí et al., 2017). Rapidly dividing facultative anaerobes from *Lactobacillaceae* and *Enterobacteriaceae* dominate in small intestine, while saccharolytic representatives of *Bacteroidales* and *Clostridiales* orders are abundant in the large intestine (Donaldson et al., 2016; Tropini et al., 2017). Mucin-utilizing species of *Akkermansia* and *Bacteroides* are followed by aerotolerant *Proteobacteria* and *Actinobacteria* in direction to the

---

Abbreviations: CSF, competence and sporulation factor; EVs, extracellular vesicles; GIT, gastrointestinal tract; NO, nitric oxide; NOS, nitric oxide synthase; RNases, ribonucleases; SCFAs, short-chain fatty acids.

epithelium (Tropini et al., 2017). *Proteobacteria* and *Firmicutes* are found in crypts and represent the stock for reseeding the colon because they are protected from the luminal flow (Tropini et al., 2017). At least 50–60% of the bacterial genera from the intestinal microbiota of a healthy individual produce spores which facilitate both microbiota persistence and transmission (Browne et al., 2016). The majority of gut bacteria are transient populations which pass through the lumen of the lower GIT (Tropini et al., 2017).

Composition of gut microbiota varies among individuals with geographic provenance, gender, age, diet, malnutrition, and intake of probiotics or antimicrobial agents (Panda et al., 2014; Haro et al., 2016; Odamaki et al., 2016; Maffei et al., 2017; Martí et al., 2017; Singh et al., 2017). Alterations in the composition of the gut microbiota and reductions in microbial diversity lead to different disorders such as inflammatory conditions of the intestine (inflammatory bowel disease, irritable bowel syndrome, colorectal cancer) (Gagnière et al., 2016; Ghoshal et al., 2017; Rapozo et al., 2017), type 2 diabetes, obesity, anorexia nervosa, forms of severe acute malnutrition, cardiovascular diseases (atherosclerosis, hypertension, heart failure) (Tang et al., 2017), neurobehavioral diseases (autism spectrum disorder, major depression) (Clemente et al., 2012). The microbiota is increasingly recognized for its ability to maintain homeostasis in health and disease influencing host appetite, function of the nervous system and several complex host behaviors (Sharon et al., 2016; Winek et al., 2016; van de Wouw et al., 2017; Vuong et al., 2017). A healthy gut microbiota can be defined by the presence of the various microbial species that enhance metabolism, resistance to infection and inflammation, prevention against cancer and autoimmunity.

Lactobacilli are historically considered as integral part of human intestinal microbiota. Today, a large body of evidence indicates that only a small number of *Lactobacillus* species are true autochthonous inhabitants of the mammalian intestinal tract and that most lactobacilli present are allochthonous members derived from food or oral cavity (Reuter, 2001; Walter, 2008). *Lactobacillus* spp. content of fecal samples is characterized by temporal fluctuations and lack of stability (Walter et al., 2001; Vanhoutte et al., 2004). Attempts to divide lactobacilli into resident and transient ones are hardly legitimate since the style of nutrition significantly affects their contents in the intestine. Lactobacilli together with enterococci dominate in the duodenum and in the jejunum (Reuter, 2001; Hammes and Hertel, 2015), although their absolute number increases along the intestine from duodenum to colon (Derrien and van Hylckama Vlieg, 2015). However, they constitute only a minor fraction within the human adult fecal microbiota, i.e., around 0.01 to 0.6% of total bacterial counts (Harmsen et al., 2002; Matsuda et al., 2009).

Metagenomics widely used for study of gut microbiota is unable to detect bacteria at concentrations less than 10^5 bacteria per gram (Lagier et al., 2015). A culturing approach that uses high-throughput culture conditions in combination with matrix-assisted laser desorption/ionization-time of flight (MALDI-TOF) mass spectrometry and 16S rRNA sequencing for taxonomic identification and referred to as culturomics has allowed significant increase in a number of bacteria discovered in human GIT including species known in humans but not in the gut, species previously considered unculturable as well as new species. Considerable part of them is represented by *Firmicutes* (Lagier et al., 2016) including *Bacillus* species (Lagier et al., 2015; Mourembou et al., 2016; Senghor et al., 2017).

For a long time, the representatives of *Bacillus* genus, unlike the species of *Lactobacillus*, were not considered as a part of the normal intestinal microbiome. Being isolated from feces, *Bacillus* spp. as soil microorganisms were considered transient. Recent studies show that they are present in the GIT in the amounts significantly higher than what can be explained by their ingestion with food only. *Bacillus* spp. (*B. pumilus*, *B. licheniformis*, *B. clausii*, *B. subtilis*, *B. megaterium*, *B. mediterraneensis*, *B. thuringiensis*) have been isolated from the healthy human GIT, where they are well-adapted and are more colonizing than transient (Fakhry et al., 2008; Alou et al., 2016; Lopetuso et al., 2016). In environment, the vegetative forms of *Bacillus* are present usually near decomposing plants and in their rhizosphere. In the soil they exist mainly in the form of spores, which germinate in the digestive tract of humans and animals. Germination of *Bacillus* spores in the human small intestine and transient colonization should be considered as a part of the life cycle of human-associated *Bacillus* species (Hong et al., 2009). In the GIT, spores not only germinate but also are formed again from vegetative cells during a time shorter than in the laboratory (Tam et al., 2006; Ghelardi et al., 2015).

Thus, it can be concluded that GIT microbiota including *Bacillus* and *Lactobacillus* species undergoes constant dynamic change. In our opinion, distinguishing between the resident and transient intestinal inhabitants is less relevant issue compared to the study of molecular pool released by them. Most of bacteria absorbed in the body can supplement the gastrointestinal microbiome (Derrien and van Hylckama Vlieg, 2015). The challenge of identifying the "spheres of influence" of the transient microbiota in the human body has not been solved, and has not even been formulated, with the exception of some aspects of the pathogen entry into the body. Its bottleneck is the lack of data on the complexes secreted by this microbiota, their components, functions and the interaction between components, namely, the composition and biological role of the secretome.

We consciously narrowed the spectrum of secretome producers observed here to two representatives of the *Bacilli* class, genera *Lactobacillus* and *Bacillus*, due to their wide distribution and high probability of entering the human body. The ingestion of microorganisms occurs with food, water and bacterial probiotics. Facultative aerobic bacilli represent a smaller proportion of the intestinal microbiota than anaerobic bacteria (Rajilić-Stojanović and de Vos, 2014), but they actively influence the microbial community of GIT and also the whole organism thanks to the great diversity of secreted compounds. Our studies of biopsies taken during surgical intervention in patients with diagnosed colorectal cancer revealed the presence of *Bacilli* closely associated with intestinal epithelium, traditionally considered as transient ones (Siraj et al., 2015). Since secretory components can be studied only in culturable microorganisms, the insufficiency of genomic analysis of intestinal microbiota and the transition to functional analysis became evident (Derrien and van Hylckama Vlieg, 2015; Lagier et al., 2015). In this regard, the identification, characterization, and elucidation of the functional role of the components secreted by the minority of the intestinal microbial community, namely representatives of the *Bacilli* class in GIT, is an actual task. The modern concept of a gut–brain axis (McKay et al., 2017) must be detailed and refined taking into account the spectra of compounds secreted by *Bacilli*, namely low- and high-molecular components of the secretome and EVs, which affect the whole body and shape human health.

BENEFICIAL EFFECTS OF *Lactobacillus* AND *Bacillus*

Historically, species of *Lactobacillus* and *Bacillus* are found in the traditional fermented food products possessing beneficial properties for the intestinal function (Nithya et al., 2012; Satish Kumar et al., 2013; Lee et al., 2016; Sornplang and Piyadeatsoontorn, 2016; Marco et al., 2017) and are widely used as components of commercially available probiotics: DE111 (Deerland Enzymes, United States), Enterogermina (Sanofi Winthrop, Italy), Biosubtyl (Biophar, Vietnam), Biosporin (Biopharma, Russia), BioSpora (Klaire Labs, United States), Blicheni and Zhengchangsheng (Northeast Pharmaceutical Group, China), GanedenBC 30 (Ganeden, United States), Lactobacterin (Microgen, Russia), HOWARU or DR20 (Danisco, United States), Yakult (Yakult, Japan), PCC (Probiomics, Australia). In food industry, lactobacilli are applied as starter cultures in the production of fermented milk products, cheese, sausages, bread, kimchi, pickles, and yogurts, the latter accounting for the largest share of sales (Giraffa et al., 2010; Tamang et al., 2016). The administration of probiotics has been shown to favorably alter the intestinal microbiota balance, enhance intestinal integrity and motility, inhibit the growth of harmful bacteria and increase resistance to infections (Tamang et al., 2016).

As a part of GIT microbiota *Bacilli* participate in metabolism of dietary components, xenobiotics and drugs helping to maintain intestinal homeostasis and host health (Jandhyala et al., 2015; Rowland et al., 2017). The beneficial effect of probiotics on GIT is mediated by influence on composition, diversity and function of the intestinal microbiota as well as whole human organism. Probiotics suppress pathogenic bacteria and favor beneficial ones via competition for nutrients, especially for shared limited resource like iron, competitive attachment to the epithelium, formation of substrates for growth, production of waste products and antimicrobial compounds, strengthening of the barrier function of the epithelium, and modulation of innate immunity (Thomas and Versalovic, 2010; Bermudez-Brito et al., 2012; Stubbendieck and Straight, 2016). For example, consumption of *B. coagulans* was shown to increase beneficial groups of bacteria in the gut of 65–80 years old humans and production of anti-inflammatory cytokines (Nyangale et al., 2015).

The efficacy of *Lactobacillus* and *Bacillus* in the prevention and/or treatment of intestinal diseases such as diarrhea, colitis, irritable bowel syndrome, irritable bowel disease, and colorectal cancer was demonstrated (Camilleri, 2006; Sazawal et al., 2006; Rafter et al., 2007; Pillai and Nelson, 2008; Ghouri et al., 2014; Urgesi et al., 2014; Choi et al., 2015; Matsuoka and Kanai, 2015; Majeed et al., 2016; Zhang et al., 2016). In particular, treatment of colorectal colitis in mice with probiotic *B. subtilis* restored balance in gut microflora: beneficial species of *Bifidobacterium*, *Lactobacillus*, and *Butyricicoccus* spp. were increased, while gut damage-promoting species of *Acinetobacter* sp., *Ruminococcus* sp., *Clostridium* spp., and *Veillonella* sp. were decreased (Zhang et al., 2016). *B. subtilis* also retained gut barrier integrity, decreased the endotoxin concentration and reduced gut inflammation (Zhang et al., 2016; Bene et al., 2017). Sporulation of *B. subtilis* plays a major role in the development of GALT – gut lymphoid tissue associated with the gastrointestinal mucosa - and in the diversity of the primary antibody population ("preimmune" repertoire) in rabbits (Rhee et al., 2004). *Bacillus* spp. like other strains isolated from human stool were able to bind the human norovirus strains, the cause of acute viral gastroenteritis and foodborne diseases, around the outer cell surfaces and pili structures (Almand et al., 2017). The interaction between virus and bacteria is hypothesized to help the host immune system to better recognize infectious particles.

The ratio between the two major phyla inhabiting the human GIT, *Firmicutes* and *Bacteroidetes*, reflects the GIT status during the life and diseases. It is significantly decreased in infants and elderly individuals as compared to adults (0.4, 0.6, and 10.9, respectively) (Mariat et al., 2009) and lowers upon antibiotic-associated diarrhea, coeliac disease, Crohn's disease, and ulcerative colitis (Ott et al., 2004; Panda et al., 2014; Carding et al., 2015; Quagliariello et al., 2016). A decrease in populations of *Ruminococcus* and *Lactobacillus* was observed in a rat model of colorectal cancer (Zhu et al., 2014). Microbial content of the patients with diagnosed colorectal cancer and healthy individuals differed significantly. *Firmicutes* and *Fusobacteria* were over-represented whereas *Proteobacteria* were under-represented in patients. In addition, *Lactococcus* and *Fusobacterium* exhibited a relatively higher abundance while *Pseudomonas* and *Escherichia–Shigella* were reduced in cancerous tissues compared to adjacent non-cancerous ones (Gao et al., 2015). *Bacilli* were shown to decrease quantitatively upon type 2 diabetes (Sankar et al., 2015). The possibility of using probiotics in the therapy of diseases, namely allergy, asthma, diabetes, cardiovascular diseases is discussed (Ebel et al., 2014).

Viability is by definition a prerequisite for probiotic effectiveness as it is essential for colonization of intestinal mucosa, displacement of pathogens and immunomodulation. Viable bacteria demonstrate adhesive and antagonistic properties and produce a large number of extracellular enzymes and biologically active compounds (Shobharani and Halami, 2014). Nevertheless, there is increasing evidence that isolated bacteria-derived molecules and surface components (e.g., cell wall components, cell wall associated proteins, S-layer proteins) potentiate probiotic benefits attributed earlier to viable probiotic bacteria (Lahtinen, 2012; Ruiz et al., 2014).

Despite more than a century of active use of probiotics, initiated by I. Mechnikov in 1907, the majority of modern reviews assessing the effectiveness of these drugs confirm the need for further studies to determine the exact mechanisms of positive effects of probiotics on the human body. Both live probiotic bacterial cells and their metabolites can be useful in treatment of intestinal diseases (Okamoto et al., 2012). The molecular basis for the effectiveness of probiotics remains unexplored or only partially studied. The future study aimed at deciphering the mechanisms that determine the probiotic properties of bacteria will certainly allow expanding the areas of scientifically proven probiotic use in medicine.

MICROBIOTA–HUMAN METABOLIC INTERACTION

Between the gut microbiota and host organism there is an extremely complex relationship that affects the human metabolism, immunity and health (Marchesi et al., 2016). This crosstalk is mediated by nutrients, metabolites, antimicrobial compounds. It was demonstrated that the psychological and physical stress of a host affects its gut microbiota and, in turn, gut microflora can modulate host's mood and appetite (Sandrini et al., 2015). Gut microbiota is regulated by the host through production of non-specific antimicrobial peptides such as defensins (Nakamura et al., 2016), secreted IgA which provides the selection and the maintenance of the commensal bacteria (Fransen et al., 2015), and miRNAs specifically regulating bacterial transcripts and affecting bacterial growth (Liu and Weiner, 2016). It was proved that host genetic background affects the composition and function of the gut microbiota, altering the production of microbial metabolites and intestinal inflammation (Lamas et al., 2016). For example, the microbiota of mice deficient in caspase recruitment domain family member 9 (*CARD9*) failed to metabolize tryptophan that increased host susceptibility to colitis (Lamas et al., 2016).

Microbial species are recognized by host's immune system. Commensal bacteria have immunomodulatory properties that allow them inducing tolerogenic immune responses against themselves and contributing to host protective immune responses against pathogens (Bene et al., 2017; Guo et al., 2017; Shi et al., 2017). It is known that probiotics affect key signaling pathways, such as NFκB and MAPK, through the pattern-recognition receptors (TLR, NOD) (Bermudez-Brito et al., 2012) enhancing the production of anti-inflammatory cytokines (Nyangale et al., 2015) and reducing the emergence of proinflammatory ones (Selvam et al., 2009). The gut microbiota is able to influence host antigen production by human monocyte-derived dendritic cell populations in a species-specific manner (Bene et al., 2017).

Gut microbiota affects host physiology by releasing bioactive metabolites including antibiotics, enzymes, vitamins and amino acids (choline, methionine, vitamin B), minerals (cobalt, iodine, selenium, and zinc) and energy metabolites (SAM, acetyl-CoA, NAD^+, α-KG, and ATP), SCFAs (acetate, propionate, butyrate, caproate, and valerate), neurotransmitters [acetylcholine, dopamine, noradrenaline, serotonin, and γ-aminobutyric acid (GABA)], hormones, bacterial antigens, pathogen-associated molecular patterns, and toxins (Donia et al., 2014; Luber and Kostic, 2017). These molecules enter host circulation thereby mediating the link between the gut and other organs (brain, lung, liver, muscle) (Shukla et al., 2017) and modulate physiological pathways and even behavior (van de Wouw et al., 2017; Vuong et al., 2017). The influence of gut microbiota on the epigenetic regulation of host genes via DNA methylation and histone modifications has been demonstrated (Ye et al., 2017). Contact-independent metabolic exchange helps signal dispersal among neighboring cells as well as its blockage when needed.

Bacteria produce a lot of chemically diverse metabolites with poorly understood function. *Bacillus* species are among the most frequent producers of bioactive secondary metabolites (800 compounds), while lactobacilli produce 100s of compounds (Bérdy, 2005). Known to date, the results of the study of representatives of the *Bacilli* class colonizing the human GIT mostly refer to ascertaining their positive, less often negative, impact on the body. We tried to systematize the available knowledge about compounds and complexes produced by these bacteria which serve as effectors triggering certain processes in the body (**Figure 1**), and identify the stage responsible for actually registered "influence." *Bacilli* introduced into the GIT through the consumption of fermented food do integrate the resident microbiome (Derrien and van Hylckama Vlieg, 2015) and contribute to its regulatory and health promoting action producing a variety of substances ranging from low molecular weight regulatory agents to proteins and peptides with antimicrobial and antitumor effects. Metabolites secreted by bacteria form a coat around the cells which contributes to nutrient supply, communication, and protection from damage caused by direct interaction with other species or their metabolites. Due to diffusion, the concentration of extracellular metabolites decreases with distance. To ensure that secreted components will reach their targets bacteria utilize membranous vesicles for their transportation.

TOP-APPRECIATED COMPONENTS OF *Bacilli* SECRETOME

It is well-appreciated that complex of **enzymes** (proteases, amylases, cellulases, lipases) secreted by *Bacilli* aid in digestion of food components in GIT (Khochamit et al., 2015; Keller et al., 2017). Bile salt hydrolases of lactobacilli reduce blood cholesterol and diminish the risk for cardiovascular diseases (Patel et al., 2010; Kumar et al., 2012). Recently, an antagonistic role of *L. johnsonii* La1 extracellular bile salt hydrolase against intestinal protozoan parasite *Giardia duodenalis* was revealed (Travers et al., 2016). Other enzymes like *N*-acylated homoserine lactone (AHL)-lactonase help to modulate the microbiota content by decreasing the number of quorum-sensing pathogenic bacteria in the GIT through direct disruption of their signal molecules (Vinoj et al., 2014; Zhou et al., 2016). Moreover, many enzymes are involved in the formation of metabolites which possess their own biological activities. For instance, during fermentation of milk and other proteinaceous products lactobacilli are able to release biologically active peptides with angiotensin I-converting enzyme (ACE)-inhibitory activity. Among these antihypertensive

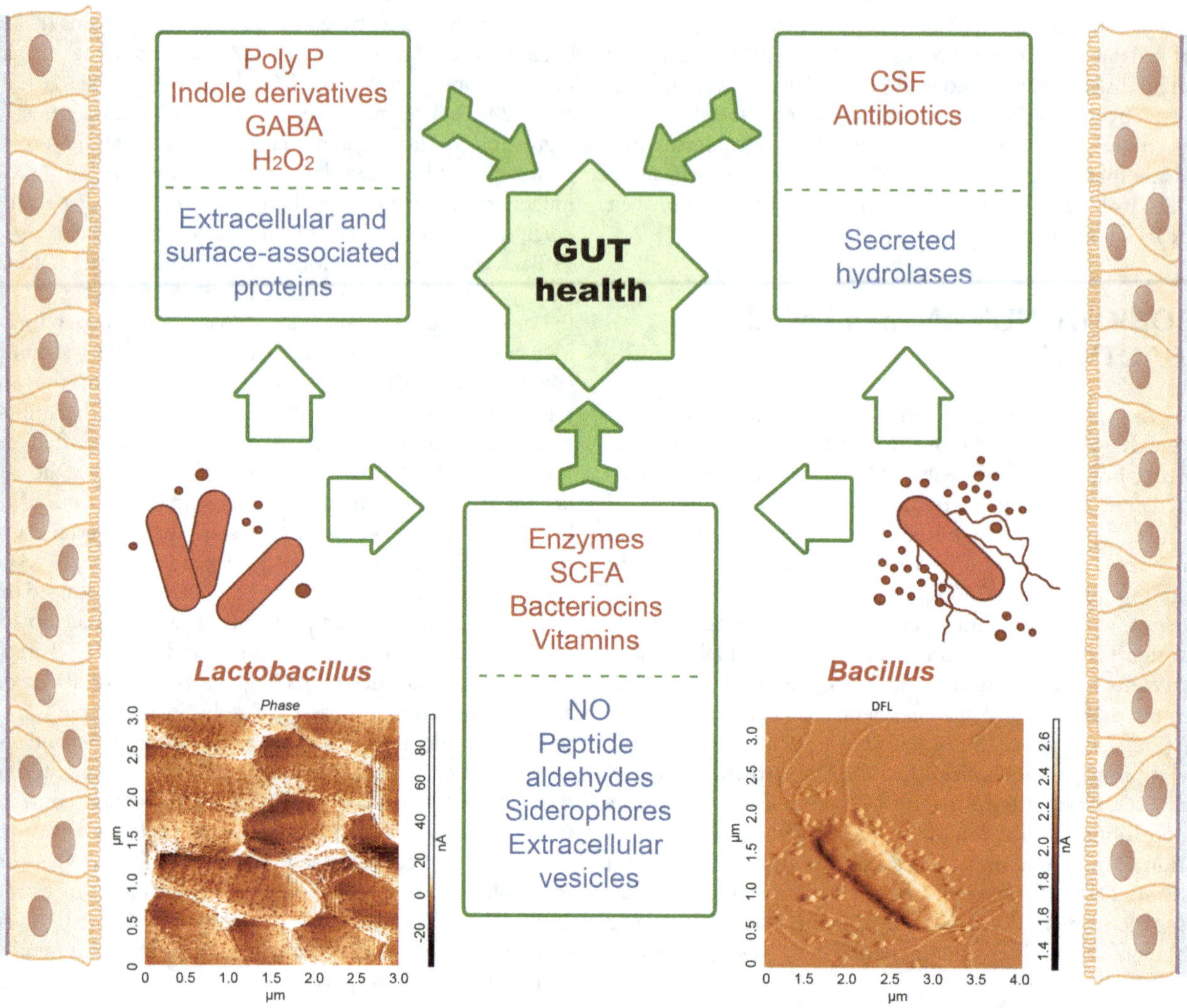

FIGURE 1 | Compounds secreted by the representatives of *Lactobacillus* and *Bacillus* mediating their beneficial effects in the GIT. Top-appreciated compounds are shown in upper part of panels, under-appreciated compounds – in lower parts. Both *Lactobacillus* and *Bacillus* are minor part of GIT microbiota. Of them, *Lactobacillus* spp. dominate quantitatively secreting a few compounds, while *Bacillus* spp. are less abundant but produce a variety of secreted substances with a wide spectrum of activities. Representatives of the *Bacilli* class were isolated from colon epithelia biopsy of the patients with diagnosed colorectal cancer. Atomic force microscopy images of *L. plantarum* (photo provided by Dr. *Dina Yarullina*) and *B. pumilus* (photo kindly provided by Dr. *Galina Yakovleva*) were obtained in air (contact mode) of stationary phase cells that were deposited on glass and dried prior analysis. Bacteria were identified using MALDI-TOF technique and 16S RNA sequencing. Representative AFM images show nanoscale structures on the cell surface and around the cells attributed to EVs.

peptides β-casein-derived tripeptides (lactotripeptides) are most studied (Hayes et al., 2007; Fekete et al., 2015).

Short-chain fatty acids are formed upon dietary carbohydrates fermentation by both *Bacilli* genera, studied in this review. The most common SCFA is lactate followed by acetic, propionic, butyric acids and minor isobutyrate, 2-methylpropionate, valerate, isovalerate, hexanoate. SCFAs are one of the most important gut microbial products affecting a range of host processes including energy utilization, host-microbe signaling, and control of colonic pH. Decrease of a luminal pH creates an environment favoring beneficial species like *Faecalibacterium prausnitzii* and inappropriate for many others bacteria and yeasts (Nyangale et al., 2015). SCFAs positively influence the gut motility (Yang and Chiu, 2017) and intestinal secretion (Bhattarai et al., 2017), inhibit proliferation of tumor cells by apoptosis induction, stimulate production of insulin-like growth factor 1 promoting bone growth and remodeling (Yan et al., 2016), cause epigenetic modifications, regulate blood pressure and inflammation (Natarajan and Pluznick, 2014). The multifaceted roles of SCFAs nominate them for the key molecular link between diet, the microbiome and health.

Lactate produced by *Lactobacillus* provides an unfavorable environment for the growth of many pathogenic bacteria, it also acts as a permeabilizer of the Gram-negative bacterial outer membrane, thus increasing the susceptibility of pathogens to antimicrobial molecules, e.g., bacteriocins or host lysozyme (Alakomi et al., 2000). Strains of *B. licheniformis* and *B. coagulans* also ferment different sugars with formation of lactic acid (Wang et al., 2011; Nyangale et al., 2015). Butyrate is the local energy source for colonocytes (LeBlanc et al., 2017); also it plays an important role in maintenance of the gut barrier function through stimulation of tight junction integrity and mucin production (Peng et al., 2009; Jung et al., 2015). The SCFAs produced by the human gut microbiota are transported from the gut lumen with the bloodstream to a variety of different organs, where they are used in lipid and energy metabolism, particularly by the hepatocyte cells of the liver, which use propionate for gluconeogenesis, whilst acetate and butyrate are mostly involved in lipid biosynthesis (den Besten et al., 2013a). Besides, SCFAs appear to exert regulatory effects on gluconeogenesis and lipogenesis mediated by peroxisome proliferator-activated receptor gamma (PPARγ) (den Besten et al., 2015) and protein kinases, such as AMP-activated protein kinase (Peng et al., 2009; den Besten et al., 2015) or mitogen-activated protein kinases (MAPK) (Jung et al., 2015). SCFAs have been reported to represent the natural ligands for free fatty acid receptors 2 and 3 (FFAR 2/3) (former G protein-coupled receptors, GPR43 and GPR41), involved in the regulation of lipid and glucose metabolism and found on a wide range of cell types, including enteroendocrine and immune cells (den Besten et al., 2013b). Moreover, as far as these receptors are expressed on neurons of the peripheral, autonomic and somatic nervous systems, SCFAs can modulate neuronal activity and visceral reflexes (Nøhr et al., 2015). SCFAs are considered as promising for the prevention and treatment of the metabolic syndrome, certain types of cancer, bowel disorders, such as ulcerative colitis, Crohn's disease, and antibiotic-associated diarrhea (den Besten et al., 2013b; Ríos-Covián et al., 2016).

Hydrogen peroxide (H_2O_2) production by lactobacilli has been suggested to be a non-specific antimicrobial defense mechanism. *L. jensenii, L. crispatus, L. gasseri,* and *L. acidophilus* are the most common H_2O_2-producing lactobacilli inhabiting the human intestine and are often applied as probiotic supplements in the food industry (Martín and Suárez, 2010; Hertzberger et al., 2014). In gastrointestinal environment, SCFAs and bacteriocins have been considered as key antimicrobial factors, whereas the impact of H_2O_2 production remains underappreciated. However, H_2O_2, like other reactive oxygen species, exerts strong cytotoxicity against microorganisms. Although H_2O_2 itself is not highly reactive, it can readily diffuse across cellular membrane and through the Fenton reaction form highly reactive hydroxyl radicals, which cause oxidative damage to major biological macromolecules, e.g., oxidation of protein thiols, peroxidation of lipids, DNA base damage, and strand breakage of nucleic acids (Imlay, 2003; Valko et al., 2005). The role for H_2O_2 in the anti-*Salmonella* activity of *L. johnsonii* NCC533, the human intestinal isolate and a probiotic strain, was revealed *in vitro* (Pridmore et al., 2008). *L. delbrueckii* VI1007 produces at least three growth-inhibiting factors, other than lactic acid, one of which has been identified as H_2O_2 (Van De Guchte et al., 2001). H_2O_2 may contribute to the maintenance of the normal microbiota. Especially for the vaginal microbiota, strong evidence exists that colonization with H_2O_2-producing lactobacilli is associated with lower rates of bacterial vaginosis and HIV acquisition (Wilks et al., 2004; Balkus et al., 2012). Moreover, H_2O_2 may exert immunomodulatory properties. It was showed that H_2O_2, produced by *L. crispatus* M247, acts as a signal transducing molecule activating peroxisome proliferator activated receptor γ (PPAR-γ), which plays a central role in regulation of intestinal inflammation and homeostasis (Voltan et al., 2008). *L. johnsonii*-derived H_2O_2 has been shown to affect the activity of indoleamine 2,3-dioxygenase, an important immune modulator, both *in vitro* and in the rat model of type 1 diabetes (Valladares et al., 2013).

Poly P, a linear polymer of over 700 phosphate residues, is synthesized by *Lactobacillus* with the help of polyphosphate kinase (Alcántara et al., 2014). It suppresses the oxidant-induced intestinal permeability inducing cytoprotective heat shock proteins in mouse small intestine through activation of integrin β1-p38 MAPK pathway (Segawa et al., 2011). Poly P was shown to improve the inflammation grade and survival rate in mice model of colitis (Segawa et al., 2011) and to inhibit viability of colon cancer cells via apoptosis through activation of the ERK pathway (Sakatani et al., 2016).

Indole derivatives formed from tryptophan by *Lactobacillus* cells act on the aryl hydrocarbon receptor in intestinal immune cells increasing IL-22 production which, in turns, beneficially impacts the immune system, enhances antifungal resistance and protection of mucosa from damage (Zelante et al., 2013; Lamas et al., 2016; Etienne-Mesmin et al., 2017). The main inhibitory neurotransmitter in the brain, **GABA,** is produced with the help of glutamate decarboxylase expressed by multiple strains of *Lactobacillus* (Barrett et al., 2012; Yunes et al., 2016).

Bacilli synthesize B-group **vitamins** including folate and biotin during the fermentation of foods in GIT and can exchange them, thereby enabling the survival of organisms that do not synthesize those (Magnúsdóttir et al., 2015).

A number of **peptide and lipopeptide antibiotics and bacteriocins** are produced by *Bacilli* both involving ribosomes and non-ribosomally (Zacharofa and Lovitt, 2012; Sumi et al., 2015; Zhao and Kuipers, 2016). These structurally diverse compounds suppress the growth of competing species and pathogens through different mechanisms primarily connected to membrane permeabilization (Fiedler and Heerklotz, 2015; Shobharani et al., 2015). Antimicrobial peptides of *Bacilli* were shown to be active against pathogenic bacteria such as *Staphylococcus aureus*, methicillin resistant *S. aureus, Clostridium perfringens, Klebsiella* sp., and common food spoilage bacteria such as *B. cereus, Escherichia coli, Listeria monocytogenes, Pseudomonas aeruginosa, Aeromonas* sp., *Serratia marcescens, Pasteurella haemolytica, Salmonella enteritidis,* and *S. gallinarum* (Ahmadova et al., 2013; Martinez et al., 2013; Berić et al., 2014; Ayed et al., 2015; Khochamit et al., 2015; Shobharani et al., 2015; Collins et al., 2016; Lim et al., 2016; Chauhan et al., 2017; Perez et al., 2017). Bacteriocins attract great interest with regard to their potential use as food preservatives (De Vuyst and Leroy, 2007; Kaškonienė et al., 2017) and are regarded as a promising alternative to prevent gastrointestinal infections (Dobson et al., 2012).

Lactobacillus produces a number of bacteriocins usually active against closely related Gram-positive bacteria which are likely to reside in the same ecological niche. Most *Lactobacillus* bacteriocins are small, heat-stable cationic peptides which form pores in the cytoplasmic membrane of sensitive bacteria and thus cause leaking of target cells (Oscariz and Pisabarro, 2001). Other bacteriocins interrupt production of peptidoglycan or act by interfering with essential enzyme activities in susceptible bacteria (Servin, 2004). Bacteriocins from *Lactobacillus* are generally recognized as being inactive against Gram-negative organisms. However, it has been reported that bacteriocin from *L. plantarum* TN635 is active against *Salmonella enterica* ATCC43972, *Pseudomonas aeruginosa* ATCC 49189, *Hafnia* sp. and *Serratia* sp. (Smaoui et al., 2010). Moreover, a small bacteriocin (<6.5 kDa) produced by *L. acidophilus* IBB 801 and designated as acidophilin 801, displayed bactericidal activity against *E. coli* Row and *Salmonella panama* 1467 (Zamfir et al., 1999). Bacteriocin OR-7 produced by *L. salivarius* NRRL B-30514 resulted in reduction of *Campylobacter jejuni* colonization in chicken GI tracts when was added into feed. Interestingly, OR-7 had high sequence similarity to acidocin A, which was previously identified from *L. acidophilus* and had activity only to Gram-positive bacteria (Stern et al., 2006).

Bacillus is considered to be the second most important bacteriocin producer following lactic acid bacteria which differs from the latter by broad antimicrobial spectrum (Abriouel et al., 2011; Ayed et al., 2015). Bacteriocins and bacteriocin-like inhibitory substances produced by *Bacillus* exhibit antibacterial activity toward Gram-positive and Gram-negative bacteria as well as fungi, however, activity against Gram-positives is comparatively higher (Hyronimus et al., 1998; Rey et al., 2004; Arias et al., 2013; Berić et al., 2014; Chopra et al., 2014; Barbosa et al., 2015; Shobharani et al., 2015; Lee et al., 2016; Lim et al., 2016; Liu et al., 2017; Perez et al., 2017). Species of *Bacillus* differ by their antimicrobial potential (Perez et al., 2017). Non-ribosomal peptide antibiotics produced by *Bacillus* (bacitracin, proticin, lichenicidin, bacillaene) are essential for the protection of these bacteria from predation and antibiotics produced by other species (Rey et al., 2004; Barger et al., 2012; Alvarez-Ordóñez et al., 2014; Müller et al., 2014). *Bacillus* spp. were shown to produce a mixture of different lipopeptides with antimicrobial activities (Huang et al., 2006). *B. subtilis* produces surfactins, fengycins and iturins in a ratio of 6:37:57 (Fiedler and Heerklotz, 2015; Perez et al., 2017). The less abundant surfactins unlike other types of *Bacillus* lipopeptides exhibit a broad range of antimicrobial activities and possess antiviral action (Huang et al., 2006). They protect bacilli against extracellular antibiotic-containing vesicles of other species (Brown et al., 2014) and inhibit phospholipase A2 resulting in subsequent downregulation of pro-inflammatory cytokines and upregulation of anti-inflammatory cytokines (Selvam et al., 2009).

Probiotic effect of *B. subtilis* was shown to be connected to **competence and sporulation factor**, a small quorum-sensing peptide involved in bacteria communication, proliferation and sporulation (Okamoto et al., 2012). CSF activates the Akt and p38 MAPK pathways and exerts its anti-inflammatory effect by downregulation of pro-inflammatory mediators (IL-4, IL-6, and CXCL-1), the upregulation of anti-inflammatory IL-10, and the induction of cytoprotective heat shock protein Hsp27 in the intestinal epithelia (Okamoto et al., 2012). The similar effects were observed for two peptides secreted by *B. megaterium* isolated from human ileal biopsies of healthy volunteers (Di Luccia et al., 2016). Effects of CSF depend on its uptake by an organic cation transporter-2 in intestine which helps the host to monitor and respond to changes in the behavior or composition of colonic microbiota (Fujiya et al., 2007).

UNDER-APPRECIATED COMPONENTS OF *Bacilli* SECRETOME

Extracellular and surface-associated proteins secreted by commensal bacteria play an important role in gut colonization and persistence. Moreover, some of them can interact directly with mucosal cells, activating signaling pathways that lead to different cytokine secretion and gene expression profiles (Tsilingiri and Rescigno, 2013). For instance, two secreted proteins p75 and p40 (also known as Msp1 and Msp2) of *L. rhamnosus* GG have been demonstrated to prevent cytokine-induced cell apoptosis by activating the antiapoptotic protein kinase B and by inhibiting the pro-apoptotic MAPK (Yan and Polk, 2002; Yan et al., 2007), reduce TNF induced epithelial damage in the colon and as a result promote epithelial homeostasis (Yan et al., 2007). Homologs of genes that encode for p40 and p75 were also found in the genomes of *L. casei* and *L. rhamnosus*; the proteins from *L. casei* BL23 were demonstrated to elicit similar host responses (Bäuerl et al., 2010).

Secreted hydrolytic enzymes contribute to probiotic effects of *Bacilli* due to their ability to decompose food polymers releasing digestive discomfort. However, accumulating data indicate that these proteins might be involved in a complex interaction with host and its microbiota. Hydrolases demonstrate direct antimicrobial activity. Proteases, glycoside hydrolases and DNases participate in dispersal of bacterial biofilms and inhibition of biofilm formation (Chen et al., 2013; Nguyen and Burrows, 2014; Watters et al., 2016; Fleming and Rumbaugh, 2017). Extracellular nuclease, NucB, from *B. licheniformis*, was shown to digest extracellular DNA in biofilms of staphylococci and streptococci associated with chronic rhinosinusitis proving enzyme effectiveness in eradicating biofilms of multidrug-resistant bacteria (Shields et al., 2013). Secretion of low-molecular-weight guanyl-preferring ribonucleases (RNases) is a distinct feature of some *Bacillus* species (Ulyanova et al., 2016). A well-studied representative of these RNases, binase from *B. pumilus*, has manifested antitumor (Ulyanova et al., 2011; Cabrera-Fuentes et al., 2013; Mitkevich et al., 2013) and antiviral activities (Shah Mahmud and Ilinskaya, 2013; Ilinskaya and Shah Mahmud, 2014; Shah Mahmud et al., 2016, 2017; Müller et al., 2017). KRAS which has mutations in about 40% of patients with colorectal cancer (Prior et al., 2012) was shown to be a direct target for antitumor binase (Ilinskaya et al., 2016). 2′,3′-cGMP generated by binase upon RNA cleavage (Sokurenko et al., 2015) may also contribute to modulation of host cells physiology, since it is able to duplicate its counterpart 3′,5′-cGMP (Boadu et al., 2001) and can exhibit its own regulatory functions. Extracellular cGMP enhances extracellular adenosine and reduces uric acid levels which may render tissue protective effect upon injury (Jackson et al., 2013). Guanylate cyclase which catalyzes the synthesis of cGMP from GTP is represented in the cell membranes along the intestine. The cGMP signaling regulates intestinal fluid and electrolyte balance, epithelial homeostasis, mucosal barrier integrity, visceral sensation through ERK and AKT pathways (Han et al., 2011; Lin et al., 2012; Hannig et al., 2014; Lan et al., 2016). Increased cGMP levels in the colon epithelium activate antioxidant gene expression (Wang et al., 2017). cGMP expression is significantly decreased upon ulcerative colitis and colon cancer (Lin et al., 2012; Lan et al., 2016; Pattison et al., 2016). cGMP and ways for enhancement of its production are considered for treatment of irritable bowel syndrome by decreasing of gastrointestinal pain and abdominal sensory symptoms (Lan et al., 2016) and as a tool for tumor suppression (Pattison et al., 2016).

Recently, gut *Firmicutes* were shown to produce **peptide aldehydes**, cell-permeable protease inhibitors with a half-life of hours, which target cathepsins in the host lysosome blocking immune recognition of these mutualistic species and enabling them to reside in gut epithelial (Guo et al., 2017).

Nitric oxide is a well-known ubiquitous molecular mediator produced in mammals by the NOS isoforms at a catalytic site comprising a heme associated with a biopterin cofactor. Genome sequencing has shown the presence of genes encoding for proteins that are highly homologous to the oxygenase domain of mammalian NOS in bacteria, including those of the class *Bacilli*: *S. aureus* (Bird et al., 2002; Salard et al., 2006), *B. subtilis* (Adak et al., 2002), *B. anthracis* (Midha et al., 2005; Salard et al., 2006), *Geobacillus stearothermophilus* (Sudhamsu and Crane, 2006), *L. fermentum* (Morita et al., 1997), and *L. plantarum* (Adawi et al., 1997; Iarullina et al., 2006; Iarullina and Ilinskaia, 2007; Yarullina et al., 2015). So, intestinal *Bacilli* have NOS that is evolutionary related to the mammalian enzymes. Moreover, as bacteria have the most ancient version of NOS, it was hypothesized that Eukaryotes acquired NOS from bacteria by horizontal gene transfer (Gusarov et al., 2013). Recently, the conservation of NOS-derived NO-heme receptor signaling between bacteria and mammals was proved (Kinkel et al., 2016). NO as reactive oxygen molecule is widely considered as important participant in the immune system of different organisms to confront microbial infections. Thus, inhibition of bacterial NOS has the potential to improve the efficacy of antimicrobials used to treat infections by Gram-positive pathogens *S. aureus* and *B. anthracis* possessing this enzyme (Holden et al., 2015). Commensal microbiota-derived NO has been shown to influence host physiology. NO synthesized by *L. plantarum* takes part in the regulation of intestinal motility in rat (Yarullina et al., 2016). Being a signaling molecule, NO released by *B. subtilis* in the intestine of *Caenorhabditis elegans* initiates a signaling cascade that results in the induction of 65 genes, including *hsp*s and several other genes that have been implicated in longevity and stress resistance (Gusarov et al., 2013). Involvement of bacterial NO in human cardiovascular system is under investigation (Cabrera-Fuentes et al., 2016).

Ferrichrome of *L. casei* was identified as a tumor-suppressive molecule on colon cancer cells which induces apoptosis via activation of c-jun N-terminal kinase (JNK) (Konishi et al., 2016). Many siderophore-binding proteins were found in EVs of *B. subtilis* (Dubois et al., 2009; Brown et al., 2014). Siderophores can endow bacilli advantage in competition for low-available iron with pathogenic bacteria. Iron cations are potent crosslinkers of the biofilm matrix (Chen and Stewart, 2002) and their chelation causes dispersal of biofilms (Sobke et al., 2012).

Over the last decade, **extracellular vesicles** have emerged as prominent vehicles of biological signals. Intense research on that topic revealed that EVs play important roles in bacterial physiology and pathogenesis, ranging from secretion and delivery of biomolecules (for example, toxins, DNA, or quorum sensing molecules) over stress response and biofilm formation to immunomodulation and adherence to host cells (Roier et al., 2016). Both *Bacillus* and *Lactobacillus* species were reported to produce EVs, spherical membranous structures of 20–150 nm in diameter (Brown et al., 2014, 2015; Avila-Calderón et al., 2015; Behzadi et al., 2017; Li et al., 2017). EVs are formed both in planktonic cultures and bacterial biofilms where they help to maintain biofilm cohesion. The quantity of EVs varies with the strain (Brown et al., 2014), conditions and stage of growth (Kim et al., 2016). Thus, EVs can be produced by Bacilli in GIT.

The EVs are enriched with proteins, lipids, nucleic acids, and metabolites which exhibit biological activities. Release of vesicular cargo is achieved by direct intercellular transfer mediated by the membranes fusion (Kim et al., 2016; Stubbendieck and Straight, 2016) or by production of special molecules like lipopeptide surfactin which disrupts EVs unspecifically (Brown et al., 2014). Therefore, proteins with specific biological activities can be directly delivered inside EVs into other cells ensuring their penetration. In Gram-positive bacteria, proteins secreted via specific pathways are believed to be important for nutrient acquisition, detoxification, competitive survival, and communication (Brown et al., 2015). Recent findings support the importance of EVs for interaction of bacteria with each other and the host cells (Kim et al., 2016).

Extracellular vesicles carry hydrolytic enzymes for nutrient acquisition from extracellular complex substrates or key nutrients to feed sibling cells and contain specific agents for antagonizing competing species. In EV important for survival compounds are protected from damage retaining activities much longer and can be transported in concentrated amounts for long distances from producing cells. Among these compounds are antibiotics and hydrolytic enzymes including peptidoglycan-degrading hydrolases (Mashburn and Whiteley, 2005; Alves et al., 2016; Stubbendieck and Straight, 2016). EVs isolated from *B. subtilis* contain proteins which are mostly associated with metabolic pathways including biosynthesis of secondary metabolites (Brown et al., 2014; Kim et al., 2016). Proteins with oxidoreductase and nucleotide binding activities are abundant in vegetative EVs, while proteins with hydrolytic, nucleic acid binding, and structural activity are predominant in sporulating EV (Kim et al., 2016). In EVs of sporulating *B. subtilis* superoxide dismutase, alkaline phosphatase III, polyketide synthase PKsM (associated with antibiotic activity) were identified (Kim et al., 2016). Sunl protein which confers self-immunity to antibiotic sublancin and many siderophore-binding proteins were found in EVs of *B. subtilis* (Dubois et al., 2009; Brown et al., 2014). The targeted lysis of EVs by surfactin of *B. subtilis* is hypothesized to guard bacilli from alien EVs and disrupt cell signaling by means of EVs in competing populations (Stubbendieck and Straight, 2016). EVs were also shown to adsorb phages (Biller et al., 2014).

Interaction of EVs with the host is specific to the microorganism from which the EVs were produced and is based on the lipid content and cargo of the EVs (Brown et al., 2015). Gram-positive bacterial EVs are composed of various fatty acids which might have a positive effect on host organism (Rivera et al., 2010). EVs were shown to elicit protective immune response in host (Vargas et al., 2015). For example, treatment of *C. elegans* with EVs originated from *L. plantarum* WCFS1 led to increased transcription of host defense genes, *cpr-1* and *clec-60*, and thus provided protection against vancomycin-resistant *Enterococcus faecium*. Moreover, in human Caco-2 cells these EVs had similar effect, leading to the upregulation of *REG3G*, which is functionally similar to *clec-60*, and *CTSB*, the human ortholog of *cpr-1* (Li et al., 2017). The EVs from *B. lentus* isolated from Korean soybean fermented food induced apoptosis of human colon carcinoma cells HCT116 (Yang et al., 2016). EVs derived from *L. rhamnosus* GG are likely to be implicated in the anti-cancer activity as they induce apoptosis in the hepatic adenocarcinoma cell line HepG2 via augmentation of the expression ratio between pro- and anti-apoptotic genes *bax/bcl-2* (Behzadi et al., 2017).

CONCLUSION AND FURTHER PERSPECTIVES

Now, it has become clear that studies on phylotype profiling are limited to the identification of microbial constituents, where information is lacking about the molecular interaction of bacterial communities with the host. Lactobacilli are well-represented in the human GIT and secrete a number of compounds which have direct and indirect effects on the health of GIT and organism as a whole. Species of *Bacillus* genus are much less abundant but are capable of producing several times more extracellular molecules than lactobacilli. Many of them still require exploration. Further deep studies are needed for better understanding of the complex interactions between human organism and its microbiota, clarification of the particular mechanisms underlying remarkable beneficial properties of probiotic *Bacilli*, and the specific action of innumerous secreted low- and high-molecular weight compounds and their vesicular transportation.

AUTHOR CONTRIBUTIONS

The basis of this review was the experimental work of the group led by ONI, in which a variety of biological activities of bacilli and lactobacilli secretome was established. ONI developed the main idea of this review, collected literature data, verified the text and coordinated it with co-authors carrying out the general guidance of the review. The part of the review devoted to the properties of representatives of the genus *Bacillus* and the components of their secretome belongs to VVU. She structured the review and created the scheme summarizing the main idea of the review on the diversity of components secreted by the representatives of Bacilli class. DRY, being a specialist in the field of probiotic activity of lactobacilli, analyzed data on the influence of *Lactobacillus* and their metabolites on intestinal functions and microbiota, and host organism. IGG collected literature data on the microflora of the human intestine. On the basis of his analysis of epithelial biopsy samples obtained during the operations of patients with diagnosed colorectal cancer, a conclusion about the contribution of Bacilli class to the microbiota closely associated with the epithelium was made.

FUNDING

The research was performed within the Russian Government Program of Competitive Growth of Kazan Federal University and supported by the Russian Science Foundation grant No 14-14-00522.

ACKNOWLEDGMENTS

Authors are thankful to Anna Makeeva for contribution to the Figure and to Galina Yakovleva for providing AFM image of *B. pumilus*.

REFERENCES

Abriouel, H., Franz, C. M. A. P., Omar, N. B., and Galvez, A. (2011). Diversity and applications of *Bacillus* bacteriocins. *FEMS Microbiol. Rev.* 35, 201–232. doi: 10.1111/j.1574-6976.2010.00244.x

Adak, S., Aulak, K. S., and Stuehr, D. J. (2002). Direct evidence for nitric oxide production by a nitric-oxide synthase-like protein from *Bacillus subtilis*. *J. Biol. Chem.* 277, 16167–16171. doi: 10.1074/jbc.M201136200

Adawi, D., Kasravi, F. B., Molin, G., and Jeppsson, B. (1997). Effect of *Lactobacillus* supplementation with and without arginine on liver damage and bacterial translocation in an acute liver injury model in the rat. *Hepatology* 25, 642–647. doi: 10.1002/hep.510250325

Ahmadova, A., Todorov, S. D., Hadji-Sfaxi, I., Choiset, Y., Rabesona, H., Messaoudi, S., et al. (2013). Antimicrobial and antifungal activities of *Lactobacillus curvatus* strain isolated from homemade Azerbaijani cheese. *Anaerobe* 20, 42–49. doi: 10.1016/j.anaerobe.2013.01.003

Alakomi, H. L., Skytta, E., Saarela, M., Mattila-Sandholm, T., Latva-Kala, K., and Helander, I. M. (2000). Lactic acid permeabilizes gram-negative bacteria by disrupting the outer membrane. *Appl. Environ. Microbiol.* 66, 2001–2005. doi: 10.1128/AEM.66.5.2001-2005.2000

Alcántara, C., Blasco, A., Zúñiga, M., and Monedero, V. (2014). Accumulation of polyphosphate in *Lactobacillus* spp. and its involvement in stress resistance. *Appl. Environ. Microbiol.* 80, 1650–1659. doi: 10.1128/AEM.03997-13

Almand, E. A., Moore, M. D., Outlaw, J., and Jaykus, L. A. (2017). Human norovirus binding to select bacteria representative of the human gut microbiota. *PLoS ONE* 12:e0173124. doi: 10.1371/journal.pone.0173124

Alou, M. T., Fournier, P. E., and Raoult, D. (2016). "*Bacillus mediterraneensis*," a new bacterial species isolated from human gut microbiota. *New Microbes New Infect.* 12, 86–87. doi: 10.1016/j.nmni.2016.05.006

Alvarez-Ordóñez, A., Begley, M., Clifford, T., Deasy, T., Considine, K., O'Connor, P., et al. (2014). Investigation of the antimicrobial activity of *Bacillus licheniformis* strains isolated from retail powdered infant milk formulae. *Probiotics Antimicrob. Proteins* 6, 32–40. doi: 10.1007/s12602-013-9151-1

Alves, N. J., Turner, K. B., Medintz, I. L., and Walper, S. A. (2016). Protecting enzymatic function through directed packaging into bacterial outer membrane vesicles. *Sci. Rep.* 6:24866. doi: 10.1038/srep24866

Arias, A. A., Ongena, M., Devreese, B., Terrak, M., Joris, B., and Fickers, P. (2013). Characterization of amylolysin, a novel lantibiotic from *Bacillus amyloliquefaciens* GA1. *PLoS ONE* 8:e83037. doi: 10.1371/journal.pone.0083037

Avila-Calderón, E. D., Araiza-Villanueva, M. G., Cancino-Diaz, J. C., López-Villegas, E. O., Sriranganathan, N., Boyle, S. M., et al. (2015). Roles of bacterial membrane vesicles. *Arch. Microbiol.* 197, 1–10. doi: 10.1007/s00203-014-1042-7

Ayed, H. B., Maalej, H., Hmidet, N., and Nasri, M. (2015). Isolation and biochemical characterisation of a bacteriocin-like substance produced by *Bacillus amyloliquefaciens* An6. *J. Glob. Antimicrob. Resist.* 3, 255–261. doi: 10.1016/j.jgar.2015.07.001

Balkus, J. E., Mitchell, C., Agnew, K., Liu, C., Fiedler, T., Cohn, S. E., et al. (2012). Detection of hydrogen peroxide-producing *Lactobacillus* species in the vagina: a comparison of culture and quantitative PCR among HIV-1 seropositive women. *BMC Infect. Dis.* 12:188. doi: 10.1186/1471-2334-12-188

Barbosa, J., Caetano, T., and Mendo, S. (2015). Class I and class II lanthipeptides produced by *Bacillus* spp. *J. Nat. Prod.* 78, 2850–2866. doi: 10.1021/np500424y

Barger, S. R., Hoefler, B. C., Cubillos-Ruiz, A., Russell, W. K., Russell, D. H., and Straight, P. D. (2012). Imaging secondary metabolism of *Streptomyces* sp. Mg1 during cellular lysis and colony degradation of competing *Bacillus subtilis*. *Antonie Van Leeuwenhoek* 102, 435–445. doi: 10.1007/s10482-012-9769-0

Barrett, E., Ross, R. P., O'Toole, P. W., Fitzgerald, G. F., and Stanton, C. (2012). γ-Aminobutyric acid production by culturable bacteria from the human intestine. *J. Appl. Microbiol.* 113, 411–417. doi: 10.1111/j.1365-2672.2012.05344.x

Bäuerl, C., Perez-Martinez, G., Yan, F., Polk, D. B., and Monedero, V. (2010). Functional analysis of the p40 and p75 proteins from *Lactobacillus casei* BL23. *J. Mol. Microbiol. Biotechnol.* 19, 231–241. doi: 10.1159/000322233

Behzadi, E., Hosseini, H. M., and Imani Fooladi, A. A. (2017). The inhibitory impacts of *Lactobacillus rhamnosus* GG-derived extracellular vesicles on the growth of hepatic cancer cells. *Microb. Pathog.* doi: 10.1016/j.micpath.2017.06.016 [Epub ahead of print].

Bene, K., Varga, Z., Petrov, V. O., Boyko, N., and Rajnavolgyi, E. (2017). Gut microbiota species can provoke both inflammatory and tolerogenic immune responses in human dendritic cells mediated by retinoic acid receptor alpha ligation. *Front. Immunol.* 8:427. doi: 10.3389/fimmu.2017.00427

Bérdy, J. (2005). Bioactive microbial metabolites. *J. Antibiot.* 58, 1–26. doi: 10.1038/ja.2005.1

Berić, T., Stanković, S., Draganić, V., Kojić, M., Lozo, J., and Fira, D. (2014). Novel antilisterial bacteriocin licheniocin 50.2 *from Bacillus licheniformis* VPS50.2 isolated from soil sample. *J. Appl. Microbiol.* 116, 502–510. doi: 10.1111/jam.12393

Bermudez-Brito, M., Plaza-Díaz, J., Muñoz-Quezada, S., Gómez-Llorente, C., and Gil, A. (2012). Probiotic mechanisms of action. *Ann. Nutr. Metab.* 61, 160–174. doi: 10.1159/000342079

Bhattarai, Y., Schmidt, B. A., Linden, D. R., Larson, E. D., Grover, M., Beyder, A., et al. (2017). Human derived gut microbiota modulates colonic secretion in mice by regulating 5-HT3 receptor expression via acetate production. *Am. J. Physiol. Gastrointest. Liver Physiol.* 313, G80–G87. doi: 10.1152/ajpgi.00448.2016

Biller, S. J., Schubotz, F., Roggensack, S. E., Thompson, A. W., Summons, R. E., and Chisholm, S. W. (2014). Bacterial vesicles in marine ecosystems. *Science* 343, 183–186. doi: 10.1126/science.1243457

Bird, L. E., Ren, J., Zhang, J., Foxwell, N., Hawkins, A. R., Charles, I. G., et al. (2002). Crystal structure of SANOS, a bacterial nitric oxide synthase oxygenase protein from *Staphylococcus aureus*. *Structure* 10, 1687–1696. doi: 10.1016/S0969-2126(02)00911-5

Boadu, E., Vaskinn, S., Sundkvist, E., Jaeger, R., and Sager, G. (2001). Inhibition by guanosine cyclic monophosphate (cGMP) analogues of uptake of [(3)H]3',5'-cGMP without stimulation of ATPase activity in human erythrocyte inside-out vesicles. *Biochem. Pharmacol.* 62, 425–429. doi: 10.1016/S0006-2952(01)00682-7

Brown, L., Kessler, A., Cabezas-Sanchez, P., Luque-Garcia, J. L., and Casadevall, A. (2014). Extracellular vesicles produced by the Gram-positive bacterium *Bacillus subtilis* are disrupted by the lipopeptide surfactin. *Mol. Microbiol.* 93, 183–198. doi: 10.1111/mmi.12650

Brown, L., Wolf, J. M., Prados-Rosales, R., and Casadevall, A. (2015). Through the wall: extracellular vesicles in Gram-positive bacteria, mycobacteria and fungi. *Nat. Rev. Microbiol.* 13, 620–630. doi: 10.1038/nrmicro3480

Browne, H. P., Forster, S. C., Anonye, B. O., Kumar, N., Neville, B. A., Stares, M. D., et al. (2016). Culturing of 'unculturable' human microbiota reveals novel taxa and extensive sporulation. *Nature* 533, 543–546. doi: 10.1038/nature17645

Cabrera-Fuentes, H. A., Alba-Alba, C., Aragones, J., Bernhagen, J., Boisvert, W. A., Bøtker, H. E., et al. (2016). Meeting report from the 2nd International Symposium on New Frontiers in Cardiovascular Research. Protecting the cardiovascular system from ischemia: between bench and bedside. *Basic Res. Cardiol.* 111, 7. doi: 10.1007/s00395-015-0527-0

Cabrera-Fuentes, H. A., Aslam, M., Saffarzadeh, M., Kolpakov, A., Zelenikhin, P., Preissner, K. T., et al. (2013). Internalization of *Bacillus intermedius* ribonuclease (BINASE) induces human alveolar adenocarcinoma cell death. *Toxicon* 69, 219–226. doi: 10.1016/j.toxicon.2013.03.015

Camilleri, M. (2006). Probiotics and irritable bowel syndrome: rationale, putative mechanisms, and evidence of clinical efficacy. *J. Clin. Gastroenterol.* 40, 264–269. doi: 10.1097/00004836-200603000-00020

Carding, S., Verbeke, K., Vipond, D. T., Corfe, B. M., and Owen, L. J. (2015). Dysbiosis of the gut microbiota in disease. *Microb. Ecol. Health Dis.* 26:26191. doi: 10.3402/mehd.v26.26191

Chauhan, A. K., Maheshwari, D. K., and Bajpai, V. K. (2017). Isolation and preliminary characterization of a bacteriocin-producer *Bacillus* strain inhibiting methicillin resistant *Staphylococcus aureus*. *Acta Biol. Hung.* 68, 208–219. doi: 10.1556/018.68.2017.2.8

Chen, C., Krishnan, V., Macon, K., Manne, K., Narayana, S. V. L., and Schneewind, O. (2013). Secreted proteases control autolysin-mediated biofilm growth of *Staphylococcus aureus*. *J. Biol. Chem.* 288, 29440–29452. doi: 10.1074/jbc.M113.502039

Chen, X., and Stewart, P. S. (2002). Role of electrostatic interactions in cohesion of bacterial biofilms. *Appl. Microbiol. Biotechnol.* 59, 718–720. doi: 10.1007/s00253-002-1044-2

Choi, C. H., Kwon, J. G., Kim, S. K., Myung, S. J., Park, K. S., Sohn, C. I., et al. (2015). Efficacy of combination therapy with probiotics and mosapride in patients with IBS without diarrhea: a randomized, double-blind, placebo-controlled, multicenter, Phase II trial. *Neurogastroenterol. Motil.* 27, 705–716. doi: 10.1111/nmo.12544

Chopra, L., Singh, G., Choudhary, V., and Sahoo, D. K. (2014). Sonorensin: an antimicrobial peptide, belonging to the heterocycloanthracin subfamily of bacteriocins, from a new marine isolate, *Bacillus sonorensis* MT93. *Appl. Environ. Microbiol.* 80, 2981–2990. doi: 10.1128/AEM.04259-13

Clemente, J. C., Ursell, L. K., Parfrey, L. W., and Knight, R. (2012). The impact of the gut microbiota on human health: an integrative view. *Cell* 148, 1258–1270. doi: 10.1016/j.cell.2012.01.035

Collins, F. W., O'Connor, P. M., O'Sullivan, O., Rea, M. C., Hill, C., and Ross, R. P. (2016). Formicin – a novel broad-spectrum two-component lantibiotic produced by *Bacillus paralicheniformis* APC 1576. *Microbiology* 162, 1662–1671. doi: 10.1099/mic.0.000340

De Vuyst, L., and Leroy, F. (2007). Bacteriocins from lactic acid bacteria: production, purification, and food applications. *J. Mol. Microbiol. Biotechnol.* 13, 194–199. doi: 10.1159/000104752

den Besten, G., Bleeker, A., Gerding, A., van Eunen, K., Havinga, R., van Dijk, T. H., et al. (2015). Short-chain fatty acids protect against high-fat diet-induced obesity via a PPARγ-dependent switch from lipogenesis to fat oxidation. *Diabetes Metab. Res. Rev.* 64, 2398–2408. doi: 10.2337/db14-1213 den Besten, G., Lange, K., Havinga, R., van Dijk, T. H., Gerding, A., van Eunen, K., et al. (2013a). Gut-derived short-chain fatty acids are vividly assimilated into host carbohydrates and lipids. *Am. J. Physiol. Gastrointest. Liver Physiol.* 305, G900–G910. doi: 10.1152/ajpgi.00265.2013

den Besten, G., van Eunen, K., Groen, A. K., Venema, K., Reijngoud, D. J., and Bakker, B. M. (2013b). The role of short-chain fatty acids in the interplay between diet, gut microbiota, and host energy metabolism. *J. Lipid Res.* 54, 2325–2340. doi: 10.1194/jlr.R036012

Derrien, M., and van Hylckama Vlieg, J. E. (2015). Fate, activity, and impact of ingested bacteria within the human gut microbiota. *Trends Microbiol.* 23, 354–366. doi: 10.1016/j.tim.2015.03.002

Dethlefsen, L., Huse, S., Sogin, M. L., and Relman, D. A. (2008). The pervasive effects of an antibiotic on the human gut microbiota, as revealed by deep 16S rRNA sequencing. *PLoS Biol.* 6:e280. doi: 10.1371/journal.pbio.0060280

Di Luccia, B., D'Apuzzo, E., Varriale, F., Baccigalupi, L., Ricca, E., and Pollice, A. (2016). *Bacillus megaterium* SF185 induces stress pathways and affects the cell cycle distribution of human intestinal epithelial cells. *Benef. Microbes* 7, 609–620. doi: 10.3920/BM2016.0020

Dobson, A., Cotter, P. D., Ross, R. P., and Hill, C. (2012). Bacteriocin production: a probiotic trait? *Appl. Environ. Microbiol.* 78, 1–6. doi: 10.1128/AEM.05576-11

Donaldson, G. P., Lee, S. M., and Mazmanian, S. K. (2016). Gut biogeography of the bacterial microbiota. *Nat. Rev. Microbiol.* 14, 20–32. doi: 10.1038/nrmicro3552

Donia, M. S., Cimermancic, P., Schulze, C. J., Wieland Brown, L. C., Martin, J., Mitreva, M., et al. (2014). A systematic analysis of biosynthetic gene clusters in the human microbiome reveals a common family of antibiotics. *Cell* 158, 1402–1414. doi: 10.1016/j.cell.2014.08.032

Dubois, J. Y., Kouwen, T. R., Schurich, A. K., Reis, C. R., Ensing, H. T., Trip, E. N., et al. (2009). Immunity to the bacteriocin sublancin 168 is determined by the SunI (YolF) protein of *Bacillus subtilis*. *Antimicrob. Agents Chemother.* 53, 651–661. doi: 10.1128/AAC.01189-08

Ebel, B., Lemetais, G., Beney, L., Cachon, R., Sokol, H., Langella, P., et al. (2014). Impact of probiotics on risk factors for cardiovascular diseases. A review. *Crit. Rev. Food Sci. Nutr.* 54, 175–189. doi: 10.1080/10408398.2011.579361

Etienne-Mesmin, L., Chassaing, B., and Gewirtz, A. T. (2017). Tryptophan: a gut microbiota-derived metabolites regulating inflammation. *World J. Gastrointest. Pharmacol. Ther.* 8, 7–9. doi: 10.4292/wjgpt.v8.i1.7

Fakhry, S., Sorrentini, I., Ricca, E., De Felice, M., and Baccigalupi, L. (2008). Characterization of spore forming Bacilli isolated from the human gastrointestinal tract. *J. Appl. Microbiol.* 105, 2178–2186. doi: 10.1111/j.1365-2672.2008.03934.x

Fekete, Á. A., Givens, D. I., and Lovegrove, J. A. (2015). Casein-derived lactotripeptides reduce systolic and diastolic blood pressure in a meta-analysis of randomised clinical trials. *Nutrients* 7, 659–681. doi: 10.3390/nu7010659

Fiedler, S., and Heerklotz, H. (2015). Vesicle leakage reflects the target selectivity of antimicrobial lipopeptides from *Bacillus subtilis*. *Biophys. J.* 109, 2079–2089. doi: 10.1016/j.bpj.2015.09.021

Fleming, D., and Rumbaugh, K. P. (2017). Approaches to dispersing medical biofilms. *Microorganisms* 5:E15. doi: 10.3390/microorganisms5020015

Fransen, F., Zagato, E., Mazzini, E., Fosso, B., Manzari, C., El Aidy, S., et al. (2015). BALB/c and C57BL/6 mice differ in polyreactive IgA abundance, which impacts the generation of antigen-specific IgA and microbiota diversity. *Immunity* 43, 527–540. doi: 10.1016/j.immuni.2015.08.011

Fujiya, M., Musch, M. W., Nakagawa, Y., Hu, S., Alverdy, J., Kohgo, Y., et al. (2007). The *Bacillus subtilis* quorum-sensing molecule CSF contributes to intestinal homeostasis via OCTN2, a host cell membrane transporter. *Cell Host Microbe* 1, 299–308. doi: 10.1016/j.chom.2007.05.004

Gagnière, J., Raisch, J., Veziant, J., Barnich, N., Bonnet, R., Buc, E., et al. (2016). Gut microbiota imbalance and colorectal cancer. *World J. Gastroenterol.* 22, 501–518. doi: 10.3748/wjg.v22.i2.501

Gao, Z., Guo, B., Gao, R., Zhu, Q., and Qin, H. (2015). Microbiota disbiosis is associated with colorectal cancer. *Front. Microbiol.* 6:20. doi: 10.3389/fmicb.2015.00020

Ghelardi, E., Celandroni, F., Salvetti, S., Gueye, S. A., Lupetti, A., and Senesi, S. (2015). Survival and persistence of *Bacillus clausii* in the human gastrointestinal tract following oral administration as spore-based probiotic formulation. *J. Appl. Microbiol.* 119, 552–559. doi: 10.1111/jam.12848

Ghoshal, U. C., Shukla, R., and Ghoshal, U. (2017). Small intestinal bacterial overgrowth and irritable bowel syndrome: a bridge between functional organic dichotomy. *Gut Liver* 11, 196–208. doi: 10.5009/gnl16126

Ghouri, Y. A., Richards, D. M., Rahimi, E. F., Krill, J. T., Jelinek, K. A., Dupont, A. W., et al. (2014). Systematic review of randomized controlled trials of probiotics, prebiotics, and synbiotics in inflammatory bowel disease. *Clin. Exp. Gastroenterol.* 7, 473–487. doi: 10.2147/CEG.S27530

Giraffa, G., Chanishvili, N., and Widyastuti, Y. (2010). Importance of lactobacilli in food and feed biotechnology. *Res. Microbiol.* 161, 480–487. doi: 10.1016/j.resmic.2010.03.001

Guo, C. J., Chang, F. Y., Wyche, T. P., Backus, K. M., Acker, T. M., Funabashi, M., et al. (2017). Discovery of reactive microbiota-derived metabolites that inhibit host proteases. *Cell* 168, 517.e18–526.e18. doi: 10.1016/j.cell.2016.12.021

Gusarov, I., Gautier, L., Smolentseva, O., Shamovsky, I., Eremina, S., Mironov, A., et al. (2013). Bacterial nitric oxide extends the lifespan of *C. elegans*. *Cell* 152, 818–830. doi: 10.1016/j.cell.2012.12.043

Hammes, W. P., and Hertel, C. (2015). "*Lactobacillus*," in *Bergey's Manual of Systematics of Archaea and Bacteria*, ed. W. B. Whitman (Hoboken, NJ: John Wiley & Sons), 1–76. doi: 10.1002/9781118960608.gbm00604

Han, X., Mann, E., Gilbert, S., Guan, Y., Steinbrecher, K. A., Montrose, M. H., et al. (2011). Loss of guanylyl cyclase C (GCC) signaling leads to dysfunctional intestinal barrier. *PLoS ONE* 6:e16139. doi: 10.1371/journal.pone.0016139

Hannig, G., Tchernychev, B., Kurtz, C. B., Bryant, A. P., Currie, M. G., and Silos-Santiago, I. (2014). Guanylate cyclase-C/cGMP: an emerging pathway in the regulation of visceral pain. *Front. Mol. Neurosci.* 7:31. doi: 10.3389/fnmol.2014.00031

Harmsen, H. J., Raangs, G. C., He, T., Degener, J. E., and Welling, G. W. (2002). Extensive set of 16S rRNA-based probes for detection of bacteria in human feces. *Appl. Environ. Microbiol.* 68, 2982–2990. doi: 10.1128/AEM.68.6.2982-2990.2002

Haro, C., Rangel-Zuniga, O. A., Alcala-Diaz, J. F., Gomez-Delgado, F., Perez-Martinez, P., Delgado-Lista, J., et al. (2016). Intestinal microbiota is influenced by gender and body mass index. *PLoS ONE* 11:e0154090. doi: 10.1371/journal.pone.0154090

Hayes, M., Stanton, C., Slattery, H., O'Sullivan, O., Hill, C., Fitzgerald, G. F., et al. (2007). Casein fermentate of *Lactobacillus animalis* DPC6134 contains a range of novel propeptide angiotensin-converting enzyme inhibitors. *Appl. Environ. Microbiol.* 73, 4658–4667. doi: 10.1128/AEM.00096-07

Hertzberger, R., Arents, J., Dekker, H. L., Pridmore, R. D., Gysler, C., Kleerebezem, M., et al. (2014). H_2O_2 production in species of the *Lactobacillus acidophilus* group: a central role for a novel NADH-dependent flavin reductase. *Appl. Environ. Microbiol.* 80, 2229–2239. doi: 10.1128/AEM.04272-13

Holden, J. K., Kang, S., Hollingsworth, S. A., Li, H., Lim, N., Chen, S., et al. (2015). Structure-based design of bacterial nitric oxide synthase inhibitors. *J. Med. Chem.* 58, 994–1004. doi: 10.1021/jm501723p

Hong, H. A., To, E., Fakhry, S., Baccigalupi, L., Ricca, E., and Cutting, S. M. (2009). Defining the natural habitat of *Bacillus* spore-formers. *Res. Microbiol.* 160, 375–379. doi: 10.1016/j.resmic.2009.06.006

Huang, X., Lu, Z., and Yang, S. (2006). Antiviral activity of antimicrobial lipopeptide from *Bacillus subtilis* fmbj against pseudorabies virus, porcine parvovirus, newcastle disease virus and infectious bursal disease virus *in vitro*. *Int. J. Pept. Res. Ther.* 12, 373–377. doi: 10.1007/s10989-006-9041-4

Hyronimus, B., Le Marrec, C., and Urdaci, M. C. (1998). Coagulin, a bacteriocin-like inhibitory substance produced by *Bacillus coagulans* I4. *J. Appl. Microbiol.* 85, 42–50. doi: 10.1046/j.1365-2672.1998.00466.x

Iarullina, D. R., and Ilinskaia, O. N. (2007). Genomic determinants of nitric oxide biosynthesis by *Lactobacillus plantarum*: potential opportunities and reality. *Mol. Biol.* 41, 900–907. doi: 10.1134/S0026893307050159

Iarullina, D. R., Ilinskaia, O. N., Aganov, A. V., Silkin, N. I., and Zverev, D. G. (2006). Alternative pathways of nitric oxide formation in lactobacilli: EPR evidence for nitric oxide synthase activity. *Mikrobiologiia* 75, 731–736. doi: 10.1134/S0026261706060026

Ilinskaya, O. N., and Shah Mahmud, R. (2014). Ribonucleases as antiviral agents. *Mol. Biol.* 48, 707–717. doi: 10.1134/S0026893314040050

Ilinskaya, O. N., Singh, I., Dudkina, E., Ulyanova, V., Kayumov, A., and Barreto, G. (2016). Direct inhibition of oncogenic KRAS by *Bacillus pumilus* ribonuclease (binase). *Biochim. Biophys. Acta* 1863, 1559–1567. doi: 10.1016/j.bbamcr.2016.04.005

Imlay, J. A. (2003). Pathways of oxidative damage. *Annu. Rev. Microbiol.* 57, 395–418. doi: 10.1146/annurev.micro.57.030502.090938

Jackson, E. K., Cheng, D., Jackson, T. C., Verrier, J. D., and Gillespie, D. G. (2013). Extracellular guanosine regulates extracellular adenosine levels. *Am. J. Physiol. Cell Physiol.* 304, C406–C421. doi: 10.1152/ajpcell.00212.2012

Jandhyala, S. M., Talukdar, R., Subramanyam, C., Vuyyuru, H., Sasikala, M., and Reddy, D. N. (2015). Role of the normal gut microbiota. *World J. Gastroenterol.* 21, 8787–8803. doi: 10.3748/wjg.v21.i29.8787

Jung, T. H., Park, J. H., Jeon, W. M., and Han, K. S. (2015). Butyrate modulates bacterial adherence on LS174T human colorectal cells by stimulating mucin secretion and MAPK signaling pathway. *Nutr. Res. Pract.* 9, 343–349. doi: 10.4162/nrp.2015.9.4.343

Kaškonienė, V., Stankevičius, M., Bimbiraitė-Survilienė, K., Naujokaitytė, G., Šernienė, L., Mulkytė, K., et al. (2017). Current state of purification, isolation and analysis of bacteriocins produced by lactic acid bacteria. *Appl. Microbiol. Biotechnol.* 101, 1323–1335. doi: 10.1007/s00253-017-8088-9

Keller, D., Van Dinter, R., Cash, H., Farmer, S., and Venema, K. (2017). *Bacillus coagulans* GBI-30, 6086 increases plant protein digestion in a dynamic, computer-controlled in vitro model of the small intestine (TIM-1). *Benef. Microbes* 8, 491–496. doi: 10.3920/BM2016.0196

Khochamit, N., Siripornadulsil, S., Sukon, P., and Siripornadulsil, W. (2015). Antibacterial activity and genotypic-phenotypic characteristics of bacteriocin-producing *Bacillus subtilis* KKU213: potential as a probiotic strain. *Microbiol. Res.* 170, 36–50. doi: 10.1016/j.micres.2014.09.004

Kim, Y., Edwards, N., and Fenselau, C. (2016). Extracellular vesicle proteomes reflect developmental phases of *Bacillus subtilis*. *Clin. Proteomics* 13, 6. doi: 10.1186/s12014-016-9107-z

Kinkel, T. L., Ramos-Montañez, S., Pando, J. M., Tadeo, D. V., Strom, E. N., Libby, S. J., et al. (2016). An essential role for bacterial nitric oxide synthase in *Staphylococcus aureus* electron transfer and colonization. *Nat. Microbiol.* 2:16224. doi: 10.1038/nmicrobiol.2016.224

Konishi, H., Fujiya, M., Tanaka, H., Ueno, N., Moriichi, K., Sasajima, J., et al. (2016). Probiotic-derived ferrichrome inhibits colon cancer progression via JNK-mediated apoptosis. *Nat. Commun.* 7:12365. doi: 10.1038/ncomms 12365

Kumar, R., Grover, S., and Batish, V. K. (2012). Bile salt hydrolase (Bsh) activity screening of lactobacilli: *in vitro* selection of indigenous *Lactobacillus* strains with potential bile salt hydrolysing and cholesterol-lowering ability. *Probiotics Antimicrob. Proteins* 4, 162–172. doi: 10.1007/s12602-012-9101-3

Lagier, J. C., Hugon, P., Khelaifia, S., Fournier, P. E., La Scola, B., and Raoult, D. (2015). The rebirth of culture in microbiology through the example of culturomics to study human gut microbiota. *Clin. Microbiol. Rev.* 28, 237–264. doi: 10.1128/CMR.00014-14

Lagier, J. C., Khelaifia, S., Alou, M. T., Ndongo, S., Dione, N., Hugon, P., et al. (2016). Culture of previously uncultured members of the human gut microbiota by culturomics. *Nat. Microbiol.* 1:16203. doi: 10.1038/nmicrobiol.2016.203

Lahtinen, S. J. (2012). Probiotic viability – does it matter? *Microb. Ecol. Health Dis.* 23, 10–14. doi: 10.3402/mehd.v23i0.18567

Lamas, B., Richard, M. L., Leducq, V., Pham, H. P., Michel, M. L., Da Costa, G., et al. (2016). CARD9 impacts colitis by altering gut microbiota metabolism of tryptophan into aryl hydrocarbon receptor ligands. *Nat. Med.* 22, 598–605. doi: 10.1038/nm.4102

Lan, D., Niu, J., Miao, J., Dong, X., Wang, H., Yang, G., et al. (2016). Expression of guanylate cyclase-C, guanylin, and uroguanylin is downregulated proportionally to the ulcerative colitis disease activity index. *Sci. Rep.* 6:25034. doi: 10.1038/srep25034

LeBlanc, J. G., Chain, F., Martín, R., Bermúdez-Humarán, L. G., Courau, S., and Langella, P. (2017). Beneficial effects on host energy metabolism of short-chain fatty acids and vitamins produced by commensal and probiotic bacteria. *Microb. Cell Fact.* 16, 79. doi: 10.1186/s12934-017-0691-z

Lee, M. H., Lee, J., Nam, Y. D., Lee, J. S., Seo, M. J., and Yi, S. H. (2016). Characterization of antimicrobial lipopeptides produced by *Bacillus* sp. LM7 isolated from chungkookjang, a Korean traditional fermented soybean food. *Int. J. Food Microbiol.* 221, 12–18. doi: 10.1016/j.ijfoodmicro.2015.12.010

Li, M., Lee, K., Hsu, M., Nau, G., Mylonakis, E., and Ramratnam, B. (2017). *Lactobacillus*-derived extracellular vesicles enhance host immune responses against vancomycin-resistant enterococci. *BMC Microbiol.* 17:66. doi: 10.1186/ s12866-017-0977-7

Lim, K. B., Balolong, M. P., Kim, S. H., Oh, J. K., Lee, J. Y., and Kang, D. K. (2016). Isolation and characterization of a broad spectrum bacteriocin from *Bacillus amyloliquefaciens* RX7. *Biomed Res. Int.* 2016:8521476. doi: 10.1155/ 2016/8521476

Lin, J. E., Snook, A. E., Li, P., Stoecker, B. A., Kim, G. W., Magee, M. S., et al. (2012). GUCY2C opposes systemic genotoxic tumorigenesis by regulating AKT-dependent intestinal barrier integrity. *PLoS ONE* 7:e31686. doi: 10.1371/ journal.pone.0031686

Liu, G., Kong, Y., Fan, Y., Geng, C., Peng, D., and Sun, M. (2017). Whole-genome sequencing of *Bacillus velezensis* LS69, a strain with a broad inhibitory spectrum against pathogenic bacteria. *J. Biotechnol.* 249, 20–24. doi: 10.1016/j.jbiotec. 2017.03.018

Liu, S., and Weiner, H. L. (2016). Control of the gut microbiome by fecal microRNA. *Microb. Cell* 3, 176–177. doi: 10.15698/mic2016.04.492

Lopetuso, L. R., Scaldaferri, F., Franceschi, F., and Gasbarrini, A. (2016). *Bacillus clausii* and gut homeostasis: state of the art and future perspectives. *Expert Rev. Gastroenterol. Hepatol.* 10, 943–948. doi: 10.1080/17474124.2016. 1200465

Luber, J. M., and Kostic, A. D. (2017). Gut microbiota: small molecules modulate host cellular functions. *Curr. Biol.* 27, R307–R310. doi: 10.1016/j.cub.2017. 03.026

Maffei, V. J., Kim, S., Blanchard, E., Luo, M., Jazwinski, S. M.,Taylor, C. M., et al. (2017). Biological aging and the human gut microbiota. *J. Gerontol. A Biol. Sci. Med. Sci.* doi: 10.1093/gerona/glx042 [Epub ahead of print].

Magnúsdóttir, S., Ravcheev, D., de Crécy-Lagard, V., and Thiele, I. (2015). Systematic genome assessment of B-vitamin biosynthesis suggests co-operation among gut microbes. *Front. Genet.* 6:148. doi: 10.3389/fgene.2015.00148

Majeed, M., Nagabhushanam, K., Natarajan, S., Sivakumar, A., Ali, F., Pande, A., et al. (2016). *Bacillus coagulans* MTCC 5856 supplementation in the management of diarrhea predominant Irritable Bowel Syndrome: a double blind randomized placebo controlled pilot clinical study. *Nutr. J.* 15, 21. doi: 10.1186/s12937-016-0140-6

Marchesi, J. R., Adams, D. H., Fava, F., Hermes, G. D., Hirschfield, G. M., Hold, G., et al. (2016). The gut microbiota and host health: a new clinical frontier. *Gut* 65, 330–339. doi: 10.1136/gutjnl-2015-309990

Marco, M. L., Heeney, D., Binda, S., Cifelli, C. J., Cotter, P. D., Foligné, B., et al. (2017). Health benefits of fermented foods: microbiota and beyond. *Curr. Opin. Biotechnol.* 44, 94–102. doi: 10.1016/j.copbio.2016.11.010

Mariat, D., Firmesse, O., Levenez, F., Guimarães, V., Sokol, H., Doré, J., et al. (2009). The *Firmicutes/Bacteroidetes* ratio of the human microbiota changes with age. *BMC Microbiol.* 9:123. doi: 10.1186/1471-2180-9-123

Martí, J. M., Martínez-Martínez, D., Rubio, T., Gracia, C., Peña, M., Latorre, A., et al. (2017). Health and disease imprinted in the time variability of the human microbiome. *mSystems* 2:e00144-16. doi: 10.1128/mSystems.00144-16

Martín, R., and Suárez, J. E. (2010). Biosynthesis and degradation of H_2O_2 by vaginal lactobacilli. *Appl. Environ. Microbiol.* 76, 400–405. doi: 10.1128/AEM. 01631-09

Martinez, R. C., Wachsman, M., Torres, N. I., LeBlanc, J. G., Todorov, S. D., and Franco, B. D. (2013). Biochemical, antimicrobial and molecular characterization of a noncytotoxic bacteriocin produced by *Lactobacillus plantarum* ST71KS. *Food Microbiol.* 34, 376–381. doi: 10.1016/j.fm.2013.01.011

Mashburn, L. M., and Whiteley, M. (2005). Membrane vesicles traffic signals and facilitate group activities in a prokaryote. *Nature* 437, 422–425. doi: 10.1038/ nature03925

Matsuda, K., Tsuji, H., Asahara, T., Matsumoto, K., Takada, T., and Nomoto, K. (2009). Establishment of an analytical system for the human fecal microbiota, based on reverse transcription-quantitative PCR targeting of multicopy rRNA molecules. *Appl. Environ. Microbiol.* 75, 1961–1969. doi: 10.1128/AEM.01 843-08

Matsuoka, K., and Kanai, T. (2015). The gut microbiota and inflammatory bowel disease. *Semin. Immunopathol.* 37, 47–55. doi: 10.1007/s00281-014-0454-4

McKay, K. A., Kowalec, K., Brinkman, F., Finlay, B. B., Horwitz, M., Manges, A. R., et al. (2017). From bugs to brains: the microbiome in neurological health. *Mult. Scler. Relat. Disord.* 12, 1–3. doi: 10.1016/j.msard.2016.12.007

Midha, S., Mishra, R., Aziz, M. A., Sharma, M., Mishra, A., Khandelwal, P., et al. (2005). Cloning, expression and characterization of recombinant nitric oxide synthase-like protein from *Bacillus anthracis*. *Biochem. Biophys. Res. Commun.* 336, 346–356. doi: 10.1016/j.bbrc.2005.08.083

Mitkevich, V. A., Kretova, O. V., Petrushanko, I. Y., Burnysheva, K. M., Sosin, D. V., Simonenko, O. V., et al. (2013). Ribonuclease binase apoptotic signature in leukemic Kasumi-1 cells. *Biochimie* 95, 1344–1349. doi: 10.1016/j.biochi.2013.02.016

Morita, H., Yoshikawa, H., Sakata, R., Nagata, Y., and Tanaka, H. (1997). Synthesis of nitric oxide from the two equivalent guanidino nitrogens of L-arginine by *Lactobacillus fermentum*. *J. Bacteriol.* 179, 7812–7815. doi: 10.1128/jb.179.24.7812-7815.1997

Mourembou, G., Ndjoyi-Mbiguino, A., Lekana-Douki, J. B., Fournier, P. E., Raoult, D., and Bittar, F. (2016). Discovery of a new species within *Bacillus* genus in a stool sample from Gabon: "*Bacillus massiliogabonensis*" sp. nov. *New Microbes New Infect.* 15, 3–5. doi: 10.1016/j.nmni.2016.09.013

Müller, C., Ulyanova, V., Ilinskaya, O., Pleschka, S., and Shah Mahmud, R. (2017). A novel antiviral strategy against MERS-CoV and HCoV-229E using binase to target viral genome replication. *BioNanoScience* 7, 294–299. doi: 10.1007/s12668-016-0341-7

Müller, S., Strack, S. N., Hoefler, B. C., Straight, P. D., Kearns, D. B., and Kirby, J. R. (2014). Bacillaene and sporulation protect *Bacillus subtilis* from predation by *Myxococcus xanthus*. *Appl. Environ. Microbiol.* 80, 5603–5610. doi: 10.1128/AEM.01621-14

Nakamura, K., Sakuragi, N., Takakuwa, A., and Ayabe, T. (2016). Paneth cell α-defensins and enteric microbiota in health and disease. *Biosci. Microbiota Food Health* 35, 57–67. doi: 10.12938/bmfh.2015-019

Natarajan, N., and Pluznick, J. L. (2014). From microbe to man: the role of microbial short chain fatty acid metabolites in host cell biology. *Am. J. Physiol. Cell Physiol.* 307, C979–C985. doi: 10.1152/ajpcell.00228.2014

Nava, G. M., and Stappenbeck, T. S. (2011). Diversity of the autochthonous colonic microbiota. *Gut Microbes* 2, 99–104. doi: 10.4161/gmic.2.2.15416

Nguyen, U. T., and Burrows, L. L. (2014). DNase I and proteinase K impair *Listeria monocytogenes* biofilm formation and induce dispersal of pre-existing biofilms. *Int. J. Food Microbiol.* 187, 26–32. doi: 10.1016/j.ijfoodmicro.2014.06.025

Nithya, V., Muthukumar, S. P., and Halami, P. M. (2012). Safety assessment of *Bacillus licheniformis* Me1 isolated from milk for probiotic application. *Int. J. Toxicol.* 31, 228–237. doi: 10.1177/1091581812443388

Nøhr, M. K., Egerod, K. L., Christiansen, S. H., Gille, A., Offermanns, S., Schwartz, T. W., et al. (2015). Expression of the short chain fatty acid receptor GPR41/FFAR3 in autonomic and somatic sensory ganglia. *Neuroscience* 290, 126–137. doi: 10.1016/j.neuroscience.2015.01.040

Nyangale, E. P., Farmer, S., Cash, H. A., Keller, D., Chernoff, D., and Gibson, G. R. (2015). *Bacillus coagulans* GBI-30, 6086 modulates *Faecalibacterium prausnitzii* in older men and women. *J. Nutr.* 145, 1446–1452. doi: 10.3945/jn.114.199802

Odamaki, T., Kato, K., Sugahara, H., Hashikura, N., Takahashi, S., Xiao, J. Z., et al. (2016). Age-related changes in gut microbiota composition from newborn to centenarian: a cross-sectional study. *BMC Microbiol.* 16:90. doi: 10.1186/s12866-016-0708-5

Okamoto, K., Fujiya, M., Nata, T., Ueno, N., Inaba, Y., Ishikawa, C., et al. (2012). Competence and sporulation factor derived from *Bacillus subtilis* improves epithelial cell injury in intestinal inflammation via immunomodulation and cytoprotection. *Int. J. Colorectal Dis.* 27, 1039–1046. doi: 10.1007/s00384-012-1416-8

Oscariz, J. C., and Pisabarro, A. G. (2001). Classification and mode of action of membrane-active bacteriocins produced by gram-positive bacteria. *Int. Microbiol.* 4, 13–19.

Ott, S. J., Musfeldt, M., Wenderoth, D. F., Hampe, J., Brant, O., Fölsch, U. R., et al. (2004). Reduction in diversity of the colonic mucosa associated bacterial microflora in patients with active inflammatory bowel disease. *Gut* 53, 685–693. doi: 10.1136/gut.2003.025403

Panda, S., El khader, I., Casellas, F., López Vivancos, J., García Cors, M., Santiago, A., et al. (2014). Short-term effect of antibiotics on human gut microbiota. *PLoS ONE* 9:e95476. doi: 10.1371/journal.pone.0095476

Patel, A. K., Singhania, R. R., Pandey, A., and Chincholakar, S. B. (2010). Probiotic bile salt hydrolase: current development and perspectives. *Appl. Biochem. Biotechnol.* 162, 166–180. doi: 10.1007/s12010-009-8738-1

Pattison, A. M., Merlino, D. J., Blomain, E. S., and Waldman, S. A. (2016). Guanylyl cyclase C signaling axis and colon cancer prevention. *World J. Gastroenterol.* 22, 8070–8077. doi: 10.3748/wjg.v22.i36.8070

Peng, L., Li, Z. R., Green, R. S., Holzman, I. R., and Lin, J. (2009). Butyrate enhances the intestinal barrier by facilitating tight junction assembly via activation of AMP-activated protein kinase in Caco-2 cell monolayers. *J. Nutr.* 139, 1619–1625. doi: 10.3945/jn.109.104638

Perez, K. J., Viana, J. D., Lopes, F. C., Pereira, J. Q., Dos Santos, D. M., Oliveira, J. S., et al. (2017). *Bacillus* spp. isolated from puba as a source of biosurfactants and antimicrobial lipopeptides. *Front. Microbiol.* 8:61. doi: 10.3389/fmicb.2017.00061

Pillai, A., and Nelson, R. (2008). Probiotics for treatment of *Clostridium difficile*-associated colitis in adults. *Cochrane Database Syst. Rev.* 23, CD004611. doi: 10.1002/14651858.CD004611.pub2

Pridmore, R. D., Pittet, A. C., Praplan, F., and Cavadini, C. (2008). Hydrogen peroxide production by *Lactobacillus johnsonii* NCC 533 and its role in anti-*Salmonella* activity. *FEMS Microbiol. Lett.* 283, 210–215. doi: 10.1111/j.1574-6968.2008.01176.x

Prior, I. A., Lewis, P. D., and Mattos, C. (2012). A comprehensive survey of Ras mutations in cancer. *Cancer Res.* 72, 2457–2467. doi: 10.1158/0008-5472.CAN-11-2612

Quagliariello, A., Aloisio, I., Bozzi Cionci, N., Luiselli, D., D'Auria, G., Martinez-Priego, L., et al. (2016). Effect of *Bifidobacterium breve* on the intestinal microbiota of coeliac children on a gluten free diet: a pilot study. *Nutrients* 8:660. doi: 10.3390/nu8100660

Rafter, J., Bennett, M., Caderni, G., Clune, Y., Hughes, R., Karlsson, P. C., et al. (2007). Dietary synbiotics reduce cancer risk factors in polypectomized and colon cancer patients. *Am. J. Clin. Nutr.* 85, 488–496.

Rajilić-Stojanović, M., and de Vos, W. M. (2014). The first 1000 cultured species of the human gastrointestinal microbiota. *FEMS Microbiol. Rev.* 38, 996–1047. doi: 10.1111/1574-6976.12075

Rapozo, D. C., Bernardazzi, C., and de Souza, H. S. (2017). Diet and microbiota in inflammatory bowel disease: the gut in disharmony. *World J. Gastroenterol.* 23, 2124–2140. doi: 10.3748/wjg.v23.i12.2124

Reuter, G. (2001). The *Lactobacillus* and *Bifidobacterium* microflora of the human intestine: composition and succession. *Curr. Issues Intest. Microbiol.* 2, 43–53.

Rey, M. W., Ramaiya, P., Nelson, B. A., Brody-Karpin, S. D., Zaretsky, E. J., Tang, M., et al. (2004). Complete genome sequence of the industrial bacterium *Bacillus licheniformis* and comparisons with closely related *Bacillus* species. *Genome Biol.* 5:R77. doi: 10.1186/gb-2004-5-10-r77

Rhee, K. J., Sethupathi, P., Driks, A., Lanning, D. K., and Knight, K. L. (2004). Role of commensal bacteria in development of gut-associated lymphoid tissues and preimmune antibody repertoire. *J. Immunol.* 172, 1118–1124. doi: 10.4049/jimmunol.172.2.1118

Ríos-Covián, D., Ruas-Madiedo, P., Margolles, A., Gueimonde, M., de Los Reyes-Gavilán, C. G., and Salazar, N. (2016). Intestinal short chain fatty acids and their link with diet and human health. *Front. Microbiol.* 7:185. doi: 10.3389/fmicb.2016.00185

Rivera, J., Cordero, R. J., Nakouzi, A. S., Frases, S., Nicola, A., and Casadevall, A. (2010). *Bacillus anthracis* produces membrane-derived vesicles containing biologically active toxins. *Proc. Natl. Acad. Sci. U.S.A.* 107, 19002–19007. doi: 10.1073/pnas.1008843107

Roier, S., Zingl, F. G., Cakar, F., and Schild, S. (2016). Bacterial outer membrane vesicle biogenesis: a new mechanism and its implications. *Microb. Cell* 3, 257–259. doi: 10.15698/mic2016.06.508

Rowland, I., Gibson, G., Heinken, A., Scott, K., Swann, J., Thiele, I., et al. (2017). Gut microbiota functions: metabolism of nutrients and other food components. *Eur. J. Nutr.* doi: 10.1007/s00394-017-1445-8 [Epub ahead of print].

Ruiz, L., Hevia, A., Bernardo, D., Margolles, A., and Sanchez, B. (2014). Extracellular molecular effectors mediating probiotic attributes. *FEMS Microbiol. Lett.* 359, 1–11. doi: 10.1111/1574-6968.12576

Sakatani, A., Fujiya, M., Ueno, N., Kashima, S., Sasajima, J., Moriichi, K., et al. (2016). Polyphosphate derived from Lactobacillus brevis inhibits colon cancer progression through induction of cell apoptosis. *Anticancer. Res.* 36, 591–598.

Salard, I., Mercey, E., Rekka, E., Boucher, J.-L., Nioche, P., Mikula, I., et al. (2006). Analogies and surprising differences between recombinant nitric oxide synthase-like proteins from *Staphylococcus aureus* and *Bacillus anthracis* in their interactions with L-arginine analogs and iron ligands. *J. Inorg. Biochem.* 100, 2024–2033. doi: 10.1016/j.jinorgbio.2006.09.017

Sandrini, S., Aldriwesh, M., Alruways, M., and Freestone, P. (2015). Microbial endocrinology: host-bacteria communication within the gut microbiome. *J. Endocrinol.* 225, R21–R34. doi: 10.1530/JOE-14-0615

Sankar, S. A., Lagier, J. C., Pontarotti, P., Raoult, D., and Fournier, P. E. (2015). The human gut microbiome, a taxonomic conundrum. *Syst. Appl. Microbiol.* 38, 276–286. doi: 10.1016/j.syapm.2015.03.004

Satish Kumar, R., Kanmani, P., Yuvaraj, N., Paari, K. A., Pattukumar, V., and Arul, V. (2013). Traditional Indian fermented foods: a rich source of lactic acid bacteria. *Int. J. Food Sci. Nutr.* 64, 415–428. doi: 10.3109/09637486.2012.746288

Sazawal, S., Hiremath, G., Dhingra, U., Malik, P., Deb, S., and Black, R. E. (2006). Efficacy of probiotics in prevention of acute diarrhea: a meta-analysis of masked, randomized, placebo-controlled trials. *Lancet Infect. Dis.* 6, 374–382. doi: 10.1016/S1473-3099(06)70495-9

Segawa, S., Fujiya, M., Konishi, H., Ueno, N., Kobayashi, N., Shigyo, T., et al. (2011). Probiotic-derived polyphosphate enhances the epithelial barrier function and maintains intestinal homeostasis through integrin-p38 MAPK pathway. *PLoS ONE* 6:e23278. doi: 10.1371/journal.pone.0023278

Selvam, R., Maheswari, P., Kavitha, P., Ravichandran, M., Sas, B., and Ramchand, C. N. (2009). Effect of *Bacillus subtilis* PB6, a natural probiotic on colon mucosal inflammation and plasma cytokines levels in inflammatory bowel disease. *Indian J. Biochem. Biophys.* 46, 79–85.

Senghor, B., Seck, E. H., Khelaifia, S., Bassène, H., Sokhna, C., Fournier, P. E., et al. (2017). Description of '*Bacillus dakarensis*' sp. nov., '*Bacillus sinesaloumensis*' sp. nov., '*Gracilibacillus timonensis*' sp. nov., '*Halobacillus massiliensis*' sp. nov., '*Lentibacillus massiliensis*' sp. nov., '*Oceanobacillus senegalensis*' sp. nov., '*Oceanobacillus timonensis*' sp. nov., '*Virgibacillus dakarensis*' sp. nov. and '*Virgibacillus marseillensis*' sp. nov., nine halophilic new species isolated from human stool. *New Microbes New Infect.* 17, 45–51. doi: 10.1016/j.nmni.2017.01.010

Servin, A. L. (2004). Antagonistic activities of lactobacilli and bifidobacteria against microbial pathogens. *FEMS Microbiol. Rev.* 28, 405–440. doi: 10.1016/j.femsre.2004.01.003

Shah Mahmud, R., Efimova, M., Mostafa, A., Ulyanova, V., and Ilinskaya, O. (2016). Antiviral activity of bacterial extracellular ribonuclease against single-, double stranded RNA and DNA containing viruses in cell cultures. *BioNanoScience* 6, 561–563. doi: 10.1007/s12668-016-0279-9

Shah Mahmud, R., and Ilinskaya, O. N. (2013). Antiviral activity of binase against the pandemic influenza A (H1N1) virus. *Acta Nat.* 5, 44–51.

Shah Mahmud, R., Müller, C., Romanova, Y., Mostafa, A., Ulyanova, V., Pleschka, S., et al. (2017). Ribonuclease from *Bacillus* acts as an antiviral agent against negative- and positive-sense single stranded human respiratory RNA viruses. *Biomed Res. Int.* 2017:5279065. doi: 10.1155/2017/5279065

Sharon, G., Sampson, T. R., Geschwind, D. H., and Mazmanian, S. K. (2016). The central nervous system and the gut microbiome. *Cell* 167, 915–932. doi: 10.1016/j.cell.2016.10.027

Shi, N., Li, N., Duan, X., and Niu, H. (2017). Interaction between the gut microbiome and mucosal immune system. *Mil. Med. Res.* 4, 14. doi: 10.1186/s40779-017-0122-9

Shields, R. C., Mokhtar, N., Ford, M., Hall, M. J., Burgess, J. G., ElBadawey, M. R., et al. (2013). Efficacy of a marine bacterial nuclease against biofilm forming microorganisms isolated from chronic rhinosinusitis. *PLoS ONE* 8:e55339. doi: 10.1371/journal.pone.0055339

Shobharani, P., and Halami, P. M. (2014). Cellular fatty acid profile and H^+-ATPAse activity to assess acid tolerance of *Bacillus* sp. for potential probiotic functional attributes. *Appl. Microbiol. Biotechnol.* 98, 9045–9058. doi: 10.1007/s00253-014-5981-3

Shobharani, P., Padmaja, R. J., and Halami, P. M. (2015). Diversity in the antibacterial potential of probiotic cultures *Bacillus licheniformis* MCC2514 and *Bacillus licheniformis* MCC2512. *Res. Microbiol.* 166, 546–554. doi: 10.1016/j.resmic.2015.06.003

Shukla, S. D., Budden, K. F., Neal, R., and Hansbro, P. M. (2017). Microbiome effects on immunity, health and disease in the lung. *Clin. Transl. Immunol.* 6, e133. doi: 10.1038/cti.2017.6

Singh, R. K., Chang, H. W., Yan, D., Lee, K. M., Ucmak, D., Wong, K., et al. (2017). Influence of diet on the gut microbiome and implications for human health. *J. Transl. Med.* 15, 73. doi: 10.1186/s12967-017-1175-y

Siraj, Y., Nguen, N., Zelenikhin, P. V., Sokolova, E. V., Gataullin, I. G., and Ilinskaya, O. N. (2015). Dysbiosis of cultivable aerobic microbiota tightly associated with colon cancer epithelial cells. *RJPBCS* 6, 1658–1663.

Smaoui, S., Elleuch, L., Bejar, W., Karray-Rebai, I., Ayadi, I., Jaouadi, B., et al. (2010). Inhibition of fungi and gram-negative bacteria by bacteriocin BacTN635 produced by *Lactobacillus plantarum* sp. TN635. *Appl. Biochem. Biotechnol.* 162, 1132–1146. doi: 10.1007/s12010-009-8821-7

Sobke, A., Klinger, M., Hermann, B., Sachse, S., Nietzsche, S., Makarewicz, O., et al. (2012). The urinary antibiotic 5-nitro-8-hydroxyquinoline (Nitroxoline) reduces the formation and induces the dispersal of *Pseudomonas aeruginosa* biofilms by chelation of iron and zinc. *Antimicrob. Agents Chemother.* 56, 6021–6025. doi: 10.1128/AAC.01484-12

Sokurenko, J. V., Zelenikhin, P. V., Ulyanova, V. V., Kolpakov, A. I., Muler, D., and Ilinskaya, O. N. (2015). Identification of 2',3'-cGMP as an intermediate of RNA catalytic cleavage by binase and evaluation of its biological action. *Russ. J. Bioorg. Chem.* 41, 31–36. doi: 10.1134/S1068162015010136

Sornplang, P., and Piyadeatsoontorn, S. (2016). Probiotic isolates from unconventional sources: a review. *J. Anim. Sci. Technol.* 58, 26. doi: 10.1186/s40781-016-0108-2

Stern, N. J., Svetoch, E. A., Eruslanov, B. V., Perelygin, V. V., Mitsevich, E. V., Mitsevich, I. P., et al. (2006). Isolation of a *Lactobacillus salivarius* strain and purification of its bacteriocin, which is inhibitory to *Campylobacter jejuni* in the chicken gastrointestinal system. *Antimicrob. Agents Chemother.* 50, 3111–3116. doi: 10.1128/AAC.00259-06

Stubbendieck, R. M., and Straight, P. D. (2016). Multifaceted interfaces of bacterial competition. *J. Bacteriol.* 198, 2145–2155. doi: 10.1128/JB.00275-16

Sudhamsu, J., and Crane, B. R. (2006). Structure and reactivity of a thermostable prokaryotic nitric-oxide synthase that forms a long-lived oxy-heme complex. *J. Biol. Chem.* 281, 9623–9632. doi: 10.1074/jbc.M510062200

Sumi, C. D., Yang, B. W., Yeo, I. C., and Hahm, Y. T. (2015). Antimicrobial peptides of the genus *Bacillus*: a new era for antibiotics. *Can. J. Microbiol.* 61, 93–103. doi: 10.1139/cjm-2014-0613

Tam, N. K., Uyen, N. Q., Hong, H. A., Duc, L. H., Hoa, T. T., Serra, C. R., et al. (2006). The intestinal life cycle of *Bacillus subtilis* and close relatives. *J. Bacteriol.* 188, 2692–2700. doi: 10.1128/JB.188.7.2692-2700.2006

Tamang, J. P., Shin, D. H., Jung, S. J., and Chae, S. W. (2016). Functional properties of microorganisms in fermented foods. *Front. Microbiol.* 7:578. doi: 10.3389/fmicb.2016.00578

Tang, W. H., Kitai, T., and Hazen, S. L. (2017). Gut microbiota in cardiovascular health and disease. *Circ. Res.* 120, 1183–1196. doi: 10.1161/CIRCRESAHA.117.309715

Thomas, C., and Versalovic, J. (2010). Probiotics-host communication: modulation of signaling pathways in the intestine. *Gut Microbes* 1, 148–163. doi: 10.4161/gmic.1.3.11712

Travers, M. A., Sow, C., Zirah, S., Deregnaucourt, C., Chaouch, S., Queiroz, R. M., et al. (2016). Deconjugated bile salts produced by extracellular bile-salt hydrolase-like activities from the probiotic *Lactobacillus johnsonii* La1 inhibit Giardia duodenalis in vitro growth. *Front. Microbiol.* 7:1453. doi: 10.3389/fmicb.2016.01453

Tropini, C., Earle, K. A., Huang, K. C., and Sonnenburg, J. L. (2017). The Gut microbiome: connecting spatial organization to function. *Cell Host Microbe* 21, 433–442. doi: 10.1016/j.chom.2017.03.010

Tsilingiri, K., and Rescigno, M. (2013). Postbiotics: What else? *Benef. Microbes* 4, 101–107. doi: 10.3920/BM2012.0046

Ulyanova, V., Shah Mahmud, R., Dudkina, E., Vershinina, V., Domann, E., and Ilinskaya, O. (2016). Phylogenetic distribution of extracellular guanyl-preferring ribonucleases renews taxonomic status of two *Bacillus* strains. *J. Gen. Appl. Microbiol.* 62, 181–188. doi: 10.2323/jgam.2016.02.005

Ulyanova, V., Vershinina, V., and Ilinskaya, O. (2011). Barnase and binase: twins with distinct fates. *FEBS J.* 278, 3633–3643. doi: 10.1111/j.1742-4658.2011.08294.x

Urgesi, R., Casale, C., Pistelli, R., Rapaccini, G. L., and de Vitis, I. (2014). A randomized double-blind placebo-controlled clinical trial on efficacy and safety of association of simethicone and *Bacillus coagulans* (Colinox®) in patients with irritable bowel syndrome. *Eur. Rev. Med. Pharmacol. Sci.* 18, 1344–1353.

Valko, M., Morris, H., and Cronin, M. T. (2005). Metals, toxicity and oxidative stress. *Curr. Med. Chem.* 12, 1161–1208. doi: 10.2174/0929867053764635

Valladares, R., Bojilova, L., Potts, A. H., Cameron, E., Gardner, C., Lorca, G., et al. (2013). *Lactobacillus johnsonii* inhibits indoleamine 2,3-dioxygenase and alters tryptophan metabolite levels in BioBreeding rats. *FASEB J.* 27, 1711–1720. doi: 10.1096/fj.12-223339

Van De Guchte, M., Ehrlich, S. D., and Maguin, E. (2001). Production of growth-inhibiting factors by *Lactobacillus delbrueckii*. *J. Appl. Microbiol.* 91, 147–153. doi: 10.1046/j.1365-2672.2001.01369.x

van de Wouw, M., Schellekens, H., Dinan, T. G., and Cryan, J. F. (2017). Microbiota-gut-brain axis: modulator of host metabolism and appetite. *J. Nutr.* 147, 727–745. doi: 10.3945/jn.116.240481

Vanhoutte, T., Huys, G., De Brandt, E., and Swings, J. (2004). Temporal stability analysis of the microbiota in human feces by denaturing gradient gel electrophoresis using universal and group-specific 16S rRNA gene primers. *FEMS Microbiol. Ecol.* 48, 437–446. doi: 10.1016/j.femsec.2004.03.001

Vargas, G., Rocha, J. D., Oliveira, D. L., Albuquerque, P. C., Frases, S., Santos, S. S., et al. (2015). Compositional and immunobiological analyses of extracellular vesicles released by *Candida albicans*. *Cell. Microbiol.* 17, 389–407. doi: 10.1111/cmi.12374

Vinoj, G., Vaseeharan, B., Thomas, S., Spiers, A. J., and Shanthi, S. (2014). Quorum-quenching activity of the AHL-lactonase from *Bacillus licheniformis* DAHB1 inhibits *Vibrio* biofilm formation *in vitro* and reduces shrimp intestinal colonisation and mortality. *Mar. Biotechnol.* 16, 707–715. doi: 10.1007/s10126-014-9585-9

Voltan, S., Martines, D., Elli, M., Brun, P., Longo, S., Porzionato, A., et al. (2008). *Lactobacillus crispatus* M247-derived H_2O_2 acts as a signal transducing molecule activating peroxisome proliferator activated receptor-gamma in the intestinal mucosa. *Gastroenterology* 135, 1216–1227. doi: 10.1053/j.gastro.2008.07.007

Vuong, H. E., Yano, J. M., Fung, T. C., and Hsiao, E. Y. (2017). The microbiome and host behavior. *Annu. Rev. Neurosci.* 40, 21–49. doi: 10.1146/annurev-neuro-072116-031347

Walter, J. (2008). Ecological role of lactobacilli in the gastrointestinal tract: implications for fundamental and biomedical research. *Appl. Environ. Microbiol.* 74, 4985–4996. doi: 10.1128/AEM.00753-08

Walter, J., Hertel, C., Tannock, G. W., Lis, C. M., Munro, K., and Hammes, W. P. (2001). Detection of *Lactobacillus*, *Pediococcus*, *Leuconostoc*, and *Weissella* species in human feces by using group-specific PCR primers and denaturing gradient gel electrophoresis. *Appl. Environ. Microbiol.* 67, 2578–2585. doi: 10.1128/AEM.67.6.2578-2585.2001

Wang, Q., Zhao, X., Chamu, J., and Shanmugam, K. T. (2011). Isolation, characterization and evolution of a new thermophilic *Bacillus licheniformis* for lactic acid production in mineral salts medium. *Bioresour. Technol.* 102, 8152–8158. doi: 10.1016/j.biortech.2011.06.003

Wang, R., Islam, B. N., Bridges, A., Sharman, S. K., Hu, M., Hou, Y., et al. (2017). cGMP signaling increases antioxidant gene expression by activating forkhead box O3A in the colon epithelium. *Am. J. Pathol.* 187, 377–389. doi: 10.1016/j.ajpath.2016.10.016

Watters, C. M., Burton, T., Kirui, D. K., and Millenbaugh, N. J. (2016). Enzymatic degradation of *in vitro Staphylococcus aureus* biofilms supplemented with human plasma. *Infect. Drug Resist.* 9, 71–78. doi: 10.2147/IDR.S103101

Wilks, M., Wiggins, R., Whiley, A., Hennessy, E., Warwick, S., Porter, H., et al. (2004). Identification and H_2O_2 production of vaginal lactobacilli from pregnant women at high risk of preterm birth and relation with outcome. *J. Clin. Microbiol.* 42, 713–717. doi: 10.1128/JCM.42.2.713-717.2004

Winek, K., Dirnagl, U., and Meisel, A. (2016). The gut microbiome as therapeutic target in central nervous system diseases: implications for stroke. *Neurotherapeutics* 13, 762–774. doi: 10.1007/s13311-016-0475-x

Yan, F., Cao, H., Cover, T. L., Whitehead, R., Washington, M. K., and Polk, D. B. (2007). Soluble proteins produced by probiotic bacteria regulate intestinal epithelial cell survival and growth. *Gastroenterology* 132, 562–575. doi: 10.1053/j.gastro.2006.11.022

Yan, F., and Polk, D. B. (2002). Probiotic bacterium prevents cytokine-induced apoptosis in intestinal epithelial cells. *J. Biol. Chem.* 277, 50959–50965. doi: 10.1074/jbc.M207050200

Yan, J., Herzog, J. W., Tsang, K., Brennan, C. A., Bower, M. A., Garrett, W. S., et al. (2016). Gut microbiota induce IGF-1 and promote bone formation and growth. *Proc. Natl. Acad. Sci. U.S.A.* 113, E7554–E7563. doi: 10.1073/pnas.1607235113

Yang, M., Jang, I. T., Kim, H. J., and Park, J. K. (2016). *Bacillus* spp. or *Bacillus* spp.-derived membrane vesicles induce the intrinsic pathways of apoptosis of human colon cancer cell lines. *J. Bacteriol. Virol.* 46, 84–92. doi: 10.4167/jbv.2016.46.2.84

Yang, N. J., and Chiu, I. M. (2017). Bacterial signaling to the nervous system through toxins and metabolites. *J. Mol. Biol.* 429, 587–605. doi: 10.1016/j.jmb.2016.12.023

Yang, Y., and Jobin, C. (2014). Microbial imbalance and intestinal pathologies: connections and contributions. *Dis. Model Mech.* 7, 1131–1142. doi: 10.1242/dmm.016428

Yarullina, D. R., Beuerlein, K., Silkin, N. I., and Ilinskaya, O. N. (2015). Nitric oxide production in probiotic *Lactobacillus plantarum*: revision of the origin. *JMRR* 1, 5–14.

Yarullina, D. R., Mikheeva, R. O., Sabirullina, G. I., Zelenikhin, P. V., Ilinskaya, O. N., and Sitdikova, G. F. (2016). Role of nitric oxide produced by lactobacilli in relaxation of intestinal smooth muscles. *Bull. Exp. Biol. Med.* 160, 343–346. doi: 10.1007/s10517-016-3166-z

Ye, J., Wu, W., Li, Y., and Li, L. (2017). Influences of the gut microbiota on DNA methylation and histone modification. *Dig. Dis. Sci.* 62, 1155–1164. doi: 10.1007/s10620-017-4538-6

Yunes, R. A., Poluektova, E. U., Dyachkova, M. S., Klimina, K. M., Kovtun, A. S., Averina, O. V., et al. (2016). GABA production and structure of *gadB*/*gadC* genes in *Lactobacillus* and *Bifidobacterium* strains from human microbiota. *Anaerobe* 42, 197–204. doi: 10.1016/j.anaerobe.2016.10.011

Zacharofa, M. P., and Lovitt, R. W. (2012). Bacteriocins produced by lactic acid bacteria. A review article. *APCBEE Proc.* 2, 50–56.

Zamfir, M., Callewaert, R., Cornea, P. C., Savu, L., Vatafu, I., and De Vuyst, L. (1999). Purification and characterization of a bacteriocin produced by *Lactobacillus acidophilus* IBB 801. *J. Appl. Microbiol.* 87, 923–931. doi: 10.1046/j.1365-2672.1999.00950.x

Zelante, T., Iannitti Rossana, G., Cunha, C., De Luca, A., Giovannini, G., Pieraccini, G., et al. (2013). Tryptophan catabolites from microbiota engage aryl hydrocarbon receptor and balance mucosal reactivity via interleukin-22. *Immunity* 39, 372–385. doi: 10.1016/j.immuni.2013.08.003

Zhang, H. L., Li, W. S., Xu, D. N., Zheng, W. W., Liu, Y., Chen, J., et al. (2016). Mucosa-reparing and microbiota-balancing therapeutic effect of *Bacillus subtilis* alleviates dextrate sulfate sodium-induced ulcerative colitis in mice. *Exp. Ther. Med.* 12, 2554–2562. doi: 10.3892/etm.2016.3686

Zhao, X., and Kuipers, O. P. (2016). Identification and classification of known and putative antimicrobial compounds produced by a wide variety of *Bacillales* species. *BMC Genomics* 17:882. doi: 10.1186/s12864-016-3224-y

Zhou, S., Zhang, A., Yin, H., and Chu, W. (2016). *Bacillus* sp. QSI-1 modulate quorum sensing signals reduce *Aeromonas hydrophila* level and alter gut microbial community structure in fish. *Front. Cell. Infect. Microbiol.* 6:184. doi: 10.3389/fcimb.2016.00184

Zhu, Q., Jin, Z., Wu, W., Gao, R., Guo, B., Gao, Z., et al. (2014). Analysis of the intestinal lumen microbiota in an animal model of colorectal cancer. *PLoS ONE* 9:e90849. doi: 10.1371/journal.pone.0090849

3

Regulation of the Interferon Response by lncRNAs in HCV Infection

Saba Valadkhan[1] and Puri Fortes[2]**

[1] Department of Molecular Biology and Microbiology, Case Western Reserve University School of Medicine, Cleveland, OH, United States, [2] Center for Applied Medical Research, Department of Gene Therapy and Hepatology, Navarra Institute for Health Research (IdiSNA), University of Navarra, Pamplona, Spain

Correspondence:
Saba Valadkhan
saba.valadkhan@case.edu
Puri Fortes
pfortes@unav.es

The interferon (IFN) response is a critical component of the innate immunity antiviral pathways in mammalians. IFN signaling results in increased expression of cellular factors that block key steps in the viral replication cycle. Many IFN-induced antiviral factors act through decreasing viral entry, replication, transcription, translation, packaging and release. However, these effects are also deleterious for the viability of the cell, which necessitates a tight control over the magnitude and duration of the IFN response. This is partially achieved through the IFN-mediated activation of negative regulatory factors that help in termination of the IFN response and return to a normal homeostatic state. Such built-in negative regulatory mechanisms are frequently hijacked by viruses such as the Hepatitis C virus (HCV) to increase viral replication and productive infections. We and others have shown that long non-coding RNAs (lncRNAs) play prominent roles in regulation of the IFN response. Activation of the IFN cascade alters the expression of a large number of lncRNAs, many of which are directly induced by the JAK/STAT pathway and thus, resemble the well-studied protein-coding interferon-stimulated genes (ISGs). While only a handful of IFN- and virally induced lncRNAs have been characterized, recent studies have identified several lncRNAs that act as positive or negative regulators of expression of ISGs during the IFN response. A number of such regulatory lncRNAs have multiple ISG targets, while others act on a single neighboring ISG. Another group of studied lncRNAs act further upstream and regulate the expression of IFN genes or factors that sense the presence of viral genome or replication products. The large number of unstudied IFN- and virally induced lncRNAs makes it highly likely that future studies will reveal a much greater share for this class of transcripts in regulation of the antiviral response. In addition to their physiological roles, the expression of such lncRNAs is frequently modulated by virally encoded factors to interfere with the antiviral response and promote viral replication, thus making them ideal targets for therapeutic intervention.

Keywords: type I IFN, lncRNAs, HCV, proviral, antiviral, IFN response

LONG NON-CODING RNAs AS A NEW CLASS OF REGULATORY MOLECULES

High throughput transcriptome studies in the last decade have led to the discovery of 1000s of novel RNA molecules that do not appear to code for functional peptides. These transcripts, named the long non-coding RNAs (lncRNAs), can be found in both eukaryotes and prokaryotes. However, they are especially abundant in more complex eukaryotes including animals and plants (Rinn and Chang, 2012; Morris and Mattick, 2014). Interestingly, their abundance seems to correlate with the level of complexity of the organism, for example while protein-coding sequences constitute < 2% of the human genome, a significantly larger fraction of our genomes is coding for lncRNAs (ENCODE Project Consortium, 2012; Clark et al., 2013). lncRNAs have diverse modes of biogenesis and mechanism of action and constitute a heterogeneous group of transcripts. Many of them are transcribed by RNA polymerase II and are spliced and polyadenylated, although on average they contain fewer introns compared to protein-coding genes (Carninci et al., 2005; Derrien et al., 2012; Niazi and Valadkhan, 2012). However, several studied lncRNAs are RNA polymerase I and III transcripts and a significant fraction of lncRNAs are not polyadenylated (Carninci et al., 2005; Derrien et al., 2012; Djebali et al., 2012). Similarly, they show a wide heterogeneity in size and can range from a couple of hundred to tens of thousands of nucleotides in length. An arbitrary lower length limit of 200 nucleotides which has been proposed for this class of RNAs should not be applied too strictly, as it mainly serves as a general guideline for distinguishing lncRNAs from the small non-coding RNA such as small nuclear and nucleolar RNAs, microRNAs, etc. (Clark and Mattick, 2011; Rinn and Chang, 2012; Mattick and Rinn, 2015).

Despite intense research in recent years, the sheer number and diversity of lncRNAs have limited our understanding of the scope of function of lncRNAs in higher eukaryotes. Evidence emerging from existing research indicate that the expression of many lncRNAs is strongly dependent on the cell type and cellular state and is tightly controlled by various cellular signals (Rinn and Chang, 2012; Amaral et al., 2013). Thus, it is likely that many lncRNAs remain to be described and annotated as more cellular states are probed with high throughput transcriptomic studies. Even among the annotated lncRNAs, the vast majority remain unstudied. Finally, many alternatively processed unstudied isoforms of protein-coding RNAs do not have a significant protein-coding capacity and thus, can potentially affect the cellular function as non-coding RNAs (Carninci et al., 2005; Djebali et al., 2012; ENCODE Project Consortium, 2012). Therefore, it is likely that future research will elucidate a much larger share for lncRNAs in cellular function than currently assumed.

Nonetheless, data from the small number of lncRNAs currently studied indicate their involvement in diverse aspects of cellular function (Wapinski and Chang, 2011; Moran et al., 2012; Rinn and Chang, 2012; Amaral et al., 2013; Ulitsky and Bartel, 2013; Yang et al., 2014). Emerging data suggest that a major functional mechanism of lncRNAs involves regulation of nuclear events, including transcriptional regulation and control of the epigenetic state of chromatin (Rinn and Chang, 2012; Amaral et al., 2013; Rinn, 2014). Accordingly, localization of a lncRNA to the nuclear compartment and association with chromatin modifying complexes or transcription factors serve as potential clues into the function of a lncRNA.

Another potential indicator of the function of a lncRNA is the genomic locus from which it originates (**Figure 1**). Genes coding for lncRNAs frequently overlap protein-coding genes or other lncRNA genes in the sense or antisense orientation with the lncRNA initiating from a different promoter. In many cases, such promoters are located within or near the 3′ UTR of protein-coding genes (Carninci et al., 2005; Derrien et al., 2012; Djebali et al., 2012). Further, many lncRNAs result from selective stabilization of a certain region of a protein-coding gene, such as the 3′ UTR (Mercer et al., 2011). Such overlapping genes may affect the biogenesis and/or function of the other genes in the locus via several potential mechanisms, ranging from epigenetic regulation of the activity of the locus, to transcriptional interference, to masking or competing with functionally critical elements of the other transcripts arising from the overlapped locus through base-pairing (Valadkhan and Nilsen, 2010). Over 10% of human genes originate from the so-called bidirectional promoters, and in many cases at least one of the two promoter-sharing genes is a lncRNA (**Figure 1**) (Adachi and Lieber, 2002; Wakano et al., 2012; Uesaka et al., 2014). Data from studied examples has shown that in such loci, one member of the pair can regulate the expression of the other transcript which originates from the same promoter (Wei et al., 2011; Uesaka et al., 2014). Another subclass of lncRNAs, those originating from promoters in enhancer loci, are thought to be crucial for the function of the enhancers from which they are transcribed (**Figure 1**) (Lam et al., 2014). Finally, many lncRNAs are located in vicinity of other genes without overlapping them or sharing architectural elements with them (**Figure 1**). Such intergenic vicinal lncRNAs can potentially affect the expression of their nearby genes via transcriptional interference or epigenetic regulation (Valadkhan and Nilsen, 2010; Rinn and Chang, 2012; Mattick and Rinn, 2015). It should, however, be mentioned that many functional lncRNAs are located far away from their target genes and thus, locus proximity or even overlap is not necessarily a requirement for a regulatory relationship. On the other hand, some lncRNAs may function in cis to regulate the expression of genes located far in the genome but in the same nuclear territory (Hacisuleyman et al., 2014).

As mentioned above, current evidence point to the involvement of lncRNAs in virtually every aspect of cellular function. Several pioneering studies in recent years have provided evidence for the critical role of lncRNAs in regulation of diverse aspects of the immune response, including both innate and adaptive immunity (Fitzgerald and Caffrey, 2014; Heward and Lindsay, 2014; Imamura and Akimitsu, 2014; Stachurska et al., 2014; Marques-Rocha et al., 2015; Satpathy and Chang, 2015; Sigdel et al., 2015; Yu A.D. et al., 2015; Yu Q. et al., 2015). While the main focus of this review is on the host-derived lncRNAs involved in the interferon arm of the antiviral response, recent research has revealed that a number of virally coded lncRNAs also affect the IFN response (summarized in Valadkhan

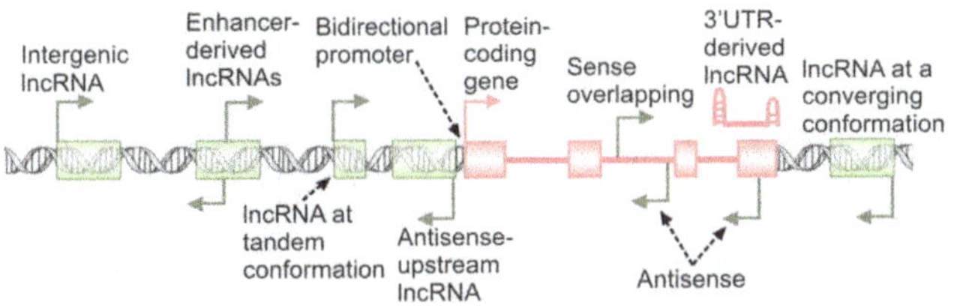

FIGURE 1 | The genomic origins of lncRNAs. The broken arrows indicate the location of transcription start sites and direction of transcription. The protein-coding gene is shown in pink, with green rectangles marking the loci of non-overlapping lncRNA genes. A 3′ UTR-derived lncRNA originating from stabilization of degradation products of the protein-coding RNA is shown.

and Gunawardane, 2015). The following sections include a discussion of the host-derived lncRNAs induced by and/or affecting the interferon response, followed by a more focused overview of the role of lncRNAs in hepatitis C infection as a well-studied example of a viral infection. Comprehensive reviews on the role of lncRNAs in development and function of the immune response are included elsewhere (Valadkhan and Gunawardane, 2015; Carpenter, 2016; Atianand et al., 2017).

THE INTERFERON ARM OF THE ANTIVIRAL RESPONSE

A crucial and nearly ubiquitous component of the innate immune response against viruses and many other microbial pathogens is mediated through the interferon (IFN) signaling cascade. IFNs are traditionally divided into three major groups (I, II, and III). While binding distinct receptors, type I (IFN-α, -β, -κ, -ε, and -ω) and type II (IFN-γ) IFNs show extensive overlap in their downstream signaling cascades and regulated genes (Hertzog et al., 2011; Pollard et al., 2013; Rusinova et al., 2013; Bolen et al., 2014). Similarly, type III IFNs (IFN-λ1, IFN-λ2, IFN-λ3, also called IL-29, IFN-λ4, IL-28A, and IL-28B, respectively), which are predominantly expressed in plasmacytoid dendritic cells in addition to a number of other cell types, bind a distinct receptor but show downstream overlap with type I IFNs (Meyer, 2009; Pollard et al., 2013; Bolen et al., 2014). The IFN response is initiated through the induction of expression of IFNs via activation of a class of cellular factors that act as the initial sensors of pathogen-associated molecular patterns. Among them, RNA sensors such as retinoic acid inducible gene I (RIG-I), melanoma differentiation-associated gene-5 (MDA5) and membrane-bound Toll-like receptors (TLR 3, 7, or 8) are particularly relevant to antiviral response against RNA viruses, although cells also contain several DNA sensors (**Figure 2**) (Hertzog and Williams, 2013; Ivashkiv and Donlin, 2014; Schneider et al., 2014). Activation of the sensor molecules, in turn, leads to signal transduction cascades and ultimately induction of the expression of genes with specific inhibitory functions against micro-organisms.

In the case of the type I IFN response, recognition of pathogen-associated patterns by RIG-I and MDA5 leads to activation of the IFN-β promoter stimulator 1 (IPS-1), while TLR3 and TLR7/TLR8 induce signaling via TRIF and MyD88, respectively (Hertzog and Williams, 2013; Ivashkiv and Donlin, 2014; Schneider et al., 2014). The activation of these pathways, in turn, will result in phosphorylation and dimerization of transcription factors including the interferon regulatory factor 3 (IRF-3), and IRF-7 followed by their nuclear translocation (**Figure 2**). Next, together with NF-κB and ATF-2/c-jun, they nucleate the formation of active transcriptional complexes through interactions with several transcription factors and regulatory proteins such as the transcriptional cofactor (CREB)-binding protein (CBP)/p300 (Kawai and Akira, 2006; Hiscott, 2007; Randall and Goodbourn, 2008; Takeuchi and Akira, 2009; Onomoto et al., 2010; Jensen and Thomsen, 2012). This, in turn, results in induction of the expression of antiviral cytokines including type I IFNs (IFN-α and IFN-β). While IFN-β is produced in most cells, IFN-α is predominantly produced in hematopoietic cells such as monocyte/macrophages and dendritic cells, especially the plasmacytoid dendritic cells. IFN-γ is induced in response to different extracellular signals, including interleukins IL2, IL12, and IL18, preferentially, in NK and T cells (Green et al., 2017). These cytokines activate JAK/STAT, NF-κB, JNK, ERK and p38 MAPK pathways, depending on the cell line, and induce transcription of IFN-γ in response to NFAT, NF-κB, STAT and AP1 transcription factors.

IFN-α and -β bind to the IFN-α/β receptor (IFNAR) in an autocrine and paracrine manner, triggering the induction of the Janus kinase/signal transducers and activators of transcription (JAK/STAT) signaling cascade (**Figure 2**) (Hertzog and Williams, 2013; Ivashkiv and Donlin, 2014; Schneider et al., 2014). The outcome is recruitment, followed by phosphorylation, dimerization and finally nuclear translocation of STAT1 and STAT2. Once in the nucleus, the complex of STAT1 and STAT2 is bound to IRF9/p48, forming the IFN-stimulated gene factor 3 (ISGF3) complex which induces the transcription of hundreds of IFN-stimulated genes (ISGs) (**Figure 2**) (Hertzog and Williams, 2013; Ivashkiv and Donlin, 2014; Schneider et al., 2014). In a highly analogous manner, IFN-γ, the sole member of the type II IFN family, binds the IFN-γ receptor and activates signaling through the JAK/STAT pathway resulting in STAT1 phosphorylation followed by nuclear translocation (Hu and Ivashkiv, 2009). Once activated, STAT1 binds the gamma-activated sequence (GAS) close to its target genes as a homodimer, triggering the transcriptional induction of STAT1-regulated genes. As mentioned above, the majority of IFN-γ-regulated genes are also induced by type I IFNs and thus, type I and type II IFN response show significant overlap in terms of the downstream effects (Hu and Ivashkiv, 2009; Pollard et al., 2013).

The final outcome of the IFN signaling is the induction of ISGs, many of which exert antimicrobial activity via regulation of different steps of cellular gene expression in addition to direct antimicrobial effects. For example, several ISGs including IFIT-1, IFIT-2, IFITM3, ISG15, ISG20, RNase L, PKR, viperin and

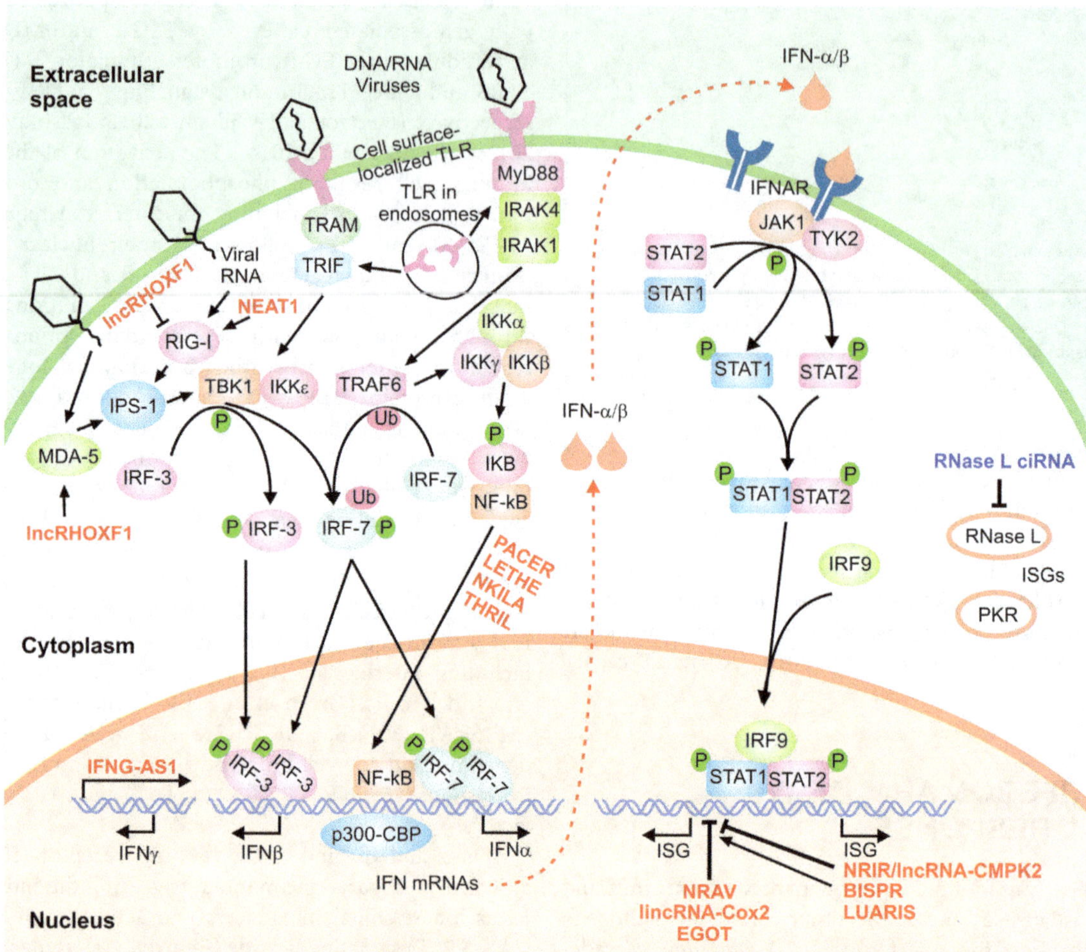

FIGURE 2 | The IFN signaling cascade. A highly simplified scheme of the type I IFN signaling cascade is shown. The host-encoded regulatory lncRNAs are shown in red font. Phosphorylation and ubiquitination events are indicated by small green circles and pink ovals, respectively.

BST2/Tetherin are known to have antiviral activity (Randall and Goodbourn, 2008). Thus, activation of the IFN response results in the induction of a cell-intrinsic antimicrobial state in both the infected and the neighboring cells which limits the spread of infectious agents. Further, these potent cytokines also affect both the innate and adaptive immune response through promoting antigen presentation, natural killer cell function, production of antibody in B cells and T cell effector function (Ivashkiv and Donlin, 2014). As mentioned above, most cells are able to launch the type I IFN response, however, cell type and context have a strong effect on the magnitude of the induced response and the specific subsets of effector genes activated (Hertzog and Williams, 2013; Ivashkiv and Donlin, 2014; Schneider et al., 2014). On the other hand, the IFN response itself is subject to negative feedback regulation by a number of ISGs and other cellular signaling pathways (Yoshimura et al., 2007; Hertzog and Williams, 2013; Ivashkiv and Donlin, 2014; Schneider et al., 2014; Porritt and Hertzog, 2015).

While the IFN cascade is mainly activated in response to the presence of exogenous viral RNAs, a group of long non-coding cellular RNAs, namely the retrotransposon-derived transcripts, also activate the IFN response (Yu Q. et al., 2015). It has been shown that activation of the Long Interspersed Element-1 (LINE-1) retroelements results in induction of the expression of IFN-β and ISGs (Yu Q. et al., 2015). Prior treatment of cells with IFN leads to suppression of LINE-1 replication, and mutations that inactivate different steps of the IFN signaling pathway cause an increase in LINE-1 replication (Yu Q. et al., 2015). Although the mechanism behind the induction of the IFN response by LINE-1 replication is not known, it is likely that the replication state of LINE elements and other retrotransposons are detected by either the same or similar sensors to those that detect the presence of exogenous viral RNA in the cell. Existing data suggest that the replication of another class of retrotransposons, the Small Interspersed Elements (SINEs) similarly results in activation of the IFN response (Leonova et al., 2013). Interestingly, it has been suggested that LINE-1 elements may contribute to the pathogenesis of autoimmune disorders such as Systemic Lupus Erythematosus (SLE) (Crow, 2010; Nakkuntod et al., 2011), which is known to involve activation of the IFN response (Bronson et al., 2012; Elkon and Wiedeman, 2012). Additional studies of the connection between autoimmunity and the replication state of cellular repeat elements will likely provide novel insight into the mechanistic basis of development of autoimmune diseases.

lncRNAs AS CRUCIAL REGULATORY FACTORS IN THE IFN RESPONSE

A number of high throughput transcriptomic analyses in both human and mouse have revealed the presence of strong changes in the expression of lncRNAs during the IFN response (Peng et al., 2010; Carnero et al., 2014; Josset et al., 2014; Kambara et al., 2014, 2015; Barriocanal et al., 2015). In the mouse studies, which were performed in both mouse lung tissue and cultured mouse embryonic fibroblasts, a significant fraction of the differentially expressed genes belonged to lncRNAs, which were either up or down-regulated after interferon stimulation and infection with respiratory viruses (Peng et al., 2010; Josset et al., 2014). Interestingly, promoter analysis and expression correlation studies raised the possibility that a significant fraction of the induced lncRNAs may be novel ISGs that were directly induced through the IFN signaling cascade (Peng et al., 2010; Josset et al., 2014).

The results obtained in the murine models were closely analogous to those obtain using human cells. In one such study, primary human hepatocytes from five donors of different ages and genders were subjected to high throughput transcriptome analysis before and at three time points of 3, 9, and 24 h after treatment with IFN-α (Kambara et al., 2014). Similar to what had been observed in the mouse, IFN stimulation resulted in both induction and repression of expression of a large number of lncRNAs. Many of the induced lncRNAs were likely direct targets of the JAK-STAT signaling pathway and thus, novel ISGs. While the majority of the induced lncRNAs remained upregulated for the three time points analyzed in this study, a fraction of them showed a shorter duration of induction and were limited to the earlier time points of the study (Kambara et al., 2014).

A third set of high throughput studies in HuH7 human hepatocytes focused on changes in gene expression observed at later time points (after 72 h) of treatment with a high dose of IFN-α2 using both microarray analysis (Carnero et al., 2014) and RNA-seq (Barriocanal et al., 2015). Interestingly, similar to the results of the study by Kambara et al. (2014), the lncRNAs that showed differential expression were almost equally divided between upregulated and downregulated ones in both microarray and RNA-seq-based datasets, while almost all differentially expressed protein coding genes were upregulated. In addition, both sets of studies revealed a significant number of differentially expressed lncRNAs which were either vicinal to or overlapped protein-coding genes that function in the immune response (Carnero et al., 2014; Kambara et al., 2014, 2015; Barriocanal et al., 2015). As mentioned above, in some cases the function of a lncRNA depends on its genomic locus and thus, these studies potentially point to the presence of an IFN-activated regulatory network of lncRNAs which may function in fine-tuning the immune response.

Regulation of the Expression of IFNs by lncRNAs

Induction of transcription of IFN genes by external or internal stimuli constitutes a key step in the IFN response and is known to be regulated by several protein-mediated mechanisms (Hertzog and Williams, 2013; Ivashkiv and Donlin, 2014; Schneider et al., 2014). Interestingly, recent evidence point to the presence of a number of lncRNA-mediated regulatory mechanisms acting on this step. At the IFNG/IFN-γ locus, lncRNA IFNG-AS1 (IFNG-antisense-1), also known as Tmevpg1 (Vigneau et al., 2003; Collier et al., 2012; Collier, 2014) and NeST (Gomez et al., 2013), is located downstream of the IFNG genic region and in human, overlaps this locus. The expression of IFNG-AS1, which is present in CD4+ and CD8+ T cells in addition to natural killer (NK) cells, shows a strong positive correlation with that of IFNG (Vigneau et al., 2003; Collier et al., 2012; Collier, 2014). The expression of IFNG-AS1 contributes to the induction of IFNG expression in CD4+ cells during their differentiation into Th1 polarization (Collier et al., 2014) and in CD8+ T cells after stimulation with PMA (phorbol 12-myristate 13-acetate) and ionomycin (Gomez et al., 2013). Mechanistic studies have shown that IFNG-AS1 acts in *trans* via interacting with WDR5, a subunit of the MLL/SET1 histone H3 lysine 4 methyltransferase complex, potentially recruiting the complex to the IFNG locus to change its methylation state (Gomez et al., 2013).

A more recent study in human trophectoderm progenitors suggested that knock down of a novel lncRNA, lncRHOXF1, which is expressed in trophectoderm and primitive endoderm cells in human blastocyst-stage embryos, may lead to upregulation of MDA5, RIG-I and IFN-β (Penkala et al., 2016). While the mechanism of the observed gene expression changes is not yet determined, the above data suggest a repressive role for lncRHOXF1 in the IFN response. NEAT1, a well-studied lncRNA with a structural role in paraspeckles, also regulates IFN-β production and RIG-I function, albeit in the opposite direction (Ma et al., 2017). Studies in the human umbilical vein endothelial cells indicated that upon infection with Hantaan virus, transcription of NEAT1 was induced through activation of RIG-I/IRF7 pathway. NEAT1, in turn, mediated the relocation of the splicing factor proline- and glutamine-rich protein (SFPQ) to paraspeckles, thus removing its transcriptional inhibitory effect on the expression of RIG-I and DDX60 leading to IFN-β production (Ma et al., 2017). In this manner, NEAT1 acts as a positive feedback regulator of RIG-I activation during viral infections. It is likely that future studies will reveal additional lncRNAs which regulate the signaling steps upstream of the expression of IFN genes, thus acting as global regulators of the IFN response.

lncRNAs Governing the Expression of IFN-Stimulated Genes

As mentioned above, high throughput transcriptomic studies have revealed the presence of a large number of lncRNAs that show differential expression in response to IFN stimulation (see **Table 1** for some functionally studied examples). One such RNA, which was identified in primary human hepatocytes by Kambara et al. (2014), originated from a locus downstream of the protein-coding ISG CMPK2 and showed a strong upregulation after IFN stimulation in additional cell types from both human and mouse. The induction of this RNA, similar to protein-coding ISGs, was dependent on the JAK-STAT signaling pathway. Knock down studies on this lncRNA, which was named lncRNA-CMPK2/NRIR (Negative Regulator of the IFN Response), resulted in a strong reduction in HCV replication in IFN-stimulated hepatocytes. Additional analyses indicated that knockdown of NRIR led to upregulation of both basal and IFN-stimulated transcription of a number of protein-coding antiviral ISGs, which could be best explained by loss of transcriptional inhibition in knockdown cells. While the mechanism of function of NRIR has not been determined, its nuclear localization together with its ability to affect the transcription of its target genes were consistent with either an epigenetic or transcriptional regulatory mechanism. Together, these data provided evidence for the presence of a lncRNA-mediated negative regulatory mechanism during the IFN response (Kambara et al., 2014). As NRIR and likely many other unstudied lncRNAs that regulate the IFN response are themselves bona-fide ISGs, it is plausible that at least some such lncRNAs may affect their own expression in addition to that of other target genes, thus creating an additional layer of self-regulatory loops. However, to our knowledge this possibility has remained unstudied.

Shortly after the discovery of NRIR, another lncRNA named NRAV (Negative Regulator of Antiviral Response) was described in a study focusing on genes differentially expressed in response to influenza virus H1N1 infection in A549 human alveolar epithelium cell line (Ouyang et al., 2014). NRAV originated from what is likely a bidirectional promoter that also gave rise to the main isoform of the dynein light chain gene DYNLL1 and was both spliced and polyadenylated. The level of NRAV was markedly reduced following infection with influenza virus and a number of other viruses in several cell lines. Importantly, forced overexpression and knock down experiments revealed that the expression level of NRAV directly correlated with the extent of viral reproduction. A microarray study of NRAV-overexpressing cell lines showed the reduction of the level of a significant number of ISGs, and additional experiments indicated that NRAV, similar to NRIR (Kambara et al., 2014), has the ability to partially block induction of the expression of its target ISGs in response to IFN stimulation (Ouyang et al., 2014).

Another lncRNA with a negative regulatory function in the IFN response is EGOT (Eosinophil Granule Ontogeny

TABLE 1 | Summary of the mode of induction and action of the lncRNAs involved in regulation of the IFN response.

lncRNA	Known mode of induction	Known mechanism of induction	Locus	Known mode of action	Known mechanism of action
NRIR (lncRNA-CMPK2)	Induced by IFN-α, β and γ	JAK-STAT pathway (ISG)	hg38 chr2:6,828,880–6,833,531	Acts in trans	Transcriptional downregulation of several target genes including other ISGs
NRAV	Downregulated after infection with influenza and other viruses	Not known	hg38 chr12:120,490,328–120,495,940	Acts in trans	Downregulation of several target genes including other ISGs through binding ZONAB
BISPR	Induced by IFN-α, β and γ	JAK-STAT pathway (ISG)	hg38 chr19:17,405,743–17,415,738	Acts in cis/trans	Transcriptional regulation of expression of its promoter-sharing ISG neighbor BST2
EGOT	Induced by IFN-α, poly(I:C) or infection with HCV, SFV or inflyuenza virus	NF-κB pathway	hg38 chr3:4,749,192–4,751,590	Acts in cis	Transcriptional downregulation of several target genes including other ISGs
LUARIS	Downregulated after IFN-β or poly(I:C) treatment	IRF3-mediated downregulation	hg38 chr7:43,508,728–43,522,542	Acts in trans	Through binding to ATF2 positively regulates the expression of several target genes including other ISGs
IFNG-AS1 (Tmevpg1, NeST)	Th1 CD4+ T cell development	Induced by TBX21 (TBET), NF-kB and ETS1	hg38 chr12:67,989,529–68,234,686	Acts in trans	Changes the methylation status of IFNG locus through interacting with WDR5, leading to induction of IFNG gene
lncRHOXF1 (RHOXF1P1)	Not known	Not known	hg38 chrX:120,010,717–120,015,551	Not known	Negative regulation of expression of MDA5, RIG-I and IFN-β
NEAT1	Induced upon Hantaan virus infection	RIG-I/IRF7 pathway	hg38 chr11:65,422,798–65,445,540	Acts in trans	Sequesters SFPQ, leading to induction of RIG-I and DDX60 and thus, IFN-β production.

Transcript). EGOT is a structured polyadenylated nuclear lncRNA conserved, at least, in all placental mammals (Rose and Stadler, 2011). Interestingly, EGOT genomic locus shows enhancer marks with high histone 3 lysine 4 monomethylation and low trimethylation, indicating that EGOT could be an enhancer RNA (Heintzman et al., 2007). EGOT overlaps an intron of the inositol 1,4,5-trisphosphate receptor 1 (ITRP1) gene in antisense orientation but EGOT depletion does not affect ITRP1 cellular levels (Prior et al., unpublished observation). EGOT was first described as a lncRNA expressed in eosinophils during development and maturation and is thought to function in mature eosinophils in regulating the levels of toxic molecules, such as the major basic protein and the eosinophil derived neurotoxin (Wagner et al., 2007). However, GTEx studies show that the highest levels of EGOT are found in non-hematopoietic tissues such as breast, vagina, pancreas, pituitary and kidney cortex (GTEx Consortium, 2013). A recent study in HuH7 cells indicated that the level of EGOT shows a dramatic increase after infection with HCV and other RNA viruses (see below) (Carnero et al., 2016). EGOT was also induced in response to very high doses of IFN-α, but at much lower levels compared to what is observed after infection with RNA viruses. Knock down of EGOT in HCV infected cells led to an increase in the expression of a subset of ISGs including GBP1, ISG15, Mx1, BST2, ISG56, IFI6, and IFITM1, resulting in reduced viral replication (Carnero et al., 2016). Taken together, these results indicate that although EGOT is not a bona fide ISG itself, it is yet another lncRNA with a negative regulatory impact on ISG induction and thus, the IFN response.

Considering the rather small number of lncRNAs that have been studied in the context of the IFN response, the discovery of the negative regulatory roles of NRIR, NRAV and EGOT on the transcriptional induction of ISGs suggests that lncRNAs may play a prominent role in negative feedback loops controlling the IFN response and possibly other signaling cascades in the immune response. Interestingly, several protein factors involved in negative regulation of IFN response have been identified (Yoshimura et al., 2007; Hertzog and Williams, 2013; Ivashkiv and Donlin, 2014; Schneider et al., 2014; Porritt and Hertzog, 2015). Defining the interaction of the negative regulatory lncRNAs with the positive and negative regulatory proteins in the context of IFN response will yield a unified picture of the feedback mechanisms which mediate the termination of IFN signaling cascade.

While the above described lncRNAs had a negative regulatory impact on the IFN response, a recent study has provided evidence for lncRNA-mediated positive regulation of the IFN cascade. A screen for IRF3-dependent genes in HuS immortalized human hepatocytes led to the identification of an annotated but unstudied lncRNA (LOC100506895/AC011738.4/ENST00000436105.1) that was down-regulated in an IRF3-dependent manner after poly(I:C) treatment (Nishitsuji et al., 2016). This transcript, which was dubbed lncRNA#32 and was later renamed LUARIS (lncRNA upregulator of antiviral response interferon signaling), overlaps introns 21 and 22 and exon 22 of the protein-coding gene HECW1 in antisense orientation (hg38 chr7:43,508,728-43,522,542). Unlike NRIR, the level of LUARIS was reduced after stimulation with IFN-β. Interestingly, both in the presence and absence of IFN stimulation, knock down and overexpression of LUARIS led to dramatic reduction and upregulation of expression of several ISGs, respectively. Indeed, forced overexpression of LUARIS led to suppression of replication of a number of viral pathogens including HCV, further proving that it acts as a positive regulator of the IFN response (Nishitsuji et al., 2016). Mechanistic studies indicated that the transcriptional stimulatory action of this lncRNA was likely mediated through its binding to the activating transcription factor 2 (ATF2) (Nishitsuji et al., 2016). Why should a positive regulator of the IFN response be downregulated by IFNs? It is likely that the expression level of LUARIS is used to adjust the magnitude of the IFN response through the action of multiple regulatory pathways that control its transcription or stability. Defining the identity of additional signaling pathways that control the expression of this and other similarly acting lncRNAs will provide crucial insights into the complex network of interactions that regulate the antiviral response.

While the lncRNAs described above regulated a number of ISG targets, another IFN-induced lncRNA named BISPR (BST2 IFN-Stimulated Positive Regulator) seems to affect the expression of a single target gene. Independent studies from two groups (Carnero et al., 2014; Kambara et al., 2014, 2015; Barriocanal et al., 2015) identified BISPR as a lncRNA that was induced in response to IFN-α stimulation through the JAK/STAT pathway in multiple cell lines including the THP1 monocytes (Kambara et al., 2015) and HuH7 human hepatocytes (Carnero et al., 2014; Barriocanal et al., 2015). BISPR originated from a bidirectional promoter that also gave rise to BST2/Tetherin, a well-studied protein-coding ISG. RNAi-mediated knockdown of BISPR reduced the IFN-mediated induction of BST2 expression (Barriocanal et al., 2015; Kambara et al., 2015) pointing to the potential presence of a regulatory mechanism for coordinating the expression of BISPR with that of its promoter sharing gene BST2. Interestingly, after stimulation by IFN-α, the increase in cellular level of BISPR preceded the rise in the level of BST2, suggesting that expression of BISPR either induced or facilitated the initiation of transcription of BST2 (Kambara et al., 2015). Confirming these findings, forced overexpression of the spliced BISPR RNA from a transgene led to up-regulation of BST2, indicating that BISPR controls BST2 expression via interactions mediated through the BISPR RNA itself, rather than by impacting the local chromatin environment through its transcription (Kambara et al., 2015). As a number of protein-coding ISGs and immunity-related protein-coding genes originate from bidirectional promoters which also give rise to lncRNAs, it is plausible that a regulatory mechanism similar to the one described above may be present in at least a subset of them. Taken together, despite the small number of studied lncRNAs, existing data points to a critical role for this class of transcripts in regulation of the IFN response and the antiviral activity against human pathogens such as the hepatitis C virus, which is a well-studied disease model for the impact of IFNs on human pathogens. Future studies are likely to identify many additional lncRNAs that regulate different steps of this key aspect of the innate immune response.

INTERACTION OF THE NON-CODING TRANSCRIPTOME AND RNA VIRUSES: THE EXAMPLE OF HEPATITIS C VIRUS

Hepatitis C (HCV) is a deadly virus that affects ~2% of the world's population (60–170 million people) (Manns et al., 2017). About 500,000 people die every year from HCV-related diseases (Webster et al., 2015; Bukh, 2016). After the initial infection, most patients develop an asymptomatic chronic infection that causes liver damage and therefore, may progress to liver steatosis, fibrosis, cirrhosis and hepatocellular carcinoma (HCC). In the course of 30 years of HCV infection, ~20% of patients will develop cirrhosis. In fact, HCV infection is nowadays one of the major inducers of liver cirrhosis. As HCV infection induces the expression of several oncogenic factors and liver cirrhosis is a niche for HCC, ~3–7% of cirrhotic patients will develop liver tumors every year (Llovet and Villanueva, 2016).

In spite of the efforts of many groups, an effective vaccine to prevent HCV infection has not yet been developed. Recently, several inhibitors that target different viral proteins have been approved for the treatment of HCV infection (D'Ambrosio et al., 2017). The efficacy of these treatments grazes a complete sustained viral response, allowing the claim that HCV infection can be cured (Bourlière et al., 2017). A fraction of the small number of patients that resist the treatment and do not show viral clearance have high levels of liver cirrhosis. Some of the patients with HCV infection and HCC show a transient response with a later relapse of the virus, probably because HCC architecture and/or composition impairs drug penetration and serves as a reservoir for infected cells (Prenner et al., 2017). Some authors have observed an increased risk of HCC recurrence in patients that have cleared HCV infection (Llovet and Villanueva, 2016; Reig et al., 2016). In spite of this, there are good reasons for optimism. After sustained viral responses, liver fibrosis can regress, the risk of cirrhosis-related complications, including HCC, is reduced and the overall survival of the patients increases (van der Meer and Berenguer, 2016; Nahon et al., 2017; van der Meer et al., 2017). However, there is still a long way to achieve the goal of HCV cure. Patients cured of chronic HCV infection are at risk for reinfection if exposed. Work toward the development of an effective vaccine to prevent HCV infection must be intensified to cure the disease (Bukh, 2016). Research about HCV infection should not stop and a rigorous epidemiological follow up should be carried out given the high prevalence of HCV infection and the ability of HCV to generate escape mutants resistant to the treatments (Ramirez et al., 2016).

HCV Infection

The seven genotypes of HCV share similar characteristics. HCV viral particle is enveloped, small (40–80 nm) and encloses the genome coated by the core protein (Gastaminza et al., 2010; Catanese et al., 2013). The genome is an RNA molecule of 9.6 Kb of length and positive polarity that may function as messenger RNA (mRNA). Multiple coding regions of the viral genome and the 5′ and 3′ untranslated regions (UTRs) are highly structured, well-conserved and required for replication and encapsidation (Piñeiro and Martinez-Salas, 2012; Pirakitikulr et al., 2016; Shi et al., 2016). The structure located at the 5′ end contains an internal ribosome entry site (IRES) that allows viral RNA cap-independent translation. Translation synthesizes a polyprotein that can be cleaved by viral and cellular proteases co- or post-transcriptionally. Cleavage releases three major structural proteins (core, and the two envelope glycoproteins, E1 and E2) and seven non-structural proteins (p7, NS2, NS3, NS4A, NS4B, NS5A, and NS5B). These proteins are required for polyprotein cleavage, cellular antiviral response blockade, viral replication, assembly and release (Carnero and Fortes, 2016).

The majority of HCV virions are transported in the blood embedded into very low or low-density lipoproteins (VLDLs and LDLs) formed by triglycerides, apolipoproteins and cholesterol or phospholipids (Bassendine et al., 2013). This coat may help virions to escape from neutralizing antibodies and aids hepatocyte infection. LDL Receptor (LDLR), claudin-1 (CLDN1) and occludin (OCLN) are some of the several receptors identified to play a role in viral entry into hepatocytes (Ploss et al., 2009; Zeisel et al., 2011). After endocytosis, the virion uncoats in response to the acidic pH of the endosome by fusing the viral envelope with the endosome and releasing the viral genome into the cytoplasm. Viral RNA translation occurs in the rough endoplasmic reticulum (ER). There, a membranous web (MW) is formed by double-membrane vesicles, the replication complex is assembled and viral replication takes place (Romero-Brey et al., 2012; Meyers et al., 2016). Replication is carried out by NS5B, the viral RNA-dependent RNA polymerase. The positive-stranded RNAs are used as templates to produce negative-strand RNAs which are then used as guides to synthesize large quantities of new viral genomes. The low fidelity of HCV RNA-dependent RNA polymerase produces a highly variable progeny (Geller et al., 2016). Thus, in every infected patient, the incoming viruses generate a collection of descendants with related but non-identical HCV genomes, known as quasi-species (Martell et al., 1992).

The new viral genomes can be used for translation of new viral proteins, replication to produce new viral genomes or packaging into new viral particles. Assembly takes place close to lipid droplets (LDs) bound to ER membranes. NS5A molecules from the replication complex bind simultaneously to the newly synthesized RNA and core protein, helping the interaction between core protein and viral RNA which will lead to formation of a nucleocapsid bound to a LD (Masaki et al., 2008). The envelope is acquired after budding through the ER and the particle is released bound to LDL or VLDLs through the secretory pathway (Lindenbach and Rice, 2003; Bayer et al., 2016; Syed et al., 2017). Thus, inhibition of the synthesis of lipid components blocks viral assembly (Bassendine et al., 2013).

HCV and the Antiviral IFN Response

HCV-Infection and Protein Coding Genes That Regulate the IFN Response

Successful replication requires inactivation of the antiviral response, which is initiated soon after infection (Loo et al., 2006; Saito et al., 2008). RIG-I canonical sensor may recognize the incoming viral genome. Non-canonical sensors such as protein kinase R (PKR) and the DEAD box helicase DDX3X also recognize the 5′UTR and the 3′UTR of HCV genome, respectively (Arnaud et al., 2010, 2011; Li et al., 2013). Later, RIG-I and TLR3 can sense viral dsRNAs produced during replication (Binder et al., 2011; Li et al., 2012). Sensor activation induces NF-κB and IRFs via MAVS and TRIF and the synthesis of several subtypes of IFN (**Figure 2**). While type III IFNλ signaling has a special impact on HCV infection (Ge et al., 2009; Thomas et al., 2009; Boisvert and Shoukry, 2016), type I IFNα has been traditionally used to cure the disease (McHutchison et al., 1998). IFN signaling is a potent activator of the expression of several ISGs that limit HCV replication. They function by reinforcing IFN signaling (STAT1, STAT2, IRF1, 3, 7 and 9, PKR, OAS or RNase L) and blocking every step of the viral cycle: viral entry (IFITM, TRIM, Mx, CH25H), RNA replication, translation and stability (OAS, IFIT, GBP1), assembly and release (tetherin/BST2, viperin) (Carnero and Fortes, 2016). Viperin binds to NS5A in the replication complex and the LDs, blocking NS5A function in viral replication and assembly (Helbig et al., 2005, 2011). BST2 or tetherin impedes the budding of viral particles by attaching virions to the cell surface and allowing their degradation by the lysosomes (Neil et al., 2008; Dafa-Berger et al., 2012). Interestingly, a strong antiviral response is only achieved by the cooperative function of several ISGs and not by their individual actions (Metz et al., 2012).

To combat the antiviral response, HCV has evolved to express viral proteins that block IFN synthesis and signaling and interfere with the functionality of antiviral molecules. NS3-NS4A protease cleaves MAVS and TRIF impeding sensor signaling (Foy et al., 2005; Li et al., 2005; Meylan et al., 2005). In addition, RIG-I signaling may be affected by HCV-mediated induction of autophagy (Ke and Chen, 2011). NS4A/B precursor blocks MHC Class I transport to the cell surface. Finally, core protein blocks IFN signaling by upregulating the expression of SOCS3 or the protein phosphatase PP2Ac, which are negative regulators of STAT1 transcription factor (Bode et al., 2003; Duong et al., 2004; Kawaguchi et al., 2004; Walsh et al., 2006).

The blockade of IFN signaling induced by the virus explains why many patients fail to respond to IFN treatment (Chen et al., 2005; Sarasin-Filipowicz et al., 2008). Surprisingly, many non-responder patients have increased ISG mRNA levels both in infected and uninfected hepatocytes (Hedegaard et al., 2017). One way to explain why these patients fail to respond to IFN in spite of expressing high levels of ISG mRNAs is that these mRNAs are not efficiently translated into antiviral proteins. Interestingly, it is also possible that some ISG mRNAs are translated into proteins that exert proviral functions in HCV infected cells. Both possibilities may turn out to be correct. DsRNA-activated PKR phosphorylates eukaryotic translation initiation factor eIF2α, leading to inhibition of cap-dependent translation. This does not affect HCV protein translation, which is IRES-mediated and eIF2α-independent (Garaigorta and Chisari, 2009). However, translation of ISG mRNAs is likely to be drastically affected, leading to HCV-infected cells with high levels of ISG mRNAs that are not translated into antiviral proteins. Therefore, PKR is an ISG with a proviral function in HCV infection. Other proviral ISGs include those that function as negative regulators of the antiviral response allowing cells to return to homeostasis after IFN induction and non-canonical sensors such as DDX3X. After viral genome sensing, DDX3X activates IKKα, which induces the expression of lipogenic genes essential for viral assembly (Li et al., 2013; Pène et al., 2015).

A paradigm for an ISG that promotes HCV replication is ISG15 (Broering et al., 2010). ISG15 is an ubiquitin-like moiety cotranslationally attached to proteins by the IFN-induced ISGylation machinery. Therefore, after HCV infection, the IFN response induces ISGylation of new proteins, which are viral proteins and cellular antiviral factors (Durfee et al., 2010). ISGylation may affect the functionality of targeted proteins by modifying their structure and/or stability. IRF3 is stabilized by ISGylation-mediated inhibition of polyubiquitination (Shi et al., 2010). However, RIG-I ISGylation blocks ubiquitination and functionality, leading to decreased levels of IFN and increased replication of HCV (**Figure 2**) (Kim et al., 2008; Broering et al., 2010). Therefore, in HCV infection, ISG15 functions as a proviral ISG. In fact, upregulation of ISG15 is associated with poor response to IFN treatment and poor prognosis in HCV-infected patients (Chen et al., 2011).

The combined action of PKR and the ISGylation and ubiquitination pathways in HCV-infected cells results in decreased cap-dependent protein translation and increased protein modification that leads to protein malfunction and destabilization. Under such a protein-hostile environment it must be challenging to maintain proper cell functionality and virus replication. Therefore, it is conceivable that both cells and viruses have evolved to achieve functionality under these conditions through the expression of functional non-coding RNAs, which are at least partially immune to protein-hostile conditions (Fortes and Morris, 2016).

Effects of HCV Infection on the Non-coding Genome

Hepatitis C virus infection causes a deregulation in the expression of the non-coding genome, which may function either to facilitate or to block viral viability. This has been best studied for miRNAs. Several cellular miRNAs have been described to target the HCV genome to help or prevent viral replication or to regulate the expression of cellular factors required for the virus cell cycle or the antiviral response. Generally, virus replication-related factors induce proviral and reduce antiviral miRNAs while the innate immune response plays the opposite effect. The interplay of HCV infection and miRNAs has been reviewed elsewhere (Singaravelu et al., 2014, 2015).

In contrast, the world of infection-induced lncRNAs is widely unexplored and HCV-related lncRNAs are not an exception. The few studies performed clearly indicate that, similar to what has been described for miRNAs, several cellular lncRNAs are deregulated in response to HCV replication or to the antiviral response induced by viral infection (Barriocanal and Fortes, 2017). The function of some of them has been studied. These lncRNAs affect HCV replication by regulating cell metabolism, proliferation and the antiviral response. HCV could also express viral lncRNAs generated by XRN1 exonuclease-mediated 5′ to 3′ degradation of the viral genome. These subgenomic RNAs have lost the initial sequences of the IRES and therefore they most likely fall into the category of lncRNAs (Moon et al., 2015).

Studies performed so far to identify HCV-deregulated cellular lncRNAs have employed infected cultured cells or liver tissue from infected patients. In the latter case, it is difficult to establish whether the deregulation of the lncRNAs indeed results purely from HCV infection, as the evaluated tissue has also developed liver cirrhosis and/or HCC. Comparison of the level of lncRNAs in these tissues versus healthy liver identifies the lncRNAs that are deregulated by HCV infection, liver cirrhosis or HCC alone or in all possible combinations. In line with this, some of the lncRNAs deregulated in HCV-infected livers have been shown to play a role in the development of liver cirrhosis and/or HCC (Yuan et al., 2014; Fu et al., 2017). This has been recently reviewed (Barriocanal and Fortes, 2017). Other lncRNAs studied in patients with HCV-derived HCC could be bona-fide HCV-induced lncRNAs. This is the case for UCA1, which is also upregulated in liver and serum of patients with HCC. UCA1 serum levels correlate significantly with HCV antibodies and increase in tissue culture cells infected with HCV (Carnero et al., 2016; Kamel et al., 2016; Barriocanal and Fortes, 2017).

Infection with HCV or expression of the core protein in cultured cells has led to the identification of additional HCV-induced oncogenic lncRNAs such as PVT1, CASC15 and HOTAIR (Carnero et al., 2016; Li et al., 2016). The induction of lncRNA HOTAIR by the core protein may in turn lead to increased viral replication by silencing SIRT1 promoter and affecting glucose and lipid metabolism (Li et al., 2016). HCV-induced lncRNAs such as UCA1, PVT1 or CASC15 are upregulated in response to viral replication and not after activation of the antiviral response. Thus, these lncRNAs do not increase when cells are treated with IFN or pathogen associated molecular patterns (PAMPs) such as poly(I:C) or LPS, or in cells infected with other viruses such as HBV, influenza, adenovirus or Semliki Forest Virus (SFV), which replicate in the nucleus or in the cytoplasm, have DNA or RNA viral genomes and lead to acute or chronic infections (Carnero et al., 2016). Instead, it has been proposed that HCV replication may induce specific pathways for the activation of these lncRNAs. For example, viral protein NS5A induces MYC, which in turn activates PVT-1 transcription (Carramusa et al., 2007). Similarly, HCV-induced reactive oxygen species (ROS) is likely to induce the activation of the expression of UCA1 in HCV infected cells. Indeed, ROS inhibits C/EBPα, a negative regulator of UCA1, and stabilizes the UCA1 inducer HIF-1α, leading to UCA1 induction (Miura et al., 2008; Nishina et al., 2008).

On the other hand, several lncRNAs have been described that are upregulated both in HCV-infected cells and in cells treated with IFN or PAMPs such as poly(I:C), or when cells are infected with viruses different than HCV. Therefore, they can be considered to be lncRNAs upregulated by the antiviral response.

As described above, several IFN-induced lncRNAs have been identified after comparing the transcriptome of cells treated with IFN and controls (Carnero et al., 2014; Kambara et al., 2014, 2015; Barriocanal et al., 2015). This is the case for NRIR and BISPR (see above), ISR2 (IFN-stimulated lncRNA2), ISR8 and lncISG15 (Carnero et al., 2014; Barriocanal et al., 2015). Interestingly, the loci of the above lncRNAs are neighboring those of ISGs that play a key role in HCV infection (CMPK2 and Viperin, BST2, GBP1, IRF1 and ISG15, respectively). As detailed above, NRIR, which is a negative regulator of the IFN response, is significantly upregulated in the liver of HCV-infected patients compared to healthy controls (Kambara et al., 2014). Therefore, HCV may use NRIR to increase replication. Similarly, ISR2, ISR8, lncISG15 and BISPR are upregulated in liver and cultured cells infected with HCV compared to controls (Carnero et al., 2014; Barriocanal et al., 2015). Unexpectedly, HCV-induction of ISR2 and ISR8 is higher than induction with other viruses such as influenza, adenovirus or SFV, or mutant versions that allow induction of a strong antiviral response (Carnero et al., 2014). This suggests that HCV may have an additional mechanism distinct from the IFN response for inducing the expression of these lncRNAs. Although their cellular function has not yet been described, guilt-by-association studies predict that ISR8 is an antiviral factor that induces the immune system and the antiviral response and ISR2 regulates the action of antiviral sensors and IFN activation (Carnero et al., 2014). In the case of BISPR,

TABLE 2 | List of lncRNAs induced by HCV and poly(I:C).

Name	Position	Name	Alternative name	Fold induction by IFN	Fold induction by pI:C	Fold induction by HCV
CSR3	chrl2:93936239-93965544R	SOCS2-AS1	lnc-UBE2N-2		2.6	64
CSR6	chrl5:95819690-95832714R	CTD-253611.1	lnc-AC016251.1-8		6.7	24
CSR7	chrl7:70399463-70588479R	LINC00673	lnc-SLC39A11-1		3.6	34
CSR20	chr6:53493178-53496192F	RP11-345L23.1	LINC01564 lnc-LRRCI-3		16.2	111
CSR31	chr2:97163383-97173846R	NEURL3		12.0	30.8	1941
CSR32	chr3:4790876-4793274R	EGOT	lnc-AC018816.3.1	3.5	6.2	797

The genomic position, name and alternative names are indicated. The fold induction has been quantified in cells treated with IFN, poly(I:C) or in cells infected with HCV versus untreated cells.

increased expression by IFN leads to higher levels of BST2 and decreased virion release (Neil et al., 2008; Dafa-Berger et al., 2012; Barriocanal et al., 2015; Kambara et al., 2015). Thus, induction of IFN-induced lncRNAs may have positive effects (in the case of NRIR) or negative effects (in the case of BISPR) on HCV replication.

STAT3 transcription factor, a negative regulator of the IFN pathway, can be induced by IFN, growth factors, stress, several cytokines such as IL6 and by HCV infection (Wang et al., 2011). HCV core and other viral proteins induce ROS and activate STAT3 by several mechanisms (Yoshida et al., 2002; Waris et al., 2005; Machida et al., 2006). STAT3 activation, in turn, favors viral replication by blocking type I IFN pathway and through positive regulation of microtubule dynamics (McCartney et al., 2013). More recently, it has been shown that several lncRNAs are induced by STAT3 activation, including lncIGF2-AS and lnc7SK, which help MW formation by increasing the level of phosphatidylinositol 4-phosphate kinase (Xiong et al., 2015). Therefore, in this manner, both the IFN response and HCV infection benefit viral replication via STAT3-mediated induction of expression of lncRNAs.

Finally, a group of lncRNAs are induced 3–30 fold by IFN or PAMPs such as poly(I:C) and up to 100 times more by HCV infection (Carnero et al., 2016) (**Table 2**). These lncRNAs were identified by transcriptome analysis of cultured liver cells with and without HCV infection and were named CSRs, after H<u>C</u>V <u>S</u>timulated lnc<u>R</u>NAs.

As mentioned above, the highest upregulation of these CSRs has been observed when cells are infected with HCV. However, it has been shown that infection with other viruses also leads to the induction of their expression. DNA viruses such as adenovirus and RNA viruses such as influenza, SFV, HCV or mutant versions of influenza that allow IFN induction, upregulate CSR3, 7 and 31. On the other hand, CSR6 is only induced by adenovirus, CSR20 by influenza virus infections. Similarly, CSR32/EGOT is upregulated in response to RNA viruses (HCV, influenza, SFV) but not DNA viruses (adenovirus or HBV). Existing data suggest that the expression of EGOT (see above) is upregulated through sensing of HCV viral RNA in the cytoplasm. Therefore, increased levels of EGOT are detected shortly after infection even when UV inactivated non-replicative viruses are used (Carnero et al., 2016). Later in the infectious cycle, EGOT levels are increased in response to viral replication. Several sensor molecules are required for EGOT induction, including RIG-I and the non-canonical sensor PKR, which induce transcription through IRF3 and NF-κB, with the latter being required for EGOT transcription. Indeed, there is a good correlation between the levels of TNFα, which induces NF-κB, and cellular level of EGOT in liver tissues derived from HCV-infected patients, suggesting that TNFα could be a major driver of EGOT expression in the liver (Carnero et al., 2016).

As expected from a negative regulator of the IFN response (see above), EGOT depletion leads to decreased levels of viral genome and proteins and viral titers in HCV and SFV-infected cells (Carnero et al., 2016), likely due to increased levels of ISGs, such as GBP1, ISG15, Mx1, BST2, ISG56, IFI6 and IFITM1. Interestingly, some of the ISG targets of EGOT have been described as inhibitors of HCV or SFV entry, replication or release (Landis et al., 1998; Itsui et al., 2009; Raychoudhuri et al., 2011; Wilkins et al., 2013; Amet et al., 2014; Ooi et al., 2015). Kinetic experiments show that EGOT silencing leads first to increased levels of ISGs and then to decreased replication of HCV or SFV genomes. As discussed above, this repressive role of EGOT resembles what has been described for the lncRNAs NRIR and NRAV, negative regulators of the IFN pathway which are induced by IFN or infection (Kambara et al., 2014; Ouyang et al., 2014). Similar to what has been described for EGOT, downregulation of lncCMPK2/NRIR or NRAV lncRNA activates ISG transcription and inhibits HCV or influenza replication, respectively.

CONCLUSION

In vitro studies on the role of lncRNAs in the IFN response in the absence of pathogens point to the presence of a strong perturbation in the expression of the non-coding transcriptome following IFN stimulation. From the very small number of studies on the role of lncRNAs in the antiviral response, it is evident that changes in the expression of this class of cellular effectors do play a critical role in negative regulation of the downstream steps of the IFN response. Together with proteins that act as negative regulators, this class of lncRNAs create a complex, decentralized regulatory network with overlapping and likely partially redundant functions which allows for extreme fine tuning of the magnitude and duration of the IFN response. However, in the presence of pathogens such as HCV, such negative feedback loops can favor viral replication and in some cases are actively hijacked by the virus to help in viral survival. There are two possible scenarios that can explain this from an evolutionary perspective. One possibility is that the co-evolution of the IFN response and pathogens has tipped in favor of viral survival due to the faster rate of viral evolution, with the viruses gaining the ability to exploit the immune response. Alternatively, it is plausible that at least in the case of some chronic infections, such a reduction in the magnitude of the immune response may be beneficial for the organism through limiting the damage incurred on the infected tissue. Future studies, by providing a more complete picture of the interplay of lncRNAs and viral infections, will shed additional light on the highly complex interplay of the antiviral response and pathogens.

AUTHOR CONTRIBUTIONS

SV and PF wrote and reviewed the manuscript. PF built the table and SV the figures.

FUNDING

This work was supported by grants from the MINECO/FEDER, EU (SAF2012-40003, SAF2015-70971-R), Instituto de Salud Carlos III (ISCIII)/FEDER (PI16/0845), grant Ortiz de Landazuri from the Government of Navarra, Fundacio La Marato de TV3 (20132132), and by the project RNAREG [CSD2009-00080], funded by the MINECO under the program CONSOLIDER INGENIO 2010 to PF and NIH grants 1R01AI120204-01 and 1R21AI127252-01 to SV.

REFERENCES

Adachi, N., and Lieber, M. R. (2002). Bidirectional gene organization: a common architectural feature of the human genome. *Cell* 109, 807–809. doi: 10.1016/S0092-8674(02)00758-4

Amaral, P. P., Dinger, M. E., and Mattick, J. S. (2013). Non-coding RNAs in homeostasis, disease and stress responses: an evolutionary perspective. *Brief. Funct. Genomics* 12, 254–278. doi: 10.1093/bfgp/elt016

Amet, T., Byrd, D., Hu, N., Sun, Q., Li, F., Zhao, Y., et al. (2014). BST-2 expression in human hepatocytes is inducible by all three types of interferons and restricts production of hepatitis C virus. *Curr. Mol. Med.* 14, 349–360. doi: 10.2174/1566524013666131118111719

Arnaud, N., Dabo, S., Akazawa, D., Fukasawa, M., Shinkai-Ouchi, F., Hugon, J., et al. (2011). Hepatitis C virus reveals a novel early control in acute immune response. *PLoS Pathog.* 7:e1002289. doi: 10.1371/journal.ppat.1002289

Arnaud, N., Dabo, S., Maillard, P., Budkowska, A., Kalliampakou, K. I., Mavromara, P., et al. (2010). Hepatitis C virus controls interferon production through PKR activation. *PLoS ONE* 5:e10575. doi: 10.1371/journal.pone.0010575

Atianand, M. K., Caffrey, D. R., and Fitzgerald, K. A. (2017). Immunobiology of long noncoding RNAs. *Annu. Rev. Immunol.* 35, 177–198. doi: 10.1146/annurev-immunol-041015-055459

Barriocanal, M., Carnero, E., Segura, V., and Fortes, P. (2015). Long non-coding RNA BST2/BISPR is induced by IFN and regulates the expression of the antiviral factor tetherin. *Front. Immunol.* 5:655. doi: 10.3389/fimmu.2014.00655

Barriocanal, M., and Fortes, P. (2017). Long non-coding RNAs in hepatitis C virus-infected cells. *Front. Microbiol.* 8:1833. doi: 10.3389/fmicb.2017.01833

Bassendine, M. F., Sheridan, D. A., Bridge, S. H., Felmlee, D. J., and Neely, R. D. (2013). Lipids and HCV. *Semin. Immunopathol.* 35, 87–100. doi: 10.1007/s00281-012-0356-2

Bayer, K., Banning, C., Bruss, V., Wiltzer-Bach, L., and Schindler, M. (2016). Hepatitis C virus is released via a noncanonical secretory route. *J. Virol.* 90, 10558–10573. doi: 10.1128/JVI.01615-16

Binder, M., Eberle, F., Seitz, S., Mücke, N., Hüber, C. M., Kiani, N., et al. (2011). Molecular mechanism of signal perception and integration by the innate immune sensor retinoic acid-inducible gene-I (RIG-I). *J. Biol. Chem.* 286, 27278–27287. doi: 10.1074/jbc.M111.256974

Bode, J. G., Ludwig, S., Ehrhardt, C., Albrecht, U., Erhardt, A., Schaper, F., et al. (2003). IFN-alpha antagonistic activity of HCV core protein involves induction of suppressor of cytokine signaling-3. *FASEB J.* 17, 488–490. doi: 10.1096/fj.02-0664fje

Boisvert, M., and Shoukry, N. H. (2016). Type III interferons in hepatitis C virus infection. *Front. Immunol.* 7:628. doi: 10.3389/fimmu.2016.00628

Bolen, C. R., Ding, S., Robek, M. D., and Kleinstein, S. H. (2014). Dynamic expression profiling of type I and type III interferon-stimulated hepatocytes reveals a stable hierarchy of gene expression. *Hepatology* 59, 1262–1272. doi: 10.1002/hep.26657

Bourlière, M., Gordon, S. C., Flamm, S. L., Cooper, C. L., Ramji, A., Tong, M., et al. (2017). Sofosbuvir, velpatasvir, and voxilaprevir for previously treated HCV infection. *N. Engl. J. Med.* 376, 2134–2146. doi: 10.1056/NEJMoa1613512

Broering, R., Zhang, X., Kottilil, S., Trippler, M., Jiang, M., Lu, M., et al. (2010). The interferon stimulated gene 15 functions as a proviral factor for the hepatitis C virus and as a regulator of the IFN response. *Gut* 59, 1111–1119. doi: 10.1136/gut.2009.195545

Bronson, P. G., Chaivorapol, C., Ortmann, W., Behrens, T. W., and Graham, R. R. (2012). The genetics of type I interferon in systemic lupus erythematosus. *Curr. Opin. Immunol.* 24, 530–537. doi: 10.1016/j.coi.2012.07.008

Bukh, J. (2016). The history of hepatitis C virus (HCV): basic research reveals unique features in phylogeny, evolution and the viral life cycle with new perspectives for epidemic control. *J. Hepatol.* 65, S2–S21. doi: 10.1016/j.jhep.2016.07.035

Carnero, E., Barriocanal, M., Prior, C., Pablo Unfried, J., Segura, V., Guruceaga, E., et al. (2016). Long noncoding RNA EGOT negatively affects the antiviral response and favors HCV replication. *EMBO Rep.* 17, 1013–1028. doi: 10.15252/embr.201541763

Carnero, E., Barriocanal, M., Segura, V., Guruceaga, E., Prior, C., Börner, K., et al. (2014). Type I interferon regulates the expression of long non-coding RNAs. *Front. Immunol.* 5:548. doi: 10.3389/fimmu.2014.00548

Carnero, E., and Fortes, P. (2016). HCV infection, IFN response and the coding and non-coding host cell genome. *Virus Res.* 212, 85–102. doi: 10.1016/j.virusres.2015.10.001

Carninci, P., Kasukawa, T., Katayama, S., Gough, J., Frith, M. C., Maeda, N., et al. (2005). The transcriptional landscape of the mammalian genome. *Science* 309, 1559–1563. doi: 10.1126/science.1112014

Carpenter, S. (2016). Long noncoding RNA: novel links between gene expression and innate immunity. *Virus Res.* 212, 137–145. doi: 10.1016/j.virusres.2015.08.019

Carramusa, L., Contino, F., Ferro, A., Minafra, L., Perconti, G., Giallongo, A., et al. (2007). The PVT-1 oncogene is a Myc protein target that is overexpressed in transformed cells. *J. Cell. Physiol.* 213, 511–518. doi: 10.1002/jcp.21133

Catanese, M. T., Uryu, K., Kopp, M., Edwards, T. J., Andrus, L., et al. (2013). Ultrastructural analysis of hepatitis C virus particles. *Proc. Natl. Acad. Sci. U.S.A.* 110, 9505–9510. doi: 10.1073/pnas.1307527110

Chen, L., Borozan, I., Feld, J., Sun, J., Tannis, L. L., Coltescu, C., et al. (2005). Hepatic gene expression discriminates responders and nonresponders in treatment of chronic hepatitis C viral infection. *Gastroenterology* 128, 1437–1444. doi: 10.1053/j.gastro.2005.01.059

Chen, L., Li, S., and McGilvray, I. (2011). The ISG15/USP18 ubiquitin-like pathway (ISGylation system) in hepatitis C virus infection and resistance to interferon therapy. *Int. J. Biochem. Cell Biol.* 43, 1427–1431. doi: 10.1016/j.biocel.2011.06.006

Clark, M. B., Choudhary, A., Smith, M. A., Taft, R. J., and Mattick, J. S. (2013). The dark matter rises: the expanding world of regulatory RNAs. *Essays Biochem.* 54, 1–16. doi: 10.1042/bse0540001

Clark, M. B., and Mattick, J. S. (2011). Long noncoding RNAs in cell biology. *Semin. Cell Dev. Biol.* 22, 366–376. doi: 10.1016/j.semcdb.2011.01.001

Collier, S. P. (2014). *TMEVPG1, A Long Noncoding RNA within the Immune System.* Available at: http://etd.library.vanderbilt.edu/available/etd-03182014-144429/ [accessed June 29, 2015].

Collier, S. P., Collins, P. L., Williams, C. L., Boothby, M. R., and Aune, T. M. (2012). Cutting edge: influence of Tmevpg1, a long intergenic noncoding RNA, on the expression of Ifng by Th1 cells. *J. Immunol.* 189, 2084–2088. doi: 10.4049/jimmunol.1200774

Collier, S. P., Henderson, M. A., Tossberg, J. T., and Aune, T. M. (2014). Regulation of the Th1 genomic locus from Ifng through Tmevpg1 by T-bet. *J. Immunol.* 193, 3959–3965. doi: 10.4049/jimmunol.1401099

Crow, M. K. (2010). Long interspersed nuclear elements (LINE-1): potential triggers of systemic autoimmune disease. *Autoimmunity* 43, 7–16. doi: 10.3109/08916930903374865

Dafa-Berger, A., Kuzmina, A., Fassler, M., Yitzhak-Asraf, H., Shemer-Avni, Y., and Taube, R. (2012). Modulation of hepatitis C virus release by the interferon-induced protein BST-2/tetherin. *Virology* 428, 98–111. doi: 10.1016/j.virol.2012.03.011

D'Ambrosio, R., Degasperi, E., Colombo, M., and Aghemo, A. (2017). Direct-acting antivirals: the endgame for hepatitis C? *Curr. Opin. Virol.* 24, 31–37. doi: 10.1016/j.coviro.2017.03.017

Derrien, T., Johnson, R., Bussotti, G., Tanzer, A., Djebali, S., Tilgner, H., et al. (2012). The GENCODE v7 catalog of human long noncoding RNAs: analysis of their gene structure, evolution, and expression. *Genome Res.* 22, 1775–1789. doi: 10.1101/gr.132159.111

Djebali, S., Davis, C. A., Merkel, A., Dobin, A., Lassmann, T., Mortazavi, A., et al. (2012). Landscape of transcription in human cells. *Nature* 489, 101–108. doi: 10.1038/nature11233

Duong, F. H. T., Filipowicz, M., Tripodi, M., La Monica, N., and Heim, M. H. (2004). Hepatitis C virus inhibits interferon signaling through up-regulation of protein phosphatase 2A. *Gastroenterology* 126, 263–277. doi: 10.1053/j.gastro.2003.10.076

Durfee, L. A., Lyon, N., Seo, K., and Huibregtse, J. M. (2010). The ISG15 conjugation system broadly targets newly synthesized proteins: implications for the antiviral function of ISG15. *Mol. Cell* 38, 722–732. doi: 10.1016/j.molcel.2010.05.002

Elkon, K. B., and Wiedeman, A. (2012). Type I IFN system in the development and manifestations of SLE. *Curr. Opin. Rheumatol.* 24, 499–505. doi: 10.1097/BOR.0b013e3283562c3e

ENCODE Project Consortium (2012). An integrated encyclopedia of DNA elements in the human genome. *Nature* 489, 57–74. doi: 10.1038/nature11247

Fitzgerald, K. A., and Caffrey, D. R. (2014). Long noncoding RNAs in innate and adaptive immunity. *Curr. Opin. Immunol.* 26, 140–146. doi: 10.1016/j.coi.2013.12.001

Fortes, P., and Morris, K. V. (2016). Long noncoding RNAs in viral infections. *Virus Res.* 212, 1–11. doi: 10.1016/j.virusres.2015.10.002

Foy, E., Li, K., Sumpter, R. Jr., Loo, Y. M., Johnson, C. L., Wang, C., et al. (2005). Control of antiviral defenses through hepatitis C virus disruption of retinoic acid-inducible gene-I signaling. *Proc. Natl. Acad. Sci. U.S.A.* 102, 2986–2991. doi: 10.1073/pnas.0408707102

Fu, N., Zhao, S. X., Kong, L. B., Du, J. H., Ren, W. G., Han, F., et al. (2017). LncRNA-ATB/microRNA-200a/β-catenin regulatory axis involved in the progression of HCV-related hepatic fibrosis. *Gene* 618, 1–7. doi: 10.1016/j.gene.2017.03.008

Garaigorta, U., and Chisari, F. V. (2009). Hepatitis C virus blocks interferon effector function by inducing protein kinase R phosphorylation. *Cell Host Microbe* 6, 513–522. doi: 10.1016/j.chom.2009.11.004

Gastaminza, P., Dryden, K. A., Boyd, B., Wood, M. R., Law, M., Yeager, M., et al. (2010). Ultrastructural and biophysical characterization of hepatitis C virus particles produced in cell culture. *J. Virol.* 84, 10999–11009. doi: 10.1128/JVI.00526-10

Ge, D., Fellay, J., Thompson, A. J., Simon, J. S., Shianna, K. V., Urban, T. J., et al. (2009). Genetic variation in IL28B predicts hepatitis C treatment-induced viral clearance. *Nature* 461, 399–401. doi: 10.1038/nature08309

Geller, R., Estada, Ú., Peris, J. B., Andreu, I., Bou, J. V., Garijo, R., et al. (2016). Highly heterogeneous mutation rates in the hepatitis C virus genome. *Nat. Microbiol.* 1:16045. doi: 10.1038/nmicrobiol.2016.45

Gomez, J. A., Wapinski, O. L., Yang, Y. W., Bureau, J.-F., Gopinath, S., Monack, D. M., et al. (2013). The NeST long ncRNA controls microbial susceptibility and epigenetic activation of the interferon-γ locus. *Cell* 152, 743–754. doi: 10.1016/j.cell.2013.01.015

Green, D. S., Young, H. A., and Valencia, J. C. (2017). Current prospects of type II interferon γ signaling and autoimmunity. *J. Biol. Chem.* 292, 13925–13933. doi: 10.1074/jbc.R116.774745

GTEx Consortium (2013). The genotype-tissue expression (GTEx) project. *Nat. Genet.* 45, 580–585. doi: 10.1038/ng.2653

Hacisuleyman, E., Goff, L. A., Trapnell, C., Williams, A., Henao-Mejia, J., Sun, L., et al. (2014). Topological organization of multichromosomal regions by the long intergenic noncoding RNA Firre. *Nat. Struct. Mol. Biol.* 21, 198–206. doi: 10.1038/nsmb.2764

Hedegaard, D. L., Tully, D. C., Rowe, I. A., Reynolds, G. M., Bean, D. J., Hu, K., et al. (2017). High resolution sequencing of hepatitis C virus reveals limited intra-hepatic compartmentalization in end-stage liver disease. *J. Hepatol.* 66, 28–38. doi: 10.1016/j.jhep.2016.07.048

Heintzman, N. D., Stuart, R. K., Hon, G., Fu, Y., Ching, C. W., Hawkins, R. D., et al. (2007). Distinct and predictive chromatin signatures of transcriptional promoters and enhancers in the human genome. *Nat. Genet.* 39, 311–318. doi: 10.1038/ng1966

Helbig, K. J., Eyre, N. S., Yip, E., Narayana, S., Li, K., Fiches, G., et al. (2011). The antiviral protein viperin inhibits hepatitis C virus replication via interaction with nonstructural protein 5A. *Hepatology* 54, 1506–1517. doi: 10.1002/hep.24542

Helbig, K. J., Lau, D. T., Semendric, L., Harley, H. A., and Beard, M. R. (2005). Analysis of ISG expression in chronic hepatitis C identifies viperin as a potential antiviral effector. *Hepatology* 42, 702–710. doi: 10.1002/hep.20844

Hertzog, P., Forster, S., and Samarajiwa, S. (2011). Systems biology of interferon responses. *J. Interferon Cytokine Res.* 31, 5–11. doi: 10.1089/jir.2010.0126

Hertzog, P. J., and Williams, B. R. G. (2013). Fine tuning type I interferon responses. *Cytokine Growth Factor Rev.* 24, 217–225. doi: 10.1016/j.cytogfr.2013.04.002

Heward, J. A., and Lindsay, M. A. (2014). Long non-coding RNAs in the regulation of the immune response. *Trends Immunol.* 35, 408–419. doi: 10.1016/j.it.2014.07.005

Hiscott, J. (2007). Triggering the innate antiviral response through IRF-3 activation. *J. Biol. Chem.* 282, 15325–15329. doi: 10.1074/jbc.R700002200

Hu, X., and Ivashkiv, L. B. (2009). Cross-regulation of signaling pathways by interferon-gamma: implications for immune responses and autoimmune diseases. *Immunity* 31, 539–550. doi: 10.1016/j.immuni.2009.09.002

Imamura, K., and Akimitsu, N. (2014). Long non-coding RNAs involved in immune responses. *Front. Immunol.* 5:573. doi: 10.3389/fimmu.2014.00573

Itsui, Y., Sakamoto, N., Kakinuma, S., Nakagawa, M., Sekine-Osajima, Y., Tasaka-Fujita, M., et al. (2009). Antiviral effects of the interferon-induced protein guanylate binding protein 1 and its interaction with the hepatitis C virus NS5B protein. *Hepatology* 50, 1727–1737. doi: 10.1002/hep.23195

Ivashkiv, L. B., and Donlin, L. T. (2014). Regulation of type I interferon responses. *Nat. Rev. Immunol.* 14, 36–49. doi: 10.1038/nri3581

Jensen, S., and Thomsen, A. R. (2012). Sensing of RNA viruses: a review of innate immune receptors involved in recognizing RNA virus invasion. *J. Virol.* 86, 2900–2910. doi: 10.1128/JVI.05738-11

Josset, L., Tchitchek, N., Gralinski, L. E., Ferris, M. T., Eisfeld, A. J., Green, R. R., et al. (2014). Annotation of long non-coding RNAs expressed in collaborative cross founder mice in response to respiratory virus infection reveals a new class of interferon-stimulated transcripts. *RNA Biol.* 11, 875–890. doi: 10.4161/rna.29442

Kambara, H., Gunawardane, L., Zebrowski, E., Kostadinova, L., Jobava, R., Krokowski, D., et al. (2015). Regulation of interferon-stimulated gene BST2 by a lncRNA transcribed from a shared bidirectional promoter. *Front. Immunol.* 5:676. doi: 10.3389/fimmu.2014.00676

Kambara, H., Niazi, F., Kostadinova, L., Moonka, D. K., Siegel, C. T., Post, A. B., et al. (2014). Negative regulation of the interferon response by an interferon-induced long non-coding RNA. *Nucleic Acids Res.* 42, 10668–10680. doi: 10.1093/nar/gku713

Kamel, M. M., Matboli, M., Sallam, M., Montasser, I. F., Saad, A. S., and El-Tawdi, A. H. F. (2016). Investigation of long noncoding RNAs expression profile as potential serum biomarkers in patients with hepatocellular carcinoma. *Transl. Res.* 168, 134–145. doi: 10.1016/j.trsl.2015.10.002

Kawaguchi, T., Yoshida, T., Harada, M., Hisamoto, T., Nagao, Y., Ide, T., et al. (2004). Hepatitis C virus down-regulates insulin receptor substrates 1 and 2 through up-regulation of suppressor of cytokine signaling 3. *Am. J. Pathol.* 165, 1499–1508. doi: 10.1016/S0002-9440(10)63408-6

Kawai, T., and Akira, S. (2006). Innate immune recognition of viral infection. *Nat. Immunol.* 7, 131–137. doi: 10.1038/ni1303

Ke, P.-Y., and Chen, S. S.-L. (2011). Activation of the unfolded protein response and autophagy after hepatitis C virus infection suppresses innate antiviral immunity in vitro. *J. Clin. Invest.* 121, 37–56. doi: 10.1172/JCI41474

Kim, M. J., Hwang, S. Y., Imaizumi, T., and Yoo, J. Y. (2008). Negative feedback regulation of RIG-I-mediated antiviral signaling by interferon-induced ISG15 conjugation. *J. Virol.* 82, 1474–1483. doi: 10.1128/JVI.01650-07

Lam, M. T. Y., Li, W., Rosenfeld, M. G., and Glass, C. K. (2014). Enhancer RNAs and regulated transcriptional programs. *Trends Biochem. Sci.* 39, 170–182. doi: 10.1016/j.tibs.2014.02.007

Landis, H., Simon-Jödicke, A., Klöti, A., Di Paolo, C., Schnorr, J. J., Schneider-Schaulies, S., et al. (1998). Human MxA protein confers resistance to Semliki Forest virus and inhibits the amplification of a Semliki Forest virus-based replicon in the absence of viral structural proteins. *J. Virol.* 72, 1516–1522.

Leonova, K. I., Brodsky, L., Lipchick, B., Pal, M., Novototskaya, L., Chenchik, A. A., et al. (2013). p53 cooperates with DNA methylation and a suicidal interferon response to maintain epigenetic silencing of repeats and noncoding RNAs. *Proc. Natl. Acad. Sci. U.S.A.* 110, E89–E98. doi: 10.1073/pnas.1216922110

Li, K., Foy, E., Ferreon, J. C., Nakamura, M., Ferreon, A. C., Ikeda, M., et al. (2005). Immune evasion by hepatitis C virus NS3/4A protease-mediated cleavage of the Toll-like receptor 3 adaptor protein TRIF. *Proc. Natl. Acad. Sci. U.S.A.* 102, 2992–2997. doi: 10.1073/pnas.0408824102

Li, K., Li, N. L., Wei, D., Pfeffer, S. R., Fan, M., and Pfeffer, L. M. (2012). Activation of chemokine and inflammatory cytokine response in hepatitis C virus-infected hepatocytes depends on Toll-like receptor 3 sensing of hepatitis C virus double-stranded RNA intermediates. *Hepatology* 55, 666–675. doi: 10.1002/hep.24763

Li, Q., Pène, V., Krishnamurthy, S., Cha, H., and Liang, T. J. (2013). Hepatitis C virus infection activates an innate pathway involving IKK-α in lipogenesis and viral assembly. *Nat. Med.* 19, 722–729. doi: 10.1038/nm.3190

Li, Z.-Q., Gu, X. Y., Hu, J. X., Ping, Y., Li, H., Yan, J. Y., et al. (2016). Hepatitis C virus core protein impairs metabolic disorder of liver cell via HOTAIR-Sirt1 signalling. *Biosci. Rep.* 36:e00336. doi: 10.1042/BSR20160088

Lindenbach, B. D., and Rice, C. M. (2003). Evasive maneuvers by hepatitits C virus. *Hepatology* 38, 769–771. doi: 10.1002/hep.510380327

Llovet, J. M., and Villanueva, A. (2016). Liver cancer: effect of HCV clearance with direct-acting antiviral agents on HCC. *Nat. Rev. Gastroenterol. Hepatol.* 13, 561–562. doi: 10.1038/nrgastro.2016.140

Loo, Y. M., Owen, D. M., Li, K., Erickson, A. K., Johnson, C. L., Fish, P. M., et al. (2006). Viral and therapeutic control of IFN-beta promoter stimulator 1 during hepatitis C virus infection. *Proc. Natl. Acad. Sci. U.S.A.* 103, 6001–6006. doi: 10.1073/pnas.0601523103

Ma, H., Han, P., Ye, W., Chen, H., Zheng, X., Cheng, L., et al. (2017). The long noncoding RNA NEAT1 exerts antihantaviral effects by acting as positive feedback for RIG-I signaling. *J. Virol.* 91, 2250–2216. doi: 10.1128/JVI.02250-16

Machida, K., Cheng, K. T., Lai, C. K., Jeng, K. S., Sung, V. M., and Lai, M. M. (2006). Hepatitis C virus triggers mitochondrial permeability transition with production of reactive oxygen species, leading to DNA damage and STAT3 activation. *J. Virol.* 80, 7199–7207. doi: 10.1128/JVI.00321-06

Manns, M. P., Buti, M., Gane, E., Pawlotsky, J. M., Razavi, H., Terrault, N., et al. (2017). Hepatitis C virus infection. *Nat. Rev. Dis. Primers* 3:17006. doi: 10.1038/nrdp.2017.6

Marques-Rocha, J. L., Samblas, M., Milagro, F. I., Bressan, J., Martínez, J. A., and Marti, A. (2015). Noncoding RNAs, cytokines, and inflammation-related diseases. *FASEB J.* 29, 3595–3611. doi: 10.1096/fj.14-260323

Martell, M., Esteban, J. I., Quer, J., Genescà, J., Weiner, A., Esteban, R., et al. (1992). Hepatitis C virus (HCV) circulates as a population of different but closely related genomes: quasispecies nature of HCV genome distribution. *J. Virol.* 66, 3225–3229.

Masaki, T., Suzuki, R., Murakami, K., Aizaki, H., Ishii, K., Murayama, A., et al. (2008). Interaction of hepatitis C virus nonstructural protein 5A with core protein is critical for the production of infectious virus particles. *J. Virol.* 82, 7964–7976. doi: 10.1128/JVI.00826-08

Mattick, J. S., and Rinn, J. L. (2015). Discovery and annotation of long noncoding RNAs. *Nat. Struct. Mol. Biol.* 22, 5–7. doi: 10.1038/nsmb.2942

McCartney, E. M., Helbig, K. J., Narayana, S. K., Eyre, N. S., Aloia, A. L., and Beard, M. R. (2013). Signal transducer and activator of transcription 3 is a proviral host factor for hepatitis C virus. *Hepatology* 58, 1558–1568. doi: 10.1002/hep.26496

McHutchison, J. G., Gordon, S. C., Schiff, E. R., Shiffman, M. L., Lee, W. M., Rustgi, V. K., et al. (1998). Interferon Alfa-2b alone or in combination with ribavirin as initial treatment for chronic hepatitis C. *N. Engl. J. Med.* 339, 1485–1492. doi: 10.1056/NEJM199811193392101

Mercer, T. R., Wilhelm, D., Dinger, M. E., Soldà, G., Korbie, D. J., Glazov, E. A., et al. (2011). Expression of distinct RNAs from 3' untranslated regions. *Nucleic Acids Res.* 39, 2393–2403. doi: 10.1093/nar/gkq1158

Metz, P., Dazert, E., Ruggieri, A., Mazur, J., Kaderali, L., Kaul, A., et al. (2012). Identification of type I and type II interferon-induced effectors controlling hepatitis C virus replication. *Hepatology* 56, 2082–2093. doi: 10.1002/hep.25908

Meyer, O. (2009). Interferons and autoimmune disorders. *Joint Bone Spine* 76, 464–473. doi: 10.1016/j.jbspin.2009.03.012

Meyers, N. L., Fontaine, K. A., Kumar, G. R., and Ott, M. (2016). Entangled in a membranous web: ER and lipid droplet reorganization during hepatitis C virus infection. *Curr. Opin. Cell Biol.* 41, 117–124. doi: 10.1016/j.ceb.2016.05.003

Meylan, E., Curran, J., Hofmann, K., Moradpour, D., Binder, M., Bartenschlager, R., et al. (2005). Cardif is an adaptor protein in the RIG-I antiviral pathway and is targeted by hepatitis C virus. *Nature* 437, 1167–1172. doi: 10.1038/nature04193

Miura, K., Taura, K., Kodama, Y., Schnabl, B., and Brenner, D. A. (2008). Hepatitis C virus-induced oxidative stress suppresses hepcidin expression through increased histone deacetylase activity. *Hepatology* 48, 1420–1429. doi: 10.1002/hep.22486

Moon, S. L., Blackinton, J. G., Anderson, J. R., Dozier, M. K., Dodd, B. J., Keene, J. D., et al. (2015). XRN1 stalling in the 5' UTR of hepatitis C virus and bovine viral diarrhea virus is associated with dysregulated host mRNA stability. *PLoS Pathog.* 11:e1004708. doi: 10.1371/journal.ppat.1004708

Moran, V. A., Perera, R. J., and Khalil, A. M. (2012). Emerging functional and mechanistic paradigms of mammalian long non-coding RNAs. *Nucleic Acids Res.* 40, 6391–6400. doi: 10.1093/nar/gks296

Morris, K. V., and Mattick, J. S. (2014). The rise of regulatory RNA. *Nat. Rev. Genet.* 15, 423–437. doi: 10.1038/nrg3722

Nahon, P., Bourcier, V., Layese, R., Audureau, E., Cagnot, C., Marcellin, P., et al. (2017). Eradication of hepatitis C virus infection in patients with cirrhosis reduces risk of liver and non-liver complications. *Gastroenterology* 152, 142.e2–156.e2. doi: 10.1053/j.gastro.2016.09.009

Nakkuntod, J., Avihingsanon, Y., Mutirangura, A., and Hirankarn, N. (2011). Hypomethylation of LINE-1 but not Alu in lymphocyte subsets of systemic lupus erythematosus patients. *Clin. Chim. Acta* 412, 1457–1461. doi: 10.1016/j.cca.2011.04.002

Neil, S. J. D., Zang, T., and Bieniasz, P. D. (2008). Tetherin inhibits retrovirus release and is antagonized by HIV-1 Vpu. *Nature* 451, 425–430. doi: 10.1038/nature06553

Niazi, F., and Valadkhan, S. (2012). Computational analysis of functional long noncoding RNAs reveals lack of peptide-coding capacity and parallels with 3' UTRs. *RNA* 18, 825–843. doi: 10.1261/rna.029520.111

Nishina, S., Hino, K., Korenaga, M., Vecchi, C., Pietrangelo, A., Mizukami, Y., et al. (2008). Hepatitis C virus-induced reactive oxygen species raise hepatic iron level in mice by reducing hepcidin transcription. *Gastroenterology* 134, 226–238. doi: 10.1053/j.gastro.2007.10.011

Nishitsuji, H., Ujino, S., Yoshio, S., Sugiyama, M., Mizokami, M., Kanto, T., et al. (2016). Long noncoding RNA #32 contributes to antiviral responses by controlling interferon-stimulated gene expression. *Proc. Natl. Acad. Sci. U.S.A.* 113, 10388–10393. doi: 10.1073/pnas.1525022113

Onomoto, K., Onoguchi, K., Takahasi, K., and Fujita, T. (2010). Type I interferon production induced by RIG-I-like receptors. *J. Interferon Cytokine Res.* 30, 875–881. doi: 10.1089/jir.2010.0117

Ooi, Y. S., Dubé, M., and Kielian, M. (2015). BST2/tetherin inhibition of alphavirus exit. *Viruses* 7, 2147–2167. doi: 10.3390/v7042147

Ouyang, J., Zhu, X., Chen, Y., Wei, H., Chen, Q., Chi, X., et al. (2014). NRAV, a long noncoding RNA, modulates antiviral responses through suppression of interferon-stimulated gene transcription. *Cell Host Microbe* 16, 616–626. doi: 10.1016/j.chom.2014.10.001

Pène, V., Li, Q., Sodroski, C., Hsu, C. S., and Liang, T. J. (2015). Dynamic interaction of stress granules, DDX3X, and IKK-α mediates multiple functions in hepatitis C virus infection. *J. Virol.* 89, 5462–5477. doi: 10.1128/JVI.03197-14

Peng, X., Gralinski, L., Armour, C. D., Ferris, M. T., Thomas, M. J., Proll, S., et al. (2010). Unique signatures of long noncoding RNA expression in response to virus infection and altered innate immune signaling. *mBio* 1:e00206-10. doi: 10.1128/mBio.00206-10

Penkala, I., Wang, J., Syrett, C. M., Goetzl, L., López, C. B., and Anguera, M. C. (2016). lncRHOXF1, a long noncoding RNA from the X chromosome that suppresses viral response genes during development of the early human placenta. *Mol. Cell. Biol.* 36, 1764–1775. doi: 10.1128/MCB.01098-15

Piñeiro, D., and Martinez-Salas, E. (2012). RNA structural elements of hepatitis C virus controlling viral RNA translation and the implications for viral pathogenesis. *Viruses* 4, 2233–2250. doi: 10.3390/v4102233

Pirakitikulr, N., Kohlway, A., Lindenbach, B. D., and Pyle, A. M. (2016). The coding region of the HCV genome contains a network of regulatory RNA structures. *Mol. Cell* 62, 111–120. doi: 10.1016/j.molcel.2016.01.024

Ploss, A., Evans, M. J., Gaysinskaya, V. A., Panis, M., You, H., de Jong, Y. P., et al. (2009). Human occludin is a hepatitis C virus entry factor required for infection of mouse cells. *Nature* 457, 882–886. doi: 10.1038/nature07684

Pollard, K. M., Cauvi, D. M., Toomey, C. B., Morris, K. V., and Kono, D. H. (2013). Interferon-gamma and systemic autoimmunity. *Discov. Med.* 16, 123–131.

Porritt, R. A., and Hertzog, P. J. (2015). Dynamic control of type I IFN signalling by an integrated network of negative regulators. *Trends Immunol.* 36, 150–160. doi: 10.1016/j.it.2015.02.002

Prenner, S. B., VanWagner, L. B., Flamm, S. L., Salem, R., Lewandowski, R. J., and Kulik, L. (2017). Hepatocellular carcinoma decreases the chance of successful hepatitis C virus therapy with direct-acting antivirals. *J. Hepatol.* 66, 1173–1181. doi: 10.1016/j.jhep.2017.01.020

Ramirez, S., Mikkelsen, L. S., Gottwein, J. M., and Bukh, J. (2016). Robust HCV genotype 3a infectious cell culture system permits identification of escape variants with resistance to sofosbuvir. *Gastroenterology* 151, 973.e2–985.e2. doi: 10.1053/j.gastro.2016.07.013

Randall, R. E., and Goodbourn, S. (2008). Interferons and viruses: an interplay between induction, signalling, antiviral responses and virus countermeasures. *J. Gen. Virol.* 89, 1–47. doi: 10.1099/vir.0.83391-0

Raychoudhuri, A., Shrivastava, S., Steele, R., Kim, H., Ray, R., and Ray, R. B. (2011). ISG56 and IFITM1 proteins inhibit hepatitis C virus replication. *J. Virol.* 85, 12881–12889. doi: 10.1128/JVI.05633-11

Reig, M., Mariño, Z., Perelló, C., Iñarrairaegui, M., Ribeiro, A., Lens, S., et al. (2016). Unexpected high rate of early tumor recurrence in patients with HCV-related HCC undergoing interferon-free therapy. *J. Hepatol.* 65, 719–726. doi: 10.1016/j.jhep.2016.04.008

Rinn, J. L. (2014). lncRNAs: linking RNA to chromatin. *Cold Spring Harb. Perspect. Biol.* 6:a018614. doi: 10.1101/cshperspect.a018614

Rinn, J. L., and Chang, H. Y. (2012). Genome regulation by long noncoding RNAs. *Annu. Rev. Biochem.* 81, 145–166. doi: 10.1146/annurev-biochem-051410-092902

Romero-Brey, I., Merz, A., Chiramel, A., Lee, J. Y., Chlanda, P., Haselman, U., et al. (2012). Three-dimensional architecture and biogenesis of membrane structures associated with hepatitis C virus replication. *PLoS Pathog.* 8:e1003056. doi: 10.1371/journal.ppat.1003056

Rose, D., and Stadler, P. F. (2011). Molecular evolution of the non-coding eosinophil granule ontogeny transcript. *Front. Genet.* 2:69. doi: 10.3389/fgene.2011.00069

Rusinova, I., Forster, S., Yu, S., Kannan, A., Masse, M., Cumming, H., et al. (2013). Interferome v2.0: an updated database of annotated interferon-regulated genes. *Nucleic Acids Res.* 41, D1040–D1046. doi: 10.1093/nar/gks1215

Saito, T., Owen, D. M., Jiang, F., Marcotrigiano, J., and Gale, M. Jr. (2008). Innate immunity induced by composition-dependent RIG-I recognition of hepatitis C virus RNA. *Nature* 454, 523–527. doi: 10.1038/nature07106

Sarasin-Filipowicz, M., Oakeley, E. J., Duong, F. H., Christen, V., Terracciano, L., Filipowicz, W., et al. (2008). Interferon signaling and treatment outcome in chronic hepatitis C. *Proc. Natl. Acad. Sci. U.S.A.* 105, 7034–7039. doi: 10.1073/pnas.0707882105

Satpathy, A. T., and Chang, H. Y. (2015). Long noncoding RNA in hematopoiesis and immunity. *Immunity* 42, 792–804. doi: 10.1016/j.immuni.2015.05.004

Schneider, W. M., Chevillotte, M. D., and Rice, C. M. (2014). Interferon-stimulated genes: a complex web of host defenses. *Annu. Rev. Immunol.* 32, 513–545. doi: 10.1146/annurev-immunol-032713-120231

Shi, G., Ando, T., Suzuki, R., Matsuda, M., Nakashima, K., Ito, M., et al. (2016). Involvement of the 3' untranslated region in encapsidation of the hepatitis C virus. *PLoS Pathog.* 12:e1005441. doi: 10.1371/journal.ppat.1005441

Shi, H. X., Yang, K., Liu, X., Liu, X. Y., Wei, B., Shan, Y. F., et al. (2010). Positive regulation of interferon regulatory factor 3 activation by Herc5 via ISG15 modification. *Mol. Cell. Biol.* 30, 2424–2436. doi: 10.1128/MCB.01466-09

Sigdel, K. R., Cheng, A., Wang, Y., Duan, L., and Zhang, Y. (2015). The emerging functions of long noncoding RNA in immune cells: autoimmune diseases. *J. Immunol. Res.* 2015:848790. doi: 10.1155/2015/848790

Singaravelu, R., O'Hara, S., Jones, D. M., Chen, R., Taylor, N. G., Srinivasan, P., et al. (2015). MicroRNAs regulate the immunometabolic response to viral infection in the liver. *Nat. Chem. Biol.* 11, 988–993. doi: 10.1038/nchembio.1940

Singaravelu, R., Russell, R. S., Tyrrell, D. L., and Pezacki, J. P. (2014). Hepatitis C virus and microRNAs: miRed in a host of possibilities. *Curr. Opin. Virol.* 7, 1–10. doi: 10.1016/j.coviro.2014.03.004

Stachurska, A., Zorro, M. M., van der Sijde, M. R., and Withoff, S. (2014). Small and long regulatory RNAs in the immune system and immune diseases. *Front. Immunol.* 5:513. doi: 10.3389/fimmu.2014.00513

Syed, G. H., Khan, M., Yang, S., and Siddiqui, A. (2017). Hepatitis C virus lipoviroparticles assemble in the endoplasmic reticulum (ER) and bud off from the ER to the golgi compartment in COPII vesicles. *J. Virol.* 91:e00499-17. doi: 10.1128/JVI.00499-17

Takeuchi, O., and Akira, S. (2009). Innate immunity to virus infection. *Immunol. Rev.* 227, 75–86. doi: 10.1111/j.1600-065X.2008.00737.x

Thomas, D. L., Thio, C. L., Martin, M. P., Qi, Y., Ge, D., O'Huigin, C., et al. (2009). Genetic variation in IL28B and spontaneous clearance of hepatitis C virus. *Nature* 461, 798–801. doi: 10.1038/nature08463

Uesaka, M., Nishimura, O., Go, Y., Nakashima, K., Agata, K., and Imamura, T. (2014). Bidirectional promoters are the major source of gene activation-associated non-coding RNAs in mammals. *BMC Genomics* 15:35. doi: 10.1186/1471-2164-15-35

Ulitsky, I., and Bartel, D. P. (2013). lincRNAs: genomics, evolution, and mechanisms. *Cell* 154, 26–46. doi: 10.1016/j.cell.2013.06.020

Valadkhan, S., and Gunawardane, L. S. (2015). lncRNA-mediated regulation of the interferon response. *Virus Res.* 212, 127–136. doi: 10.1016/j.virusres.2015.09.023

Valadkhan, S., and Nilsen, T. W. (2010). Reprogramming of the non-coding transcriptome during brain development. *J. Biol.* 9:5. doi: 10.1186/jbio l197

van der Meer, A. J., and Berenguer, M. (2016). Reversion of disease manifestations after HCV eradication. *J. Hepatol.* 65, S95–S108. doi: 10.1016/j.jhep.2016.07.039

van der Meer, A. J., Feld, J. J., Hofer, H., Almasio, P. L., Calvaruso, V., Fernández-Rodríguez, C. M., et al. (2017). Risk of cirrhosis-related complications in patients with advanced fibrosis following hepatitis C virus eradication. *J. Hepatol.* 66, 485–493. doi: 10.1016/j.jhep.2016.10.017

Vigneau, S., Rohrlich, P.-S., Brahic, M., and Bureau, J.-F. (2003). Tmevpg1, a candidate gene for the control of Theiler's virus persistence, could be implicated in the regulation of gamma interferon. *J. Virol.* 77, 5632–5638. doi: 10.1128/JVI.77.10.5632-5638.2003

Wagner, L. A., Christensen, C. J., Dunn, D. M., Spangrude, G. J., Georgelas, A., Kelley, L., et al. (2007). EGO, a novel, noncoding RNA gene, regulates eosinophil granule protein transcript expression. *Blood* 109, 5191–5198. doi: 10.1182/blood-2006-06-027987

Wakano, C., Byun, J. S., Di, L.-J., and Gardner, K. (2012). The dual lives of bidirectional promoters. *Biochim. Biophys. Acta* 1819, 688–693. doi: 10.1016/j.bbagrm.2012.02.006

Walsh, M. J., Jonsson, J. R., Richardson, M. M., Lipka, G. M., Purdie, D. M., Clouston, A. D., et al. (2006). Non-response to antiviral therapy is associated with obesity and increased hepatic expression of suppressor of cytokine signalling 3 (SOCS-3) in patients with chronic hepatitis C, viral genotype 1. *Gut* 55, 529–535. doi: 10.1136/gut.2005.069674

Wang, W.-B., Levy, D. E., and Lee, C.-K. (2011). STAT3 negatively regulates type I IFN-mediated antiviral response. *J. Immunol.* 187, 2578–2585. doi: 10.4049/jimmunol.1004128

Wapinski, O., and Chang, H. Y. (2011). Long noncoding RNAs and human disease. *Trends Cell Biol.* 21, 354–361. doi: 10.1016/j.tcb.2011.04.001

Waris, G., Turkson, J., Hassanein, T., and Siddiqui, A. (2005). Hepatitis C virus (HCV) constitutively activates STAT-3 via oxidative stress: role of STAT-3 in HCV replication. *J. Virol.* 79, 1569–1580. doi: 10.1128/JVI.79.3.1569-1580.2005

Webster, D. P., Klenerman, P., and Dusheiko, G. M. (2015). Hepatitis C. *Lancet* 385, 1124–1135. doi: 10.1016/S0140-6736(14)62401-6

Wei, W., Pelechano, V., Järvelin, A. I., and Steinmetz, L. M. (2011). Functional consequences of bidirectional promoters. *Trends Genet.* 27, 267–276. doi: 10.1016/j.tig.2011.04.002

Wilkins, C., Woodward, J., Lau, D. T., Barnes, A., Joyce, M., McFarlane, N., et al. (2013). IFITM1 is a tight junction protein that inhibits hepatitis C virus entry. *Hepatology* 57, 461–469. doi: 10.1002/hep.26066

Xiong, Y., Yuan, J., Zhang, C., Zhu, Y., Kuang, X., Lan, L., et al. (2015). STAT3-regulated long non-coding RNAs lnc-7SK and lnc-IGF2-AS promote hepatitis C virus replication. *Mol. Med. Rep.* 12, 6738–6744. doi: 10.3892/mmr.2015.4278

Yang, L., Froberg, J. E., and Lee, J. T. (2014). Long noncoding RNAs: fresh perspectives into the RNA world. *Trends Biochem. Sci.* 39, 35–43. doi: 10.1016/j.tibs.2013.10.002

Yoshida, T., Hanada, T., Tokuhisa, T., Kosai, K., Sata, M., Kohara, M., et al. (2002). Activation of STAT3 by the hepatitis C virus core protein leads to cellular transformation. *J. Exp. Med.* 196, 641–653. doi: 10.1084/jem.20012127

Yoshimura, A., Naka, T., and Kubo, M. (2007). SOCS proteins, cytokine signalling and immune regulation. *Nat. Rev. Immunol.* 7, 454–465. doi: 10.1038/nri2093

Yu, A. D., Wang, Z., and Morris, K. V. (2015). Long noncoding RNAs: a potent source of regulation in immunity and disease. *Immunol. Cell Biol.* 93, 277–283. doi: 10.1038/icb.2015.2

Yu, Q., Carbone, C. J., Katlinskaya, Y. V., Zheng, H., Zheng, K., Luo, M., et al. (2015). Type I interferon controls propagation of long interspersed element-1. *J. Biol. Chem.* 290, 10191–10199. doi: 10.1074/jbc.M114.612374

Yuan, J. H., Yang, F., Wang, F., Ma, J. Z., Guo, Y. J., Tao, Q. F., et al. (2014). A long noncoding RNA activated by TGF-β promotes the invasion-metastasis cascade in hepatocellular carcinoma. *Cancer Cell* 25, 666–681. doi: 10.1016/j.ccr.2014.03.010

Zeisel, M. B., Fofana, I., Fafi-Kremer, S., and Baumert, T. F. (2011). Hepatitis C virus entry into hepatocytes: molecular mechanisms and targets for antiviral therapies. *J. Hepatol.* 54, 566–576. doi: 10.1016/j.jhep.2010.10.014

4

Cesarean or Vaginal Birth does not Impact the Longitudinal Development of the Gut Microbiome in a Cohort of Exclusively Preterm Infants

Christopher J. Stewart[1], Nicholas D. Embleton[2], Elizabeth Clements[3], Pamela N. Luna[4], Daniel P. Smith[1], Tatiana Y. Fofanova[1], Andrew Nelson[5], Gillian Taylor[3], Caroline H. Orr[3], Joseph F. Petrosino[1], Janet E. Berrington[2] and Stephen P. Cummings[3]*

[1] Alkek Center for Metagenomics and Microbiome Research, Department of Molecular Virology and Microbiology, Baylor College of Medicine, Houston, TX, United States, [2] Newcastle Neonatal Service, Royal Victoria Infirmary, Newcastle upon Tyne, United Kingdom, [3] School of Science and Engineering, Teesside University, Middlesbrough, United Kingdom, [4] Department of Statistics, Rice University, Houston, TX, United States, [5] Faculty of Health and Life Sciences, Northumbria University, Newcastle upon Tyne, United Kingdom

***Correspondence:**
Christopher J. Stewart
christopher.stewart@bcm.edu

The short and long-term impact of birth mode on the developing gut microbiome in neonates has potential implications for the health of infants. In term infants, the microbiome immediately following birth across multiple body sites corresponds to birth mode, with increased *Bacteroides* in vaginally delivered infants. We aimed to determine the impact of birth mode of the preterm gut microbiome over the first 100 days of life and following neonatal intensive care unit (NICU) discharge. In total, 867 stool samples from 46 preterm infants (21 cesarean and 25 vaginal), median gestational age 27 weeks, were sequenced (V4 region 16S rRNA gene, Illumina MiSeq). Of these, 776 samples passed quality filtering and were included in the analysis. The overall longitudinal alpha-diversity and within infant beta-diversity was comparable between cesarean and vaginally delivered infants. Vaginally delivered infants kept significantly more OTUs from 2 months of life and following NICU discharge, but OTUs lost, gained, and regained were not different based on birth mode. Furthermore, the temporal progression of dominant genera was comparable between birth modes and no significant difference was found for any genera following adjustment for covariates. Lastly, preterm gut community types (PGCTs) showed some moderate differences in very early life, but progressed toward a comparable pattern by week 5. No PGCT was significantly associated with cesarean or vaginal birth. Unlike term infants, birth mode was not significantly associated with changes in microbial diversity, composition, specific taxa, or overall microbial development in preterm infants. This may result from the dominating effects of NICU exposures including the universal use of antibiotics immediately following birth and/or the lack of *Bacteroides* colonizing preterm infants.

Keywords: birth mode, cesarean, vaginal, gut microbiome, preterm infants, 16S rRNA sequencing

---

Abbreviations: LOS, late onset sepsis; NEC, necrotising enterocolitis; NICU, neonatal intensive care unit; OTU, operational taxonomic unit; PCoA, principal coordinates analysis; PGCT, preterm gut community type.

INTRODUCTION

Immediately following birth, a neonate encounters large numbers of viable microbes. Despite emerging evidence suggesting the potential for prenatal exposure to microorganisms during the fetal stages (Jiménez et al., 2008; Aagaard et al., 2014; Collado et al., 2016), the main colonisation event occurs at birth, where for term infants birth mode shapes what microbes are passed from the mother to the offspring (Aagaard et al., 2016). Within the first 24 h of life, the microbiome of multiple distinct sites across the neonate reflect the route of delivery, with vaginally delivered neonates harboring vaginally derived organisms (typically *Lactobacillus*) and cesarean delivered neonates harboring skin-like microbes (typically increased *Staphylococcus*) (Dominguez-Bello et al., 2010). In the subsequent days and weeks following birth, the microbes colonizing different body sites begin to show more distinction (Chu et al., 2017). In infants delivered at term, the impact of birth mode has been studied in several longitudinal studies, most showing infants delivered vaginally have increased *Bacteroides* throughout the 1st year of life (Azad et al., 2013; Jakobsson et al., 2014; Bäckhed et al., 2015; Bokulich et al., 2016; Yassour et al., 2016). Contrary to these reports, no difference in the overall microbial community or in specific taxa between vaginal and cesarean infants at 6 weeks of life has also been reported (Chu et al., 2017). Differences between cohorts and methods (e.g., sequencing depth) may account for these discrepancies.

In preterm infants, studies directly exploring associations between birth mode and the temporal microbiome are lacking, although evidence suggests other factors such as feeding practices, postnatal age, and diseases like sepsis or necrotizing enterocolitis (NEC) likely have a bigger association with the microbiome (Stewart et al., 2013a, 2015b, 2016; La Rosa et al., 2014; Cong et al., 2016; Hill et al., 2017). A recent meta-analysis in preterm infants found reduced Bacteroides and increased Firmicutes in cesarean infants (Pammi et al., 2017). Infants delivered by cesarean have increased risks of later life obesity (Yuan et al., 2016), allergy (Roduit et al., 2009), and asthma (Thavagnanam et al., 2008; Sevelsted et al., 2014). Notably, while the microbiome has been suggested to be involved in the pathobiology of these diseases, direct causality has not been demonstrated.

In the current study we combined our existing publically available datasets (Abdulkadir et al., 2016; Stewart et al., 2016) and our previously unpublished data to directly explore how the birth mode impacts the temporal development of preterm infants while on the NICU and following discharge.

MATERIALS AND METHODS

Ethics Statement

Ethical approval was obtained from the County Durham and Tees Valley Research Ethics Committee. Parental written informed consent was given.

Participants and Study Design

The study design, setting, participants, and methods of data collection have been reported previously (Stewart et al., 2012, 2013b; Abdulkadir et al., 2016). Briefly, all infants were cared for in a single NICU with standardized feeding, antibiotic and antifungal guidelines. Due to a change in NICU practice in 2013 infants born after this routinely received the probiotic Infloran® (*Bifidobacterium bifidum*-ATCC15696 and *Lactobacillus acidophilus*-NCIMB701748) soon after initial introduction of feeds, where half an Infloran capsule was given twice daily (125 mg b.d. at 10 9 organisms per dose). Infants contributing a minimum of seven samples in their first 100 days were included in the study.

16S rRNA Gene Bacterial Profiling

Nucleic acid extraction was carried out on 100 mg of stool using the PowerLyzer™ PowerSoil® DNA Isolation Kit (MoBio, CA, United States) in accordance with the manufacturer's instructions. The V4 region of the 16S rRNA gene was amplified by PCR using barcoded Illumina adapter-containing primers 515F and 806R (Caporaso et al., 2012) and sequenced on the MiSeq platform (Illumina; San Diego, CA, United States) by NU-OMICS using the 2 × 250 bp paired-end protocol yielding pair-end reads that overlap almost completely. Sequencing read pairs were demultiplexed based on the unique molecular barcodes, and reads were merged using USEARCH v7.0.1090 (Edgar, 2010). Merging allowed zero mismatches and a minimum overlap of 50 bases, and merged reads were trimmed at the first base with a $Q \leq 5$. In addition, a quality filter was applied to the resulting merged reads and those containing above 0.05% expected errors were discarded. Sequences were stepwise clustered into OTUs at a similarity cutoff value of 97% using the UPARSE algorithm (Edgar, 2013). Chimeras were removed using USEARCH v7.0.1090. OTUs were determined by mapping the centroids to the SILVA database (Quast et al., 2013) containing only the 16S rDNA V4 region to determine taxonomies. A custom script constructed a rarefied OTU table (rarefaction was performed at only one sequence depth) from the output files generated in the previous two steps for downstream analyses. We utilized multiple quality control measures, including the use of non-template controls during microbial DNA extraction and 16S rRNA gene amplification. Resulting OTU tables were rarified to 4300 reads per sample.

Bioinformatic and Statistical Analysis

Data analysis was conducted in R version 3.3 using ggplot2 (R Core Team, 2014). Alpha diversity analyses, specifically observed OTUs and Shannon diversity, are presented between infants. Weighted and unweighted UniFrac distances (Lozupone et al., 2011) were performed within infants based on consecutive samples. The number of OTUs kept (retained from one sample to the next), OTUs lost (present in the previous but not current sample), OTUs regained (any OTU detected in the current sample and previously detected within the infant, but not the preceding sample), and new OTUs gained (OTU detected in an infant for the first time) was performed within infants based on consecutive samples.

Inferred metabolic capacity of the bacterial community was determined by Tax4Fun (Asshauer et al., 2015). FishTaco was then performed at the pathway level using genomic content inference to determine which species attenuated and drove the significantly altered functions (Manor and Borenstein, 2017).

Preterm gut community types were determined based on a publically available script for linear mixed-effects modeling, medoid-based clustering, and Markov chain modeling (DiGiulio et al., 2015). Weighted UniFrac (Lozupone et al., 2011) was used to calculate the distance between all samples and this was denoised by extraction of the most significant PCoA eigenvectors before applying the PAM algorithm. Gap statistic was used to determine the appropriate number of clusters based on the section of the plot where the curve markedly flattens (i.e., the elbow phenomenon).

Cross-sectional analyses were performed at discrete time points (1, 3, 5, and 8 weeks of age) to overcome bias of repeated measures in longitudinal analyses. At a given time point, samples within ±10 week days included, where the sample nearest to the specific week were chosen, giving preference to samples collected prior to the time point. Significance of categorical variables were determined using the non-parametric Mann–Whitney test for two category comparisons or the Kruskal–Wallis test when comparing three or more categories (Kruskal and Wallis, 1952). All *P*-values were adjusted for multiple comparisons using the false discovery rate (FDR) algorithm (Benjamini and Hochberg, 1995). Linear regression models adjusted for age (day of life), sex, birth weight, gestational age, diagnosis of NEC and/or LOS, receipt of expressed breast milk, and antibiotics ($<$ or $>$10 days of antibiotics while on the NICU).

RESULTS

Study Population

In total, 63,592,993 sequencing reads from 867 samples (46 patients) mapped to the database, with 776 (760 NICU and 16 post discharge) samples remaining in the analysis following rarefication to 4300 reads. Of these 46 infants, 25 infants were delivered vaginally and 21 infants were delivery by cesarean section (**Table 1**). All infants received at least 48 h of antibiotics immediately following birth and the total number of days of antibiotic treatment while on the NICU was comparable between birth modes. Due to a change in unit practice, probiotics were administered in 4/21 of the cesarean infants born after 2013 and no vaginal infants received probiotics ($P = 0.07$). Use of probiotics was associated with increased relative abundance in only the genera contained within the probiotic (Infloran; *Bifidobacterium* and *Lactobacillus*), but not in other taxa (Supplementary Figure 1). Nonetheless, receipt of probiotics (along with other important covariates – see Materials and Methods) were also adjusted for in all significance testing of taxa.

TABLE 1 | Characteristics of 46 preterm infants born by either vaginal or cesarean delivery.

	Vaginal	Caesarean	*P*-value
Infants	25	21	–
NICU samples*	439	321	–
Post discharge samples*	10	6	–
Birth weight in grams, median (IQR)	910 (750–1180)	950 (840–1150)	0.18
Gestational age in weeks, median (IQR)	26 (25–28)	27 (26–28)	0.18
Male sex	14 (56%)	16 (76%)	0.13
Received expressed breast milk	24 (96%)	20 (95%)	0.47
Received probiotics	0	4 (19%)	0.07
Number of days of antibiotics	8 (4–17)	6 (2–12)	0.35
NEC and/or LOS	7 (28%)	6 (29%)	1

**Samples remaining after QC and rarefaction.*
NICU, neonatal intensive care unit; NEC, necrotising enterocolitis; LOS, late onset sepsis.

Longitudinal Alpha and Beta Diversity Was Comparable between Cesarean and Vaginally Delivered Infants

The number of observed OTUs of samples decreased initially following birth, then increased from 11 OTUs on day 12 to 17 OTUs on day 100 of life. While vaginal infants had slightly more observed OTUs, there was no significant difference between cesarean and vaginally delivered infants (Mann–Whitney cross-sectional comparison at each week *P*-value was 0.43 or higher) (**Figure 1A**). The Shannon diversity increased from around 0.75 in the days following birth to 1.25 at NICU discharge, with comparable development between cesarean and vaginally delivered infants (Mann–Whitney cross-sectional comparison at each week *P*-value was 0.49 or higher) (**Figure 1B**). The observed OTUs and Shannon diversity continued to increase following discharge but no significant difference between cesarean and vaginally delivered infants occurred in post discharge samples (observed OTUs $P = 0.212$; Shannon $P = 0.428$) (Supplementary Figures 2A,B). Birth mode was also comparable between weighted and unweighted UniFrac distance between consecutive samples during NICU sampling (**Figures 1C,D**) and post discharge (weighted UniFrac $P = 1$; unweighted UniFrac $P = 0.875$) (Supplementary Figures 2C,D). Comparing the cross-sectional weighted UniFrac distance between birth modes at weeks 1, 3, 5, 8, and post discharge showed no significant difference at any time point (Supplementary Figure 3).

Vaginally Delivered Infants Have Increased OTU Stability, But Comparable OTU Acquisition While on the NICU and Following Discharge

The individual OTUs were tracked through time in consecutive samples, showing that vaginally delivered infants kept significantly more OTUs from month 2 of life ($P < 0.001$)

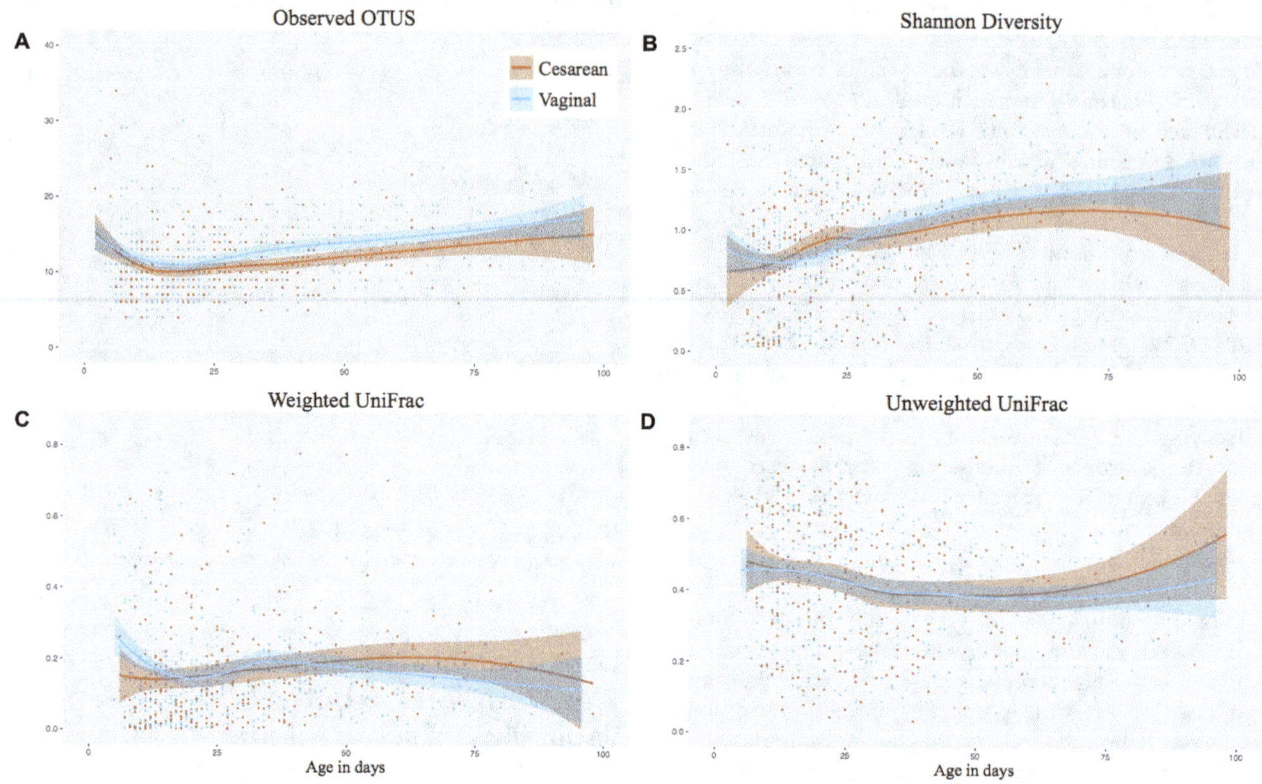

FIGURE 1 | Longitudinal development of alpha and beta diversity by birth mode. Post discharge samples omitted from the analysis. Shaded bars represent the 95% confidence interval. **(A)** Observed OTUs (richness). **(B)** Shannon Diversity. **(C)** Weighted UniFrac based on consecutive samples. **(D)** Unweighted UniFrac based on consecutive samples.

than those delivered by cesarean (**Figure 2A**). The number of OTUs kept in month 1 of life was comparable between birth modes ($P = 0.947$). The microbiome stabilized rapidly from birth to week 4 of life, where the number of 'OTUs lost' and 'new OTUs gained' declined, but the 'OTUs regained' (previously present but not in the preceding sample) increased (**Figure 2**). However, there was no difference in birth mode between OTUs lost, regained, or newly gained during the first 100 days while on the NICU. Following discharge, vaginally delivered infants continued to have significantly ($P = 0.021$) increased kept OTUs compared to cesarean, relative to the last NICU sample collected (Supplementary Figure 2E). As with the NICU samples, no significant difference between OTUs lost, regained, or newly gained was found for post discharge samples, relative to the last NICU sample (Supplementary Figures 2F–H).

Bacterial Genera Were Comparable between Cesarean and Vaginally Delivered Infants

Klebsiella (28% overall relative abundance in NICU samples), *Escherichia* (22% overall relative abundance), *Enterococcus* (15%), *Staphylococcus* (14%), and *Bifidobacterium* (5%) dominated NICU samples, accounting for 84% of the total relative abundance in the first 100 days of life (**Figure 3**). *Klebsiella* and *Enterococcus* remained relatively consistent during the NICU period, *Staphylococcus* and *Escherichia* declined from birth, and *Bifidobacterium* gradually increased through the NICU period. To determine significant differences in the relative abundance of genera through the NICU, while accounting for repeated measures, the first sample from each infant in weeks 1, 3, 5, 8, and 10+ were included. This cross-sectional comparison showed no significant difference between cesarean and vaginal infants in any genera at any time point (Supplementary Table 1). *Bacteroides* was the 8th most abundant genera from all NICU samples (Supplementary Figure 4), but was 3rd most abundant in the post discharge samples (Supplementary Figure 5). Despite associations in term infants, the relative abundance of *Bacteroides* was comparable between cesarean and vaginal infants during NICU and following discharge in this preterm population. Comparing delivery mode in the post discharge period also showed the relative abundance of predominant genera was comparable (Supplementary Figure 5).

Preterm Gut Community Type Development Is Comparable between Different Birth Modes

Using Partitioning Around Medoids (PAM) clustering based on weighted UniFrac, the early preterm microbiome was defined by six distinct clusters, termed PGCTs (**Figure 4A**). With the exception of PGCTs 1 and 4, all PGCTs had significantly different

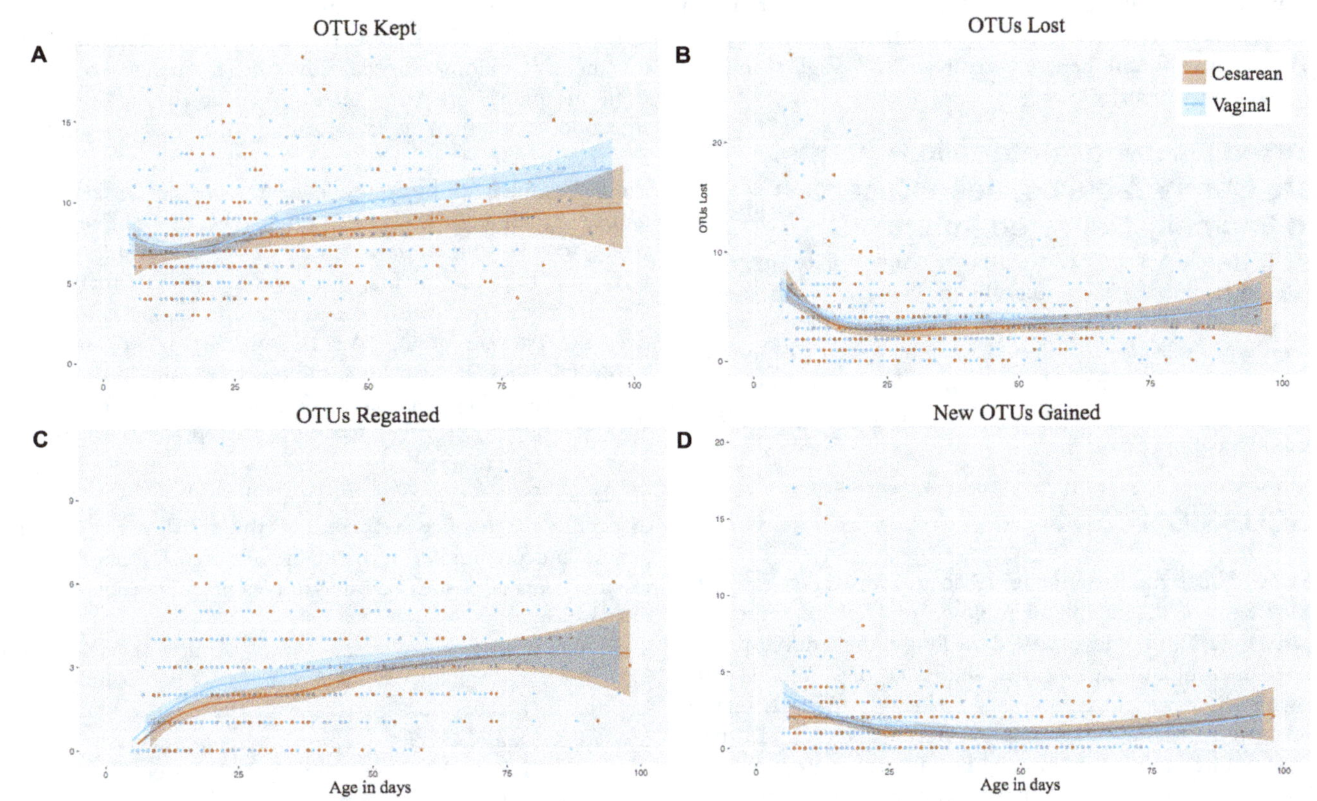

FIGURE 2 | Longitudinal OTU tracker analysis of the gut microbiome in preterm infants by birth mode. Post discharge samples omitted from the analysis. Shaded bars represent the 95% confidence interval. **(A)** OTUs kept. **(B)** OTUs lost. **(C)** OTUs regained (previously detected in the infant). **(D)** New OTUs gained (not previously detected in the infant).

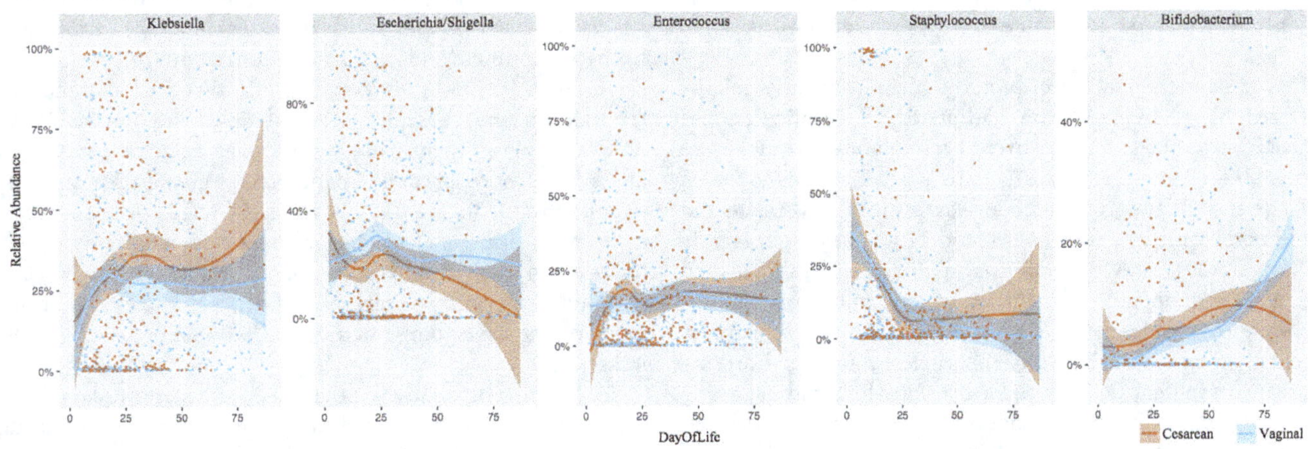

FIGURE 3 | Longitudinal development of the dominant bacterial taxa by birth mode. Top five dominant taxa representing 84% of the overall relative abundance of NICU samples are shown. Each point represents an individual sample. Shaded bars represent the 95% confidence interval.

Shannon diversity, with PGCTs 2 and 4 showing higher Shannon diversity and PGCT 6 (*Staphylococcus* dominant) showing the lowest Shannon diversity (**Figure 4B**). Birth mode showed moderate differences in the PGCTs detected over the initial weeks of life (**Figures 4C,D**). Most notable was the increase of PGCT 3 in cesarean delivery and PGCT 4 in vaginal delivery at week 1 of life. PGCT 4 continued to be increased in vaginal infants at week 3 of life, but by week 5 of life and thereafter the PGCTs detected in cesarean and vaginal infants were comparable. Despite these trends in PGCT development, the trajectory of gut microbiome development was highly variable within and between infants and no significant difference ($P = 0.125$) in PGCTs was found between cesarean and vaginal infants (Supplementary Figure 6).

Inferred Bacterial Metabolic Potential Were Comparable between Cesarean and Vaginally Delivered Infants

Tax4Fun (Asshauer et al., 2015) was employed to infer the metabolic potential of the microbiome between birth modes. FishTaco (Manor and Borenstein, 2017) was performed to determine significance of inferred function at each time point (weeks 1, 3, 5, 8, and post discharge), finding no pathway was significantly altered between cesarean and vaginally delivered infants at any time point.

DISCUSSION

The role of birth mode on the initial acquisition and subsequent development of the infant microbiome remains an important research question. We investigated the longitudinal development of the microbiome during the first 100 days of life and following discharge. In a cohort of exclusively preterm infants (24–31 weeks gestation), sampled during NICU and post discharge, birth mode was not significantly associated with the alpha- or beta- diversity (both within and between patients). Furthermore, birth mode had no significant association with the relative abundance of any bacterial genera or PGCTs. A novel analysis temporally tracking OTUs within infants in consecutive samples showed vaginally delivered infants retain more OTUs from month 2 of life and post discharge, suggesting increased microbiome stability associated with vaginal delivery.

In a large meta-analysis of preterm gut microbiome, infants delivered by cesarean section had increased Firmicutes and reduced Bacteroides, but the overall microbiome profiles were comparable (Pammi et al., 2017). In a recent study of term and preterm infants, birth mode was associated with altered stool microbiome at weeks 1, 4, 8, and 24 for term infants only (Hill et al., 2017). While only four preterm infants delivered vaginally were included in the study by Hill et al. (2017), microbiome profiles of NICU and post discharge samples appeared comparable between the preterm infants born by cesarean or vaginal delivery. In a previous longitudinal study of 58 preterm infants, postconceptional age was associated with the gut microbiome, with delivery mode reported to have minimal influences (La Rosa et al., 2014). Furthermore, in a study of 29 preterm infants, gender and feeding were more associated with the gut microbiome development compared to other demographics, including birth mode (Cong et al., 2016). While no clear associations in preterm infants have been reported, birth mode has been associated with significantly altered gut microbiome in term infants in the 1st year of life (Azad et al., 2013; Jakobsson et al., 2014; Bäckhed et al., 2015; Bokulich et al., 2016; Yassour et al., 2016). The discrepancy between term and preterm infants may result from the greater use of antibiotics in preterm populations (Berrington et al., 2012), or other NICU practices that have a dominant effect on the microbiome. Specifically, the frequency with which preterm infants are considered to be at risk of early onset infection, and thereby determining the use of antibiotics for the first 48 h of life, may supersede perinatal maternal influences such as birth mode or reasons for preterm labor and/or expedited delivery. Alternatively, the difference may relate to the differential abundance of *Bacteroides* between term and preterm infants. *Bacteroides* is the primary genera significantly altered between cesarean and vaginal term infants over the 1st year of life (Azad et al., 2013; Jakobsson et al., 2014; Bäckhed et al., 2015; Bokulich et al., 2016; Yassour et al., 2016). However, *Bacteroides* was not dominant in the current study, nor previous studies of preterm populations during NICU (Taft et al., 2014; Stewart et al., 2015b; Ward et al., 2016; Warner et al., 2016; Hill et al., 2017). Following discharge, *Bacteroides* represented the third most abundant genera and was higher in vaginally delivered infants. However, low numbers of post discharge samples preclude robust analysis of significance.

Previous studies collecting samples immediately at birth have shown vaginally delivered term born neonates have increased *Lactobacillus* and cesarean delivered neonates have increased *Staphylococcus*, *Propionibacterium*, and *Streptococcus* across multiple body sites (Dominguez-Bello et al., 2010; Chu et al., 2017). The earliest sample collected in the current study was on day 2 of life, at which stage the infant had received antibiotics (most commonly penicillin and gentamicin). This may account for why no specific bacterial genera or PGCT was significantly associated with the birth mode. It is also noteworthy that samples collected within the initial hours of life generally reflect (viable and non-viable) microbes transmitted from the mother, and not true colonization *per se* (Aagaard et al., 2016). Thus, it is also possible that no difference was reported in the current cohort because the non-viable and non-colonizing organisms are no longer detected by day 2 of life. Furthermore, preterm infants have a greater exposure time to microbes in the NICU environment (e.g., surfaces, bedside equipment, and staff), which are also responsible for shaping the preterm microbiome (Brooks et al., 2014; Hartz et al., 2015), and might add to the discrepancies between the effects of birth mode on the developing microbiome between preterm and term infants.

In the current study a novel OTU tracker was applied to determine the OTUs kept, lost, gained, or regained through consecutive samples. This was the only analysis that found a significant association, showing that vaginal infants had an increased number of kept OTUs in consecutive NICU samples from month 2 of life, which remained in samples collected post discharge. This is potentially reflective of increased gut microbiome stability in vaginal infants, compared to cesarean (Bäckhed et al., 2015). No difference in kept OTUs was found in the 1st month of life, reflecting the dynamic nature of the microbiome in both cesarean and vaginal infants during this phase (Koenig et al., 2010; Stewart et al., 2016). Notably, the number of new OTUs gained

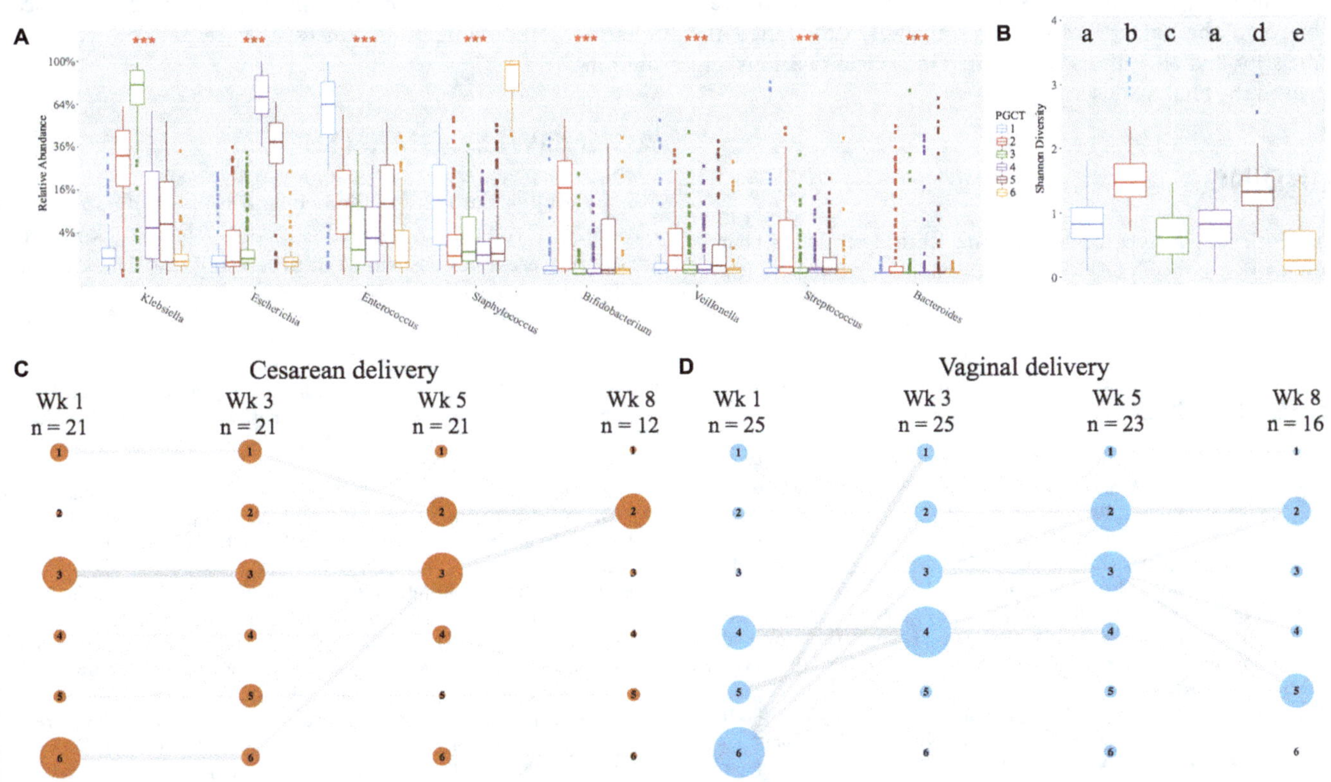

FIGURE 4 | Preterm gut community type (PGCT) development in NICU samples. PGCT clustering based on weighted UniFrac. **(A)** Box plots showing the eight most significant genera between the six PGCTs. *** denotes a *P*-value of >0.001. **(B)** Box plots showing the Shannon Diversity of each PGCT. Lower case letters denote the significance, where a unique letter represents the Shannon diversity of that PGCT is significantly different from all other groups. Only 'a' exists more then once, demonstrating PGCT 1 and 4 are not significantly different to each other, but are significantly different to all other PGCTs. **(C,D)** PGCT transition model showing the progression of cesarean **(C)** and vaginal **(D)** infants through four distinct time points over the first 8 weeks of life. Nodes and edges are sized based on the total counts. See Supplementary Figure 6 for full trajectory plots of all samples.

while on the NICU was typically low (usually a single OTU per consecutive sample), but regained OTUs increased through NICU stay. This is likely a consequence of NICU practices, with limited environmental microbial exposure (e.g., use of sterile incubators, use of hand sanitizer, minimal skin-to-skin contact) restricting the introduction of new OTUs.

The current study has several limitations. First, a larger cohort comprised of preterm infants from multiple NICUs may reveal novel associations not seen in this single unit study. Second, collection of post discharge samples was challenging, with additional costs for sample collection and variable response rates to sampling requests, resulting in inclusion of post discharge samples from only 35% (16/46) of infants. Further study of post discharge samples is needed to determine the long-term associations of birth mode and specifically if *Bacteroides* establishes in higher relative abundance in vaginal infants (Azad et al., 2013; Jakobsson et al., 2014; Bäckhed et al., 2015; Bokulich et al., 2016; Yassour et al., 2016). Third, the universal use of antibiotics in this cohort prevents direct analysis on the role of antibiotics in superseding birth mode effects. Either much larger cohorts, or additional experimentation utilising animal models will be necessary to determine if antibiotics alone account for the discrepancies between preterm and term infants. Finally, the current analysis was performed only on 16S rRNA gene sequencing data, but differences in microbiome and host function may occur between vaginal and cesarean infants, requiring the use of proteomics and metabolomics to explore these elements further (Stewart et al., 2015a).

In summary, in a single NICU preterm population exposed to antibiotics postpartum, birth mode was not significantly associated with the diversity or composition of the microbiome. Vaginal infants tended to have greater stability following month 2 of life and post discharge. These findings highlight key differences between preterm and term infants. The long-term effects on host immune development from the transfer of microbes during delivery and the subsequent risk of obesity, autoimmunity, and allergy warrant further investigation.

AUTHOR CONTRIBUTIONS

CS, NE, GT, CO, JB, and SC were responsible for the study concept and design. CS and AN were responsible for extraction and sequencing of samples. CS, EC, PL, DS, TF, and JP were involved in the data processing and analysis. CS drafted the manuscript and all authors contributed to critical revisions and approved the final manuscript.

FUNDING

This work was supported by funding from Tiny Lives charity (Newcastle upon Tyne, United Kingdom), Newcastle upon Tyne Hospitals NHS Charity and the Newcastle Healthcare Charity. The content is solely the responsibility of the authors.

ACKNOWLEDGMENTS

We gratefully acknowledge the help and support of parents who have helped with this and our other studies. We also acknowledge Jonathan Geselle for assistance in processing raw data and biom file formation.

REFERENCES

Aagaard, K., Ma, J., Antony, K. M., Ganu, R., Petrosino, J., and Versalovic, J. (2014). The placenta harbors a unique microbiome. *Sci. Transl. Med.* 6:237ra65. doi: 10.1126/scitranslmed.3008599

Aagaard, K., Stewart, C. J., and Chu, D. (2016). Una destinatio, viae diversae: Does exposure to the vaginal microbiota confer health benefits to the infant, and does lack of exposure confer disease risk? *EMBO Rep.* 17, 1679–1684.

Abdulkadir, B., Nelson, A., Skeath, T., Marrs, E. C. L., Perry, J. D., Cummings, S. P., et al. (2016). Routine use of probiotics in preterm infants: longitudinal impact on the microbiome and metabolome. *Neonatology* 109, 239–247. doi: 10.1159/000442936

Asshauer, K. P., Wemheuer, B., Daniel, R., and Meinicke, P. (2015). Tax4Fun: predicting functional profiles from metagenomic 16S rRNA data. *Bioinformatics* 31, 2882–2884. doi: 10.1093/bioinformatics/btv287

Azad, M. B., Konya, T., Maughan, H., Guttman, D. S., Field, C. J., Chari, R. S., et al. (2013). Gut microbiota of healthy Canadian infants: profiles by mode of delivery and infant diet at 4 months. *CMAJ* 185, 385–394. doi: 10.1503/cmaj.121189

Bäckhed, F., Roswall, J., Peng, Y., Feng, Q., Jia, H., Kovatcheva-Datchary, P., et al. (2015). Dynamics and stabilization of the human gut microbiome during the first year of life. *Cell Host Microbe* 17, 690–703. doi: 10.1016/j.chom.2015.04.004

Benjamini, Y., and Hochberg, Y. (1995). Controlling the false discovery rate: a practical and powerful approach to multiple testing. *J. R. Stat. Soc. Ser. B* 57, 289–300. doi: 10.2307/2346101

Berrington, J. E., Stewart, C. J., Embleton, N. D., and Cummings, S. P. (2012). Gut microbiota in preterm infants: assessment and relevance to health and disease. *Arch. Dis. Child. Fetal Neonatal Ed.* 98, F286–F290. doi: 10.1136/archdischild-2012-302134

Bokulich, N. A., Chung, J., Battaglia, T., Henderson, N., Jay, M., Li, H., et al. (2016). Antibiotics, birth mode, and diet shape microbiome maturation during early life. *Sci. Transl. Med.* 8:343ra82. doi: 10.1126/scitranslmed.aad7121

Brooks, B., Firek, B. A., Miller, C. S., Sharon, I., Thomas, B. C., Baker, R., et al. (2014). Microbes in the neonatal intensive care unit resemble those found in the gut of premature infants. *Microbiome* 2:1. doi: 10.1186/2049-2618-2-1

Caporaso, J. G., Lauber, C. L., Walters, W. A., Berg-Lyons, D., Huntley, J., Fierer, N., et al. (2012). Ultra-high-throughput microbial community analysis on the Illumina HiSeq and MiSeq platforms. *ISME J.* 6, 1621–1624. doi: 10.1038/ismej.2012.8

Chu, D. M., Ma, J., Prince, A. L., Antony, K. M., Seferovic, M. D., and Aagaard, K. M. (2017). Maturation of the infant microbiome community structure and function across multiple body sites and in relation to mode of delivery. *Nat. Med.* 23, 314–326. doi: 10.1038/nm.4272

Collado, M. C., Rautava, S., Aakko, J., Isolauri, E., and Salminen, S. (2016). Human gut colonisation may be initiated in *utero* by distinct microbial communities in the placenta and amniotic fluid. *Sci. Rep.* 6:23129. doi: 10.1038/srep23129

Cong, X., Xu, W., Janton, S., Henderson, W. A., Matson, A., McGrath, J. M., et al. (2016). Gut microbiome developmental patterns in early life of preterm infants: impacts of feeding and gender. *PLoS ONE* 11:e0152751. doi: 10.1371/journal.pone.0152751

DiGiulio, D. B., Callahan, B. J., McMurdie, P. J., Costello, E. K., Lyell, D. J., Robaczewska, A., et al. (2015). Temporal and spatial variation of the human microbiota during pregnancy. *Proc. Natl. Acad. Sci. U.S.A.* 112, 11060–11065. doi: 10.1073/pnas.1502875112

Dominguez-Bello, M. G., Costello, E. K., Contreras, M., Magris, M., Hidalgo, G., Fierer, N., et al. (2010). Delivery mode shapes the acquisition and structure of the initial microbiota across multiple body habitats in newborns. *Proc. Natl. Acad. Sci. U.S.A.* 107, 11971–11975. doi: 10.1073/pnas.1002601107

Edgar, R. C. (2010). Search and clustering orders of magnitude faster than BLAST. *Bioinformatics* 26, 2460–2461. doi: 10.1093/bioinformatics/btq461

Edgar, R. C. (2013). UPARSE: highly accurate OTU sequences from microbial amplicon reads. *Nat. Methods* 10, 996–998. doi: 10.1038/nmeth.2604

Hartz, L. E., Bradshaw, W., and Brandon, D. H. (2015). Potential NICU environmental influences on the neonate's microbiome: a systematic review. *Adv. Neonatal Care* 15, 324–335. doi: 10.1097/ANC.0000000000000220

Hill, C. J., Lynch, D. B., Murphy, K., Ulaszewska, M., Jeffery, I. B., O'Shea, C. A., et al. (2017). Evolution of gut microbiota composition from birth to 24 weeks in the INFANTMET cohort. *Microbiome* 5:21. doi: 10.1186/s40168-016-0213-y

Jakobsson, H. E., Abrahamsson, T. R., Jenmalm, M. C., Harris, K., Quince, C., Jernberg, C., et al. (2014). Decreased gut microbiota diversity, delayed Bacteroidetes colonisation and reduced Th1 responses in infants delivered by caesarean section. *Gut* 63, 559–566. doi: 10.1136/gutjnl-2012-303249

Jiménez, E., Marín, M. L., Martín, R., Odriozola, J. M., Olivares, M., Xaus, J., et al. (2008). Is meconium from healthy newborns actually sterile? *Res. Microbiol.* 159, 187–193. doi: 10.1016/j.resmic.2007.12.007

Koenig, J. E., Spor, A., Scalfone, N., Fricker, A. D., Stombaugh, J., Knight, R., et al. (2010). Succession of microbial consortia in the developing infant gut microbiome. *Proc. Natl. Acad. Sci. U.S.A.* 108, 4578–4585. doi: 10.1073/pnas.1000081107

Kruskal, W. H., and Wallis, W. A. (1952). Use of ranks in one-criterion variance analysis. *J. Am. Stat. Assoc.* 47, 583–621.

La Rosa, P. S., Warner, B. B., Zhou, Y., Weinstock, G. M., Sodergren, E., Hall-Moore, C. M., et al. (2014). Patterned progression of bacterial populations in the premature infant gut. *Proc. Natl. Acad. Sci. U.S.A.* 111, 12522–12527. doi: 10.1073/pnas.1409497111

Lozupone, C., Lladser, M. E., Knights, D., Stombaugh, J., and Knight, R. (2011). UniFrac: an effective distance metric for microbial community comparison. *ISME J.* 5, 169–172. doi: 10.1038/ismej.2010.133

Manor, O., and Borenstein, E. (2017). Systematic characterization and analysis of the taxonomic drivers of functional shifts in the human microbiome. *Cell Host Microbe* 21, 254–267. doi: 10.1016/j.chom.2016.12.014

Pammi, M., Cope, J., Tarr, P. I., Warner, B. B., Morrow, A. L., Mai, V., et al. (2017). Intestinal dysbiosis in preterm infants preceding necrotizing enterocolitis: a systematic review and meta-analysis. *Microbiome* 5:31. doi: 10.1186/s40168-017-0248-8

Quast, C., Pruesse, E., Yilmaz, P., Gerken, J., Schweer, T., Yarza, P., et al. (2013). The SILVA ribosomal RNA gene database project: improved data processing and web-based tools. *Nucleic Acids Res.* 41, D590–D596. doi: 10.1093/nar/gks1219

R Core Team (2014). *R: A Language and Environment for Statistical Computing.* Available at: http://www.r-project.org/

Roduit, C., Scholtens, S., de Jongste, J. C., Wijga, A. H., Gerritsen, J., Postma, D. S., et al. (2009). Asthma at 8 years of age in children born by caesarean section. *Thorax* 64, 107–113. doi: 10.1136/thx.2008.100875

Sevelsted, A., Stokholm, J., Bonnelykke, K., and Bisgaard, H. (2014). Cesarean section and chronic immune disorders – editorial comment. *Pediatrics* 135, e92–e98. doi: 10.1542/peds.2014-0596

Stewart, C. J., Embleton, N. D., Marrs, E. C. L., Smith, D. P., Nelson, A., Abdulkadir, B., et al. (2016). Temporal bacterial and metabolic development of the preterm gut reveals specific signatures in health and disease. *Microbiome* 4:67. doi: 10.1186/s40168-016-0216-8

Stewart, C. J., Marrs, E. C. L., Magorrian, S., Nelson, A., Lanyon, C., Perry, J. D., et al. (2012). The preterm gut microbiota: changes associated with necrotizing enterocolitis and infection. *Acta Paediatr. Int. J. Paediatr.* 101, 1121–1127. doi: 10.1111/j.1651-2227.2012.02801.x

Stewart, C. J., Marrs, E. C. L., Nelson, A., Lanyon, C., Perry, J. D., Embleton, N. D., et al. (2013a). Development of the preterm gut microbiome in twins at risk of necrotising enterocolitis and sepsis. *PLoS ONE* 8:e73465. doi: 10.1371/journal.pone.0073465

Stewart, C. J., Nelson, A., Scribbins, D., Marrs, E. C. L., Perry, J. D., Embleton, N. D., et al. (2013b). Bacterial and fungal viability in the preterm gut: NEC and sepsis. *Arch. Dis. Child. Fetal Neonatal Ed.* 98, F298–F303. doi: 10.1136/archdischild-2012-302119

Stewart, C. J., Nelson, A., Treumann, A., Skeath, T., Cummings, S. P., Embleton, N. D., et al. (2015a). Metabolomic and proteomic analysis of serum from preterm infants with necrotising entercolitis and late-onset sepsis. *Pediatr. Res.* 79, 425–431. doi: 10.1038/pr.2015.235

Stewart, C. J., Skeath, T., Nelson, A., Fernstad, S., Marrs, E., Perry, J., et al. (2015b). Preterm gut microbiota and metabolome following discharge from intensive care. *Sci. Rep.* 5:17141. doi: 10.1038/srep17141

Taft, D. H., Ambalavanan, N., Schibler, K. R., Yu, Z., Newburg, D. S., Ward, D. V., et al. (2014). Intestinal microbiota of preterm infants differ over time and between hospitals. *Microbiome* 2:36. doi: 10.1186/2049-2618-2-36

Thavagnanam, S., Fleming, J., Bromley, A., Shields, M. D., and Cardwell, C. R. (2008). A meta-analysis of the association between Caesarean section and childhood asthma. *Clin. Exp. Allergy* 38, 629–633. doi: 10.1111/j.1365-2222.2007.02780.x

Ward, D. V., Scholz, M., Zolfo, M., Taft, D. H., Schibler, K. R., Tett, A., et al. (2016). Metagenomic sequencing with strain-level resolution implicates uropathogenic *E. coli* in necrotizing enterocolitis and mortality in preterm infants. *Cell Rep.* 14, 2912–2924. doi: 10.1016/j.celrep.2016.03.015

Warner, B. B., Deych, E., Zhou, Y., Hall-Moore, C., Weinstock, G. M., Sodergren, E., et al. (2016). Gut bacteria dysbiosis and necrotising enterocolitis in very low birthweight infants: a prospective case-control study. *Lancet* 387, 1928–1936. doi: 10.1016/S0140-6736(16)00081-7

Yassour, M., Vatanen, T., Siljander, H., Hämäläinen, A.-M., Härkönen, T., Ryhänen, S. J., et al. (2016). Natural history of the infant gut microbiome and impact of antibiotic treatment on bacterial strain diversity and stability. *Sci. Transl. Med.* 8, 343–381. doi: 10.1126/scitranslmed.aad0917

Yuan, C., Gaskins, A. J., Blaine, A. I., Zhang, C., Gillman, M. W., Missmer, S. A., et al. (2016). Association between cesarean birth and risk of obesity in offspring in childhood, adolescence, and early adulthood. *JAMA Pediatr.* 64:e162385. doi: 10.1001/JAMAPEDIATRICS.2016.2385

5

Role of *Lactobacillus reuteri* in Human Health and Diseases

Qinghui Mu, Vincent J. Tavella and Xin M. Luo*

Department of Biomedical Sciences and Pathobiology, Virginia-Maryland College of Veterinary Medicine, Virginia Tech, Blacksburg, VA, United States

***Correspondence:**
Xin M. Luo
xinluo@vt.edu

Lactobacillus reuteri (*L. reuteri*) is a well-studied probiotic bacterium that can colonize a large number of mammals. In humans, *L. reuteri* is found in different body sites, including the gastrointestinal tract, urinary tract, skin, and breast milk. The abundance of *L. reuteri* varies among different individuals. Several beneficial effects of *L. reuteri* have been noted. First, *L. reuteri* can produce antimicrobial molecules, such as organic acids, ethanol, and reuterin. Due to its antimicrobial activity, *L. reuteri* is able to inhibit the colonization of pathogenic microbes and remodel the commensal microbiota composition in the host. Second, *L. reuteri* can benefit the host immune system. For instance, some *L. reuteri* strains can reduce the production of pro-inflammatory cytokines while promoting regulatory T cell development and function. Third, bearing the ability to strengthen the intestinal barrier, the colonization of *L. reuteri* may decrease the microbial translocation from the gut lumen to the tissues. Microbial translocation across the intestinal epithelium has been hypothesized as an initiator of inflammation. Therefore, inflammatory diseases, including those located in the gut as well as in remote tissues, may be ameliorated by increasing the colonization of *L. reuteri*. Notably, the decrease in the abundance of *L. reuteri* in humans in the past decades is correlated with an increase in the incidences of inflammatory diseases over the same period of time. Direct supplementation or prebiotic modulation of *L. reuteri* may be an attractive preventive and/or therapeutic avenue against inflammatory diseases.

Keywords: *Lactobacillus reuteri*, probiotic, microbiota, immune system, inflammatory diseases

INTRODUCTION

Probiotics are defined as "live microorganisms which, when administered in adequate amounts, confer a health benefit on the host" by the World Health Organization. While the idea to use probiotics for health benefits is not new, the interest has significantly increased in recent years (Islam, 2016). This may be due, in part, to the increase in antibiotic resistance particularly in the treatment of diseases in the gastrointestinal (GI) system, as well as an increasing desire by the public for natural health promotants. Those probiotic microorganisms that have been shown to have beneficial properties include *Lactobacillus spp.*, *Bifidobacterium spp.*, *Saccharomyces boulardii*, *Propionibacterium spp.*, *Streptococcus spp.*, *Bacillus spp.*, *Enterococcus spp.*, and some specific strains of *Escherichia coli* (Kechagia et al., 2013).

There are certain criteria that a probiotic must have to be considered efficacious. These include the capacity to survive in the GI tract, a high resistance to gastric acids, the lack of any transferable antibiotic resistance genes, and the capacity to exert clear benefits in the host (Montalban-Arques et al., 2015). Probiotics promote a healthy body through diverse mechanisms. A widespread generalization describing common mechanisms among studied probiotic genera includes colonizing resistance, producing acid, and short chain fatty acid (SCFA), regulating intestinal transit, normalizing perturbed microbiota, increasing enterocyte turnover, and competitive exclusion of pathogens (Hill et al., 2014). Though not widely observed, there are a lot of effects among specific probiotic species, some being strain specific. For instance, some probiotic strains can improve host food digestion by metabolizing bile salt or complementing the functions of missing digestive enzymes (Amara and Shibl, 2015; Shi et al., 2016).

Lactobacillus spp. are one of the most widely used probiotics and can be found in a large variety of food products throughout the world (Giraffa et al., 2010). The genus *Lactobacillus* comprises a large heterogeneous group of Gram-positive, nonsporulating, facultative anaerobic bacteria which include *L. acidophilus*, *L. rhamnosus*, *L. bulgaricus*, *L. casei*, and *L. reuteri*. This genus plays a very important role in food fermentation and can also be found in the GI system of humans and animals in variable amounts depending on the species, age of the host, or location within the gut (Duar et al., 2017).

Animal studies and preclinical results have shown that *Lactobacilli* may help in the prevention and treatment of numerous GI tract disorders. Among these disorders are enteric infections, antibiotic-associated diarrhea, necrotizing enterocolitis in preterm neonates, inflammatory bowel disease, colorectal cancer, and irritable bowel syndrome (Lebeer et al., 2008). Although the GI tract is the site where *Lactobacilli* are believed to show the most benefits, probiotic applications of some *Lactobacillus* strains at other sites of the body have been reported. These include the prevention and treatment of urogenital diseases and bacterial vaginosis in women, atopic disease, food hypersensitivity, and the prevention of dental caries (Lebeer et al., 2008).

One species of *Lactobacillus*, *L. reuteri* has multiple beneficial effects on host health such as prevention and/or amelioration of diverse disorders. *L. reuteri* was first isolated in 1962. It has been characterized as heterofermentative species that grows in oxygen-limited atmospheres and colonizes the GI tract of humans and animals (Kandler et al., 1980). The fact that it normally colonizes the GI tract may be the reason it confers great probiotic properties. This organism can withstand a wide variety of pH environments, employs multiple mechanisms that allow it to successfully inhibit pathogenic microorganisms, and has been shown to secrete antimicrobial intermediaries (Jacobsen et al., 1999; Valeur et al., 2004).

L. reuteri has been shown to be one of the truly indigenous bacteria of the human GI tract (Sinkiewicz, 2010). It naturally colonizes a wide range of vertebrates, including pigs, rodents, and chickens. In fact, it has gone through long-term evolution to diversify into host-adapted lineages (Oh et al., 2010; Walter et al., 2011). This organism is most typically found in the proximal digestive tract of the host (Frese et al., 2013). Several studies have assessed the safety of this organism in adults, children, infants, and even in an HIV-infected population (Wolf et al., 1998; Valeur et al., 2004; Weizman and Alsheikh, 2006; Mangalat et al., 2012; Jones et al., 2012a,c; Hoy-Schulz et al., 2016). The results showed that a dose as high as 2.9×10^9 colony-forming units (cfu)/day was still well tolerated, safe, and efficacious in humans. There have also been numerous articles enumerating the benefits of *L. reuteri* as a probiotic. These benefits include promoting health, reducing infections, improving feed tolerance, enhancing the absorption of nutrients, minerals, and vitamins, modulating host immune responses, promoting gut mucosal integrity, and reducing bacterial translocation (Tubelius et al., 2005; McFall-Ngai, 2007; Indrio et al., 2008; Spinler et al., 2008; Hou et al., 2015). In the current review, we will focus on the particular probiotic, *L. reuteri*, and discuss its beneficial functions in promoting health and preventing infections and diverse diseases.

PROBIOTIC PROPERTIES OF *L. reuteri*

There are some prerequisites for becoming potential probiotics: to survive in low pH and enzyme-enriched environments, to adhere to epithelium for host-probiotic interaction, competition with pathogenic microorganisms, and most importantly, safety. *L. reuteri* meets all of these requirements. Here, additional probiotic properties of *L. reuteri* are discussed that contribute to its diverse beneficial effects on host health and disease prevention and/or amelioration (**Figure 1**).

Gut Colonization of *L. reuteri*

Built for digestion and absorption, some sites of the GI system have developed to be harsh for microorganism colonization. Examples of this can be seen in the low pH conditions caused by gastric acids and bile salts in upper small intestine. Thus, the very first step of colonizing the GI tract is to survive in such environments. Multiple *L. reuteri* stains are resistant to low pH and bile salts (Seo et al., 2010; Krumbeck et al., 2016). This resistance is believed to be at least partially dependent on its ability to form biofilms (Salas-Jara et al., 2016).

L. reuteri is capable of attaching to mucin and intestinal epithelia, and some strains can adhere to gut epithelial cells in a range of vertebrate hosts (Li et al., 2008; Hou et al., 2014, 2015). A possible mechanism for adherence is the binding of bacterial surface molecules to the mucus layer. Mucus-binding proteins (MUBs) and MUB-like proteins, encoded by *Lactobacillales*-specific clusters of orthologous protein coding genes, serve as adherence mediators, or so-called adhesins (Roos and Jonsson, 2002; Kleerebezem et al., 2010; Gunning et al., 2016). The considerable diversity of MUBs among *L. reuteri* strains and the variation in the abundance of cell-surface MUBs significantly correlates with their mucus binding ability (Mackenzie et al., 2010). The strain-specific role of MUBs in recognizing mucus elements and/or their capability of promoting aggregation can explain the contribution of MUBs on the adherence of *L. reuteri*. Factors that mediate the attachment to the surfaces include multiple large surface proteins (Walter et al., 2005; Wang et al., 2008; Frese et al., 2011), MUB A (Jensen et al., 2014), glucosyltransferase A (GtfA) and inulosucrase (Inu) (Walter et al., 2008), and D-alanyl ester (Walter et al., 2007).

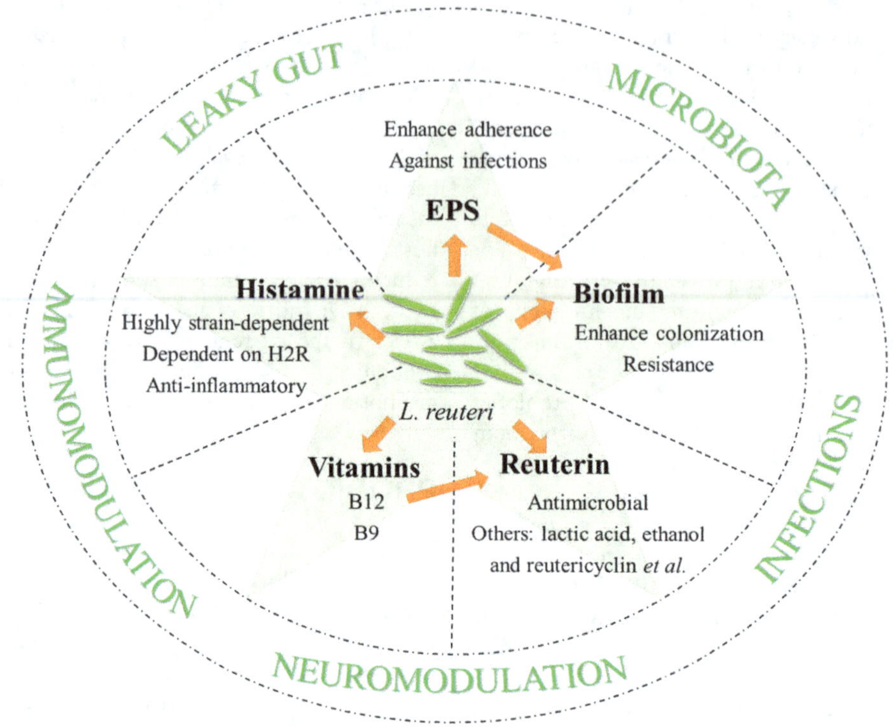

FIGURE 1 | Probiotic properties of *L. reuteri*.

As *L. reuteri* that has colonized to the host GI tract can form biofilms, efforts have been made to study the regulation of *L. reuteri* biofilm secretion and its association with the adherence of bacteria to host GI epithelium. By doing *in vitro* biofilm assay, Water, J. et al. uncovered the contribution of GtfA and Inu in the biofilm formation of *L. reuteri* TMW1.106 (Walter et al., 2008). The *in vivo* biofilm formation of *L. reuteri* strains seems to be dependent on the host origin of the strains. In one study, nine *L. reuteri* strains isolated from different hosts (human, mouse, rat, chicken, and pig) were given to germ-free mice and the biofilms were evaluated after 2 days. Interestingly, only rodent strains were able to form biofilms and adhere to the forestomach epithelium, although the luminal populations were comparable among strains of different origins (Frese et al., 2013). Another study by the same authors showed that a specialized transport pathway (the SecA2-SecY2 system) was unique in the rodent and porcine strains (Frese et al., 2011). By using a rodent strain *L. reuteri* 100-23, they compared extracellular and cell wall-associated proteins between the wild-type strain and the *secA2* mutant. Only one surface protein, *L. reuteri* 70902, was absent in the *secA2* mutant. *In vivo* colonization studies showed that the absence of *L. reuteri* 70902 leads to almost completely eliminated biofilm formation. This strongly suggests that *L. reuteri* 70902 and the SecA2-SecY2 system are key factors regulating biofilm production from *L. reuteri* 100-23 in germ-free mice (Frese et al., 2013). Another group investigated the role of two-component systems *bfrKRT* and *cemAKR* in *in vitro* biofilm formation of *L. reuteri* 100-23 (Su and Ganzle, 2014). They found the deletion of certain genes in the operons enhanced the adherence and biofilm formation. However, the contribution of the *bfrKRT* and *cemAKR* to *in vivo* biofilm formation remains to be elucidated. The role of exopolysaccharide (EPS) in assisting colonization was also examined with *L. reuteri* 100-23. The production of EPS was eliminated due to a mutation of the fructosyl transferase (*ftf*) gene (Sims et al., 2011). After administration to *Lactobacillus*-free mice, compared to the wild-type strain, the colonization of the *ftf* mutant in the forestomach and cecum was largely impaired. This indicates EPS production can enhance the colonizing ability of strain 100-23 in the gut. Interestingly, *L. reuteri* RC-14 has been demonstrated to be able to penetrate mature *E. coli* biofilm and become part of it (McMillan et al., 2011). Recently, *L. reuteri* was delivered as a biofilm on microsphere and such delivery was found to promote the adherence of *L. reuteri* to intestinal epithelium and enhance its probiotic property (Olson et al., 2016; Navarro et al., 2017).

Production of Metabolites With Health-Promoting Effect

The antimicrobial and immunomodulatory effects of *L. reuteri* strains are linked to their metabolite production profile. Here, we discuss a few well-studied metabolites with regard to the probiotic potential of *L. reuteri*.

Reuterin

Most *L. reuteri* strains of human and poultry lineage are able to produce and excrete reuterin, a well-known antimicrobial compound (Talarico et al., 1988; Talarico and Dobrogosz, 1989; Cadieux et al., 2008; Jones and Versalovic, 2009;

Mishra et al., 2012; Greifova et al., 2017). Reuterin is a mixture of different forms of 3-hydroxypropionaldehyde (3-HPA) (Talarico and Dobrogosz, 1989). It is known that *L. reuteri* can metabolize glycerol to generate 3-HPA in a coenzyme B12-dependent, glycerol dehydratase-mediated reaction (Talarico and Dobrogosz, 1990; Chen and Chen, 2013). The production of 3-HPA has also been demonstrated in a few other bacterial species (Zhu et al., 2002; Raynaud et al., 2003; Yang et al., 2007). However, *L. reuteri* is unique in its ability to produce and secrete 3-HPA in a manner more than its bioenergetics requirement (Stevens et al., 2011). Moreover, the antimicrobial activity of reuterin seems to rely on the spontaneous conversion of 3-HPA to acrolein, a cytotoxic electrophile (Stevens and Maier, 2008; Engels et al., 2016). Reuterin can inhibit a wide range of microorganisms, mainly Gram-negative bacteria (Cleusix et al., 2007). Not surprisingly, most *Lactobacillus* species are resistant to reuterin, among which *L. reuteri* strains exert the most resistance (Jones and Versalovic, 2009; Mishra et al., 2012). In addition to its antimicrobial property, reuterin is able to conjugate heterocyclic amines, which also seems to be dependent on the formation of acrolein (Engels et al., 2016). This suggests acrolein is an essential compound in the activity of reuterin.

Apart from reuterin, several other antimicrobial substances, including lactic acid, acetic acid, ethanol, and reutericyclin, have been determined as products of some *L. reuteri* strains (Ganzle and Vogel, 2003; Burge et al., 2015; Gopi et al., 2015; Yang Y. et al., 2015; Greifova et al., 2017). With the synthesis of these substances, *L. reuteri* has been shown to be effective against a variety of GI bacterial infections. These infections include *Helicobacter pylori, E. coli, Clostridium difficile*, and *Salmonella* (Reid and Burton, 2002; Cherian et al., 2015; Abhisingha et al., 2017; Genis et al., 2017). One of the more notable illustrations of the efficacy of *L. reuteri* as a probiotic against infections is the use of *L. reuteri* to treat *H. pylori. H. pylori* infection is a major cause of chronic gastritis and peptic ulcers, as well as a risk factor for gastric malignancies (Franceschi et al., 2007; Lesbros-Pantoflickova et al., 2007; Park et al., 2007). The use of *L. reuteri* against *H. pylori* has been explored in many studies (**Table 1**). It has been suggested that *L. reuteri* works by competing with *H. pylori* and inhibiting its binding to glycolipid receptors (Mukai et al., 2002). The competition reduces the bacterial load of *H. pylori* and decreases the related symptoms (Lionetti et al., 2006; Francavilla et al., 2008). Some studies have shown that *L. reuteri* has the potential to completely eradicate *H. pylori* from the intestine (Ojetti et al., 2012). Importantly, *L. reuteri* is advantageous in the treatment of *H.* pylori as the supplementation eradicates the pathogen without causing the common side effects associated with antibiotic therapies (Francavilla et al., 2014).

A considerable amount of research has been done to determine the beneficial effects of *L. reuteri* against viruses and/or fungi. There is evidence showing the benefit of *L. reuteri* against pneumoviruses, circoviruses, rotaviruses, coxsackieviruses, and papillomaviruses (Shornikova et al., 1997a,b; Preidis et al., 2012; Ang et al., 2016; Brenner et al., 2016; Piyathilake et al., 2016; Karaffova et al., 2017). It has been suggested that *L. reuteri* ameliorates viral infection by regulating the microbiota and secreting metabolites that have antiviral components (Ang et al., 2016). Furthermore, some studies suggest that *L. reuteri* may have antifungal properties as well, where *L. reuteri* antagonizes, stops the growth of, and eventually kills various species of Candida (Jorgensen et al., 2017).

Histamine

A few strains of *L. reuteri* are able to convert the amino acid L-histidine, a dietary component, to the biogenic amine histamine (Diaz et al., 2016; Greifova et al., 2017). A human commensal bacterium, *L. reuteri* 6475 was used as the model strain for studying histamine in *L. reuteri*. J. Versalovic's group reported that *L. reuteri* 6475-derived histamine suppressed tumor necrosis factor (TNF) production from stimulated human monocytes (Thomas et al., 2012). This suppression was dependent on the activation of histamine H_2 receptor, increased intracellular cAMP and protein kinase A, and the inhibition of MEK/ERK signaling. The production of histamine and subsequent *in vitro* TNF-suppressing function are regulated by a complete chromosomal histidine decarboxylase (*hdc*) gene cluster, which contains *hdcA*, *hdcB*, and *hdcP* (Rossi et al., 2011; Thomas et al., 2012). The same group of researchers also found that oral administration of hdc^+ *L. reuteri* could effectively suppress intestinal inflammation in a trinitrobenzene sulfonic acid (TNBS)-induced mouse colitis model (Gao et al., 2015). Moreover, intraperitoneal injection of *L. reuteri* 6475 culture supernatant to TNBS-treated mice resulted in similar colitis attenuation. These results strongly indicate the involvement of *L. reuteri* metabolites, including histamine, in intestinal immunomodulation (Thomas et al., 2016). Further investigations showed that a gene called *rsiR* was necessary for the expression of *hdc* gene cluster in *L. reuteri* 6475 (Hemarajata et al., 2013). Inactivation of *rsiR* gene led to reduced TNF inhibition *in vitro* and diminished anti-inflammatory function *in vivo*. Additionally, both the *in vitro* TNF suppression and the *in vivo* anti-colitis effects appear to be regulated by a gene named *folC2* (Thomas et al., 2016). Inactivation of *folC2* gene resulted in suppression of the *hdc* gene cluster and diminished histamine production. Notably, histamine production by *L. reuteri* is highly strain-dependent, and most studies have been focused on strains of human origin (Mishra et al., 2012).

Vitamins

There are 13 essential vitamins for humans due to the inability of the human body to synthesize them (Linares et al., 2017). Like many other *Lactobacillus* spp., several *L. reuteri* strains are able to produce different types of vitamins, including vitamin B12 (cobalamin) and B9 (folate). As mentioned earlier, B12 is vital in reuterin production because the reduction of glycerol to 3-HPA requires a B12-dependent coenzyme. Up to now, at least 4 *L. reuteri* strains with various origins have been found to produce B12 (Taranto et al., 2003; Santos et al., 2008b; Sriramulu et al., 2008; Gu et al., 2015). Among these strains, *L. reuteri* CRL1098 and *L. reuteri* JCM1112 are the most studied (Morita et al., 2008; Santos et al., 2008a, 2011). In one study, the administration of *L. reuteri* CRL1098 together with a diet lacking vitamin B12 was shown to ameliorate pathologies in B12-deficient pregnant

TABLE 1 | Clinical efficacies of *L. reuteri* against *H. pylori.*

Strain	Treatment	Subjects	Result	Citation
DSM 17648	14 days	Adults	Decrease in pathogen load in the stomach	Holz et al., 2015
DSM 17938	20 days	Patients	93% successful eradication of the pathogen with inhibitor-tetracycline-metronidazole – *L. reuteri* therapy	Dore et al., 2016
ATCC 55730	10 days	Infected children	Improvement of GI symptoms	Lionetti et al., 2006
–	7 days	Patients	No improvement of the standard triple therapy	Scaccianoce et al., 2008
ATCC 55730	4 weeks	Patients	Significant decrease of pathogen load and improvement of dyspeptic symptoms	Francavilla et al., 2008
SD2112	4 weeks	Patients	Decrease of pathogen density and suppression of urease activity	Imase et al., 2007
DSMZ 17648	14 days	Patients	Decrease in pathogen load	Mehling and Busjahn, 2013
DSM 17938, ATCC PTA 6475	During therapy	Patients	Reduction of antibiotic-associated side effects in eradication therapy	Francavilla et al., 2014
DSM 17938	8 weeks	Patients	Decrease of urease activity in pantoprazole therapy	Dore et al., 2014

female mice and their offspring (Molina et al., 2009). This clearly points to the potential application of *L. reuteri* in treating B12 deficiency. In addition to B12, folate can also be synthesized by some specific *L. reuteri* strains, including *L. reuteri* 6475 and *L. reuteri* JCM1112 (Santos et al., 2008b; Thomas et al., 2016).

Exopolysaccharide (EPS)

The EPS produced by *L. reuteri* is important for biofilm formation and adherence of *L. reuteri* to epithelial surfaces (Salas-Jara et al., 2016). In addition, EPS synthesized by *L. reuteri* is able to inhibit *E. coli* adhesion to porcine epithelial cells *in vitro* (Ksonzekova et al., 2016). More importantly, EPS-mediated blocking of adhesion also suppresses gene expression of pro-inflammatory cytokines that are induced by *E. coli* infection, including IL-1β and IL-6. Further *in vivo* experiments in piglets showed similar results in that EPS originated from *L. reuteri* prevented piglet diarrhea in bacterial infection by reducing the adhesion of *E. coli* (Chen et al., 2014). In addition, EPS of *L. reuteri* origin has been reported to suppress the binding of enterotoxigenic *E. coli* to porcine erythrocytes (Wang et al., 2010). EPS produced by rodent *L. reuteri* 100-23 was also demonstrated to induce Foxp3$^+$ regulatory T (Treg) cells in the spleen (Sims et al., 2011). In contrast, an *L. reuteri* 100-23 strain with the *ftf* mutation that eliminates EPS production from *L. reuteri* did not induce splenic Treg cells. This suggests that EPS is required for the *L. reuteri*-mediated induction of Treg cells and indicates the potential of using wild-type *L. reuteri* 100-23 to treat Treg deficiency.

L. reuteri-Mediated Modulation of Host Microbiota

Emerging evidence suggests that the host microbiota and immune system interact to maintain tissue homeostasis in healthy individuals (Kamada et al., 2013; Bene et al., 2017). Many diseases have been associated with perturbation of the microbiota (Mu et al., 2015), whereas restoration of the microbiota has been demonstrated to prevent or ameliorate several diseases (Scott et al., 2015). *L. reuteri* is able to influence the diversity, composition and metabolic function of the gut, oral, and vaginal microbiotas. These effects are largely strain-specific (Yang Y. et al., 2015; Garcia Rodenas et al., 2016; Galley et al., 2017; Su et al., 2017).

Gut Microbiota

Studies have shown the modulatory effects of *L. reuteri* on the microbiotas of rodents, piglets, and humans. One study assessed oral administration of a human-origin *L. reuteri* strain (DSM17938) to scurfy mice, which have gut microbial dysbiosis due to the *foxp3* gene mutation. The results indicated that this strain of *L. reuteri* was able to prolong the lifespan of the mice and reduce multi-organ inflammation while remodeling the gut microbiota (He et al., 2017). Changes of gut microbiota included increases in the phylum *Firmicutes* and the genera *Lactobacillus* and *Oscilospira*. Notably, the disease-ameliorating effect of *L. reuteri* was attributed to the remodeled gut microbiota, though the community composition was still distinct from wild-type littermates. Further investigation showed that inosine production was enhanced by the gut microbiota upon *L. reuteri* administration. Through adenosine A_{2A} receptor engagement, inosine can reduce Th1/Th2 cells and their associated cytokines. These results suggested that the *L. reuteri* – gut microbiota – inosine – adenosine A_{2A} receptor axis serves as a potential therapeutic method for Treg-deficient disorders. Moreover, oral *L. reuteri* 6475 treatment led to a higher diversity of microbiota in both jejunum and ileum in an ovariectomy-induced bone loss mouse model (Britton et al., 2014). Specifically, there were more abundant *Clostridiales* but less *Bacteriodales*. However, whether or not the changed gut microbiota was directly associated with the prevention of bone loss requires further investigation. Furthermore, *L. reuteri* C10-2-1 has been shown to modulate the diversity of gut microbiota in the ileum of rats (Wang P. et al., 2016).

Compared to vaginally delivered infants, Cesarean (C)-section delivered infants display a higher abundance of *Enterobacter* but less *Bifidobacterium* in their gut microbiota (Garcia Rodenas et al., 2016; Nagpal et al., 2016). In one study, treating C-section babies with *L. reuteri* DSM 17938 from 2 weeks to 4 months of age modulated the development of gut microbiota toward the community pattern found in vaginally delivered infants (Garcia Rodenas et al., 2016). The gut microbiota structure of vaginally born infants remained unaltered upon *L. reuteri* supplementation. In another study, treating infants with the same *L. reuteri* strain resulted in decreased anaerobic Gram-negative and increased Gram-positive bacterial counts in gut microbiota, whereas the abundances of *Enterobacteriaceae* and *Enterococci* were largely lowered by *L. reuteri* treatment (Savino et al., 2015b). The differences in infant age, duration of treatment, route of administration, and dosage may explain the differences in results from the two studies.

For human adults, *L. reuteri* NCIMB 30242 administered as delayed release capsules for 4 weeks was able to increase the ratio of *Firmicutes* to *Bacteroidetes* in healthy individuals (Martoni et al., 2015). This strain of *L. reuteri* is known to be able to activate bile salt hydrolase and its effect in increasing circulating bile acid has been reported (Jones et al., 2012b). The upregulation of circulating bile acid has been proposed as a reason for the modulated gut microbiota (Jones et al., 2012b). In type 2 diabetes patients, although 3 months of *L. reuteri* DSM 17938 supplementation did not significantly change the gut microbial structure, the disease outcome of *L. reuteri* treatment was highly correlated with the baseline gut microbiota structure of individuals (Mobini et al., 2017). Furthermore, the administration of *L. reuteri* DSM 17938 in cystic fibrosis (CF) patients rescued gut microbiota dysbiosis by reducing *Proteobacteria* while also enhancing the relative abundance of *Firmicutes* (del Campo et al., 2014). However, whether or not the modulated gut microbiota contributed to improved GI health in probiotic-treated CF patients needs to be explored further.

L. reuteri influences the gut microbial community in piglets in a strain-specific manner. For instance, oral *L. reuteri* ZLR003 administration was able to change both the diversity and the composition of the gut microbiota (Zhang et al., 2016). However, treatment with the I5007 strain did not affect colonic microbial structure in piglets (Liu H. et al., 2017). In another study, fodder fermented with *L. reuteri* changed the abundances of 6 different bacterial taxa, particularly the family *Enterobacteriacae*, in weanling pigs (Yang Y. et al., 2015). However, the major alterations including increased *Mitsuokella* and decreased a family under phylum *Bacteroidetes* could only be seen with *L. reuteri* TMW1.656 rather than *L. reuteri* LTH5794. TMW1.656 is a reutericyclin-producing strain while LTH5794 is not, suggesting the possible contribution of reutericyclin in modulating gut microbiota in piglets (Yang Y. et al., 2015).

Oral Microbiota

The phyla *Firmicutes, Bacteroidetes, Fusobacteria, Proteobacteria, and Actinobacteria* are most abundant in the human oral microbiome (Romani Vestman et al., 2015). In a randomized controlled trial, 12 weeks of daily consumption of two *L. reuteri* strains - DSM 17938 and PTA 5289 led to a shift in oral microbiota composition, though the bacterial species richness was not altered (Romani Vestman et al., 2015). The alterations disappeared 4 weeks after the treatments were terminated, suggesting the fast turnover of the oral microbiome. In another human study, oral *L. reuteri* treatment reduced the amount of periodontal pathogens in the subgingival microbiota, though no clinical impact was seen (Iniesta et al., 2012).

Vaginal Microbiota

Lactobacilli dominate the vaginal bacterial community in healthy women (Macklaim et al., 2015). One study showed that only 14 days of oral *L. reuteri* RC-14 administration could restore the normal vaginal flora in postmenopausal women (Petricevic et al., 2008). Interestingly, the relative abundance of *Lactobacilli* is largely decreased in bacterial vaginosis patients (Macklaim et al., 2015). A total of 4 weeks of oral capsule consumption of two *Lactobacilli* strains including *L. reuteri* RC-14 increased the relative abundance of *Lactobacilli*. A similar increase of *Lactobacilli* was seen when *L. reuteri* RC-14 was administered vaginally together with a *L. rhamnosus* strain (Bisanz et al., 2014). However, in pregnant women, 8 weeks of oral *L. reuteri* RC-14 treatment did not efficiently restore the normal vaginal microbiota (Gille et al., 2016). This suggests that *L. reuteri* RC-14 may not be able to act alone.

Role of *L. reuteri* in Immunomodulation

Lactobacillus reuteri is able to increase free secretory IgA (sIgA) levels in rats (Wang P. et al., 2016). However, the upregulation of sIgA was eliminated in vitamin A-deficient rats, suggesting that *L. reuteri* functions in a vitamin A-dependent manner. In pregnant women, the intake of *L. reuteri* did not alter the levels of total IgA or sIgA in breast milk (Bottcher et al., 2008). When it comes to the effect of *L. reuteri* in inducing salivary IgA, the results are controversial. Increased salivary IgA levels were reported in humans' chewing gum containing *L. reuteri* (Ericson et al., 2013). However, other studies showed that *L. reuteri* did not affect IgA concentration in saliva (Garofoli et al., 2014; Jorgensen et al., 2016; Braathen et al., 2017). The difference in the strains of *L. reuteri* used in the studies may explain the difference in results. Notably, an important commonality is that salivary *L. reuteri*-positive individuals have higher salivary IgA levels. Whether *L. reuteri* affects IgA levels by directly regulating B cells requires further investigations.

Many studies have shown that *L. reuteri* can induce anti-inflammatory Treg cells, which likely contributes to the beneficial effects of *L. reuteri* in a wide range of diseased and non-diseased conditions (**Table 2**). The Treg-inducing property of *L. reuteri* is largely strain-dependent. However, the anti-inflammatory effect of *L. reuteri* does not always rely on the induction of Treg cells. A good example is *L. reuteri*-mediated suppression of Th1/Th2 responses in Treg-deficient mice (He et al., 2017). Certain *L. reuteri* strains are able to reduce the production of many pro-inflammatory cytokines. For example, *L. reuteri* GMNL-263 can reduce serum MCP-1, TNF, and IL-6 levels in mice fed with high fat diet (Hsieh et al., 2016). Similar effects were observed in mice treated with heat-killed

TABLE 2 | *L. reuteri*-mediated induction of Treg cells under various diseased and non-diseased conditions.

Condition	Subject	Tissue	Strain	Citation
Western-diet-associated obesity	Mouse	MLN	ATCC PTA 6475	Poutahidis et al., 2013b
Wound healing	Mouse	Biopsy	ATCC PTA 6475	Poutahidis et al., 2013a
Systemic lupus erythematosus	Mouse	Kidney	ATCC PTA 6475	Mu et al., 2017c
Necrotizing enterocolitis	Mouse	Intestine, MLN	DSM 17938	Liu et al., 2013, 2014
Wild-type	Mouse	MLN, Spleen	100-23	Livingston et al., 2010; Sims et al., 2011
Wild-type	Mouse	Spleen	ATCC 23272	Karimi et al., 2009
Wild-type, IBD, atopic dermatitis	Mouse	MLN, Colon, Ear	–	Abediankenari and Ghasemi, 2009
IBD	Human	Peripheral blood	RC-14	Lorea Baroja et al., 2007

IBD, inflammatory bowel disease; MLN, mesenteric lymph node.

GMNL-263. However, in some cases, the immunomodulatory effects of *L. reuteri* appear to rely on its metabolites, as the culture supernatant of *L. reuteri* BM36301 could reduce TNF production from human myeloid THP-1 cells (Lee et al., 2016). Interestingly, tryptophan catabolites of *L. reuteri* have been recognized as ligands for aryl hydrocarbon receptor (AhR). Through activating AhR, *L. reuteri* can promote local IL-22 production from innate lymphoid cells (ILCs) (Zelante et al., 2013). In addition, the derivatives of tryptophan generated by *L. reuteri* can induce the development of regulatory $CD4^+CD8\alpha\alpha^+$ double-positive intraepithelial lymphocytes in an AhR-dependent manner (Cervantes-Barragan et al., 2017). Considering that AhR is ubiquitously expressed, *L. reuteri* and its metabolites may be able to influence many more types of immune cells beyond ILCs and T cells (Nguyen et al., 2013).

Neuromodulatory Capability of *L. reuteri*

The intestinal microbiota plays a role in the functions of the enteric nervous system (ENS) (Yoo and Mazmanian, 2017). Subjects with microbiota depletion exhibit an abnormal ENS state (Anitha et al., 2012; Brun et al., 2013, 2015; Yoo and Mazmanian, 2017). Antibiotic treatment reduces the number of neurons in the ENS. This may be related to the decrease in Glial cell line-derived neurotrophic factor (GDNF), which can be restored by TLR2 stimulation (Brun et al., 2013). Moreover, germ-free animals show defective ENS morphology and excitability, which can be reversed by microbiota colonization (McVey Neufeld et al., 2013; Collins et al., 2014). *L. reuteri*, specifically, can prevent visceral pain response mainly by reducing the enteric nerve activity during the colorectal distension pressure in mice (Kamiya et al., 2006; Ma et al., 2009). Interestingly, live, heat-killed, gamma-irradiated *L. reuteri*, or even the conditioned media all had a similar effect (Kamiya et al., 2006). *L. reuteri* can also produce gamma-aminobutyric acid (GABA), the major inhibitory neurotransmitter in the central nervous system (Su et al., 2011; Barrett et al., 2012; Pallin et al., 2016). However, the *in vivo* bioactivity of the produced GABA has not been addressed (Yoo and Mazmanian, 2017). Furthermore, *L. reuteri* can increase the excitability and the number of action potentials in rat colonic sensory neurons (Kunze et al., 2009). These distinct effects of *L. reuteri* may be due to the difference in target neurons (Lai et al., 2017).

Role of *L. reuteri* in Reversing the Leaky Gut

Physical, biochemical, and immunological barriers comprise the gut barrier function, which is required to block the entry of exterior antigens and toxins (Mu et al., 2017a). If any abnormalities occur in the intestinal barrier, the permeability may increase resulting in a leaky gut. Various probiotics are known for their abilities to enhance mucosal barrier function, of which *L. reuteri* is a well-known example (Mu et al., 2017a). In DSS-induced colitis, *L. reuteri* administration could reduce bacterial translocation from the GI tract to the mesenteric lymph nodes (MLN) (Dicksved et al., 2012). In addition, treatment of lupus-prone mice with a mixture of *Lactobacillus* species including *L. reuteri* led to a higher expression of tight junction (TJ) proteins in intestinal epithelial cells (Mu et al., 2017c). Subsequently, the translocation of pro-inflammatory molecules such as LPS was significantly suppressed, which correlated with attenuated disease. In addition to mouse studies, several strains of *L. reuteri* have been shown to possess the ability to modulate TJ protein expression and maintain intestinal barrier integrity in pigs (Yang F. et al., 2015; Wang Z. et al., 2016). Moreover, the ability of *L. reuteri* to decrease intestinal permeability has been seen in humans. In children with atopic dermatitis, where the impairment of intestinal barrier function has been positively correlated with disease pathogenesis (De Benedetto et al., 2011), treatment with *L. reuteri* DSM 12246 (and *L. rhamnosus* 19070-2) significantly reduced the frequency of GI symptoms while decreasing the lactulose to mannitol ratio (Rosenfeldt et al., 2004), which reflects the reversal of a leaky gut (Camilleri et al., 2010).

L. reuteri ATTENUATE HUMAN DISEASES

A growing body of evidences links microbiota and bacterial translocation with multiple diseases, including several autoimmune disorders (Mu et al., 2015, 2017a). Due to its strong modulatory effects on host microbiota and immune responses with almost no safety concerns, *L. reuteri* is a good candidate for disease prevention and/or treatment. Indeed, the therapeutic potential of various *L. reuteri* strains has been studied in diverse diseases and the results are promising in many cases.

TABLE 3 | Effects of *L. reuteri* on early-life diseases.

Target	Strain	Duration	Subjects	Result	Citation
Early caries lesions	DSM 17938, ATCC PTA 5289	3 months	Adolescent	No significant change in fluorescence or lesion area	Keller et al., 2014
Caries	ATCC 55730	First year life	Infants	Reduced prevalence of caries and gingivitis score when the kids were 9 years old	Stensson et al., 2014
FAP	DSM 17938	4 weeks	FAP children	Significant decrease in the frequency and intensity of functional abdominal pain	Weizman et al., 2016
FAP	DSM 17938	4 weeks	FAP children	Significant reduction of pain intensity	Romano et al., 2014
Infectious diarrhea	DSM 17938	5 days	Children	Safe and well-tolerated; decreased duration of diarrhea	Dinleyici et al., 2015
Rotavirus diarrhea	-	Up to 5 days	Young children	Shortened diarrhea duration and large decrease in the occurrence of watery diarrhea	Shornikova et al., 1997a,b
Nosocomial diarrhea	DSM 17938	During hospital stay	Children	No effect on the overall incidence of diarrhea, including that related to rotavirus infection	Wanke and Szajewska, 2012
Acute diarrhea	DSM 12246 (with 19070-2)	5 days	Children patients	Decreased duration of diarrhea; decreased period of rotavirus excretion	Rosenfeldt et al., 2002a,b
Acute diarrhea	DSM 17938	3 days	Children	Decrease in diarrhea frequency, duration, and relapse	Francavilla et al., 2012
Acute diarrhea	DSM 17938	5 days	Hospitalized children	Effective decrease of the duration of acute diarrhea	Dinleyici et al., 2014
Diarrhea	ATCC 55730	12 weeks	Infants	Fewer and shorter diarrhea episodes	Weizman et al., 2005
Diarrhea	DSM 17938	6 months	Children	Reduced incidence of diarrhea	Agustina et al., 2012
Diarrhea	DSM 17938	3 months	Children	Decrease in diarrhea episodes and duration; Benefits against respiratory infection	Gutierrez-Castrellon et al., 2014
Infant colic	DSM 17938	3 weeks	Breastfed infants	Significant reduction in crying time	Mi et al., 2015
Infant colic	DSM 17938	3 weeks	Breastfed infants	Reduction in crying and fussing time	Chau et al., 2015
Infant colic	DSM 17938	12 weeks	Newborns	Effective preventive and protective action	Savino et al., 2015a
Infant colic	ATCC 55730	28 days	Breastfed infants	Significantly improvement of colicky symptoms compared with simethicone	Savino et al., 2007
Infant colic	DSM 17938	21 days	Breastfed infants	Improved symptoms; Increase of *Lactobacilli* increase and decrease of *E. coli* in the fecal microbiota	Savino et al., 2010
Infant colic	DSM 17938	21 days	Colicky infants	No effect on the global microbiota composition	Roos et al., 2013
Infant colic	DSM 17938	21 days	Breastfed infants	Higher rate of responders and reduced median crying time	Szajewska et al., 2013
Infant colic	DSM 17938	1 month	Infants	No effect on crying time	Sung et al., 2014
Infant colic	DSM 17938	90 days	Infants	Significant reduction of the mean crying time	Indrio et al., 2014
Infant growth	DSM 17938	98 days	Healthy infants	Well-tolerated but no improvement on growth	Cekola et al., 2015
Atopic dermatitis	DSM 122460 (with 19070-2)	6 weeks	AD children	Improvement of eczema; more pronounced in allergic patients	Rosenfeldt et al., 2003, 2004
Atopic dermatitis	ATCC 55730	8 weeks	AD children	Positive modulation of cytokine pattern in the exhaled breath condensate	Miniello et al., 2010
Eczema	ATCC 55730	−1 to 12 month old	Infants with family Allergic history	No protection of the general occurrence of eczema; Prevention of IgE-associated eczema	Abrahamsson et al., 2007

(Continued)

TABLE 3 | Continued

Target	Strain	Duration	Subjects	Result	Citation
GI motility	-	30 days	Newborns	Faster gastric emptying	Indrio et al., 2009
Respiratory allergy	ATCC 55730	−1 to 12 month old	Infants	No effect on the prevalence of asthma, eczema or other allergic diseases later in life	Abrahamsson et al., 2013
Feeding intolerance	DSM 17938	Until out of NICU	Preterm infants	Decrease in feeding intolerance and duration of hospitalization	Rojas et al., 2012
Necrotising enterocolitis	DSM 17938	Until discharge	Preterm infants	No effect on NEC rate; Decrease in feeding intolerance and duration of hospital stay	Oncel et al., 2014
Regurgitation	DSM 17938	28 days	Infants	Prevention of regurgitation during the first month of life	Garofoli et al., 2014
Regurgitation	DSM 17938	90 days	Infants	Significant reduction of the mean number of regurgitation	Indrio et al., 2014

FAP, functional abdominal pain; NICU, neonatal intensive care unit; NEC, necrotising enterocolitis.

Early-Life Disorders

Taking advantage of the safety and tolerance of *L. reuteri* in infants and young children, a lot of efforts have been made to test the potential application of *L. reuteri* against disorders early in life (**Table 3**). In general, the results are promising. *L. reuteri* has been demonstrated beneficial in the prevention and/or treatment of many conditions including diarrhea, functional abdominal pain, caries, atopic dermatitis, allergy, feeding intolerance, and regurgitation. Infant colic, for example, has been the major therapeutic target of *L. reuteri* (**Table 3**). Infant colic is characterized by immoderate crying and affects 10–30% infants (Mi et al., 2015). The exact cause and efficient treatment of this condition have remained elusive. The clinical efficacy of *L. reuteri* DSM 17938 has been demonstrated as most of the clinical trials were successful (**Table 3**). The failure of some studies may be explained by the differences in the dosage of *L. reuteri*, the infant age when the studies initiated, or the baseline microbiota structure. It is worth mentioning that *L. reuteri* is naturally contained in human breast milk (Soto et al., 2014), though inconsistencies exist among individuals. The presence of *L. reuteri* in milk may complicate the results of studies that involved breastfeeding. When given during pregnancy, *L. reuteri* did not show a significant effect on allergy and eczema in infants after they were born (**Table 3**).

Systemic Lupus Erythematosus

The SLE is a multi-system autoimmune disease that involves both genetics and environment as the major disease causative factors (Tsokos, 2011; Edwards et al., 2017). The role of gut microbiota in SLE development was suggested by recent studies, and probiotics have been proposed as potential immunoregulators in SLE (Mu et al., 2015, 2017b; de Oliveira et al., 2017; Edwards et al., 2017; Esmaeili et al., 2017). We reported a significantly decreased level of *Lactobacillaceae* in lupus-prone MRL/lpr female mice compared to healthy control mice both before and after the disease initiated in MRL/lpr mice (Zhang et al., 2014). Moreover, we found that treatment with retinoic acid improved kidney disease in MRL/lpr mice, and that the improvement of lupus symptoms was associated with restoration of *Lactobacilli*. This suggests a possible beneficial effect of *Lactobacilli* in lupus. Therefore, we treated MRL/lpr mice with a mixture of five strains of *Lactobacilli* to determine their therapeutic benefit. As anticipated, increasing *Lactobacilli* in the gut improved renal function, reduced serum autoantibodies, and prolonged the survival of MRL/lpr mice (Mu et al., 2017c). Interestingly, *L. reuteri* and an uncultured *Lactobacillus* sp. accounted for > 99% of the observed effects. It suggests a central role of *L. reuteri* in attenuating lupus nephritis. Furthermore, we found that MRL/lpr mice had a "leaky" gut during disease progression, whereas *Lactobacillus* treatment enhanced the intestinal barrier function in these mice and subsequently decreased metabolic endotoxemia (Mu et al., 2017c). At the same time, the local and systemic pro- and anti-inflammatory network was rebalanced by *Lactobacillus* treatment. Specifically, IL-10 production was enhanced while the level of IL-6 was decreased systemically. Strikingly, the benefits of *Lactobacilli* were only observed in females and castrated males but not in intact males. Coincidently, the relative abundance of *Lactobacilli* in gut microbiota did not decrease as disease progressed in male MRL/lpr mice (Zhang et al., 2014). Consistent with our observations, daily consumption of *L. reuteri* BM36301 significantly lowered serum TNF level in females but not in males (Lee et al., 2016). The high serum level of testosterone in males may have led to the difference in the response to *L. reuteri*. Together, these results suggest possible interaction between sex hormones and gut microbiota in autoimmune disease development (Markle et al., 2013; Yurkovetskiy et al., 2013). Further investigation of this link is required. In another lupus mouse model, NZB/W F1, the administration of two *L. reuteri* strains, together with one *L. paracasei* strain, was shown to be effective in ameliorating lupus hepatitis (Hsu et al., 2017). Liver abnormalities, manifested as increased liver enzymes, portal inflammation and histopathological changes, have been observed in both lupus mouse models and SLE patients (Hsu et al., 2008; Grover et al., 2014). In this study, the oral *L. reuteri* treatment largely mitigated hepatic apoptosis and inflammation, suggesting a protective function of *L. reuteri* against lupus-associated liver disease (Hsu et al., 2017). The protection seems to rely on the capability of *L. reuteri* to increase antioxidant activity and reduce cytokines associated with more severe lupus, such as IL-6 and TNF (Tzang et al., 2017). Interestingly, within these two *L. reuteri* strains, only GMNL-263 can significantly promote the differentiation of Treg cells, again emphasizing the uneven immunoregulatory abilities of different *L. reuteri* strains.

Obesity

The correlation between gut microbiota and obesity is well documented (Okeke et al., 2014; Harakeh et al., 2016). The microbiota composition varies between lean and obese individuals, and a surprisingly high level of *Lactobacillus* spp. has been found in the microbiota of both obese adults and obese children (Armougom et al., 2009; Bervoets et al., 2013). Among different *Lactobacillus* spp., *L. reuteri* was specifically described to be associated with obesity (Million et al., 2012, 2013a). The association was further established when vancomycin-resistant *L. reuteri* in gut microbiota was determined as a body weight gain predictor during vancomycin treatment (Million et al., 2013b). However, in a randomized, double-blind and placebo-controlled clinical trial, the administration of *L. reuteri* JBD301 for 12 weeks significantly reduced body weight in overweight adults (Chung et al., 2016). Moreover, supplementation of infant formula with *L. reuteri* did not increase weight gain in infants (Braegger et al., 2011; Koleva et al., 2015). These conflicting results indicate that *L. reuteri* may influence the development of obesity in a strain-dependent manner. This hypothesis is partially verified in an animal study. In that study, three different strains of *L. reuteri* were used to test their influence on diet-induced obesity (Fåk and Bäckhed, 2012). It was demonstrated that only *L. reuteri* PTA 4659 efficiently reduced the body weight of mice fed with high-fat diet (HFD), whereas *L. reuteri* L6798-treated mice even gained some weight. The changes of adipose and liver weights were consistent with the body weight change.

In animal studies, several strains of *L. reuteri* have been reported to negatively regulate the development of obesity (Dahiya et al., 2017). In addition to the beneficial effect of *L. reuteri* JBD301 to human obese patients mentioned earlier, the favorable role of this strain of *L. reuteri* against weight gain was confirmed in HFD-fed mice (Chung et al., 2016). In HFD-induced obese mouse models, the beneficial role of *L. reuteri* GMNL-263 was also noted (Hsieh et al., 2016). Treatment with *L. reuteri* GMNL-263 reduced the body weight as well as the percentages of adipose tissue and liver to body weight. Interestingly, heat-killed GMNL-263 appeared to have a very similar beneficial function (Hsieh et al., 2016; Liao et al., 2016). *L. reuteri* 6475 has also been shown to be beneficial against obesity in mice (Poutahidis et al., 2013b). The function of *L. reuteri* 6475 was suggested to be largely dependent on its capability to induce Treg cells without changing the gut microbial ecology. Furthermore, the weight loss properties of some reagents have been attributed to their abilities to increase *L. reuteri* in mice. Polymannuronic acid, for example, was able to increase the relative abundance of *L. reuteri* and significantly reduce HFD-induced body weight gain (Liu F. et al., 2017). Whether the increase of *L. reuteri* is the cause of weight loss requires further investigation.

Neurodevelopmental Disorder

Exposure to maternal obesity *in utero* increases the chance of neurodevelopmental disorders, such as autism spectrum disorder, in children (Connolly et al., 2016). In a recent mouse study, maternal HFD (MHFD) was shown to induce social deficits in the offspring (Buffington et al., 2016). The impaired social ability in GF mice was restored by fecal microbiota transplantation from offspring with maternal regular diet (MRD) but not MHFD, suggesting a potential role of microbiota in this process. Further analysis showed that the abundance of *L. reuteri* was reduced more than ninefold in the gut microbiome of MHFD vs. MRD offspring. The social defects in MHFD offspring were rescued by direct *L. reuteri* administration, suggesting an effect of *L. reuteri* in regulating neurodevelopment in MHFD mice. This regulatory function of *L. reuteri* was attributed to its capability to increase the level of oxytocin (Poutahidis et al., 2013a; Buffington et al., 2016). The results of these studies suggest a potential application of *L. reuteri* in the treatment of patients who suffer from neurodevelopmental disorders.

Stressor Exposure and Enteric Infection

The composition of gut microbiota shift when the host is exposed to stressors (Bailey et al., 2010; Galley et al., 2014). In C57BL/6 males, social stressors led to an altered intestinal microbiota composition, though there was no significant change in community diversity (Galley et al., 2014). Further analysis showed stressor-induced reductions in the families *Porphyromonadaceae* and *Lactobacillaceae*, especially in the genus *Lactobacillus*. Among *Lactobacillus spp.*, *L. reuteri* was specifically measured and a lower abundance of *L. reuteri* was evident in stressor-exposed CD-1 mice but not C57BL/6 mice. In fact, the level of *L. reuteri* in C57BL/6 male mice was below the detection limit with or without stressor exposure (Galley et al., 2014). It is important to note that stressor exposure increased the severity of *Citrobacter rodentium*-induced inflammation in the gut (Bailey et al., 2010; Mackos et al., 2016). The colonization of *C. rodentium* was promoted by stressor exposure, which subsequently resulted in more severe colonic pathology and increased production of inflammatory cytokines and chemokines (Mackos et al., 2016). Further studies revealed that stressor-induced *C. rodentium* colitis was C-C motif chemokine ligand 2 (CCL2)-dependent. Interestingly, administration of *L. reuteri* ATCC 23272 was able to reverse stressor-induced *C. rodentium* infection, which also relied on CCL2 (Mackos et al., 2013, 2016). However, *L. reuteri* was not able to restore the gut microbiome altered by social stressors. This indicates that the beneficial effect of *L. reuteri* on stressor exposure and subsequent enteric infection is not microbiota-dependent (Galley et al., 2017).

CONCLUSION

There has been a decrease in the abundance of *L. reuteri* in humans in the past few decades likely caused by the modern lifestyle (Antibiotic use, western diet, improved hygiene). Such decrease coincides with higher incidences of inflammatory diseases over the same period of time. While evidence is lacking to establish the correlation, it may be helpful to increase *L. reuteri* colonization and/or facilitate its probiotic functions as a new and relatively safe strategy against inflammatory diseases. In addition, through direct regulation or indirect modulation via the host microbiota, *L. reuteri* plays an impressive role in eliminating infections and attenuating both GI diseases and diseases in remote tissues. The safety and tolerance of *L. reuteri* has been proven by the numerous clinical studies. There are multiple *L. reuteri* strains with different host origins, and many of the probiotic functions of *L. reuteri* are strain-dependent. Therefore, it may be advantageous to combine different strains of *L. reuteri* to maximize their beneficial effects.

AUTHOR CONTRIBUTIONS

QM and VT wrote the first draft of the review. XL edited and finalized the manuscript.

FUNDING

This work was funded by NIH R15AR067418 and R01AR073240.

REFERENCES

Abediankenari, S., and Ghasemi, M. (2009). Generation of immune inhibitory dendritic cells and CD4+T regulatory cells inducing by TGF-beta. *Iran. J. Allergy Asthma Immunol.* 8, 25–30.

Abhisingha, M., Dumnil, J., and Pitaksutheepong, C. (2017). Selection of potential probiotic *Lactobacillus* with inhibitory activity against *Salmonella* and fecal coliform bacteria. *Probiotics Antimicrob. Proteins* doi: 10.1007/s12602-017-9304-8 [Epub ahead of print].

Abrahamsson, T. R., Jakobsson, T., Bjorksten, B., Oldaeus, G., and Jenmalm, M. C. (2013). No effect of probiotics on respiratory allergies: a seven-year follow-up of a randomized controlled trial in infancy. *Pediatr. Allergy Immunol.* 24, 556–561. doi: 10.1111/pai.12104

Abrahamsson, T. R., Jakobsson, T., Bottcher, M. F., Fredrikson, M., Jenmalm, M. C., Bjorksten, B., et al. (2007). Probiotics in prevention of IgE-associated eczema: a double-blind, randomized, placebo-controlled trial. *J. Allergy Clin. Immunol.* 119, 1174–1180. doi: 10.1016/j.jaci.2007.01.007

Agustina, R., Kok, F. J., van de Rest, O., Fahmida, U., Firmansyah, A., Lukito, W., et al. (2012). Randomized trial of probiotics and calcium on diarrhea and respiratory tract infections in Indonesian children. *Pediatrics* 129, e1155–e1164. doi: 10.1542/peds.2011-1379

Amara, A. A., and Shibl, A. (2015). Role of probiotics in health improvement, infection control and disease treatment and management. *Saudi Pharm. J.* 23, 107–114. doi: 10.1016/j.jsps.2013.07.001

Ang, L. Y., Too, H. K., Tan, E. L., Chow, T. K., Shek, P. C., Tham, E., et al. (2016). Antiviral activity of *Lactobacillus reuteri* Protectis against Coxsackievirus A and Enterovirus 71 infection in human skeletal muscle and colon cell lines. *Virol. J.* 13:111. doi: 10.1186/s12985-016-0567-6

Anitha, M., Vijay-Kumar, M., Sitaraman, S. V., Gewirtz, A. T., and Srinivasan, S. (2012). Gut microbial products regulate murine gastrointestinal motility via Toll-like receptor 4 signaling. *Gastroenterology* 143, 1006.e4–1016.e4. doi: 10.1053/j.gastro.2012.06.034

Armougom, F., Henry, M., Vialettes, B., Raccah, D., and Raoult, D. (2009). Monitoring bacterial community of human gut microbiota reveals an increase in *Lactobacillus* in obese patients and *Methanogens* in anorexic patients. *PLoS One* 4:e7125. doi: 10.1371/journal.pone.0007125

Bailey, M. T., Dowd, S. E., Parry, N. M., Galley, J. D., Schauer, D. B., and Lyte, M. (2010). Stressor exposure disrupts commensal microbial populations in the intestines and leads to increased colonization by *Citrobacter rodentium*. *Infect. Immun.* 78, 1509–1519. doi: 10.1128/IAI.00862-09

Barrett, E., Ross, R. P., O'Toole, P. W., Fitzgerald, G. F., and Stanton, C. (2012). gamma-Aminobutyric acid production by culturable bacteria from the human intestine. *J. Appl. Microbiol.* 113, 411–417. doi: 10.1111/j.1365-2672.2012.05344.x

Bene, K., Varga, Z., Petrov, V. O., Boyko, N., and Rajnavolgyi, E. (2017). Gut microbiota species can provoke both inflammatory and tolerogenic immune responses in human dendritic cells mediated by retinoic acid receptor alpha ligation. *Front. Immunol.* 8:427. doi: 10.3389/fimmu.2017.00427

Bervoets, L., Van Hoorenbeeck, K., Kortleven, I., Van Noten, C., Hens, N., Vael, C., et al. (2013). Differences in gut microbiota composition between obese and lean children: a cross-sectional study. *Gut Pathog.* 5:10. doi: 10.1186/1757-4749-5-10

Bisanz, J. E., Seney, S., McMillan, A., Vongsa, R., Koenig, D., Wong, L., et al. (2014). A systems biology approach investigating the effect of probiotics on the vaginal microbiome and host responses in a double blind, placebo-controlled clinical trial of post-menopausal women. *PLoS One* 9:e104511. doi: 10.1371/journal.pone.0104511

Bottcher, M. F., Abrahamsson, T. R., Fredriksson, M., Jakobsson, T., and Bjorksten, B. (2008). Low breast milk TGF-beta2 is induced by *Lactobacillus reuteri* supplementation and associates with reduced risk of sensitization during infancy. *Pediatr. Allergy Immunol.* 19, 497–504. doi: 10.1111/j.1399-3038.2007.00687.x

Braathen, G., Ingildsen, V., Twetman, S., Ericson, D., and Jorgensen, M. R. (2017). Presence of *Lactobacillus reuteri* in saliva coincide with higher salivary IgA in young adults after intake of probiotic lozenges. *Benef. Microbes* 8, 17–22. doi: 10.3920/BM2016.0081

Braegger, C., Chmielewska, A., Decsi, T., Kolacek, S., Mihatsch, W., Moreno, L., et al. (2011). Supplementation of infant formula with probiotics and/or prebiotics: a systematic review and comment by the ESPGHAN committee on nutrition. *J. Pediatr. Gastroenterol. Nutr.* 52, 238–250. doi: 10.1097/MPG.0b013e3181fb9e80

Brenner, T. A., Rice, T. A., Anderson, E. D., Percopo, C. M., and Rosenberg, H. F. (2016). Immortalized MH-S cells lack defining features of primary alveolar macrophages and do not support mouse pneumovirus replication. *Immunol. Lett.* 172, 106–112. doi: 10.1016/j.imlet.2016.02.012

Britton, R. A., Irwin, R., Quach, D., Schaefer, L., Zhang, J., Lee, T., et al. (2014). Probiotic *L. reuteri* treatment prevents bone loss in a menopausal ovariectomized mouse model. *J. Cell. Physiol.* 229, 1822–1830. doi: 10.1002/jcp.24636

Brun, P., Giron, M. C., Qesari, M., Porzionato, A., Caputi, V., Zoppellaro, C., et al. (2013). Toll-like receptor 2 regulates intestinal inflammation by controlling integrity of the enteric nervous system. *Gastroenterology* 145, 1323–1333. doi: 10.1053/j.gastro.2013.08.047

Brun, P., Gobbo, S., Caputi, V., Spagnol, L., Schirato, G., Pasqualin, M., et al. (2015). Toll like receptor-2 regulates production of glial-derived neurotrophic factors in murine intestinal smooth muscle cells. *Mol. Cell. Neurosci.* 68, 24–35. doi: 10.1016/j.mcn.2015.03.018

Buffington, S. A., Di Prisco, G. V., Auchtung, T. A., Ajami, N. J., Petrosino, J. F., and Costa-Mattioli, M. (2016). Microbial reconstitution reverses maternal diet-induced social and synaptic deficits in offspring. *Cell* 165, 1762–1775. doi: 10.1016/j.cell.2016.06.001

Burge, G., Saulou-Berion, C., Moussa, M., Pollet, B., Flourat, A., Allais, F., et al. (2015). Diversity of *Lactobacillus reuteri* strains in converting glycerol into 3-hydroxypropionic acid. *Appl. Biochem. Biotechnol.* 177, 923–939. doi: 10.1007/s12010-015-1787-8

Cadieux, P., Wind, A., Sommer, P., Schaefer, L., Crowley, K., Britton, R. A., et al. (2008). Evaluation of reuterin production in urogenital probiotic *Lactobacillus reuteri* RC-14. *Appl. Environ. Microbiol.* 74, 4645–4649. doi: 10.1128/AEM.00139-08

Camilleri, M., Nadeau, A., Lamsam, J., Nord, S. L., Ryks, M., Burton, D., et al. (2010). Understanding measurements of intestinal permeability in healthy humans with urine lactulose and mannitol excretion. *Neurogastroenterol. Motil.* 22, e15–e26. doi: 10.1111/j.1365-2982.2009.01361.x

Cekola, P. L., Czerkies, L. A., Storm, H. M., Wang, M. H., Roberts, J., and Saavedra, J. M. (2015). Growth and tolerance of term infants fed formula with probiotic *Lactobacillus reuteri*. *Clin. Pediatr.* 54, 1175–1184. doi: 10.1177/0009922815574076

Cervantes-Barragan, L., Chai, J. N., Tianero, M. D., Di Luccia, B., Ahern, P. P., Merriman, J., et al. (2017). *Lactobacillus reuteri* induces gut intraepithelial CD4$^+$CD8alphaalpha$^+$ T cells. *Science* 357, 806–810. doi: 10.1126/science.aah5825

Chau, K., Lau, E., Greenberg, S., Jacobson, S., Yazdani-Brojeni, P., Verma, N., et al. (2015). Probiotics for infantile colic: a randomized, double-blind, placebo-controlled trial investigating *Lactobacillus reuteri* DSM 17938. *J. Pediatr.* 166, 74–78. doi: 10.1016/j.jpeds.2014.09.020

Chen, G., and Chen, J. (2013). A novel cell modification method used in biotransformation of glycerol to 3-HPA by *Lactobacillus reuteri*. *Appl. Microbiol. Biotechnol.* 97, 4325–4332. doi: 10.1007/s00253-013-4723-2

Chen, X. Y., Woodward, A., Zijlstra, R. T., and Ganzle, M. G. (2014). Exopolysaccharides synthesized by *Lactobacillus reuteri* protect against enterotoxigenic *Escherichia coli* in piglets. *Appl. Environ. Microbiol.* 80, 5752–5760. doi: 10.1128/AEM.01782-14

Cherian, P. T., Wu, X., Yang, L., Scarborough, J. S., Singh, A. P., Alam, Z. A., et al. (2015). Gastrointestinal localization of metronidazole by a lactobacilli-inspired tetramic acid motif improves treatment outcomes in the hamster model of *Clostridium difficile* infection. *J. Antimicrob. Chemother.* 70, 3061–3069. doi: 10.1093/jac/dkv231

Chung, H. J., Yu, J. G., Lee, I. A., Liu, M. J., Shen, Y. F., Sharma, S. P., et al. (2016). Intestinal removal of free fatty acids from hosts by *Lactobacilli* for the treatment of obesity. *FEBS Open Bio* 6, 64–76. doi: 10.1002/2211-5463.12024

Cleusix, V., Lacroix, C., Vollenweider, S., Duboux, M., and Le Blay, G. (2007). Inhibitory activity spectrum of reuterin produced by *Lactobacillus reuteri* against intestinal bacteria. *BMC Microbiol.* 7:101. doi: 10.1186/1471-2180-7-101

Collins, J., Borojevic, R., Verdu, E. F., Huizinga, J. D., and Ratcliffe, E. M. (2014). Intestinal microbiota influence the early postnatal development of the enteric nervous system. *Neurogastroenterol. Motil.* 26, 98–107. doi: 10.1111/nmo.12236

Connolly, N., Anixt, J., Manning, P., Ping-I Lin, D., Marsolo, K. A., and Bowers, K. (2016). Maternal metabolic risk factors for autism spectrum disorder-An analysis of electronic medical records and linked birth data. *Autism Res.* 9, 829–837. doi: 10.1002/aur.1586

Dahiya, D. K., Renuka, Puniya, M., Shandilya, U. K., Dhewa, T., Kumar, N., et al. (2017). Gut microbiota modulation and its relationship with obesity using prebiotic fibers and probiotics: a review. *Front. Microbiol.* 8:563. doi: 10.3389/fmicb.2017.00563

De Benedetto, A., Rafaels, N. M., McGirt, L. Y., Ivanov, A. I., Georas, S. N., Cheadle, C., et al. (2011). Tight junction defects in patients with atopic dermatitis. *J. Allergy Clin. Immunol.* 127, 771.e7–786.e7. doi: 10.1016/j.jaci.2010.10.018

de Oliveira, G. L. V., Leite, A. Z., Higuchi, B. S., Gonzaga, M. I., and Mariano, V. S. (2017). Intestinal dysbiosis and probiotic applications in autoimmune diseases. *Immunology* 152, 1–12. doi: 10.1111/imm.12765

del Campo, R., Garriga, M., Perez-Aragon, A., Guallarte, P., Lamas, A., Maiz, L., et al. (2014). Improvement of digestive health and reduction in proteobacterial populations in the gut microbiota of cystic fibrosis patients using a *Lactobacillus reuteri* probiotic preparation: a double blind prospective study. *J. Cyst. Fibros.* 13, 716–722. doi: 10.1016/j.jcf.2014.02.007

Diaz, M., Ladero, V., del Rio, B., Redruello, B., Fernandez, M., Martin, M. C., et al. (2016). Biofilm-forming capacity in biogenic amine-producing bacteria isolated from dairy products. *Front. Microbiol.* 7:591. doi: 10.3389/fmicb.2016.00591

Dicksved, J., Schreiber, O., Willing, B., Petersson, J., Rang, S., Phillipson, M., et al. (2012). *Lactobacillus reuteri* maintains a functional mucosal barrier during DSS treatment despite mucus layer dysfunction. *PLoS One* 7:e46399. doi: 10.1371/journal.pone.0046399

Dinleyici, E. C., Dalgic, N., Guven, S., Metin, O., Yasa, O., Kurugol, Z., et al. (2015). *Lactobacillus reuteri* DSM 17938 shortens acute infectious diarrhea in a pediatric outpatient setting. *J. Pediatr.* 91, 392–396. doi: 10.1016/j.jped.2014.10.009

Dinleyici, E. C., Probage Study Group, and Vandenplas, Y. (2014). *Lactobacillus reuteri* DSM 17938 effectively reduces the duration of acute diarrhoea in hospitalised children. *Acta Paediatr.* 103, e300–e305. doi: 10.1111/apa.12617

Dore, M. P., Cuccu, M., Pes, G. M., Manca, A., and Graham, D. Y. (2014). *Lactobacillus reuteri* in the treatment of *Helicobacter pylori* infection. *Intern. Emerg. Med.* 9, 649–654. doi: 10.1007/s11739-013-1013-z

Dore, M. P., Soro, S., Rocchi, C., Loria, M. F., Bibbo, S., and Pes, G. M. (2016). Inclusion of *Lactobacillus reuteri* in the treatment of *Helicobacter pylori* in Sardinian patients: a case report series. *Medicine* 95:e3411. doi: 10.1097/MD.0000000000003411

Duar, R. M., Lin, X. B., Zheng, J., Martino, M. E., Grenier, T., Perez-Munoz, M. E., et al. (2017). Lifestyles in transition: evolution and natural history of the genus *Lactobacillus*. *FEMS Microbiol. Rev.* 41(Suppl. 1), S27–S48. doi: 10.1093/femsre/fux030

Edwards, M. R., Dai, R., Heid, B., Cecere, T. E., Khan, D., Mu, Q., et al. (2017). Commercial rodent diets differentially regulate autoimmune glomerulonephritis, epigenetics and microbiota in MRL/lpr mice. *Int. Immunol.* 29, 263–276. doi: 10.1093/intimm/dxx033

Engels, C., Schwab, C., Zhang, J., Stevens, M. J., Bieri, C., Ebert, M. O., et al. (2016). Acrolein contributes strongly to antimicrobial and heterocyclic amine transformation activities of reuterin. *Sci. Rep.* 6:36246. doi: 10.1038/srep36246

Ericson, D., Hamberg, K., Bratthall, G., Sinkiewicz-Enggren, G., and Ljunggren, L. (2013). Salivary IgA response to probiotic bacteria and mutans streptococci after the use of chewing gum containing *Lactobacillus reuteri*. *Pathog. Dis.* 68, 82–87. doi: 10.1111/2049-632X.12048

Esmaeili, S. A., Mahmoudi, M., Momtazi, A. A., Sahebkar, A., Doulabi, H., and Rastin, M. (2017). Tolerogenic probiotics: potential immunoregulators in Systemic Lupus Erythematosus. *J. Cell. Physiol.* 232, 1994–2007. doi: 10.1002/jcp.25748

Fåk, F., and Bäckhed, F. (2012). *Lactobacillus reuteri* prevents diet-induced obesity, but not atherosclerosis, in a strain dependent fashion in Apoe-/- mice. *PLoS One* 7:e46837. doi: 10.1371/journal.pone.0046837

Francavilla, R., Lionetti, E., Castellaneta, S., Ciruzzi, F., Indrio, F., Masciale, A., et al. (2012). Randomised clinical trial: *Lactobacillus reuteri* DSM 17938 vs. placebo in children with acute diarrhoea–a double-blind study. *Aliment. Pharmacol. Ther.* 36, 363–369. doi: 10.1111/j.1365-2036.2012.05180.x

Francavilla, R., Lionetti, E., Castellaneta, S. P., Magista, A. M., Maurogiovanni, G., Bucci, N., et al. (2008). Inhibition of *Helicobacter pylori* infection in humans by *Lactobacillus reuteri* ATCC 55730 and effect on eradication therapy: a pilot study. *Helicobacter* 13, 127–134. doi: 10.1111/j.1523-5378.2008.00593.x

Francavilla, R., Polimeno, L., Demichina, A., Maurogiovanni, G., Principi, B., Scaccianoce, G., et al. (2014). *Lactobacillus reuteri* strain combination in *Helicobacter pylori* infection: a randomized, double-blind, placebo-controlled study. *J. Clin. Gastroenterol.* 48, 407–413. doi: 10.1097/MCG.0000000000000007

Franceschi, F., Cazzato, A., Nista, E. C., Scarpellini, E., Roccarina, D., Gigante, G., et al. (2007). Role of probiotics in patients with *Helicobacter pylori* infection. *Helicobacter* 12(Suppl. 2), 59–63. doi: 10.1111/j.1523-5378.2007.00565.x

Frese, S. A., Benson, A. K., Tannock, G. W., Loach, D. M., Kim, J., Zhang, M., et al. (2011). The evolution of host specialization in the vertebrate gut symbiont *Lactobacillus reuteri*. *PLoS Genet.* 7:e1001314. doi: 10.1371/journal.pgen.1001314

Frese, S. A., Mackenzie, D. A., Peterson, D. A., Schmaltz, R., Fangman, T., Zhou, Y., et al. (2013). Molecular characterization of host-specific biofilm formation in a vertebrate gut symbiont. *PLoS Genet.* 9:e1004057. doi: 10.1371/journal.pgen.1004057

Galley, J. D., Mackos, A. R., Varaljay, V. A., and Bailey, M. T. (2017). Stressor exposure has prolonged effects on colonic microbial community structure in *Citrobacter rodentium*-challenged mice. *Sci. Rep.* 7:45012. doi: 10.1038/srep45012

Galley, J. D., Nelson, M. C., Yu, Z., Dowd, S. E., Walter, J., Kumar, P. S., et al. (2014). Exposure to a social stressor disrupts the community structure of the colonic mucosa-associated microbiota. *BMC Microbiol.* 14:189. doi: 10.1186/1471-2180-14-189

Ganzle, M. G., and Vogel, R. F. (2003). Studies on the mode of action of reutericyclin. *Appl. Environ. Microbiol.* 69, 1305–1307. doi: 10.1128/AEM.69.2.1305-1307.2003

Gao, C., Major, A., Rendon, D., Lugo, M., Jackson, V., Shi, Z., et al. (2015). Histamine H2 Receptor-Mediated Suppression of Intestinal Inflammation by Probiotic *Lactobacillus reuteri*. *mBio* 6:e01358-15. doi: 10.1128/mBio.01358-15

Garcia Rodenas, C. L., Lepage, M., Ngom-Bru, C., Fotiou, A., Papagaroufalis, K., and Berger, B. (2016). Effect of formula containing *Lactobacillus reuteri* DSM 17938 on fecal microbiota of infants born by cesarean-section. *J. Pediatr. Gastroenterol. Nutr.* 63, 681–687. doi: 10.1097/MPG.0000000000001198

Garofoli, F., Civardi, E., Indrio, F., Mazzucchelli, I., Angelini, M., Tinelli, C., et al. (2014). The early administration of *Lactobacillus reuteri* DSM 17938 controls regurgitation episodes in full-term breastfed infants. *Int. J. Food Sci. Nutr.* 65, 646–648. doi: 10.3109/09637486.2014.898251

Genis, S., Sanchez-Chardi, A., Bach, A., Fabregas, F., and Aris, A. (2017). A combination of lactic acid bacteria regulates *Escherichia coli* infection and inflammation of the bovine endometrium. *J. Dairy Sci.* 100, 479–492. doi: 10.3168/jds.2016-11671

Gille, C., Boer, B., Marschal, M., Urschitz, M. S., Heinecke, V., Hund, V., et al. (2016). Effect of probiotics on vaginal health in pregnancy. EFFPRO, a randomized controlled trial. *Am. J. Obstet. Gynecol.* 215, 608.e1–608.e7. doi: 10.1016/j.ajog.2016.06.021

Giraffa, G., Chanishvili, N., and Widyastuti, Y. (2010). Importance of lactobacilli in food and feed biotechnology. *Res. Microbiol.* 161, 480–487. doi: 10.1016/j.resmic.2010.03.001

Gopi, G. R., Ganesh, N., Pandiaraj, S., Sowmiya, B., Brajesh, R. G., and Ramalingam, S. (2015). A study on enhanced expression of 3-hydroxypropionic acid pathway genes and impact on its production in *Lactobacillus reuteri*. *Food Technol. Biotechnol.* 53, 331–336. doi: 10.17113/ftb.53.03.15.3976

Greifova, G., Majekova, H., Greif, G., Body, P., Greifova, M., and Dubnickova, M. (2017). Analysis of antimicrobial and immunomodulatory substances produced by heterofermentative *Lactobacillus reuteri*. *Folia Microbiol.* 62, 515–524. doi: 10.1007/s12223-017-0524-9

Grover, S., Rastogi, A., Singh, J., Rajbongshi, A., and Bihari, C. (2014). Spectrum of histomorphologic findings in liver in patients with SLE: a review. *Hepat. Res. Treat.* 2014:562979. doi: 10.1155/2014/562979

Gu, Q., Zhang, C., Song, D., Li, P., and Zhu, X. (2015). Enhancing vitamin B12 content in soy-yogurt by *Lactobacillus reuteri*. *Int. J. Food Microbiol.* 206, 56–59. doi: 10.1016/j.ijfoodmicro.2015.04.033

Gunning, A. P., Kavanaugh, D., Thursby, E., Etzold, S., MacKenzie, D. A., and Juge, N. (2016). Use of atomic force microscopy to study the multi-modular interaction of bacterial adhesins to mucins. *Int. J. Mol. Sci.* 17:E1854. doi: 10.3390/ijms17111854

Gutierrez-Castrellon, P., Lopez-Velazquez, G., Diaz-Garcia, L., Jimenez-Gutierrez, C., Mancilla-Ramirez, J., Estevez-Jimenez, J., et al. (2014). Diarrhea in preschool children and *Lactobacillus reuteri*: a randomized controlled trial. *Pediatrics* 133, e904–e909. doi: 10.1542/peds.2013-0652

Harakeh, S. M., Khan, I., Kumosani, T., Barbour, E., Almasaudi, S. B., Bahijri, S. M., et al. (2016). Gut microbiota: a contributing factor to obesity. *Front. Cell. Infect. Microbiol.* 6:95. doi: 10.3389/fcimb.2016.00095

He, B., Hoang, T. K., Wang, T., Ferris, M., Taylor, C. M., Tian, X., et al. (2017). Resetting microbiota by *Lactobacillus reuteri* inhibits T reg deficiency-induced autoimmunity via adenosine A_{2A} receptors. *J. Exp. Med.* 214, 107–123. doi: 10.1084/jem.20160961

Hemarajata, P., Gao, C., Pflughoeft, K. J., Thomas, C. M., Saulnier, D. M., Spinler, J. K., et al. (2013). *Lactobacillus reuteri*-specific immunoregulatory gene rsiR modulates histamine production and immunomodulation by *Lactobacillus reuteri*. *J. Bacteriol.* 195, 5567–5576. doi: 10.1128/JB.00261-13

Hill, C., Guarner, F., Reid, G., Gibson, G. R., Merenstein, D. J., Pot, B., et al. (2014). Expert consensus document. The International Scientific Association for Probiotics and Prebiotics consensus statement on the scope and appropriate use of the term probiotic. *Nat. Rev. Gastroenterol. Hepatol.* 11, 506–514. doi: 10.1038/nrgastro.2014.66

Holz, C., Busjahn, A., Mehling, H., Arya, S., Boettner, M., Habibi, H., et al. (2015). Significant reduction in *Helicobacter pylori* load in humans with non-viable *Lactobacillus reuteri* DSM17648: a pilot study. *Probiotics Antimicrob. Proteins* 7, 91–100. doi: 10.1007/s12602-014-9181-3

Hou, C., Wang, Q., Zeng, X., Yang, F., Zhang, J., Liu, H., et al. (2014). Complete genome sequence of *Lactobacillus reuteri* I5007, a probiotic strain isolated from healthy piglet. *J. Biotechnol.* 179, 63–64. doi: 10.1016/j.jbiotec.2014.03.019

Hou, C., Zeng, X., Yang, F., Liu, H., and Qiao, S. (2015). Study and use of the probiotic *Lactobacillus reuteri* in pigs: a review. *J. Anim. Sci. Biotechnol.* 6:14. doi: 10.1186/s40104-015-0014-3

Hoy-Schulz, Y. E., Jannat, K., Roberts, T., Zaidi, S. H., Unicomb, L., Luby, S., et al. (2016). Safety and acceptability of *Lactobacillus reuteri* DSM 17938 and *Bifidobacterium longum* subspecies *infantis* 35624 in Bangladeshi infants: a phase I randomized clinical trial. *BMC Complement. Altern. Med.* 16:44. doi: 10.1186/s12906-016-1016-1

Hsieh, F. C., Lan, C. C., Huang, T. Y., Chen, K. W., Chai, C. Y., Chen, W. T., et al. (2016). Heat-killed and live *Lactobacillus reuteri* GMNL-263 exhibit similar effects on improving metabolic functions in high-fat diet-induced obese rats. *Food Funct.* 7, 2374–2388. doi: 10.1039/c5fo01396h

Hsu, T. C., Huang, C. Y., Chiang, S. Y., Lai, W. X., Tsai, C. H., and Tzang, B. S. (2008). Transglutaminase inhibitor cystamine alleviates the abnormality in liver from NZB/W F1 mice. *Eur. J. Pharmacol.* 579, 382–389. doi: 10.1016/j.ejphar.2007.10.059

Hsu, T. C., Huang, C. Y., Liu, C. H., Hsu, K. C., Chen, Y. H., and Tzang, B. S. (2017). *Lactobacillus paracasei* GMNL-32, *Lactobacillus reuteri* GMNL-89 and *L. reuteri* GMNL-263 ameliorate hepatic injuries in lupus-prone mice. *Br. J. Nutr.* 117, 1066–1074. doi: 10.1017/S0007114517001039

Imase, K., Tanaka, A., Tokunaga, K., Sugano, H., Ishida, H., and Takahashi, S. (2007). *Lactobacillus reuteri* tablets suppress *Helicobacter pylori* infection–a double-blind randomised placebo-controlled cross-over clinical study. *Kansenshogaku Zasshi* 81, 387–393. doi: 10.11150/kansenshogakuzasshi1970.81.387

Indrio, F., Di Mauro, A., Riezzo, G., Civardi, E., Intini, C., Corvaglia, L., et al. (2014). Prophylactic use of a probiotic in the prevention of colic, regurgitation, and functional constipation: a randomized clinical trial. *JAMA Pediatr.* 168, 228–233. doi: 10.1001/jamapediatrics.2013.4367

Indrio, F., Riezzo, G., Raimondi, F., Bisceglia, M., Cavallo, L., and Francavilla, R. (2008). The effects of probiotics on feeding tolerance, bowel habits, and gastrointestinal motility in preterm newborns. *J. Pediatr.* 152, 801–806. doi: 10.1016/j.jpeds.2007.11.005

Indrio, F., Riezzo, G., Raimondi, F., Bisceglia, M., Cavallo, L., and Francavilla, R. (2009). Effects of probiotic and prebiotic on gastrointestinal motility in newborns. *J. Physiol. Pharmacol.* 60(Suppl. 6), 27–31.

Iniesta, M., Herrera, D., Montero, E., Zurbriggen, M., Matos, A. R., Marin, M. J., et al. (2012). Probiotic effects of orally administered *Lactobacillus reuteri*-containing tablets on the subgingival and salivary microbiota in patients with gingivitis. A randomized clinical trial. *J. Clin. Periodontol.* 39, 736–744. doi: 10.1111/j.1600-051X.2012.01914.x

Islam, S. U. (2016). Clinical uses of probiotics. *Medicine* 95:e2658. doi: 10.1097/MD.0000000000002658

Jacobsen, C. N., Rosenfeldt Nielsen, V., Hayford, A. E., Moller, P. L., Michaelsen, K. F., Paerregaard, A., et al. (1999). Screening of probiotic activities of forty-seven strains of *Lactobacillus* spp. by in vitro techniques and evaluation of the colonization ability of five selected strains in humans. *Appl. Environ. Microbiol.* 65, 4949–4956.

Jensen, H., Roos, S., Jonsson, H., Rud, I., Grimmer, S., van Pijkeren, J. P., et al. (2014). Role of *Lactobacillus reuteri* cell and mucus-binding protein A (CmbA) in adhesion to intestinal epithelial cells and mucus in vitro. *Microbiology* 160(Pt 4), 671–681. doi: 10.1099/mic.0.073551-0

Jones, M. L., Martoni, C. J., Di Pietro, E., Simon, R. R., and Prakash, S. (2012a). Evaluation of clinical safety and tolerance of a *Lactobacillus reuteri* NCIMB 30242 supplement capsule: a randomized control trial. *Regul. Toxicol. Pharmacol.* 63, 313–320. doi: 10.1016/j.yrtph.2012.04.003

Jones, M. L., Martoni, C. J., and Prakash, S. (2012b). Cholesterol lowering and inhibition of sterol absorption by *Lactobacillus reuteri* NCIMB 30242: a randomized controlled trial. *Eur. J. Clin. Nutr.* 66, 1234–1241. doi: 10.1038/ejcn.2012.126

Jones, M. L., Martoni, C. J., Tamber, S., Parent, M., and Prakash, S. (2012c). Evaluation of safety and tolerance of microencapsulated *Lactobacillus reuteri* NCIMB 30242 in a yogurt formulation: a randomized, placebo-controlled, double-blind study. *Food Chem. Toxicol.* 50, 2216–2223. doi: 10.1016/j.fct.2012.03.010

Jones, S. E., and Versalovic, J. (2009). Probiotic *Lactobacillus reuteri* biofilms produce antimicrobial and anti-inflammatory factors. *BMC Microbiol.* 9:35. doi: 10.1186/1471-2180-9-35

Jorgensen, M. R., Keller, M. K., Kragelund, C., Hamberg, K., Ericson, D., Nielsen, C. H., et al. (2016). *Lactobacillus reuteri* supplements do not affect salivary IgA or cytokine levels in healthy subjects: a randomized, double-blind, placebo-controlled, cross-over trial. *Acta Odontol. Scand.* 74, 399–404. doi: 10.3109/00016357.2016.1169439

Jorgensen, M. R., Kragelund, C., Jensen, P. O., Keller, M. K., and Twetman, S. (2017). Probiotic *Lactobacillus reuteri* has antifungal effects on oral *Candida* species *in vitro*. *J. Oral Microbiol.* 9:1274582. doi: 10.1080/20002297.2016.1274582

Kamada, N., Seo, S. U., Chen, G. Y., and Nunez, G. (2013). Role of the gut microbiota in immunity and inflammatory disease. *Nat. Rev. Immunol.* 13, 321–335. doi: 10.1038/nri3430

Kamiya, T., Wang, L., Forsythe, P., Goettsche, G., Mao, Y., Wang, Y., et al. (2006). Inhibitory effects of *Lactobacillus reuteri* on visceral pain induced by colorectal distension in Sprague-Dawley rats. *Gut* 55, 191–196. doi: 10.1136/gut.2005.070987

Kandler, O., Stetter, K. O., and Kohl, R. (1980). *Lactobacillus reuteri* sp. nov., a new species of heterofermentative lactobacilli. *Zentralbl. Bakteriol. Hyg. I Abt Orig.* 1, 264–269. doi: 10.1016/S0172-5564(80)80007-8

Karaffova, V., Csank, T., Mudronova, D., Kiraly, J., Revajova, V., Gancarcikova, S., et al. (2017). Influence of *Lactobacillus reuteri* L26 Biocenol on immune response against porcine circovirus type 2 infection in germ-free mice. *Benef. Microbes* 8, 367–378. doi: 10.3920/BM2016.0114

Karimi, K., Inman, M. D., Bienenstock, J., and Forsythe, P. (2009). *Lactobacillus reuteri*-induced regulatory T cells protect against an allergic airway response in mice. *Am. J. Respir. Crit. Care Med.* 179, 186–193. doi: 10.1164/rccm.200806-951OC

Kechagia, M., Basoulis, D., Konstantopoulou, S., Dimitriadi, D., Gyftopoulou, K., Skarmoutsou, N., et al. (2013). Health benefits of probiotics: a review. *ISRN Nutr.* 2013:481651. doi: 10.5402/2013/481651

Keller, M. K., Nohr Larsen, I., Karlsson, I., and Twetman, S. (2014). Effect of tablets containing probiotic bacteria (*Lactobacillus reuteri*) on early caries lesions in adolescents: a pilot study. *Benef. Microbes* 5, 403–407. doi: 10.3920/BM2013.0089

Kleerebezem, M., Hols, P., Bernard, E., Rolain, T., Zhou, M., Siezen, R. J., et al. (2010). The extracellular biology of the lactobacilli. *FEMS Microbiol. Rev.* 34, 199–230. doi: 10.1111/j.1574-6976.2010.00208.x

Koleva, P. T., Bridgman, S. L., and Kozyrskyj, A. L. (2015). The infant gut microbiome: evidence for obesity risk and dietary intervention. *Nutrients* 7, 2237–2260. doi: 10.3390/nu7042237

Krumbeck, J. A., Marsteller, N. L., Frese, S. A., Peterson, D. A., Ramer-Tait, A. E., Hutkins, R. W., et al. (2016). Characterization of the ecological role of genes mediating acid resistance in *Lactobacillus reuteri* during colonization of the gastrointestinal tract. *Environ. Microbiol.* 18, 2172–2184. doi: 10.1111/1462-2920.13108

Ksonzekova, P., Bystricky, P., Vlckova, S., Patoprsty, V., Pulzova, L., Mudronova, D., et al. (2016). Exopolysaccharides of *Lactobacillus reuteri*: their influence on adherence of *E. coli* to epithelial cells and inflammatory response. *Carbohydr. Polym.* 141, 10–19. doi: 10.1016/j.carbpol.2015.12.037

Kunze, W. A., Mao, Y. K., Wang, B., Huizinga, J. D., Ma, X., Forsythe, P., et al. (2009). *Lactobacillus reuteri* enhances excitability of colonic AH neurons by inhibiting calcium-dependent potassium channel opening. *J. Cell Mol. Med.* 13, 2261–2270. doi: 10.1111/j.1582-4934.2009.00686.x

Lai, N. Y., Mills, K., and Chiu, I. M. (2017). Sensory neuron regulation of gastrointestinal inflammation and bacterial host defence. *J. Intern. Med.* 282, 5–23. doi: 10.1111/joim.12591

Lebeer, S., Vanderleyden, J., and De Keersmaecker, S. C. (2008). Genes and molecules of lactobacilli supporting probiotic action. *Microbiol. Mol. Biol. Rev.* 72, 728–764. doi: 10.1128/MMBR.00017-08

Lee, J., Yang, W., Hostetler, A., Schultz, N., Suckow, M. A., Stewart, K. L., et al. (2016). Characterization of the anti-inflammatory *Lactobacillus reuteri* BM36301 and its probiotic benefits on aged mice. *BMC Microbiol.* 16:69. doi: 10.1186/s12866-016-0686-7

Lesbros-Pantoflickova, D., Corthesy-Theulaz, I., and Blum, A. L. (2007). *Helicobacter pylori* and probiotics. *J. Nutr.* 137(3 Suppl. 2), 812S–818S. doi: 10.1093/jn/137.3.812S

Li, X. J., Yue, L. Y., Guan, X. F., and Qiao, S. Y. (2008). The adhesion of putative probiotic lactobacilli to cultured epithelial cells and porcine intestinal mucus. *J. Appl. Microbiol.* 104, 1082–1091. doi: 10.1111/j.1365-2672.2007.03636.x

Liao, P. H., Kuo, W. W., Hsieh, D. J., Yeh, Y. L., Day, C. H., Chen, Y. H., et al. (2016). Heat-killed *Lactobacillus reuteri* GMNL-263 prevents epididymal fat accumulation and cardiac injury in high-calorie diet-fed rats. *Int. J. Med. Sci.* 13, 569–577. doi: 10.7150/ijms.15597

Linares, D. M., Gomez, C., Renes, E., Fresno, J. M., Tornadijo, M. E., Ross, R. P., et al. (2017). Lactic acid bacteria and bifidobacteria with potential to design natural biofunctional health-promoting dairy foods. *Front. Microbiol.* 8:846. doi: 10.3389/fmicb.2017.00846

Lionetti, E., Miniello, V. L., Castellaneta, S. P., Magista, A. M., de Canio, A., Maurogiovanni, G., et al. (2006). *Lactobacillus reuteri* therapy to reduce side-effects during anti-*Helicobacter pylori* treatment in children: a randomized placebo controlled trial. *Aliment. Pharmacol. Ther.* 24, 1461–1468. doi: 10.1111/j.1365-2036.2006.03145.x

Liu, F., Wang, X., Shi, H., Wang, Y., Xue, C., and Tang, Q. J. (2017). Polymannuronic acid ameliorated obesity and inflammation associated with a high-fat and high-sucrose diet by modulating the gut microbiome in a murine model. *Br. J. Nutr.* 117, 1332–1342. doi: 10.1017/S0007114517000964

Liu, H., Hou, C., Wang, G., Jia, H., Yu, H., Zeng, X., et al. (2017). *Lactobacillus reuteri* I5007 modulates intestinal host defense peptide expression in the model of IPEC-J2 cells and neonatal piglets. *Nutrients* 9:E559. doi: 10.3390/nu9060559

Liu, Y., Fatheree, N. Y., Dingle, B. M., Tran, D. Q., and Rhoads, J. M. (2013). *Lactobacillus reuteri* DSM 17938 changes the frequency of Foxp3+ regulatory T cells in the intestine and mesenteric lymph node in experimental necrotizing enterocolitis. *PLoS One* 8:e56547. doi: 10.1371/journal.pone.0056547

Liu, Y., Tran, D. Q., Fatheree, N. Y., and Marc Rhoads, J. (2014). *Lactobacillus reuteri* DSM 17938 differentially modulates effector memory T cells and Foxp3+ regulatory T cells in a mouse model of necrotizing enterocolitis. *Am. J. Physiol. Gastrointest. Liver Physiol.* 307, G177–G186. doi: 10.1152/ajpgi.00038.2014

Livingston, M., Loach, D., Wilson, M., Tannock, G. W., and Baird, M. (2010). Gut commensal *Lactobacillus reuteri* 100-23 stimulates an immunoregulatory response. *Immunol. Cell Biol.* 88, 99–102. doi: 10.1038/icb.2009.71

Lorea Baroja, M., Kirjavainen, P. V., Hekmat, S., and Reid, G. (2007). Anti-inflammatory effects of probiotic yogurt in inflammatory bowel disease patients. *Clin. Exp. Immunol.* 149, 470–479. doi: 10.1111/j.1365-2249.2007.03434.x

Ma, X., Mao, Y. K., Wang, B., Huizinga, J. D., Bienenstock, J., and Kunze, W. (2009). *Lactobacillus reuteri* ingestion prevents hyperexcitability of colonic DRG neurons induced by noxious stimuli. *Am. J. Physiol. Gastrointest. Liver Physiol.* 296, G868–G875. doi: 10.1152/ajpgi.90511.2008

Mackenzie, D. A., Jeffers, F., Parker, M. L., Vibert-Vallet, A., Bongaerts, R. J., Roos, S., et al. (2010). Strain-specific diversity of mucus-binding proteins in the adhesion and aggregation properties of *Lactobacillus reuteri*. *Microbiology* 156(Pt 11), 3368–3378. doi: 10.1099/mic.0.043265-0

Macklaim, J. M., Clemente, J. C., Knight, R., Gloor, G. B., and Reid, G. (2015). Changes in vaginal microbiota following antimicrobial and probiotic therapy. *Microb. Ecol. Health Dis.* 26:27799. doi: 10.3402/mehd.v26.27799

Mackos, A. R., Eubank, T. D., Parry, N. M., and Bailey, M. T. (2013). Probiotic *Lactobacillus reuteri* attenuates the stressor-enhanced severity of *Citrobacter rodentium* infection. *Infect. Immun.* 81, 3253–3263. doi: 10.1128/IAI.00278-13

Mackos, A. R., Galley, J. D., Eubank, T. D., Easterling, R. S., Parry, N. M., Fox, J. G., et al. (2016). Social stress-enhanced severity of *Citrobacter rodentium*-induced colitis is CCL2-dependent and attenuated by probiotic *Lactobacillus reuteri*. *Mucosal Immunol.* 9, 515–526. doi: 10.1038/mi.2015.81

Mangalat, N., Liu, Y., Fatheree, N. Y., Ferris, M. J., Van Arsdall, M. R., Chen, Z., et al. (2012). Safety and tolerability of *Lactobacillus reuteri* DSM 17938 and effects on biomarkers in healthy adults: results from a randomized masked trial. *PLoS One* 7:e43910. doi: 10.1371/journal.pone.0043910

Markle, J. G., Frank, D. N., Mortin-Toth, S., Robertson, C. E., Feazel, L. M., Rolle-Kampczyk, U., et al. (2013). Sex differences in the gut microbiome drive hormone-dependent regulation of autoimmunity. *Science* 339, 1084–1088. doi: 10.1126/science.1233521

Martoni, C. J., Labbe, A., Ganopolsky, J. G., Prakash, S., and Jones, M. L. (2015). Changes in bile acids, FGF-19 and sterol absorption in response to bile salt hydrolase active *L. reuteri* NCIMB 30242. *Gut Microbes* 6, 57–65. doi: 10.1080/19490976.2015.1005474

McFall-Ngai, M. (2007). Adaptive immunity: care for the community. *Nature* 445:153. doi: 10.1038/445153a

McMillan, A., Dell, M., Zellar, M. P., Cribby, S., Martz, S., Hong, E., et al. (2011). Disruption of urogenital biofilms by lactobacilli. *Colloids Surf. B Biointerfaces* 86, 58–64. doi: 10.1016/j.colsurfb.2011.03.016

McVey Neufeld, K. A., Mao, Y. K., Bienenstock, J., Foster, J. A., and Kunze, W. A. (2013). The microbiome is essential for normal gut intrinsic primary afferent neuron excitability in the mouse. *Neurogastroenterol. Motil.* 25, e183–e188. doi: 10.1111/nmo.12049

Mehling, H., and Busjahn, A. (2013). Non-viable *Lactobacillus reuteri* DSMZ 17648 (Pylopass) as a new approach to *Helicobacter pylori* control in humans. *Nutrients* 5, 3062–3073. doi: 10.3390/nu5083062

Mi, G. L., Zhao, L., Qiao, D. D., Kang, W. Q., Tang, M. Q., and Xu, J. K. (2015). Effectiveness of *Lactobacillus reuteri* in infantile colic and colicky induced maternal depression: a prospective single blind randomized trial. *Antonie Van Leeuwenhoek* 107, 1547–1553. doi: 10.1007/s10482-015-0448-9

Million, M., Angelakis, E., Maraninchi, M., Henry, M., Giorgi, R., Valero, R., et al. (2013a). Correlation between body mass index and gut concentrations of *Lactobacillus reuteri, Bifidobacterium animalis, Methanobrevibacter smithii* and *Escherichia coli. Int. J. Obes.* 37, 1460–1466. doi: 10.1038/ijo.2013.20

Million, M., Maraninchi, M., Henry, M., Armougom, F., Richet, H., Carrieri, P., et al. (2012). Obesity-associated gut microbiota is enriched in *Lactobacillus reuteri* and depleted in *Bifidobacterium animalis* and *Methanobrevibacter smithii. Int. J. Obes.* 36, 817–825. doi: 10.1038/ijo.2011.153

Million, M., Thuny, F., Angelakis, E., Casalta, J. P., Giorgi, R., Habib, G., et al. (2013b). *Lactobacillus reuteri* and *Escherichia coli* in the human gut microbiota may predict weight gain associated with vancomycin treatment. *Nutr. Diabetes* 3:e87. doi: 10.1038/nutd.2013.28

Miniello, V. L., Brunetti, L., Tesse, R., Natile, M., Armenio, L., and Francavilla, R. (2010). *Lactobacillus reuteri* modulates cytokines production in exhaled breath condensate of children with atopic dermatitis. *J. Pediatr. Gastroenterol. Nutr.* 50, 573–576. doi: 10.1097/MPG.0b013e3181bb343f

Mishra, S. K., Malik, R. K., Manju, G., Pandey, N., Singroha, G., Behare, P., et al. (2012). Characterization of a reuterin-producing *Lactobacillus reuteri* BPL-36 strain isolated from human infant fecal sample. *Probiotics Antimicrob. Proteins* 4, 154–161. doi: 10.1007/s12602-012-9103-1

Mobini, R., Tremaroli, V., Stahlman, M., Karlsson, F., Levin, M., Ljungberg, M., et al. (2017). Metabolic effects of *Lactobacillus reuteri* DSM 17938 in people with type 2 diabetes: a randomized controlled trial. *Diabetes Obes. Metab.* 19, 579–589. doi: 10.1111/dom.12861

Molina, V. C., Medici, M., Taranto, M. P., and Font de Valdez, G. (2009). *Lactobacillus reuteri* CRL 1098 prevents side effects produced by a nutritional vitamin B deficiency. *J. Appl. Microbiol.* 106, 467–473. doi: 10.1111/j.1365-2672.2008.04014.x

Montalban-Arques, A., De Schryver, P., Bossier, P., Gorkiewicz, G., Mulero, V., Gatlin, D. M., et al. (2015). Selective manipulation of the gut microbiota improves immune status in vertebrates. *Front. Immunol.* 6:512. doi: 10.3389/fimmu.2015.00512

Morita, H., Toh, H., Fukuda, S., Horikawa, H., Oshima, K., Suzuki, T., et al. (2008). Comparative genome analysis of *Lactobacillus reuteri* and *Lactobacillus fermentum* reveal a genomic island for reuterin and cobalamin production. *DNA Res.* 15, 151–161. doi: 10.1093/dnares/dsn009

Mu, Q., Kirby, J., Reilly, C. M., and Luo, X. M. (2017a). Leaky gut as a danger signal for autoimmune diseases. *Front. Immunol.* 8:598. doi: 10.3389/fimmu.2017.00598

Mu, Q., Tavella, V. J., Kirby, J. L., Cecere, T. E., Chung, M., Lee, J., et al. (2017b). Antibiotics ameliorate lupus-like symptoms in mice. *Sci. Rep.* 7:13675. doi: 10.1038/s41598-017-14223-0

Mu, Q., Zhang, H., Liao, X., Lin, K., Liu, H., Edwards, M. R., et al. (2017c). Control of lupus nephritis by changes of gut microbiota. *Microbiome* 5:73. doi: 10.1186/s40168-017-0300-8

Mu, Q., Zhang, H., and Luo, X. M. (2015). SLE: another autoimmune disorder influenced by microbes and diet? *Front. Immunol.* 6:608. doi: 10.3389/fimmu.2015.00608

Mukai, T., Asasaka, T., Sato, E., Mori, K., Matsumoto, M., and Ohori, H. (2002). Inhibition of binding of *Helicobacter pylori* to the glycolipid receptors by probiotic *Lactobacillus reuteri. FEMS Immunol. Med. Microbiol.* 32, 105–110. doi: 10.1111/j.1574-695X.2002.tb00541.x

Nagpal, R., Tsuji, H., Takahashi, T., Kawashima, K., Nagata, S., Nomoto, K., et al. (2016). Sensitive quantitative analysis of the meconium bacterial microbiota in healthy term infants born vaginally or by cesarean section. *Front. Microbiol.* 7:1997. doi: 10.3389/fmicb.2016.01997

Navarro, J. B., Mashburn-Warren, L., Bakaletz, L. O., Bailey, M. T., and Goodman, S. D. (2017). Enhanced probiotic potential of *Lactobacillus reuteri* when delivered as a biofilm on dextranomer microspheres that contain beneficial cargo. *Front. Microbiol.* 8:489. doi: 10.3389/fmicb.2017.00489

Nguyen, N. T., Hanieh, H., Nakahama, T., and Kishimoto, T. (2013). The roles of aryl hydrocarbon receptor in immune responses. *Int. Immunol.* 25, 335–343. doi: 10.1093/intimm/dxt011

Oh, P. L., Benson, A. K., Peterson, D. A., Patil, P. B., Moriyama, E. N., Roos, S., et al. (2010). Diversification of the gut symbiont *Lactobacillus reuteri* as a result of host-driven evolution. *ISME J.* 4, 377–387. doi: 10.1038/ismej.2009.123

Ojetti, V., Bruno, G., Ainora, M. E., Gigante, G., Rizzo, G., Roccarina, D., et al. (2012). Impact of *Lactobacillus reuteri* supplementation on anti-*Helicobacter pylori* levofloxacin-based second-line therapy. *Gastroenterol. Res. Pract.* 2012:740381. doi: 10.1155/2012/740381

Okeke, F., Roland, B. C., and Mullin, G. E. (2014). The role of the gut microbiome in the pathogenesis and treatment of obesity. *Glob. Adv. Health Med.* 3, 44–57. doi: 10.7453/gahmj.2014.018

Olson, J. K., Rager, T. M., Navarro, J. B., Mashburn-Warren, L., Goodman, S. D., and Besner, G. E. (2016). Harvesting the benefits of biofilms: a novel probiotic delivery system for the prevention of necrotizing enterocolitis. *J. Pediatr. Surg.* 51, 936–941. doi: 10.1016/j.jpedsurg.2016.02.062

Oncel, M. Y., Sari, F. N., Arayici, S., Guzoglu, N., Erdeve, O., Uras, N., et al. (2014). *Lactobacillus reuteri* for the prevention of necrotising enterocolitis in very low birthweight infants: a randomised controlled trial. *Arch. Dis. Child. Fetal Neonatal Ed.* 99, F110–F115. doi: 10.1136/archdischild-2013-304745

Pallin, A., Agback, P., Jonsson, H., and Roos, S. (2016). Evaluation of growth, metabolism and production of potentially bioactive components during fermentation of barley with *Lactobacillus reuteri. Food Microbiol.* 57, 159–171. doi: 10.1016/j.fm.2016.02.011

Park, S. K., Park, D. I., Choi, J. S., Kang, M. S., Park, J. H., Kim, H. J., et al. (2007). The effect of probiotics on *Helicobacter pylori* eradication. *Hepatogastroenterology* 54, 2032–2036.

Petricevic, L., Unger, F. M., Viernstein, H., and Kiss, H. (2008). Randomized, double-blind, placebo-controlled study of oral lactobacilli to improve the vaginal flora of postmenopausal women. *Eur. J. Obstet. Gynecol. Reprod. Biol.* 141, 54–57. doi: 10.1016/j.ejogrb.2008.06.003

Piyathilake, C. J., Ollberding, N. J., Kumar, R., Macaluso, M., Alvarez, R. D., and Morrow, C. D. (2016). Cervical microbiota associated with higher grade cervical intraepithelial neoplasia in women infected with high-risk human papillomaviruses. *Cancer Prev. Res.* 9, 357–366. doi: 10.1158/1940-6207.CAPR-15-0350

Poutahidis, T., Kearney, S. M., Levkovich, T., Qi, P., Varian, B. J., Lakritz, J. R., et al. (2013a). Microbial symbionts accelerate wound healing via the neuropeptide hormone oxytocin. *PLoS One* 8:e78898. doi: 10.1371/journal.pone.0078898

Poutahidis, T., Kleinewietfeld, M., Smillie, C., Levkovich, T., Perrotta, A., Bhela, S., et al. (2013b). Microbial reprogramming inhibits Western diet-associated obesity. *PLoS One* 8:e68596. doi: 10.1371/journal.pone.0068596

Preidis, G. A., Saulnier, D. M., Blutt, S. E., Mistretta, T. A., Riehle, K. P., Major, A. M., et al. (2012). Host response to probiotics determined by nutritional status of rotavirus-infected neonatal mice. *J. Pediatr. Gastroenterol. Nutr.* 55, 299–307. doi: 10.1097/MPG.0b013e31824d2548

Raynaud, C., Sarcabal, P., Meynial-Salles, I., Croux, C., and Soucaille, P. (2003). Molecular characterization of the 1,3-propanediol (1,3-PD) operon of *Clostridium butyricum. Proc. Natl. Acad. Sci. U.S.A.* 100, 5010–5015. doi: 10.1073/pnas.0734105100

Reid, G., and Burton, J. (2002). Use of *Lactobacillus* to prevent infection by pathogenic bacteria. *Microbes Infect.* 4, 319–324. doi: 10.1016/S1286-4579(02)01544-7

Rojas, M. A., Lozano, J. M., Rojas, M. X., Rodriguez, V. A., Rondon, M. A., Bastidas, J. A., et al. (2012). Prophylactic probiotics to prevent death and nosocomial infection in preterm infants. *Pediatrics* 130, e1113–e1120. doi: 10.1542/peds. 2011-3584

Romani Vestman, N., Chen, T., Lif Holgerson, P., Ohman, C., and Johansson, I. (2015). Oral microbiota shift after 12-week supplementation with *Lactobacillus reuteri* DSM 17938 and PTA 5289; a randomized control trial. *PLoS One* 10:e0125812. doi: 10.1371/journal.pone.0125812

Romano, C., Ferrau, V., Cavataio, F., Iacono, G., Spina, M., Lionetti, E., et al. (2014). *Lactobacillus reuteri* in children with functional abdominal pain (FAP). *J. Paediatr. Child Health* 50, E68–E71. doi: 10.1111/j.1440-1754.2010.01797.x

Roos, S., Dicksved, J., Tarasco, V., Locatelli, E., Ricceri, F., Grandin, U., et al. (2013). 454 pyrosequencing analysis on faecal samples from a randomized DBPC trial of colicky infants treated with *Lactobacillus reuteri* DSM 17938. *PLoS One* 8:e56710. doi: 10.1371/journal.pone.0056710

Roos, S., and Jonsson, H. (2002). A high-molecular-mass cell-surface protein from *Lactobacillus reuteri* 1063 adheres to mucus components. *Microbiology* 148(Pt 2), 433–442. doi: 10.1099/00221287-148-2-433

Rosenfeldt, V., Benfeldt, E., Nielsen, S. D., Michaelsen, K. F., Jeppesen, D. L., Valerius, N. H., et al. (2003). Effect of probiotic *Lactobacillus* strains in children with atopic dermatitis. *J. Allergy Clin. Immunol.* 111, 389–395. doi: 10.1067/mai. 2003.389

Rosenfeldt, V., Benfeldt, E., Valerius, N. H., Paerregaard, A., and Michaelsen, K. F. (2004). Effect of probiotics on gastrointestinal symptoms and small intestinal permeability in children with atopic dermatitis. *J. Pediatr.* 145, 612–616. doi: 10.1016/j.jpeds.2004.06.068

Rosenfeldt, V., Michaelsen, K. F., Jakobsen, M., Larsen, C. N., Moller, P. L., Pedersen, P., et al. (2002a). Effect of probiotic *Lactobacillus* strains in young children hospitalized with acute diarrhea. *Pediatr. Infect. Dis. J.* 21, 411–416. doi: 10.1097/00006454-200205000-00012

Rosenfeldt, V., Michaelsen, K. F., Jakobsen, M., Larsen, C. N., Moller, P. L., Tvede, M., et al. (2002b). Effect of probiotic *Lactobacillus* strains on acute diarrhea in a cohort of nonhospitalized children attending day-care centers. *Pediatr. Infect. Dis. J.* 21, 417–419.

Rossi, F., Gardini, F., Rizzotti, L., La Gioia, F., Tabanelli, G., and Torriani, S. (2011). Quantitative analysis of histidine decarboxylase gene (hdcA) transcription and histamine production by *Streptococcus thermophilus* PRI60 under conditions relevant to cheese making. *Appl. Environ. Microbiol.* 77, 2817–2822. doi: 10.1128/AEM.02531-10

Salas-Jara, M. J., Ilabaca, A., Vega, M., and Garcia, A. (2016). Biofilm forming *Lactobacillus*: new challenges for the development of probiotics. *Microorganisms* 4:E35. doi: 10.3390/microorganisms4030035

Santos, F., Spinler, J. K., Saulnier, D. M., Molenaar, D., Teusink, B., de Vos, W. M., et al. (2011). Functional identification in *Lactobacillus reuteri* of a PocR-like transcription factor regulating glycerol utilization and vitamin B12 synthesis. *Microb. Cell Fact.* 10:55. doi: 10.1186/1475-2859-10-55

Santos, F., Vera, J. L., van der Heijden, R., Valdez, G., de Vos, W. M., Sesma, F., et al. (2008a). The complete coenzyme B12 biosynthesis gene cluster of *Lactobacillus reuteri* CRL1098. *Microbiology* 154(Pt 1), 81–93. doi: 10.1099/mic.0.2007/ 011569-0

Santos, F., Wegkamp, A., de Vos, W. M., Smid, E. J., and Hugenholtz, J. (2008b). High-Level folate production in fermented foods by the B12 producer *Lactobacillus reuteri* JCM1112. *Appl. Environ. Microbiol.* 74, 3291–3294. doi: 10.1128/AEM.02719-07

Savino, F., Ceratto, S., Poggi, E., Cartosio, M. E., Cordero di Montezemolo, L., and Giannattasio, A. (2015a). Preventive effects of oral probiotic on infantile colic: a prospective, randomised, blinded, controlled trial using *Lactobacillus reuteri* DSM 17938. *Benef. Microbes* 6, 245–251. doi: 10.3920/BM2014.0090

Savino, F., Cordisco, L., Tarasco, V., Palumeri, E., Calabrese, R., Oggero, R., et al. (2010). *Lactobacillus reuteri* DSM 17938 in infantile colic: a randomized, double-blind, placebo-controlled trial. *Pediatrics* 126, e526–e533. doi: 10.1542/ peds.2010-0433

Savino, F., Fornasero, S., Ceratto, S., De Marco, A., Mandras, N., Roana, J., et al. (2015b). Probiotics and gut health in infants: a preliminary case-control observational study about early treatment with *Lactobacillus reuteri* DSM 17938. *Clin. Chim. Acta* 451(Pt A), 82–87. doi: 10.1016/j.cca.2015.02.027

Savino, F., Pelle, E., Palumeri, E., Oggero, R., and Miniero, R. (2007). *Lactobacillus reuteri* (American Type Culture Collection Strain 55730) versus simethicone in the treatment of infantile colic: a prospective randomized study. *Pediatrics* 119, e124–e130. doi: 10.1542/peds.2006-1222

Scaccianoce, G., Zullo, A., Hassan, C., Gentili, F., Cristofari, F., Cardinale, V., et al. (2008). Triple therapies plus different probiotics for *Helicobacter pylori* eradication. *Eur. Rev. Med. Pharmacol. Sci.* 12, 251–256.

Scott, K. P., Antoine, J. M., Midtvedt, T., and van Hemert, S. (2015). Manipulating the gut microbiota to maintain health and treat disease. *Microb. Ecol. Health Dis.* 26:25877. doi: 10.3402/mehd.v26.25877

Seo, B. J., Mun, M. R., J, R. K., Kim, C. J., Lee, I., Chang, Y. H., et al. (2010). Bile tolerant *Lactobacillus reuteri* isolated from pig feces inhibits enteric bacterial pathogens and porcine rotavirus. *Vet. Res. Commun.* 34, 323–333. doi: 10.1007/ s11259-010-9357-6

Shi, L. H., Balakrishnan, K., Thiagarajah, K., Mohd Ismail, N. I., and Yin, O. S. (2016). Beneficial properties of probiotics. *Trop. Life Sci. Res.* 27, 73–90. doi: 10.21315/tlsr2016.27.2.6

Shornikova, A. V., Casas, I. A., Isolauri, E., Mykkanen, H., and Vesikari, T. (1997a). *Lactobacillus reuteri* as a therapeutic agent in acute diarrhea in young children. *J. Pediatr. Gastroenterol. Nutr.* 24, 399–404.

Shornikova, A. V., Casas, I. A., Mykkanen, H., Salo, E., and Vesikari, T. (1997b). Bacteriotherapy with *Lactobacillus reuteri* in rotavirus gastroenteritis. *Pediatr. Infect. Dis. J.* 16, 1103–1107.

Sims, I. M., Frese, S. A., Walter, J., Loach, D., Wilson, M., Appleyard, K., et al. (2011). Structure and functions of exopolysaccharide produced by gut commensal *Lactobacillus reuteri* 100-23. *ISME J.* 5, 1115–1124. doi: 10.1038/ ismej.2010.201

Sinkiewicz, G. (2010). *Lactobacillus reuteri in Health and Disease.* Doctoral dissertation, Malmö University, Malmö.

Soto, A., Martin, V., Jimenez, E., Mader, I., Rodriguez, J. M., and Fernandez, L. (2014). Lactobacilli and bifidobacteria in human breast milk: influence of antibiotherapy and other host and clinical factors. *J. Pediatr. Gastroenterol. Nutr.* 59, 78–88. doi: 10.1097/MPG.0000000000000347

Spinler, J. K., Taweechotipatr, M., Rognerud, C. L., Ou, C. N., Tumwasorn, S., and Versalovic, J. (2008). Human-derived probiotic *Lactobacillus reuteri* demonstrate antimicrobial activities targeting diverse enteric bacterial pathogens. *Anaerobe* 14, 166–171. doi: 10.1016/j.anaerobe.2008.02.001

Sriramulu, D. D., Liang, M., Hernandez-Romero, D., Raux-Deery, E., Lunsdorf, H., Parsons, J. B., et al. (2008). *Lactobacillus reuteri* DSM 20016 produces cobalamin-dependent diol dehydratase in metabolosomes and metabolizes 1,2-propanediol by disproportionation. *J. Bacteriol.* 190, 4559–4567. doi: 10. 1128/JB.01535-07

Stensson, M., Koch, G., Coric, S., Abrahamsson, T. R., Jenmalm, M. C., Birkhed, D., et al. (2014). Oral administration of *Lactobacillus reuteri* during the first year of life reduces caries prevalence in the primary dentition at 9 years of age. *Caries Res.* 48, 111–117. doi: 10.1159/000354412

Stevens, J. F., and Maier, C. S. (2008). Acrolein: sources, metabolism, and biomolecular interactions relevant to human health and disease. *Mol. Nutr. Food Res.* 52, 7–25. doi: 10.1002/mnfr.200700412

Stevens, M. J., Vollenweider, S., Meile, L., and Lacroix, C. (2011). 1,3-Propanediol dehydrogenases in *Lactobacillus reuteri*: impact on central metabolism and 3-hydroxypropionaldehyde production. *Microb. Cell Fact.* 10:61. doi: 10.1186/ 1475-2859-10-61

Su, M. S., and Ganzle, M. G. (2014). Novel two-component regulatory systems play a role in biofilm formation of *Lactobacillus reuteri* rodent isolate 100-23. *Microbiology* 160(Pt 4), 795–806. doi: 10.1099/mic.0.071399-0

Su, M. S., Schlicht, S., and Ganzle, M. G. (2011). Contribution of glutamate decarboxylase in *Lactobacillus reuteri* to acid resistance and persistence in sourdough fermentation. *Microb. Cell Fact.* 10(Suppl. 1):S8. doi: 10.1186/1475- 2859-10-S1-S8

Su, Y., Chen, X., Liu, M., and Guo, X. (2017). Effect of three lactobacilli with strain-specific activities on the growth performance, faecal microbiota and ileum mucosa proteomics of piglets. *J. Anim. Sci. Biotechnol.* 8:52. doi: 10.1186/ s40104-017-0183-3

Sung, V., Hiscock, H., Tang, M. L., Mensah, F. K., Nation, M. L., Satzke, C., et al. (2014). Treating infant colic with the probiotic *Lactobacillus reuteri*: double blind, placebo controlled randomised trial. *BMJ* 348:g2107. doi: 10.1136/bmj. g2107

Szajewska, H., Gyrczuk, E., and Horvath, A. (2013). *Lactobacillus reuteri* DSM 17938 for the management of infantile colic in breastfed infants: a randomized, double-blind, placebo-controlled trial. *J. Pediatr.* 162, 257–262. doi: 10.1016/j. jpeds.2012.08.004

Talarico, T. L., Casas, I. A., Chung, T. C., and Dobrogosz, W. J. (1988). Production and isolation of reuterin, a growth inhibitor produced by *Lactobacillus reuteri*. *Antimicrob. Agents Chemother.* 32, 1854–1858. doi: 10.1128/AAC.32.12.1854

Talarico, T. L., and Dobrogosz, W. J. (1989). Chemical characterization of an antimicrobial substance produced by *Lactobacillus reuteri*. *Antimicrob. Agents Chemother.* 33, 674–679. doi: 10.1128/AAC.33.5.674

Talarico, T. L., and Dobrogosz, W. J. (1990). Purification and characterization of glycerol dehydratase from *Lactobacillus reuteri*. *Appl. Environ. Microbiol.* 56, 1195–1197.

Taranto, M. P., Vera, J. L., Hugenholtz, J., De Valdez, G. F., and Sesma, F. (2003). *Lactobacillus reuteri* CRL1098 produces cobalamin. *J. Bacteriol.* 185, 5643–5647. doi: 10.1128/JB.185.18.5643-5647.2003

Thomas, C. M., Hong, T., van Pijkeren, J. P., Hemarajata, P., Trinh, D. V., Hu, W., et al. (2012). Histamine derived from probiotic *Lactobacillus reuteri* suppresses TNF via modulation of PKA and ERK signaling. *PLoS One* 7:e31951. doi: 10.1371/journal.pone.0031951

Thomas, C. M., Saulnier, D. M., Spinler, J. K., Hemarajata, P., Gao, C., Jones, S. E., et al. (2016). FolC2-mediated folate metabolism contributes to suppression of inflammation by probiotic *Lactobacillus reuteri*. *Microbiologyopen* 5, 802–818. doi: 10.1002/mbo3.371

Tsokos, G. C. (2011). Systemic lupus erythematosus. *N. Engl. J. Med.* 365, 2110–2121. doi: 10.1056/NEJMra1100359

Tubelius, P., Stan, V., and Zachrisson, A. (2005). Increasing work-place healthiness with the probiotic *Lactobacillus reuteri*: a randomised, double-blind placebo-controlled study. *Environ. Health* 4:25. doi: 10.1186/1476-069X-4-25

Tzang, B. S., Liu, C. H., Hsu, K. C., Chen, Y. H., Huang, C. Y., and Hsu, T. C. (2017). Effects of oral *Lactobacillus* administration on antioxidant activities and CD4+CD25+forkhead box P3 (FoxP3)+ T cells in NZB/W F1 mice. *Br. J. Nutr.* 118, 333–342. doi: 10.1017/S0007114517002112

Valeur, N., Engel, P., Carbajal, N., Connolly, E., and Ladefoged, K. (2004). Colonization and immunomodulation by *Lactobacillus reuteri* ATCC 55730 in the human gastrointestinal tract. *Appl. Environ. Microbiol.* 70, 1176–1181. doi: 10.1128/AEM.70.2.1176-1181.2004

Walter, J., Britton, R. A., and Roos, S. (2011). Host-microbial symbiosis in the vertebrate gastrointestinal tract and the *Lactobacillus reuteri* paradigm. *Proc. Natl. Acad. Sci. U.S.A.* 108(Suppl. 1), 4645–4652. doi: 10.1073/pnas.1000099107

Walter, J., Chagnaud, P., Tannock, G. W., Loach, D. M., Dal Bello, F., Jenkinson, H. F., et al. (2005). A high-molecular-mass surface protein (Lsp) and methionine sulfoxide reductase B (MsrB) contribute to the ecological performance of *Lactobacillus reuteri* in the murine gut. *Appl. Environ. Microbiol.* 71, 979–986. doi: 10.1128/AEM.71.2.979-986.2005

Walter, J., Loach, D. M., Alqumber, M., Rockel, C., Hermann, C., Pfitzenmaier, M., et al. (2007). D-alanyl ester depletion of teichoic acids in *Lactobacillus reuteri* 100-23 results in impaired colonization of the mouse gastrointestinal tract. *Environ. Microbiol.* 9, 1750–1760. doi: 10.1111/j.1462-2920.2007.01292.x

Walter, J., Schwab, C., Loach, D. M., Ganzle, M. G., and Tannock, G. W. (2008). Glucosyltransferase A (GtfA) and inulosucrase (Inu) of *Lactobacillus reuteri* TMW1.106 contribute to cell aggregation, in vitro biofilm formation, and colonization of the mouse gastrointestinal tract. *Microbiology* 154(Pt 1), 72–80. doi: 10.1099/mic.0.2007/010637-0

Wang, B., Wei, H., Yuan, J., Li, Q., Li, Y., Li, N., et al. (2008). Identification of a surface protein from *Lactobacillus reuteri* JCM1081 that adheres to porcine gastric mucin and human enterocyte-like HT-29 cells. *Curr. Microbiol.* 57, 33–38. doi: 10.1007/s00284-008-9148-2

Wang, P., Li, Y., Xiao, H., Shi, Y., Le, G. W., and Sun, J. (2016). Isolation of *lactobacillus reuteri* from Peyer's patches and their effects on sIgA production and gut microbiota diversity. *Mol. Nutr. Food Res.* 60, 2020–2030. doi: 10.1002/mnfr.201501065

Wang, Y., Ganzle, M. G., and Schwab, C. (2010). Exopolysaccharide synthesized by *Lactobacillus reuteri* decreases the ability of enterotoxigenic *Escherichia coli* to bind to porcine erythrocytes. *Appl. Environ. Microbiol.* 76, 4863–4866. doi: 10.1128/AEM.03137-09

Wang, Z., Wang, L., Chen, Z., Ma, X., Yang, X., Zhang, J., et al. (2016). In vitro evaluation of swine-derived *Lactobacillus reuteri*: probiotic properties and effects on intestinal porcine epithelial cells challenged with enterotoxigenic *Escherichia coli* K88. *J. Microbiol. Biotechnol.* 26, 1018–1025. doi: 10.4014/jmb.1510.10089

Wanke, M., and Szajewska, H. (2012). Lack of an effect of *Lactobacillus reuteri* DSM 17938 in preventing nosocomial diarrhea in children: a randomized, double-blind, placebo-controlled trial. *J. Pediatr.* 161, 40.e1–43.e1. doi: 10.1016/j.jpeds.2011.12.049

Weizman, Z., Abu-Abed, J., and Binsztok, M. (2016). *Lactobacillus reuteri* DSM 17938 for the management of functional abdominal pain in childhood: a randomized, double-blind, placebo-controlled trial. *J. Pediatr.* 174, 160.e1–164.e1. doi: 10.1016/j.jpeds.2016.04.003

Weizman, Z., and Alsheikh, A. (2006). Safety and tolerance of a probiotic formula in early infancy comparing two probiotic agents: a pilot study. *J. Am. Coll. Nutr.* 25, 415–419. doi: 10.1080/07315724.2006.10719554

Weizman, Z., Asli, G., and Alsheikh, A. (2005). Effect of a probiotic infant formula on infections in child care centers: comparison of two probiotic agents. *Pediatrics* 115, 5–9. doi: 10.1542/peds.2004-1815

Wolf, B. W., Wheeler, K. B., Ataya, D. G., and Garleb, K. A. (1998). Safety and tolerance of *Lactobacillus reuteri* supplementation to a population infected with the human immunodeficiency virus. *Food Chem. Toxicol.* 36, 1085–1094. doi: 10.1016/S0278-6915(98)00090-8

Yang, F., Wang, A., Zeng, X., Hou, C., Liu, H., and Qiao, S. (2015). *Lactobacillus reuteri* I5007 modulates tight junction protein expression in IPEC-J2 cells with LPS stimulation and in newborn piglets under normal conditions. *BMC Microbiol.* 15:32. doi: 10.1186/s12866-015-0372-1

Yang, G., Tian, J., and Li, J. (2007). Fermentation of 1,3-propanediol by a lactate deficient mutant of *Klebsiella oxytoca* under microaerobic conditions. *Appl. Microbiol. Biotechnol.* 73, 1017–1024. doi: 10.1007/s00253-006-0563-7

Yang, Y., Zhao, X., Le, M. H., Zijlstra, R. T., and Ganzle, M. G. (2015). Reutericyclin producing *Lactobacillus reuteri* modulates development of fecal microbiota in weanling pigs. *Front. Microbiol.* 6:762. doi: 10.3389/fmicb.2015.00762

Yoo, B. B., and Mazmanian, S. K. (2017). The enteric network: interactions between the immune and nervous systems of the gut. *Immunity* 46, 910–926. doi: 10.1016/j.immuni.2017.05.011

Yurkovetskiy, L., Burrows, M., Khan, A. A., Graham, L., Volchkov, P., Becker, L., et al. (2013). Gender bias in autoimmunity is influenced by microbiota. *Immunity* 39, 400–412. doi: 10.1016/j.immuni.2013.08.013

Zelante, T., Iannitti, R. G., Cunha, C., De Luca, A., Giovannini, G., Pieraccini, G., et al. (2013). Tryptophan catabolites from microbiota engage aryl hydrocarbon receptor and balance mucosal reactivity via interleukin-22. *Immunity* 39, 372–385. doi: 10.1016/j.immuni.2013.08.003

Zhang, D., Ji, H., Liu, H., Wang, S., Wang, J., and Wang, Y. (2016). Changes in the diversity and composition of gut microbiota of weaned piglets after oral administration of *Lactobacillus* or an antibiotic. *Appl. Microbiol. Biotechnol.* 100, 10081–10093. doi: 10.1007/s00253-016-7845-5

Zhang, H., Liao, X., Sparks, J. B., and Luo, X. M. (2014). Dynamics of gut microbiota in autoimmune lupus. *Appl. Environ. Microbiol.* 80, 7551–7560. doi: 10.1128/AEM.02676-14

Zhu, M. M., Lawman, P. D., and Cameron, D. C. (2002). Improving 1,3-propanediol production from glycerol in a metabolically engineered *Escherichia coli* by reducing accumulation of sn-glycerol-3-phosphate. *Biotechnol. Prog.* 18, 694–699. doi: 10.1021/bp020281

6

Epstein-Barr Virus DNA Enhances Diptericin Expression and Increases Hemocyte Numbers in *Drosophila melanogaster* via the Immune Deficiency Pathway

Nour Sherri, Noor Salloum, Carine Mouawad, Nathaline Haidar-Ahmad, Margret Shirinian and Elias A. Rahal**

Department of Experimental Pathology, Microbiology, and Immunology, American University of Beirut, Beirut, Lebanon

***Correspondence:**
Margret Shirinian
ms241@aub.edu.lb
Elias A. Rahal
er00@aub.edu.lb

Infection with the Epstein-Barr virus (EBV) is associated with several malignancies and autoimmune diseases in humans. The following EBV infection and establishment of latency, recurrences frequently occur resulting in potential viral DNA shedding, which may then trigger the activation of immune pathways. We have previously demonstrated that levels of the pro-inflammatory cytokine IL-17, which is associated with several autoimmune diseases, are increased in response to EBV DNA injection in mice. Whether other pro-inflammatory pathways are induced in EBV DNA pathobiology remains to be investigated. The complexity of mammalian immune systems presents a challenge to studying differential activities of their intricate immune pathways in response to a particular immune stimulus. In this study, we used *Drosophila melanogaster* to identify innate humoral and cellular immune pathways that are activated in response to EBV DNA. Injection of wild-type adult flies with EBV DNA induced the immune deficiency (IMD) pathway resulting in enhanced expression of the antimicrobial peptide diptericin. Furthermore, EBV DNA increased the number of hemocytes in flies. Conditional silencing of the IMD pathway decreased diptericin expression in addition to curbing of hemocyte proliferation in response to challenge with EBV DNA. Comparatively, upon injecting mice with EBV DNA, we detected enhanced expression of tumor necrosis factor-α (TNFα); this enhancement is rather comparable to IMD pathway activation in flies. This study hence indicates that *D. melanogaster* could possibly be utilized to identify immune mediators that may also play a role in the response to EBV DNA in higher systems.

Keywords: Epstein-Barr virus (EBV), human herpesvirus 4, *Drosophila melanogaster*, diptericin, immune deficiency (IMD) pathway, tumor necrosis factor-α (TNF-α), deoxyribonucleic acid (DNA), proinflammatory

INTRODUCTION

The Epstein-Bar virus (EBV) is a human pathogen that belongs to the herpes family of viruses. Like other herpes viruses, EBV establishes latency in the host after primary infection with potential future reactivation of viral replication. In addition to causing infectious mononucleosis, this virus is associated with several types of malignancies such as Burkitt and Hodgkin lymphomas, nasopharyngeal carcinoma, and post-transplant lymphoproliferative disorders (PTLD). Moreover, this virus is associated with multiple autoimmune diseases including systemic lupus erythematosus (SLE), rheumatoid arthritis (RA), and multiple sclerosis (MS) (Lünemann et al., 2007; Draborg et al., 2013). SLE patients were demonstrated to have high EBV viral loads in their peripheral blood mononuclear cells (PBMCs) (Gross et al., 2005; Yu et al., 2005). Similar observations were seen in RA patients whereby high EBV viral loads were detected in the blood, synovial fluid cells, and synovial membranes (Blaschke et al., 2000). Furthermore, various studies suggest that the risk of developing MS increases in EBV-infected individuals (Ascherio et al., 2001; Delorenze et al., 2006). A number of underlying mechanisms that link EBV to autoimmunity have been proposed; these have ranged from molecular mimicry to sequestered antigen release (reviewed in Ascherio and Munger, 2015). Nevertheless, despite these various proposed mechanisms, evidence that conclusively indicates one to mediate autoimmunity by EBV remains lacking; this likely indicates that multiple mechanisms are involved.

We have previously reported that injecting mice with EBV DNA triggers the expression of IL-17, a proinflammatory cytokine associated with autoimmune processes (Rahal et al., 2015). We also observed enhanced levels of other proinflammatory cytokines such as IL-23 and IFNγ. Others have reported that EBV DNA enhances the production of IL-8 from primary human monocytes and IFN-α from human plasmacytoid dendritic cell (Fiola et al., 2010). Owing to the fact that the latency established by EBV in the host is life-long and may result in frequent reactivations and consequent shedding of viral DNA, the proinflammatory pathways triggered by this DNA may contribute to autoimmune processes resulting in triggering or exacerbation of disease. The complexity of mammalian immune systems presents a challenge to comprehensively identify the various immune pathways triggered by EBV DNA and that may serve as potential therapeutic targets in autoimmune diseases. Hence, we attempted to establish *Drosophila melanogaster* as a relatively less complex system to detect innate immune pathways that are activated in response to EBV DNA. Furthermore, to the best of our knowledge, this is the first study examining the effect of viral DNA itself, rather than an infection, on the immune system in flies. The fly immune system is largely devoid of adaptable immune components and hence it solely relies on innate immune responses. Innate immunity in flies involves humoral as well as cellular responses. The humoral immune response involves three major pathways: the Toll, the immune deficiency (IMD), and the Janus kinase/signal transducers and activators of transcription (JAK-STAT) pathways. The production of about twenty antimicrobial peptides (AMPs) is under the control of the Toll and IMD pathways (Imler and Bulet, 2005). The expression of most of these AMPs such as attacin and cecropin may be triggered by either pathway; on the other hand, the production of drosomycin is primarily reliant on the Toll pathway while that of drosocin and diptericin is dependent on the IMD pathway. Activation of the JAK-STAT pathway has also been shown to respond to immunostimulatory challenges by triggering the expression of the stress-inducible humoral factor Turandot (TotA) (Agaisse et al., 2003). As for the cellular innate immune arm in flies it is reliant on defensive activities performed by the hemocyte compartment which 95% consists of plasmatocytes (Buchon et al., 2014). We report here that injecting EBV DNA into adult flies results in triggering the IMD pathway and in the concomitant enhancement of plasmatocyte proliferation.

MATERIALS AND METHODS

Flies

Flies were raised and crossed at 25°C; standard *Drosophila* husbandry procedures were followed. W1118 wild-type flies (Bloomington Drosophila Stock Center #3605, Bloomington, IN, United States), UAS-STAT92e (Ghiglione et al., 2002), UAS-Relish ((Ayyar et al., 2007), and UAS-Toll10b (Maxton-Kuchenmeister et al., 1999) flies were employed. The IMD-RNAi line (Vienna Stock center #9253) was obtained from the Vienna Drosophila Stock Center (Vienna, Austria). In addition, the hemocyte driver Cg25C-GAL4 (Bloomington stock center #7011) was used.

Overexpression of Relish, Toll10b, and STAT92e was attained using the following crosses, respectively: CG25C-Gal4> UAS-Relish, CG25C-Gal4> UAS-Toll10b, and CG25C-Gal4> UAS-STAT92e. Conditional silencing of IMD was performed using the following cross: CG25C-Gal4> UAS-IMD RNAi.

Fly Treatments

EBV DNA was obtained from Advanced Biotechnologies (Columbia, MD, United States) while bacterial DNA was prepared from an isolate of *Staphylococcus epidermidis* by phenol precipitation followed by extraction with ethanol.

To assess the effect of EBV DNA on the expression of drosomycin, diptericin, and TotA, 1-day-old flies were injected with various copy numbers of EBV DNA. As non-viral DNA control, fly groups received bacterial DNA in amounts equivalent to the weight of EBV DNA copy numbers administered. As negative controls, some fly groups received no injections while others received sterile water, the DNA solvent. Groups of 1-day-old flies that overexpressed Toll10b, STAT92e, and Relish were included as positive controls for Toll, JAK-STAT, and IMD pathway activation as well. To examine the effect of EBV DNA on older flies, 1-week-old flies were injected with EBV DNA or with sterile water. All injections were administered into the thorax of CO_2-anesthetized flies using a Nano-injector (World Precision Instruments, Sarasota, FL, United States) and glass capillary needles. A total volume of 55.2 nl was injected into each fly.

The copy numbers of EBV DNA injected into flies were extrapolated from our previous studies in mice (Rahal et al., 2015). The following formula was used to calculate *Drosophila* equivalent copy numbers and was modified from the Food and Drug Administration (FDA) recommended formula for dose conversions (14):

$$\text{Drosophila equivalent dose} = \text{Mouse dose} \times \frac{\text{Mouse Km}}{\text{Drosophila Km}}$$

Where

$$\text{Km} = \frac{\text{Weight (kg)}}{\text{Body surface area (m}^2)}$$

The body surface area of *D. melanogaster* was calculated using Mosteller's formula (Mosteller, 1987).

Gene Expression Studies in Flies

Ten flies were collected per group per time point for gene expression studies. RNA extraction was subsequently performed using TRIzol (Sigma-Aldrich, St. Louis, MO, United States) according to the manufacturer's specifications. Then, cDNA synthesis was carried out using the QuantiTect® Reverse Transcription Kit (QIAGEN, Hilden, Germany). Real-time reverse transcriptase PCR was then performed to analyze relative gene expression levels. Primers used for this purpose were obtained from Thermo Scientific (Ulm, Germany). Previously published primers (**Table 1**) were used to analyze the expression of the drosomycin (Tanji et al., 2007), diptericin (Avadhanula et al., 2009), and TotA (Kallio et al., 2010) genes. Primers used to assess the expression of the IMD gene were selected using the NCBI primer designing tool. Transcription of the house keeping gene RPL32, used as an internal control, was detected also using previously published primers (Hedges and Johnson, 2008). Real-time PCR reactions each consisted of 10 μl and contained 5 μl of SYBR green, 150 pmoles of the forward primer, 150 pmoles of the reverse primer, and 150 ng of cDNA. Samples were analyzed in triplicates. Real time detection was performed in a BioRad CFX96 Real Time System employing a C1000 Thermal Cycler (Munich, Germany). A PCR initial activation step of 95°C for 5 min was used followed by 40 cycles of 95°C for 15 and 30 s at the annealing temperature for each primer as published. Relative gene expression normalized to the water-injected group was calculated using the $\Delta\Delta$Cq method. Samples were analyzed in triplicates.

Hemocyte Count

Flies were examined for hemocyte counts as previously described (Ghosh et al., 2015). For this purpose, three female flies per time point from each assessed group were anesthetized with CO2 and then their wings were excised. The flies were then placed in phosphate buffered saline (PBS) using 10 μl per fly. A fine incision was used to expose the thorax of each fly and bleeding was allowed into the PBS for 20 s. Subsequently, hemocyte counts were determined by examining 10 μl of the bleed using a hemocytometer under a light microscope and employing a 40× magnification. Analysis was performed in triplicates for each time point.

TABLE 1 | Primer sequences.

Primer	Sequences	Reference
Drosomycin	F: 5′-TACTTGTTCGCCCTCTTCG-3′ R: 5′-GTATCTTCCGGACAGGCAGT-3′	Tanji et al., 2007
Diptericin	F: 5′-AAGTGGGAAGCACCTACACCTACA-3′ R: 5′-GTATCTTCCGGACAGGCAGT-3′	Avadhanula et al., 2009
TotA	F: 5′-CCCAGTTTGACCCCTGAG-3′ R: 5′-GCCCTTCACACCTGGAGA-3′	Kallio et al., 2010
IMD	F: 5′-TCAGCGACCCAAACTACAATTC-3′ R: 5′-TTGTCTGGACGTTACTGAGAGT-3′	(Using NCBI primer designing tool)
RPL32	F: 5′-GACGCTTCAAGGGACAGTATCTG-3′ R: 5′-AGGGCCACAGCATGGGTCTGT-3′	Hedges and Johnson, 2008

Analysis of TNFα Expression in Mice

Experimental procedures conducted on mice were approved by the Institutional Animal Care and Use Committee (IACUC) at the American University of Beirut (AUB). BALB/c mice, 4-6 weeks of age, were obtained from the Animal Care Facility at AUB. Mice were intraperitoneally injected with 144×10^3 copies of EBV DNA, 22.3 pg of *S. epidermidis* DNA (equivalent to the weight of 144×10^3 EBV DNA copies) or sterile water. Each injection consisted of 100 μl. Three mice per treatment were sacrificed on day 6 post-injection, their spleens were collected, pooled and then subjected to RNA extraction using TRIzol. The RNA was used for cDNA synthesis using the QuantiTect® Reverse Transcription Kit. Real-time reverse transcriptase PCR was then performed to detect relative gene expression levels of TNFα using previously published primers (Peinnequin et al., 2004). Previously published primers (Pindado et al., 2007) were also employed to detect the expression of β-actin, used as an internal control. Real-time PCR reactions were performed and relative gene expression normalized to the water-injected mice was calculated as described for fly gene expression studies described above. Analysis was conducted in triplicates.

Statistical Analysis

To analyze statistical significance unpaired *t*-tests were used to compare means and were performed using Graphpad; *p*-values less than 0.05 were considered statistically significant.

RESULTS

EBV DNA Enhances the Expression of Diptericin in Flies

To assess the effect of EBV DNA on the humoral arm of innate immunity in *D. melanogaster*, flies were intrathoracically injected with 70, 140, or 280 copies of EBV DNA. Flies were then analyzed for the expression of drosomycin, diptericin, and TotA as molecular indicators of activation of the Toll, IMD, and JAK-STAT pathways, respectively. Whereas we did not observe an increase in the expression of drosomycin (**Figure 1**) or TotA (**Figure 2**) upon EBV DNA treatment, we detected a 115-fold increase ($p = 0.0002$) in the transcriptional levels of diptericin (**Figure 3**) in the group injected with 70 copies of EBV DNA on day 1 post-injection. This level then decreased to 5.62 on day 3. No notable changes were observed upon injecting flies with 140 or 280 copies of EBV DNA.

To examine whether the observed effects are specific to EBV DNA itself, flies were injected with an amount of *S. epidermidis*

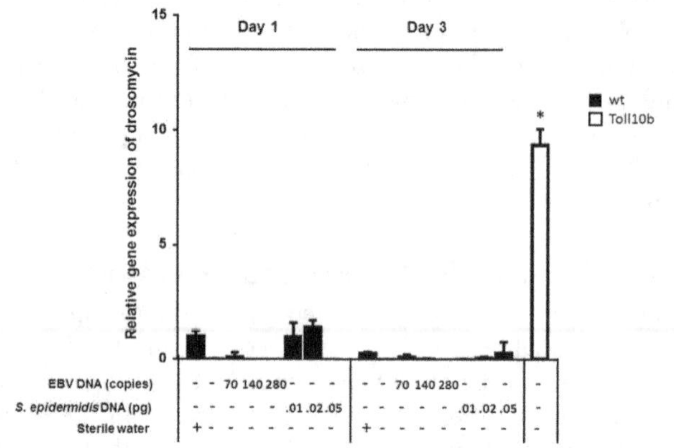

FIGURE 1 | Drosomycin relative gene expression in flies injected with EBV DNA on days 1 and 3 post-injection. Expression was assessed in W1118 wild-type (wt) flies that received no injection and wt flies injected with sterile water, EBV DNA (70, 140, or 280 copies) or *S. epidermidis* DNA (0.01, 0.02, or 0.05 pg) on days 1 and 3 post-injection. Flies overexpressing Toll10b were included as a positive control for drosomycin expression. Data is normalized to expression in water-injected flies on day 1 post-injection. *Indicates $p < 0.05$.

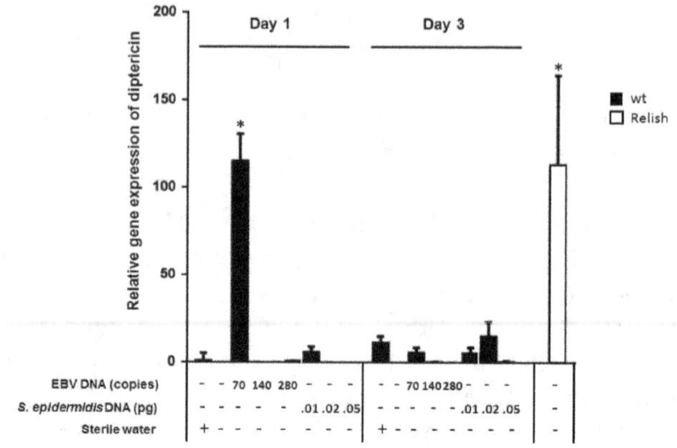

FIGURE 3 | Diptericin relative gene expression in flies injected with EBV DNA on days 1 and 3 post-injection. Expression was assessed in W1118 wild-type (wt) flies that received no injection and wt flies injected with sterile water, EBV DNA (70, 140, or 280 copies) or *S. epidermidis* DNA (0.0.1, 0.02, or 0.05 pg) on days 1 and 3 post-injection. Flies overexpressing Relish were included as positive control for diptericin expression. Data is normalized to expression in water-injected flies on day 1 post-injection. *Indicates $p < 0.05$.

DNA equivalent to the weight of the EBV DNA copy numbers employed. Treatment with this non-viral DNA control did not notably alter the expression of the humoral immunity markers assessed.

We then examined the expression of diptericin at 6, 12, 24, 48, 36, and 72 h after injection (**Figure 4A**) and included lower copy numbers of EBV DNA into the analysis. Upon injecting flies with 10 copies of EBV DNA, diptericin levels began to significantly increase after 24 h of injection and continued to elevate reaching a highest detected increase of 16-folds ($p = 0.001$) 72 h after injection. Flies injected with 35 copies of EBV DNA also demonstrated significantly increasing levels of diptericin expression after 24 h of injection with levels peaking at 48 h after injection (23-folds, $p = 0.0001$) then decreasing afterwards. Injection of 70 copies of EBV DNA resulted in a significant increase in the relative gene expression starting after 12 h of injection, peaking at 24 h and decreasing from then onwards. Hence, a time-dependent dose response is seen in the enhancement of diptericin expression by EBV DNA treatment. Injection with 140 or 280 copies did not result in any increase in the levels of diptericin expression indicating that EBV DNA may have a biphasic hormetic effect on diptericin expression in flies whereby low levels are stimulatory but high levels are inhibitory. To examine the effect of EBV DNA in older flies, 1-week-old wild-type flies were injected with 70 copies of EBV DNA; diptericin expression levels were then determined in these flies after 24 h of receiving the injection. Diptericin expression levels were reduced by about 140-folds in the 1-week-old flies upon injection with EBV DNA compared to similarly treated 1-day old flies (**Figure 4B**).

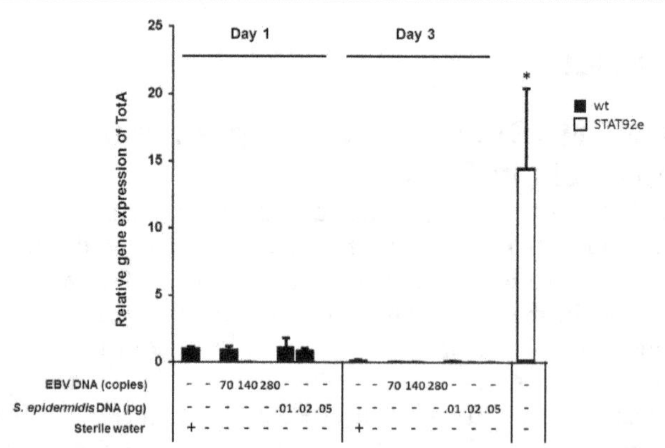

FIGURE 2 | TotA relative gene expression in flies injected with EBV DNA on days 1 and 3 post-injection. Expression was assessed in W1118 wild-type flies (wt) that received no injection and wt flies injected with sterile water, EBV DNA (70, 140, or 280 copies) or *S. epidermidis* DNA (0.01, 0.02, or 0.05 pg) on days 1 and 3 post-injection. Flies overexpressing STAT92e were included as a positive control for TotA expression. Data is normalized to expression in water-injected flies on day 1 post-injection. *Indicates $p < 0.05$.

Silencing IMD Abrogates EBV DNA-Triggered Expression of Diptericin

To establish that enhanced expression of diptericin in response to EBV DNA is the result of IMD pathway activation rather than an alternate pathway, we knocked down the expression of the IMD mediator, a key component of this pathway. Flies were then injected with 70 copies of EBV DNA and analyzed for expression of diptericin after 24 h of injection (**Figure 5A**). In contrast to wild-type flies, knocking down IMD resulted in inhibition of diptericin expression in response to EBV DNA ($p = 0.009$). Assessing the efficiency of silencing IMD demonstrated a substantial decrease in the mRNA levels (**Figure 5B**).

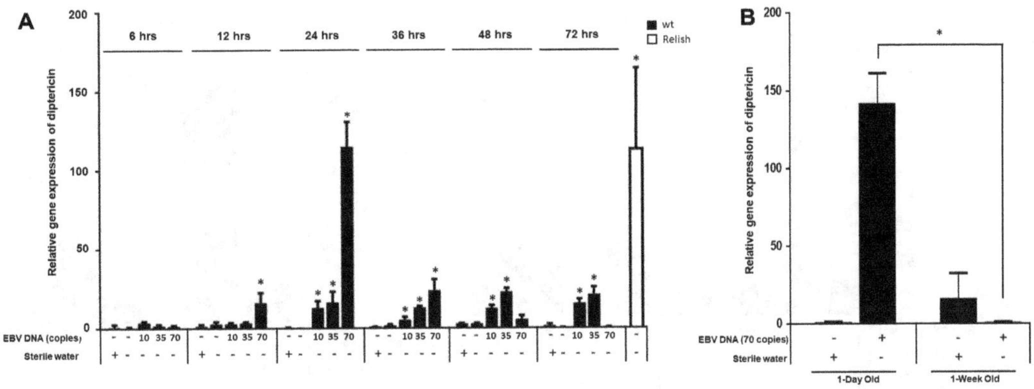

FIGURE 4 | Diptericin relative gene expression in flies injected with EBV DNA at 6, 12, 24, 36, 48, and 72 h post-injection. **(A)** Expression was assessed in W1118 wild-type (wt) flies that received no injection and wt flies injected with sterile water, EBV DNA (10, 35, or 70 copies) or *S. epidermidis* DNA (0.0.1, 0.02, or 0.05 pg) at multiple time points post-injection. Flies overexpressing Relish were included as positive control for diptericin expression. Data is normalized to expression in water-injected flies at 6 h post-injection. *Indicates $p < 0.05$. **(B)** Diptericin relative gene expression was assessed in 1-day-old and 1-week-old W1118 wild-type (wt) flies after 24 h of receiving an injection of 70 copies of EBV DNA. Flies that received injections of sterile water were included as controls. *Indicates $p < 0.05$.

EBV DNA Elevates the Number of Hemocytes in Fly Bleed

We examined the effect of EBV DNA on the cellular arm of fly immunity by injecting adult female flies with 70, 140, or 280 copies of EBV DNA and then assessing the number of hemocytes in the fly bleed on days 1 and 3 post-injection. Treatments with *S. epidermidis* DNA were included as a non-viral DNA control. We observed a sevenfold increase ($p = 0.0009$) in the number of circulating hemocytes in flies administered 70 copies of EBV DNA after 1 day of injection. This number had notably dwindled back to normal levels on day 3 after injection in this group. As for flies injected with 140 or 280 copies of EBV DNA or with *S. epidermidis* DNA no notable elevations in circulating hemocyte numbers were detected (**Figure 6A**). To examine the effect of EBV DNA in older flies, 1-week-old wild-type flies were injected with 70 copies of EBV DNA; hemocytes were then enumerated after 24 h of receiving the injection. The number of hemocytes in the bleed of 1-week-old flies upon injection with EBV DNA was about 30% lower than that in 1-day-old flies that were similarly treated (**Figure 6B**).

The IMD Pathway Plays a Role in the EBV DNA-Triggered Elevation of Hemocyte Levels

Both circulating hemocyte numbers and diptericin levels were elevated in response to 70 copies of EBV DNA after 24 h of injection but not by 140 or 280 copies of DNA or at later time points. Thus, circulating hemocyte numbers were affected by EBV

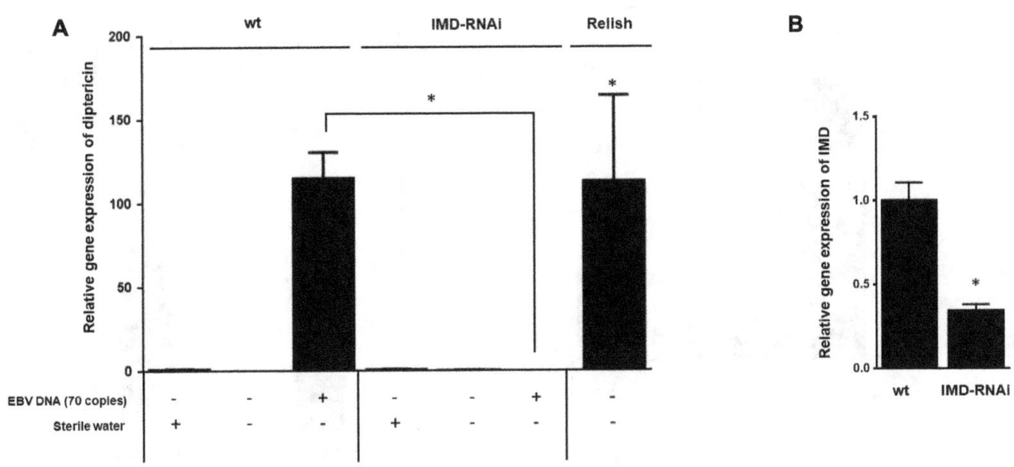

FIGURE 5 | Effect of IMD silencing on diptericin relative gene expression in flies injected with EBV DNA. **(A)** IMD relative gene expression in W1118 wild-type (wt) and IMD knock-down flies. **(B)** Diptericin expression was assessed in W1118 wild-type (wt) and IMD knock-down flies that received no injection, were injected with sterile water or with EBV DNA (70 copies). Expression was assessed on day 1 post-injection. Flies overexpressing Relish were included as a positive control for diptericin expression. *Indicates $p < 0.05$.

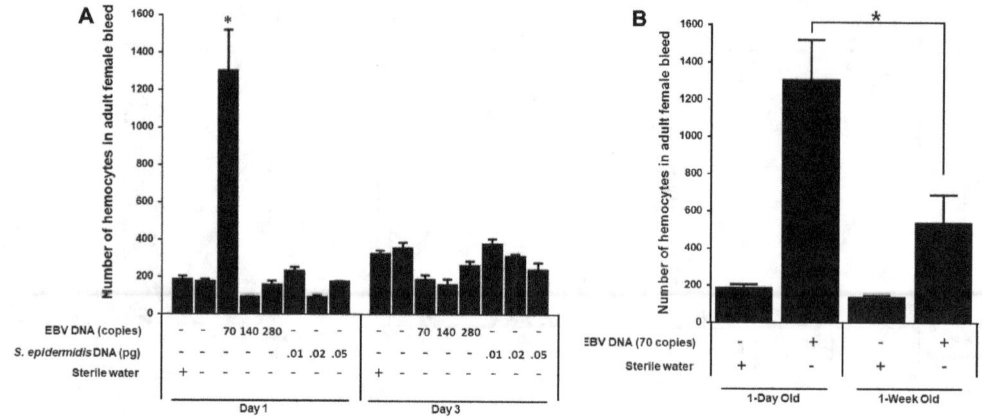

FIGURE 6 | Number of hemocytes in flies injected with EBV DNA. **(A)** Hemocytes in adult female fly bleed were enumerated in W1118 wild-type (wt) flies that received no injection and wt flies injected with sterile water, EBV DNA (70, 140, or 280 copies) or *S. epidermidis* DNA (0.0.1, 0.02, or 0.05 pg) on days 1 and 3 post-injection. *Indicates $p < 0.05$. **(B)** Hemocytes were enumerated in 1-day-old and 1-week-old W1118 wild-type (wt) flies after 24 h of receiving an injection of 70 copies of EBV DNA. Flies that received injections of sterile water were included as controls. *Indicates $p < 0.05$.

DNA in a manner that highly mirrored the observed responses in diptericin expression within EBV DNA-treated fly groups. Consequently, we analyzed whether the IMD pathway underlies this elevation in hemocytes by knocking down the IMD mediator and examining the number of hemocytes in the bleed after 24 h of injecting adult female flies with 70 copies of EBV DNA (**Figure 7**). Knocking down IMD decreased the number of hemocytes 2.5-folds ($p = 0.0035$) compared to wild-type flies upon injection with 70 copies of EBV DNA. This indicates that this pathway is a key player in the cellular responses seen upon treating flies with EBV DNA.

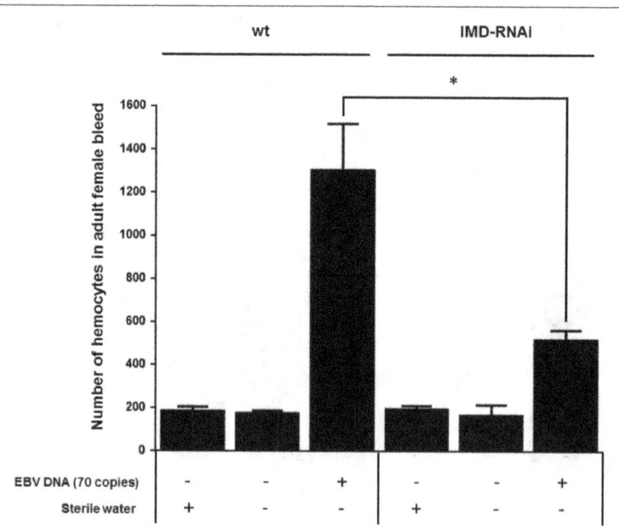

FIGURE 7 | Number of hemocytes in IMD-silenced flies injected with EBV DNA. Number of hemocytes in adult female fly bleed in W1118 wild-type (wt) and IMD knock-down flies that received no injection, were injected with sterile water or with EBV DNA (70 copies). Cells were enumerated on day 1 post-injection. *Indicates $p < 0.05$.

EBV DNA Enhances TNFα Expression in Mice

The IMD pathway is often compared to tumor necrosis Factor-α Receptor signaling (TNFR) in mammals (71). Hence, we examined whether EBV DNA triggers TNFα in a mammalian system by injecting mice with 144×10^3 copies of EBV DNA and assessing TNFα expression in mouse spleens on day 6 post-injection (**Figure 8**). We had previously detected a peak in mouse IL-17 levels on that day after injection with 144×10^3 copies of EBV DNA. Mice injected with EBV DNA showed a 3.5-fold increase in the transcription of TNFα. On the other hand, no significant changes were detected in mice injected with bacterial DNA.

DISCUSSION

Enhanced production of proinflammatory cytokines triggered by EBV DNA in mammalian systems has been reported by our

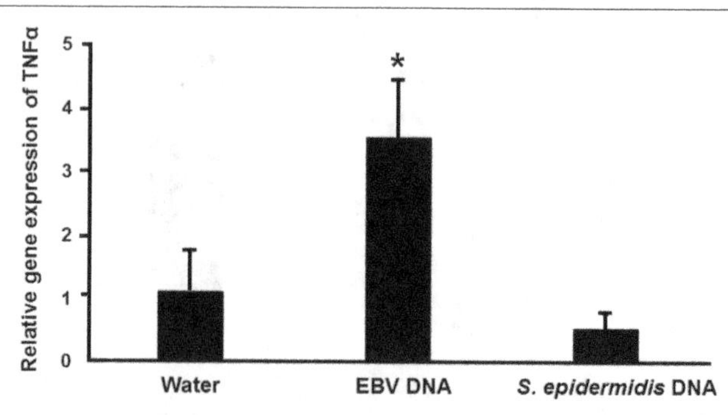

FIGURE 8 | Relative gene expression of TNFα in mice injected with EBV DNA. Expression was assessed in splenic tissue from BALB/c mice that were intraperitoneally injected with water, 144×10^3 copies of EBV DNA or 22.3 pg of *S. epidermidis* DNA on day 6 post-injection. *Indicates $p < 0.05$.

group among others (Fiola et al., 2010; Rahal et al., 2015). This raises the possibility of involvement of other immune modulators in response to EBV DNA. We thus aimed to implement a system that permits relatively simple screening of humoral and cellular responses to viral DNA. Therefore, we used the fruit fly, *D. melanogaster*, an organism with a versatile library of genetic tools to study such responses. The fruit fly has well-conserved cellular and humoral innate immune pathways in addition to the absence of adaptive immunity; this facilitates the identification of innate pathways, the basis of proinflammatory responses that may be involved in EBV DNA-triggered immune activation in higher mammalian systems.

Upon injecting 70 copies of EBV DNA into flies, the transcriptional level of diptericin, the hallmark of IMD pathway activation, was significantly increased by day 1 post-injection. In a similar manner, hemocyte numbers were significantly elevated in flies upon treatment with EBV DNA. Both diptericin expression and hemocyte proliferation effects had dwindled by day 3 post-injection. On the other hand, injections of 140 or 280 copies of EBV DNA did not result in similar increases in neither diptericin expression levels nor in hemocyte proliferation. This may indicate that EBV DNA results in a biphasic hormetic response in flies whereby lower doses induce a possibly beneficial immunostimulatory response whereas higher doses overwhelm the system and are rather inhibitory. Various agents have been previously described to have such an effect in biological systems (Calabrese and Baldwin, 1999, 2001). The particular underlying molecular etiology of such a response remains to be elucidated. Worth noting is that an injection of 144×10^3 copies of EBV DNA in mice, which we had previously reported to induce a prominent elevation of IL-17A levels and demonstrated herein to induce TNFα expression in mice, is equivalent to administration of 140 copies of EBV in flies; whereas this dose appears to be immunostimulatory in mice, a similar observation is not seen in flies. Therefore, whether higher doses of EBV DNA also have a biphasic hormetic immunomodulatory response in mice remains to be investigated. Knocking down IMD abrogated both of the humoral and cellular effects. These results suggest that cross-talk between humoral and cellular pathways may occur in response to EBV DNA injection and that IMD is a key mediator in both types of activation. The IMD pathway has been shown to induce Jun amino-terminal kinase (JNK)-dependent expression of the ligands for *Drosophila* vascular endothelial growth factor (VEGF) and platelet-derived growth factor (PDGF) receptor (PVR), PDGF- and VEGF-related factors 2 and 3 (PVF2 and PVF3) (Bond and Foley, 2009), which in turn induce hemocyte proliferation in *Drosophila* (Munier et al., 2002). Hence, the increase in diptericin expression levels and hemocyte numbers upon EBV DNA injection is likely initiated by activation of the IMD humoral immune pathway; this subsequently results in cellular responses. The observation that 70 or fewer copies of EBV DNA trigger the IMD pathway but that 140 or 280 copies do not induce such a response likely indicates that higher copy numbers exert an inhibitory effect; the particular nature of this effect was not determined by the current study. Worth noting is that the DNA within a nascent EBV virion upon release from an infected cell is linear and contains unmethylated CpG dinucleotides (Kintner and Sugden, 1981). Hence, any shed DNA in addition to that delivered into a cell upon an infection is in this form. Hence, the DNA we used in the study at hand was also linear and unmethylated.

The transcriptional levels of drosomycin and TotA, which are indicative of Toll and JAK-SAT pathway activation, respectively, were not affected by EBV DNA treatment. This may indicate that EBV DNA does not activate these pathways or that their activation occurs under other conditions than those assessed by the current study. Previous studies have indicated that unmethylated CpG DNA motifs, which are abundant in the EBV genome in a nascent viral particle (Bergbauer et al., 2010), activate innate immunity through TLR9 in mammals (Fiola et al., 2010); hence, *D. melanogaster*, as implemented for examining the immune effects of EBV DNA in the current study, may be used to assess Toll involvement in the response to EBV DNA in flies under other conditions in further studies. Worth noting is that in *D. melanogaster* endogenous accumulation of chromosomal DNA also triggers the production of diptericin (Häcker et al., 2000). Although the nature of DNA exerting this effect is not microbial, it may indicate that responses to various types of immunostimulatory DNA occur via activation of the IMD pathway in flies.

The IMD pathway in flies is considered to be comparable to signaling mediated by TNFR in mammals (Govind, 2008). We hence examined whether TNFα expression levels are affected by EBV DNA in mice. We observed elevated expression levels of this proinflammatory mediator. Hence, a congruent response was detected in mice. We have previously reported that IL-17, IL-23, and IFNγ are enhanced in mice administered EBV DNA. The detection of elevated TNFα adds to the complexity of the proinflammatory response that seems to be triggered in mammalian systems in response to EBV DNA.

CONCLUSION

EBV DNA triggers the IMD pathway in flies and enhances comparable TNFα expression in mice. This rather validates the implementation of D. melanogaster to screen for responses and mediators triggered by viral DNA. Identification of sensors of viral DNA and downstream mediators via the use of the fruit fly may reveal possible therapeutic targets of pro-inflammatory responses in humans.

AUTHOR CONTRIBUTIONS

NSh participated in the study design, performed the experiments, and contributed to analysis and writing. NSa, CM, and NH-A assisted in experimental procedures. MS and ER designed the study, supervised the work and resultant analysis. MS and ER contributed equally to this work and should both be listed as corresponding authors.

FUNDING

ER was funded by the Asmar Research Fund, the Lebanese National Council for Scientific Research (L-CNRS), and by the Medical Practice Plan (MPP) at the American University of Beirut. MS was funded by the Medical Practice Plan (MPP) at the American University of Beirut and the Lebanese National Council for Scientific Research (L-CNRS).

REFERENCES

Agaisse, H., Petersen, U. M., Boutros, M., Mathey-Prevot, B., and Perrimon, N. (2003). Signaling role of hemocytes in *Drosophila* JAK/STAT-dependent response to septic injury. *Dev. Cell* 5, 441–450. doi: 10.1016/S1534-5807(03)00244-2

Ascherio, A., and Munger, K. L. (2015). EBV and autoimmunity. *Curr. Top. Microbiol. Immunol.* 390, 365–385. doi: 10.1007/978-3-319-22822-8_15

Ascherio, A., Munger, K. L., Lennette, E. T., Spiegelman, D., Hernán, M. A., Olek, M. J., et al. (2001). Epstein-Barr virus antibodies and risk of multiple sclerosis: a prospective study. *JAMA* 286, 3083–3088. doi: 10.1001/jama.286.24.3083

Avadhanula, V., Weasner, B. P., Hardy, G. G., Kumar, J. P., and Hardy, R. W. (2009). A novel system for the launch of alphavirus RNA synthesis reveals a role for the Imd pathway in arthropod antiviral response. *PLoS Pathog.* 5:e1000582. doi: 10.1371/journal.ppat.1000582

Ayyar, S., Pistillo, D., Calleja, M., Brookfield, A., Gittins, A., Goldstone, C., et al. (2007). NF-kappaB/Rel-mediated regulation of the neural fate in *Drosophila*. *PLoS One* 2:e1178. doi: 10.1371/journal.pone.0001178

Bergbauer, M., Kalla, M., Schmeinck, A., Göbel, C., Rothbauer, U., and Eck, S. (2010). CpG-Methylation regulates a class of Epstein-Barr Virus Promoters. *PLoS Pathog.* 6:e1001114. doi: 10.1371/journal.ppat.1001114

Blaschke, S., Schwarz, G., Moneke, D., Binder, L., Müller, G., and Reuss-Borst, M. (2000). Epstein-Barr virus infection in peripheral blood mononuclear cells, synovial fluid cells, and synovial membranes of patients with rheumatoid arthritis. *J. Rheumatol.* 27, 866–873.

Bond, D., and Foley, E. A. (2009). Quantitative RNAi screen for JNK modifiers identifies Pvr as a novel regulator of *Drosophila* immune signaling. *PLoS Pathog.* 5:e1000655. doi: 10.1371/journal.ppat.1000655

Buchon, N., Silverman, N., and Cherry, S. (2014). Immunity in Drosophila melanogaster–from microbial recognition to whole-organism physiology. *Nat. Rev. Immunol.* 14, 796–810. doi: 10.1038/nri3763

Calabrese, E. J., and Baldwin, L. A. (1999). Chemical hormesis: its historical foundations as a biological hypothesis. *Toxicol. Pathol.* 27, 195–216. doi: 10.1177/019262339902700207

Calabrese, E. J., and Baldwin, L. A. (2001). Hormesis: a generalizable and unifying hypothesis. *Crit. Rev. Toxicol.* 31, 353–424. doi: 10.1080/20014091111730

Delorenze, G. N., Munger, K. L., Lennette, E. T., Orentreich, N., Vogelman, J. H., and Ascherio, A. (2006). Epstein-Barr virus and multiple sclerosis: evidence of association from a prospective study with long-term follow-up. *Arch. Neurol.* 63, 839–844. doi: 10.1001/archneur.63.6.noc50328

Draborg, A. H., Duus, K., and Houen, G. (2013). Epstein-barr virus in systemic autoimmune diseases. *Clin. Dev. Immunol.* 2013:535738. doi: 10.1155/2013/535738

Fiola, S., Gosselin, D., Takada, K., and Gosselin, J. (2010). TLR9 contributes to the recognition of EBV by primary monocytes and plasmacytoid dendritic cells. *J. Immunol.* 185, 3620–3631. doi: 10.4049/jimmunol.0903736

Ghiglione, C., Devergne, O., Georgenthum, E., Carballès, F., Médioni, C., Cerezo, D., et al. (2002). The *Drosophila* cytokine receptor Domeless controls border cell migration and epithelial polarization during oogenesis. *Development* 129, 5437–5447. doi: 10.1242/dev.00116

Ghosh, S., Singh, A., Mandal, S., and Mandal, L. (2015). Active hematopoietic hubs in *Drosophila* adults generate hemocytes and contribute to immune response. *Dev. Cell* 33, 478–488. doi: 10.1016/j.devcel.2015.03.014

Govind, S. (2008). Innate immunity in *Drosophila*: pathogens and pathways. *Insect Sci.* 15, 29–43. doi: 10.1111/j.1744-7917.2008.00185.x

Gross, A. J., Hochberg, D., Rand, W. M., and Thorley-Lawson, D. A. (2005). EBV and systemic lupus erythematosus: a new perspective. *J. Immunol.* 174, 6599–6607. doi: 10.4049/jimmunol.174.11.6599

Häcker, V. R. A., Takeuchi, O., Hoshino, K., Akira, S., and Wagner, H. (2000). Immune cell activation by bacterial CpG-DNA through myeloid differentiation marker 88 and tumor necrosis factor receptor-associated factor (TRAF)6. *J. Exp. Med.* 192, 595–600. doi: 10.1084/jem.192.4.595

Hedges, L. M., and Johnson, K. N. (2008). Induction of host defence responses by *Drosophila* C virus. *J. Gen. Virol.* 89, 1497–1501. doi: 10.1099/vir.0.83684-0

Imler, J. L., and Bulet, P. (2005). Antimicrobial peptides in Drosophila: structures, activities and gene regulation. *Chem. Immunol. Allergy* 86, 1–21. doi: 10.1159/000086648

Kallio, J., Myllymäki, H., Grönholm, J., Armstrong, M., Vanha-Aho, L. M., Mäkinen, L., et al. (2010). Eye transformer is a negative regulator of Drosophila JAK/STAT signaling. *FASEB J.* 24, 4467–4479. doi: 10.1096/fj.10-162784

Kintner, C., and Sugden, B. (1981). Conservation and progressive methylation of Epstein-Barr viral DNA sequences in transformed cells. *J. Virol.* 38, 305–316.

Lünemann, J. D., Kamradt, T., Martin, R., and Münz, C. (2007). Epstein-Barr virus: environmental trigger of multiple sclerosis? *J. Virol.* 81, 6777–6784. doi: 10.1128/JVI.00153-07

Maxton-Kuchenmeister, J., Handel, K., Schmidt-Ott, U., Roth, S., and Jäckle, H. (1999). Toll homologue expression in the beetle *Tribolium* suggests a different mode of dorsoventral patterning than in *Drosophila* embryos. *Mech. Dev.* 83, 107–114. doi: 10.1016/S0925-4773(99)00041-6

Mosteller, R. D. (1987). Simplified calculation of body-surface area. *N. Engl. J. Med.* 317:1098. doi: 10.1056/NEJM198710223171717

Munier, A. I., Doucet, D., Perrodou, E., Zachary, D., Meister, M., Hoffmann, J. A., et al. (2002). PVF2, a PDGF/VEGF-like growth factor, induces hemocyte proliferation in *Drosophila* larvae. *EMBO Rep.* 3, 1195–1200. doi: 10.1093/embo-reports/kvf242

Peinnequin, A., Mouret, C., Birot, O., Alonso, A., Mathieu, J., Clarencon, D., et al. (2004). Rat pro-inflammatory cytokine and cytokine related mRNA quantification by real-time polymerase chain reaction using SYBR green. *BMC Immunol.* 5:3. doi: 10.1186/1471-2172-5-3

Pindado, J., Balsinde, J., and Balboa, M. A. (2007). TLR3-dependent induction of nitric oxide synthase in RAW 264.7 macrophage-like cells via a cytosolic phospholipase A2/cyclooxygenase-2 pathway. *J. Immunol.* 179, 4821–4828. doi: 10.4049/jimmunol.179.7.4821

Rahal, E. A., Hajjar, H., Rajeh, M., Yamout, B., and Abdelnoor, A. M. (2015). Epstein-Barr Virus and human herpes virus 6 Type A DNA enhance IL-17 production in mice. *Viral Immunol.* 28, 297–302. doi: 10.1089/vim.2014.0129

Tanji, T., Hu, X., Weber, A., and Ip, Y. T. (2007). Toll and IMD pathways synergistically activate an innate immune response in *Drosophila* melanogaster. *Mol. Cell. Biol.* 27, 4578–4588. doi: 10.1128/MCB.01814-06

Yu, S. F., Wu, H. C., Tsai, W. C., Yen, J. H., Chiang, W., Yuo, C. Y., et al. (2005). Detecting Epstein-Barr virus DNA from peripheral blood mononuclear cells in adult patients with systemic lupus erythematosus in Taiwan. *Med. Microbiol. Immunol.* 194, 115–120. doi: 10.1007/s00430-004-0230-5

7

Herpesviral microRNAs in Cellular Metabolism and Immune Responses

Hyoji Kim, Hisashi Iizasa, Yuichi Kanehiro, Sintayehu Fekadu and Hironori Yoshiyama *

Department of Microbiology, Faculty of Medicine, Shimane University, Shimane, Japan

Correspondence:
Hironori Yoshiyama
yosiyama@med.shimane-u.ac.jp

The microRNAs (miRNAs) function as a key regulator in many biological processes through post-transcriptional suppression of messenger RNAs. Recent advancements have revealed that miRNAs are involved in many biological functions of cells. Not only host cells, but also some viruses encode miRNAs in their genomes. Viral miRNAs regulate cell proliferation, differentiation, apoptosis, and the cell cycle to establish infection and produce viral progeny. Particularly, miRNAs encoded by herpes virus families play integral roles in persistent viral infection either by regulation of metabolic processes or the immune response of host cells. The life-long persistent infection of gamma herpes virus subfamilies, such as Epstein-Barr virus and Kaposi's sarcoma-associated herpesvirus, induces host cells to malignant transformation. The unbalanced metabolic processes and evasion from host immune surveillance by viral miRNAs are induced either by direct targeting of key proteins or indirect regulation of multiple signaling pathways. We provide an overview of the pathogenic roles of viral miRNAs in cellular metabolism and immune responses during herpesvirus infection.

Keywords: microRNA, herpesvirus, oncogenesis, immune evasion, cell metabolism

INTRODUCTION

The microRNAs (miRNAs) are small non-coding RNAs consisting of 19–23 nucleotides. The primary miRNA in the nucleus is cleaved into smaller pre-miRNA consisting of around 70 nucleotides with a hairpin structure. The pre-miRNA is then exported to the cytoplasm, where it is cleaved by Dicer to form mature miRNA. The miRNA is incorporated into the RNA-induced silencing complex (RISC), which contains the essential endonuclease Argonaute 2 (Ago2). The miRNA-RISC interacts with the 3′ untranslated region (UTR) in mRNA. This complex suppresses target gene expression through the translational repression or induction of mRNA deadenylation (Winter et al., 2009). Cellular miRNAs play important parts in the regulation of cellular pathways, of which dysregulation has been linked to many disorders including cancer. Viral miRNAs were reported originally by Pfeffer et al. (2004), and now many DNA viruses are known to contain miRNAs in their genomes. More than 200 viral miRNAs are currently identified mainly in the herpesvirus family (**Table 1**).

The first report of viral miRNA was described in the herpesvirus family, especially in Epstein-Barr virus (EBV) strain B95-8 having a 12-kb deletion in *Bam*HI-A rightward transcripts (BART) region (Pfeffer et al., 2004). Subsequent studies revealed that EBV encodes 44 different mature BART miRNAs and 4 mature *Bam*HI-H rightward open reading frame 1 (BHRF1) miRNAs (Cai et al., 2006; Grundhoff et al., 2006; Zhu et al., 2009) (**Figure 1**). Rhesus lymphocryptovirus encodes miRNAs, which are orthologs of EBV miRNAs and evolutionarily conserved (Cai et al., 2006). Kaposi's sarcoma-associated herpesvirus (KSHV), the etiologic agent of Kaposi's sarcoma, encodes

TABLE 1 | The role of herpes virus-encoded miRNAs in immune evasion and cancer metabolism.

<table>
<tr><th>Viruses</th><th>miRNAs</th><th>Targets</th><th>Target sites (Upper: Target, Lower: miRNA)</th><th>Function</th><th>References</th></tr>
<tr><td>EBV</td><td>miR-BART16</td><td>LMP1</td><td>5'-AAA-AGC-CACAUUCAUAUUCUAU-3'
|| ||| |||| :| :|:|||||
3'-guucucgugugu-gg-gugagaua-5'
5'-C-A-AGC-CACACCUAACUC-AU-3'
| | ||| ||||||: |||| ||
3'-guucucgugugugg-ugagaua-5'</td><td>Latent membrane protein that mimics CD40 and induces NF-κB activation</td><td>Lo et al., 2007</td></tr>
<tr><td></td><td>miR-BART17-5p</td><td>LMP1</td><td>5'-CUUU-UAUGCCUGC-UCCUCAUCU-3'
|:|| ||||||||| ||||| | |
3'-ggaacauacggacgcaggag-a-a-5'
5'-CCUGGUGGUACUCUGUGUCCUGUUU-3'
||| || :| | |||:||||| :||
3'-ggaaca-uacg-gacgcagga-gaa-5'
5'-CUUUGCUAGAGCA-GCAGUCCUCUG-3'
|:||| || || || |||||||
3'-ggaac-au-acggacg-caggagaa-5'</td><td></td><td></td></tr>
<tr><td></td><td>miR-BART1-5p</td><td>LMP1</td><td>5'-GAGGCCCCUUACUUCCAC-AGGG-3'
: :|| | |:|||||||| |:|:
3'-ugucgugcagugaaggugauucu-5'
5'-GCGGCCUGCCCGGCUCUUCUACGGAGA-3'
:|:| | : | | | ||||:|| :|||
3'-uguc-g-u-g-cagugaaggugauucu-5'
5'-CCAGA-CGUCA-G-CAGACUAAGA-3'
||| ||||| | |||||||
3'-ugucgugcagugaag-gugauucu-5'</td><td>Latent membrane protein that mimics CD40 and induces NF-κB activation</td><td>Lo et al., 2007</td></tr>
<tr><td></td><td>miR-BART22</td><td>LMP2A</td><td>5'-CCUGUGUGACCCCUCACUUUGUAC-3'
||:: || || | ||||||||
3'-ugaugaucu-gguacugaaacauu-5'</td><td>Latent membrane protein that mimics B cell receptor</td><td>Lung et al., 2009</td></tr>
<tr><td></td><td>miR-BART2-5p</td><td>BALF5</td><td>5'-GCAAGGGCGAAUGCAGAAAAUA-3'
|||||||||||||||||||||| Antisense
3'-cguucccgcuuacgucuuuuau-5'</td><td>Viral DNA polymerase in lytic infection</td><td>Barth et al., 2008</td></tr>
<tr><td></td><td>miR-BART2-5p</td><td>MICB</td><td>5'-CUGACCUAUGAAA-CAGAAAAUA-3'
::| :|||| |||||||||
3'-cguuccc-gcuuacgucuuuuau-5'
5'-AAUACGAAGGGCUGUGGAAGAU-3'
| | |:: |:||:||
3'-cguucccgcuuacgucuuuuau-5'</td><td>Cellular stress-induced ligand for (NKG2D type II receptor NK cell, CD8 αβT cell)</td><td>Nachmani et al., 2009</td></tr>
<tr><td></td><td>miR-BART3</td><td>IPO7</td><td>5'-GUACCUGGUGACUUUGUGGUGCA-3'
::|||||||||||| |||||||
5'-uguggaccacugau-caccacgc-3'</td><td>Nuclear import receptor relating to innate immunity</td><td>Dolken et al., 2010</td></tr>
<tr><td></td><td>miR-BART15</td><td>NLRP3</td><td>5'-CGCUAUCUUUCUAUUAACTGACC-3'
| : | : |||||||
5'-g-uuccuuuguuuuggugacugg-3'</td><td>Component of inflammasome</td><td>Haneklaus et al., 2012</td></tr>
<tr><td></td><td>miR-BART20-5p</td><td>BZLF1

BRLF1</td><td>5'-UUAUUGAAACCACGCCUGCUU-3'
| ||||| || |||||||
3'-ccuuacuucuguacggacgau-5'
5'-UUUCUGCCCCUCAGCCUGCUC-3'
|| : |||||||
3'-ccuuacuucuguacggacgau-5'</td><td>Immediate-early genes that induce lytic replication</td><td>Jung et al., 2014</td></tr>
<tr><td></td><td>miR-BART6-5p</td><td>Dicer1</td><td>5'----AGGCUGUUGCUCUAACAAAUAACCUUA-3'
|| :||| | | |||||||
3'-gauacc--uaacc---ugg----uuggaau-5'
5'-UCUAUUUGAUUUUUUAAAAACCUUA-3'
: : | | ||||||||
3'-gauac-cuaa---ccugguuggaau-5'
5'-----CGAUUUGG---AACCUUA-3'
|| |||| |||||||
3'-gauaccu-aaccugguuggaau-5'
5'-------------GUAACCUUA-3'
:|||||||
3'-gauaccuaaccugguuggaau-5'</td><td>RNase III family enzyme generating miRNA from pre-miRNA</td><td>Iizasa et al., 2010</td></tr>
<tr><td></td><td>miR-BHRF1-3</td><td>CXCL11 (I-TAC)</td><td>Not defined in the reference</td><td>Chemoattractant factor for activated T cells (chemokine)</td><td>Xia et al., 2008</td></tr>
<tr><td></td><td>miR-BART1</td><td>PHGDH</td><td>Not defined in the reference</td><td>Central metabolite involved in synthesis of L-serine, cystine, and glycine</td><td>Ye et al., 2013</td></tr>
</table>

(Continued)

TABLE 1 | Continued

<table>
<tr><th>Viruses</th><th>miRNAs</th><th>Targets</th><th>Target sites (Upper: Target, Lower: miRNA)</th><th>Function</th><th>References</th></tr>
<tr><td></td><td></td><td>EHD1</td><td>Not defined in the reference</td><td>Regulator of endosomal transport of plasma membrane proteins</td><td rowspan="2">Cai et al., 2015</td></tr>
<tr><td></td><td></td><td>PTEN</td><td>5'-AACAGAUAAGUUUGCAGUUGGCUAAGAG-3'
|||| ||: |: : |||||
3'-gugucgug-caguga--aggugauucu-3'

5'------UGUGUAAUCAAGGCCAGUGCUAA-3'
||| || || ||||||
3'-cuguaucaccuau----cgc-cacgau-3'</td><td>Tumor suppressor gene antagonizing the PI3K/AKT pathway</td></tr>
<tr><td></td><td>miR-BART1-5p,3,4,5,6,7,8,10,18-3p</td><td>TGF-β Pathway
Wnt pathway</td><td>Not defined in the reference
Not defined in the reference</td><td>Metabolic reprogramming
Regulation of Warburg metabolism</td><td>Wan et al., 2015</td></tr>
<tr><td></td><td>miR-BHRF1</td><td>SUMO pathyway</td><td>Not defined in the reference</td><td>Post-translational modification involved in various cellular processes</td><td>Callegari et al., 2014</td></tr>
<tr><td>KSHV</td><td>miR-K12-7</td><td>MICB</td><td>5'-AGAGCCAGCAAGA-GGGAUCA-3'
|| |||||||| | |||||||
5'-ucgcggucguuguacccuagu-3'</td><td>Cellular stress-induced ligand for NKG2D type II receptor (NK cell, CD8 αβT cell)</td><td>Nachmani et al., 2009</td></tr>
<tr><td></td><td>KSHV miRNAs</td><td>EGLN2</td><td>Not defined in the reference</td><td>Enzyme involved in the hypoxia-inducible factor signaling pathways</td><td rowspan="2">Yogev et al., 2014</td></tr>
<tr><td></td><td></td><td>HSPA9</td><td>Not defined in the reference</td><td>Key protein in mitochondrial import machinery</td></tr>
<tr><td>HCMV</td><td>miR-UL112</td><td>MICB</td><td>Not defined in the reference</td><td>Cellular stress-induced ligand for NKG2D type II receptor (NK cell, CD8 αβT cell, γδT cell)</td><td>Nachmani et al., 2010</td></tr>
<tr><td></td><td>miR-US4-1</td><td>ERAP1</td><td>5'--GCCCUCU-CAA----AUGUUG-3'
|||:|| || ||||:|
3'-uaggggacgugcagguacagc-3'
5'-UGUCCAAACCCUGUACC-CCAUGUU-3'
:||| |||||:|| ||||||:
3'--uagg---gggacgugcagguacagc-3'</td><td>Aminopeptidase 1 processing protein to form HLA class I binding peptide</td><td>Kim et al., 2011</td></tr>
<tr><td></td><td>miR-UL148D</td><td>CCL5 (RANTES)</td><td>5'-AGGC-AAGGAGGGGAGGA-3'
|| |||:|||||||||
3'-gccacuucuuccccuccugcu-3'</td><td>Chemoattractant factor for memory T cells and eosinophils (chemokine)</td><td>Kim et al., 2012</td></tr>
<tr><td></td><td>miR-UL112-3p</td><td>TLR2</td><td>5'-AGUUGGGAUCUUUAUGUCACUA-3'
||:: ||||||: :||||||
3'-ucggaccuagaguggcagugaa-5'
5'--ACGUGGAUG-UACCGUCAUUUG-3'
| ||||| :|||||||:||
3'-ucggaccuagaguggcagugaa-5'</td><td>Receptor for peptidoglycan (lipopolysaccharide) activating inflammation</td><td>Landais et al., 2015</td></tr>
<tr><td></td><td>miR-UL112-3p</td><td>IKKA, IKKB</td><td>Not defined in the reference</td><td>Inducer of NF-κB signal, upregulation of Glut3 by mediating aerobic glycolysis</td><td rowspan="2">Hancock et al., 2017</td></tr>
<tr><td></td><td>miR-US5-1</td><td>IKKA, IKKB</td><td>Not defined in the reference</td><td>Inducer of NF-κB signal, upregulation of Glut3 by mediating aerobic glycolysis</td></tr>
<tr><td>HSV-1</td><td>miR-H8</td><td>PIGT</td><td>5'---CCUCACCUGUAGUGGCCACCUCUAUAUU-3'
|:| |||| ||| ||||||
5'-cuuggg-ggac--------ugg-gauauau-5'</td><td>Component of GPI transamidase complex</td><td>Enk et al., 2016</td></tr>
<tr><td></td><td>miR-H6</td><td>ICP4</td><td>5'-ACGCCCCGCGGCGGGAAGUU-3'
| : |:||||||||
3'-cccuaccuuccugcccuucac-5'</td><td>Transactivator of lytic infection-associated genes</td><td>Umbach et al., 2008</td></tr>
<tr><td></td><td>miR-H2</td><td>ICP0</td><td>5'-AGUCGCACUCGUCCCUGGCUGAGG-3'
|||||||||||||||||||| |||
3'-ucagcgugagcagggaccgagucc-5'</td><td>E3 ubiquitin ligase that activates viral gene transcription</td><td>Umbach et al., 2008</td></tr>
<tr><td></td><td>miR-H3</td><td>ICP34.5</td><td>5'-TCCCAACCGCACAGTCCCAG-3'
||||||||||||||||||||
3'-aggguuggcgugucaggguc-5'</td><td>Neurovirulence factor that inactivates autophagy</td><td>Umbach et al., 2008</td></tr>
</table>

(Continued)

TABLE 1 | Continued

<table>
<tr><th>Viruses</th><th>miRNAs</th><th>Targets</th><th>Target sites (Upper: Target, Lower: miRNA)</th><th>Function</th><th>References</th></tr>
<tr><td></td><td>miR-H4</td><td>ICP34.5</td><td>5'-ACTAGCGAGTTAGACAGGCAAG-3'
||||||||||||||||||||||
3'-ugaucgcucaaucuguccguuc-5'</td><td>Neurovirulence factor that inactivates autophagy</td><td>Umbach et al., 2008</td></tr>
<tr><td></td><td>miR-H4-5p</td><td>p16INK4A</td><td>5'-GGGAAGGCUAUCUCUACG-3'
| | | | ||||||
3'-acgaacaguuugagaugg-3'</td><td>Tumor suppressor gene and repressor of the PI3K/AKT pathway</td><td>Zhao et al., 2015</td></tr>
</table>

White or gray backgrounds relate to immuno evasion, and black backgrounds relate to cancer metabolism. KSHV, Kaposi's sarcoma-associated herpesvirus; HCMV, human cytomegalovirus; HSV, herpes simplex virus.

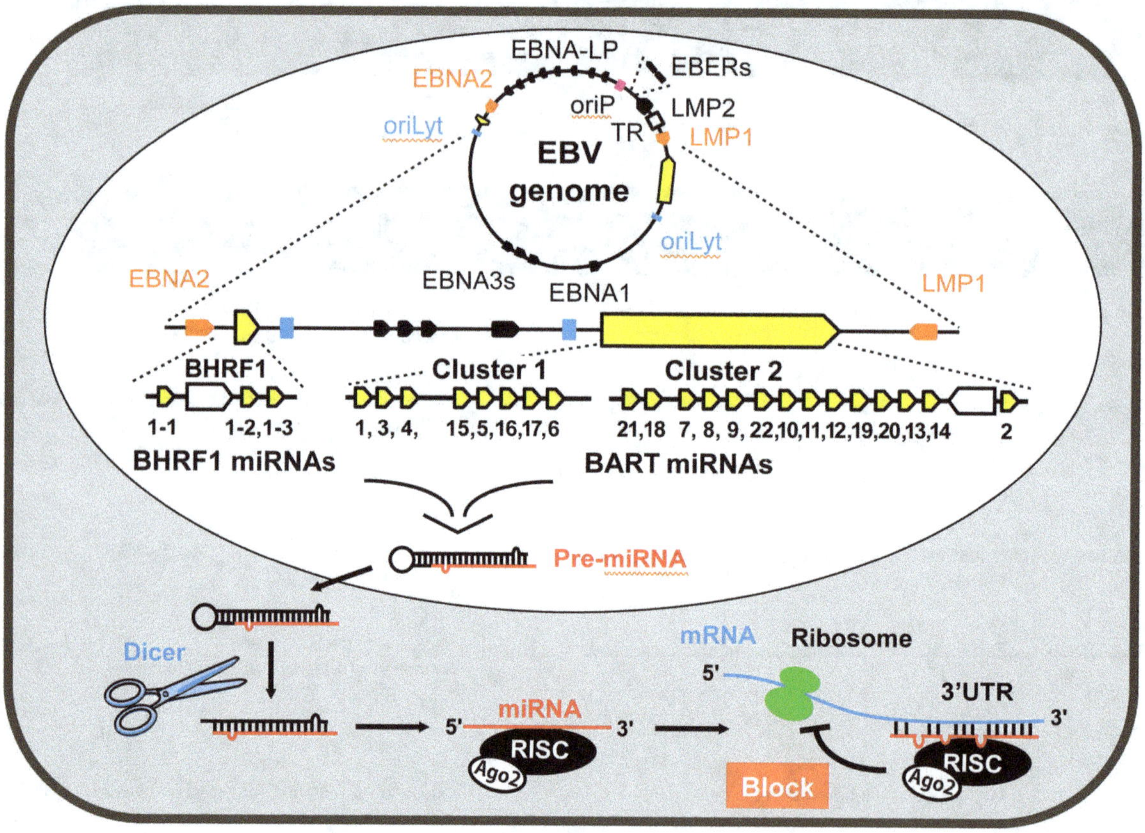

FIGURE 1 | Genome organization and location of miRNAs encoded by the Epstein-Barr virus (EBV). The EBV genome is maintained as a circular episome in latently infected cells. The relative positions of the latency-associated genes on the episomal genome are indicated. The origin of plasmid replication (oriP) and two origins of lytic replication (oriLyt) are indicated as a red and two blue squares, respectively. Orange arrows represents the coding regions of the latent membrane protein 1 (LMP1) and EBNA2 transcribed in antisense and sense orientations, respectively. EBNA-LP is transcribed from variable numbers of repetitive exons (denoted by black lines between EBNA2 and oriP). EBNA3s and EBNA1 shown by black arrows locate between two oriLyt regions. The highly transcribed non-polyadenylated EBER RNAs are represented in the right top of the diagram as black arrows. TR (represented by the white square) denotes the terminal repeats of EBV DNA. LMP2 locating between EBERs and TR is transcribed in sense. The genomic location of miRNAs encoded by EBV is enlarged and represented linearly. The regions of the BHRF cluster and BART clusters 1 and 2 are expanded to show individual miRNAs. Each miRNA is processed from pre-miRNA precursors and transported from nucleus to cytoplasm. Dicer is a part of the RNase III enzyme and cleaves pre-miRNA into short double-stranded RNA fragments called miRNA. The complex of RNA-induced silencing complex (RISC), Argonaute 2 (Ago2), and miRNA specifically inhibits transcription of the target mRNA.

13 precursor (pre)-miRNAs. These KSHV miRNAs are located in the KSHV latency-associated region (Pfeffer et al., 2005; Grundhoff et al., 2006). By sharing target genes, these KSHV miRNAs function as analogs of cellular oncomirs (Skalsky et al., 2007; Gottwein et al., 2011; Manzano et al., 2013).

This mini-review summarizes the role of viral miRNAs in cellular metabolism and the immune system of hosts to understand the pathologies of viral infection. Although viral miRNAs have also been detected in JC virus and human immunodeficiency virus, we mainly discuss miRNAs from *Herpesviridae*.

PATHOLOGICAL ROLES OF EBV MIRNAS

EBV-Encoded miRNAs

EBV is associated with many tumors, including lymphoma and epithelial carcinomas (Young and Murray, 2003; Luo et al., 2005). Detection of EBV-encoded small non-coding RNAs (EBERs) by *in situ* hybridization is used as a diagnostic hallmark of EBV infection in tumor cells. EBERs can be detected in a variety of tumors, such as nasal NK/T-cell lymphoma, post-transplant lymphoma, Burkitt's lymphoma, Hodgkin's disease, diffuse large B-cell lymphoma, nasopharyngeal carcinoma (NPC), and gastric carcinoma (Delecluse et al., 2007). Following primary infection, EBV establishes latent infection. Three latency types (I, II, III) are defined depending on the pattern of expression in viral genes (Middeldorp et al., 2003). BART miRNAs are expressed in all latency types, whereas BHRF1 miRNAs are expressed only in type III latency. BHRF1 transcripts encode four mature BHRF1 miRNAs. BART transcripts have two clusters, cluster 1 and cluster 2, which generate 44 mature BART miRNAs (**Figure 1**) (Pfeffer et al., 2004; Cai et al., 2006; Zhu et al., 2009). EBV B95-8 strain has a 12-kb deletion and lacks most of the BART miRNAs (Baer et al., 1984).

BART miRNAs are expressed more strongly in EBV-associated epithelial cells than in B lymphocytes (Chen et al., 2010). BART transcripts have two TATA-less promoter regions, designated P1 and P2 (Sadler and Raab-Traub, 1995). Although P1 supports substantial activity in epithelial cells and B lymphocytes, P2 exhibits strong activity only in epithelial cells. Several transcription factors, important for cellular metabolism and immunity, regulate BART promoter activity (Chen et al., 2005). P1 activity is negatively regulated by interferon regulatory factor 5 (IRF5) and IRF7, and P2 activity is positively regulated by c-Myc and CCAAT-enhancer-binding protein (C/EBP) family members. Relative expression between positive and negative transcription factors in EBV-infected cells probably controls the expression level of BART miRNAs. BHRF1 miRNAs are generated as part of the Cp- and/or Wp-initiated EBNA transcripts in cells showing latency III infection (Amoroso et al., 2011). The expression of miR-BHRF1-1 absolutely depends on Cp/Wp activity, because it locates at the 5′ UTR of BHRF1 mRNA and overlaps with the EBV replication-activated BHRF1 promoter (Amoroso et al., 2011). However, because miR-BHRF1-2 and miR-BHRF1-3 locate at the 3′ UTR, they are strongly expressed by an alternative promoter for lytic BHRF1 transcript during lytic replication (Kelly et al., 2009; Xing and Kieff, 2011). The expression of BART miRNAs inversely correlates with the methylation status of the promoter in EBV-infected B lymphocytes. Promoter methylation may be important in regulating the expression of BART and BHRF1 miRNAs (Kim do et al., 2011).

EBV miRNAs are transferred to adjacent cells via exosomes (Pegtel et al., 2010). The secreted viral miRNAs modify the expression of target genes in recipient cells (Haneklaus et al., 2012). Some BART miRNAs show distinctive expression between cells and exosomes. MiR-BART7 is expressed more abundantly in exosomes than in EBV-positive NPC cells (Meckes et al., 2010). However, miR-BART8-5p is expressed less abundantly in exosomes than in lymphoblastoid cell lines (Hoshina et al., 2016). These findings indicate that some EBV miRNAs are selectively packaged and transported into recipient cells via exosomes.

Immune Evasion by EBV miRNAs

EBV can establish either latent infection or lytic replication (Kenney and Mertz, 2014). In tumor cells, EBV usually maintains latent infection rather than entering into lytic replication (Cohen, 2000). During latent infection, EBV transcribes viral miRNAs to escape from the host immune system by targeting both cellular and viral genes. Lowered expression of viral proteins enables infected cells to escape antigenic recognition by the host immune system. Expression of latent membrane protein 1 (LMP1) and LMP2A is downregulated by BART cluster 1 miRNAs (miR-BART16, 17-5p, and 1-5p) (Lo et al., 2007) and miR-BART22 (Lung et al., 2009), respectively. LMP1 and LMP2A are oncogenic viral proteins that promote EBV-positive malignancies by engaging a number of signal pathways, such as the NFκB, JNK/p38-SAPK, PI3K/Akt, ERK-MAPK, and JAK/STAT pathways, followed by subsequent induction of morphological and phenotypic alterations (Young and Rickinson, 2004). LMP1 and LMP2A alter the host immune system by cooperating with environmental and host genetic factors (Dawson et al., 2012).

Viral miRNAs help maintain latent infection by expressing limited numbers of viral genes that allow EBV to evade host immune surveillance. MiR-BART20-5p suppresses lytic replication by targeting EBV immediate-early genes BZLF1 and BRLF1 (Jung et al., 2014), key regulators of the expression of EBV proteins and the production of progeny virus (Pattle and Farrell, 2006). Downregulation of Dicer by miR-BART6-5p reduces the expression of BZLF1, BRLF1, and both EBNA2 and LMP1 latent proteins in C666-1, an EBV-positive NPC cell line (Iizasa et al., 2010). Likewise, miR-BART2-5p blocks lytic replication by inhibiting expression of viral DNA polymerase BALF5 (Barth et al., 2008).

EBV miRNAs can also block immune response by reducing cytokines, chemokines, and T-cell stimulatory molecules. MiR-BHRF1-3 modulates host interferon (IFN) response by targeting CXCL11, an IFN-inducible T-cell-attracting chemokine (Xia et al., 2008). Suppression of MHC class I-related chain B (MICB) by miR-BART2-5p protects EBV-infected cells from attack by NK cells and T cells. MICB is also a target gene for other herpesvirus miRNAs, including KSHV-encoded miR-K12-1 and human cytomegalovirus (HCMV)-encoded miR-UL112 (Nachmani et al., 2009). Importin 7 (IPO7), a receptor for importing transcription factors into the nucleus, has important function for innate immunity, because loss of IPO7 in macrophages inhibits interleukin (IL)-6 secretion (Yang et al., 2009). IPO7 is a putative target for miR-BART1-3p and miR-BART3 (Dolken et al., 2010). MiR-BART15 also reduces IL-1β production from the inflammasome by targeting NLRP3 (NLR family, pyrin domain containing 3; also known as cryopyrin) at the same 3′ UTR region that host miR-223 recognizes (Haneklaus et al., 2012). These findings suggest that EBV miRNAs inhibit immune response by multiple mechanisms.

EBV miRNAs in Cancer Metabolism

Compared with normal cells, cancer cells increase metabolic autonomy, which uses nutrients and promotes metabolic processes of the host cells to support proliferation. Recent studies showed that several EBV miRNAs regulate cellular metabolic processes. MiR-BART1 is one of the metabolic regulators strongly expressed in NPC. The expression levels of phosphoglycerate dehydrogenase (PHGDH) and EH domain-containing protein 1 (EHD1) were significantly upregulated by miR-BART1 expression in an NPC cell line, CNE1 (Ye et al., 2013). PHGDH is important for the synthesis of serine and glycine, a central metabolite for a variety of biosynthetic pathways, by removing 3-phosphoglycerate during glycolysis (DeBerardinis, 2011). EHD1 regulates endosomal transport of plasma membrane proteins such as transferrin receptor and ß1 integrin (Jovic et al., 2007).

Wan et al. reported that 9 EBV miRNAs (miR-BART1-5p, 3, 4, 5, 6, 7, 8, 10, and 18-3p) are highly expressed in NPC tissues. Genome pathway analysis indicated that upregulated EBV miRNAs mainly target transforming growth factor β (TGF-β) and Wnt signaling pathways (Wan et al., 2015), which are involved in many biological processes during oncogenesis, including reprogramming of tumor cell bioenergetics (Sherwood, 2015) and the bioenergetic shift toward catabolism (Guido et al., 2012). Previous studies showed that both pathways are dysregulated in NPC (Zeng et al., 2007; Chen et al., 2009). Consistent with this result, the TGF-β signaling pathway is suppressed by upregulation of miR-BHRF1, because miR-BHRF1 targets the small ubiquitin-like modifier-regulated component SMAD3 and the transcription co-regulators JUN and FOS (Callegari et al., 2014). Recently, target genes for EBV miRNAs were identified by high-throughput sequencing of RNA isolated by the methods of crosslinking immunoprecipitation (HITS-CLIP) and photoactivatable ribonucleoside-enhanced crosslinking and immunoprecipitation (PAR-CLIP). These EBV miRNA targets include many components of the Wnt signaling pathway (Riley et al., 2012; Skalsky et al., 2012).

The PI3K/AKT/mTOR pathway is a critical regulator in cell survival, growth, protein synthesis, and glucose metabolism (Yap et al., 2008). Moreover, the AKT pathway promotes the expression of genes involved in glycolysis and lipid genesis (Wullschleger et al., 2006). In NPC cells, miR-BART1 significantly reduces phosphatase and tensin homolog (PTEN) expression while increasing the phosphorylation level of pAKT, pFAK, p130Cas, pShc, and pERK1/2 (Cai et al., 2015). PTEN inhibits the PI3K/AKT pathway by dephosphorylating PIP3 and increasing PIP2, resulting in a reduction of membrane recruitment of AKTs (Rafalski and Brunet, 2011). Thus, miR-BART1 activates migration, invasion, and metastasis of NPC cells via suppression of PTEN (Cai et al., 2015).

MiR-BART7 is expressed strongly in NPC cells and promotes cell proliferation, migration, and invasion. Pathway analysis indicates that the expression level of various genes is altered by the expression of miR-BART7. These target genes belong to the signaling pathway of calcium and the immune system, ionotropic glutamate receptor, ATP-binding cassette transporters, nuclear receptors in lipid metabolism and toxicity, the TGF-ß-signaling pathway, and metabolism of lipids and lipoproteins (Chan et al., 2012). Therefore, the aberrant expression of EBV miRNAs may contribute to metabolic abnormality and oncogenesis in EBV-infected cells by unbalancing various signaling pathways.

MIRNAS IN OTHER HERPESVIRUSES

Herpesvirus-Encoded miRNAs

Herpesviruses other than EBV and KSHV also encode miRNAs. Herpes simplex virus (HSV) has two serotypes, HSV-1 and HSV-2, which infect oral or genital mucosa. The latency-associated transcript functioning as a primary miRNA precursor is exclusively expressed during latent infection (Wagner et al., 1988; Umbach et al., 2008). Since the first report in 2006, 27 mature miRNA sequences have been identified in the HSV-1 genome (Cui et al., 2006; Jurak et al., 2010). Similarly, HSV-2 encodes 24 mature miRNAs (Umbach et al., 2010). Several miRNAs are conserved between HSV-1 and HSV-2, especially in their seed regions. These viral miRNAs have analogous functions in immune evasion and virus propagation (Jurak et al., 2010; Umbach et al., 2010).

Unlike other herpesviruses, HCMV miRNAs are not clustered in latent transcripts, but are distributed throughout the viral genome (Buck et al., 2007). Currently, 26 mature HCMV miRNA sequences are uploaded on miRBase (http://www.mirbase.org). HCMV miRNAs target multiple genes related to immune response, cell cycle control, and vesicle trafficking (Hook et al., 2014).

Varicella-zoster virus (VZV) is a pathogenic human virus that causes chicken pox and shingles. Unlike other herpesviruses examined, although many small RNA sequencing studies have been performed, VZV miRNAs have not been identified yet (Umbach et al., 2009).

Human herpesvirus 6 (HHV-6), with its two variants HHV-6A and HHV-6B, is a ubiquitous pathogen in general human populations. Both are very closely related, with nearly 90% homology at the genomic level. Deep sequencing of small RNA species identified a small non-coding RNA with the characteristics of a viral miRNA from cells harboring HHV-6A. Growth analyses of mutant viruses revealed that miR-U86 directly impacts lytic replication by targeting HHV-6A immediate-early gene U86 (Nukui et al., 2015). HHV-6B encodes four pre-miRNAs expressed from direct repeat regions located at either side of the genome. HHV-6B miR-Ro6-2 is a seed ortholog of host miR-582-5p, which targets SMAD3 to downregulate TGF-β. HHV-6B miRNAs also have the potential to regulate viral replication (Tuddenham et al., 2012).

HHV-7 is a ubiquitous T-lymphotropic virus infecting most humans. As with VZV, HHV-7-encoded miRNAs have not yet been identified (Louten et al., 2015).

Herpes Viral miRNAs in Immune Evasion

EBV miR-BART2-5p and KSHV miR-K12-7 target the 3′ UTR of MICB at different locations (Nachmani et al., 2009). HCMV miR-UL112 and cellular miR-376a synergistically downregulate MICB expression and subsequently help the virus evade innate immune recognition (Nachmani et al., 2010). Recognition of HCMV-infected cells by cytotoxic T lymphocytes is impaired due to the reduced expression of aminopeptidase ERAP1 by HCMV miR-US4-1 (Kim et al., 2011). In human fibroblast cells, HCMV clinical strain-specific miR-UL148D was shown to block the human chemokine RANTES, which attracts immune cells during inflammation and the immune response (Kim et al., 2012).

HSV-1 miR-H8 targets the glycosylphosphatidylinositol gene, which results in reduced expression of several immune-modulating proteins, viral expansion, and viral evasion from natural killer cell elimination (Enk et al., 2016). HSV miRNAs also target viral genes to maintain latency and suppress immune function. HSV-1 miR-H6 and miR-H2 reduce infected cell polypeptide 4 (ICP4) and ICP0, respectively (Umbach et al., 2008; Duan et al., 2012). Both miR-H3 and miR-H4 target ICP34.5 mRNA (Umbach et al., 2008). HSV-2 miRNAs also contribute to latency and immune evasion similarly to HSV-1 miRNAs because of the close homology of these two viruses.

In KSHV-infected primary effusion lymphoma cells, KSHV miR-K1 inhibits viral lytic replication by targeting the 3′ UTR of IκBα protein, an inhibitor of the NFκB complexes. Enhanced NFκB activity evades host immune system and promotes cell survival (Lei et al., 2010). The KSHV miRNA cluster also represses a network of targets associated with STAT3 and suppresses STAT3 activation upon IL-6 treatment. KSHV miR-K6-5 targets the 3′ UTR of PKCδ, a Ser/Thr kinase that phosphorylates and activates STAT3. KSHV miR-K921 also targets a second Ser/Tr kinase, IRAK1. Repression of BIRC5, a transcriptional target of STAT3, by KSHV miR-K12-5 promotes KSHV infection. These multiple KSHV miRNAs that repress STAT3 can weaken the innate immune responses to type-I interferons and inhibit the induction of antiviral genes, such as IRF1, IFITM1, and ISG15 (Ramalingam and Ziegelbauer, 2017).

Herpes Viral miRNAs in Cancer Metabolism

Several core cellular metabolic pathways are significantly altered by herpesvirus infection and the expression of viral miRNAs (Sanchez and Lagunoff, 2015). HSV-1 miR-H4-5p directly targets cyclin-dependent kinase inhibitor 2A (p16) mRNA in neuroblastoma cell lines. Suppression of miR-H4-5p inhibits cell proliferation, invasion, and progression of the cell cycle via the p16-mediated PI3K-AKT signaling pathway (Zhao et al., 2015). Likewise, HCMV miR-UL112-3p modulates the TLR/IRAK1/NFκB signaling pathway by targeting Toll-like receptor 2 mRNA (Landais et al., 2015). NFκB signaling is known to upregulate the expression of Glut3 in p53-deficient cells (Kawauchi et al., 2008), suggesting that inhibition of NFκB signaling by miR-UL112-3p and miR-US5-1 might suppress aerobic glycolysis (Hancock et al., 2017).

KSHV has been shown to alter host cell energy metabolism by concurrent regulation of two independent pathways. First, KSHV miRNAs stabilize and activate transcription factor HIF1α, a master regulator of cell metabolism, by targeting hypoxia-inducible factor prolyl hydroxylase, EGLN2. Second, downregulation of the mitochondrial heat shock protein A9 (HSPA9) by KSHV miRNAs reduces mitochondrial copy numbers and enhances anaerobic glycolysis (Warburg effect). Downregulation of EGLN2 and HSPA9 allows cell proliferation in a low oxygen condition (Yogev et al., 2014). KSHV miR-K12-11 and miR-K12-3 prevent lytic reactivation by reducing the expression of cellular transcription factors MYB, C/EBPα, and Ets-1, which are reported as activators of the RTA promoter (Plaisance-Bonstaff et al., 2014).

Murine gammaherpesvirus 68 (MHV-68), a natural pathogen of wild rodents, encodes for 14 pre-miRNAs. All MHV-68 miRNAs are located downstream of viral tRNA-like elements and transcribed by RNA polymerase III. Recent research showed that an MHV-68 mutant lacking the expression of all miRNAs results in a higher viral genomic load in the spleen. This report shows that MHV-68 miRNAs contribute to the maintenance of latency *in vivo* (Steer et al., 2016).

The generation and analysis of mutant viruses revealed that MHV-68 miRNAs are dispensable for short-term virus replication but are important for the establishment of lifelong infection in memory B cells. Furthermore, a lack of miRNA expression results in the complete attenuation of lethal disease in a virus-induced pneumonia model, demonstrating a key role for the viral miRNAs in pathogenesis (Feldman et al., 2014).

Similar to EBERs in EBV, MHV-68 encodes non-coding RNAs called TMERs (tRNA-miRNA-encoded RNAs), which are highly expressed in latently infected cells. TMERs harbor a predicted tRNA-like element and two downstream pre-miRNA hairpins and are processed by tRNase Z instead of Drosha, similar to cellular non-coding tRNAs, to generate mature miRNAs. Analysis of individual TMER mutant viruses has shown TMER4 to be a key mediator of virus dissemination. Interestingly, TMER4 miRNA seed sequence mutants do not compromise TMER4 function. These results demonstrate a crucial miRNA-independent function of TMER4 in hematogenous dissemination and the establishment of peripheral latency (Feldman et al., 2016).

SUMMARY AND CONCLUSIONS

Viral miRNAs play important roles in cancer development and progression by modulating immune response and metabolic circuits. Although further study is necessary to understand the pathogenic significance of viral miRNAs, viral miRNAs can be applied for the diagnosis of cancer, identification of drug targets, and therapeutic use.

AUTHOR CONTRIBUTIONS

HK wrote the manuscript. SF and YK assisted in creating the table. HI and HY edited the paper and contributed financial assistance.

FUNDING

This study was supported by KAKENHI (Grant-in-Aid for Scientific Research) from the Ministry of Education, Culture, Sports, Science, and Technology (HI: 26460465, and HY: 16H05843), and a Health Labor Sciences Research Grant from the Ministry of Health Labor and Welfare, Japan (17fk0310105h0001).

ACKNOWLEDGMENTS

The authors thank Ms. Sayuri Hamada for her support in the preparation of the figure.

REFERENCES

Amoroso, R., Fitzsimmons, L., Thomas, W. A., Kelly, G. L., Rowe, M., and Bell, A. I. (2011). Quantitative studies of Epstein-Barr virus-encoded microRNAs provide novel insights into their regulation. *J. Virol.* 85, 996–1010. doi: 10.1128/jvi.01528-10

Baer, R., Bankier, A. T., Biggin, M. D., Deininger, P. L., Farrell, P. J., Gibson, T. J., et al. (1984). DNA sequence and expression of the B95-8 Epstein-Barr virus genome. *Nature* 310, 207–211. doi: 10.1038/310207a0

Barth, S., Pfuhl, T., Mamiani, A., Ehses, C., Roemer, K., Kremmer, E., et al. (2008). Epstein-Barr virus-encoded microRNA miR-BART2 down-regulates the viral DNA polymerase BALF5. *Nucleic Acids Res.* 36, 666–675. doi: 10.1093/nar/gkm1080

Buck, A. H., Santoyo-Lopez, J., Robertson, K. A., Kumar, D. S., Reczko, M., and Ghazal, P. (2007). Discrete clusters of virus-encoded micrornas are associated with complementary strands of the genome and the 7.2-kilobase stable intron in murine cytomegalovirus. *J. Virol.* 81, 13761–13770. doi: 10.1128/jvi.01290-07

Cai, L., Ye, Y., Jiang, Q., Chen, Y., Lyu, X., Li, J., et al. (2015). Epstein-Barr virus-encoded microRNA BART1 induces tumour metastasis by regulating PTEN-dependent pathways in nasopharyngeal carcinoma. *Nat. Commun.* 6:7353. doi: 10.1038/ncomms8353

Cai, X., Schafer, A., Lu, S., Bilello, J., Desrosiers, R., Edwards, R., et al. (2006). Epstein-Barr virus microRNAs are evolutionarily conserved and differentially expressed. *PLoS Pathog.* 2:e23. doi: 10.1371/journal.ppat.0020023

Callegari, S., Gastaldello, S., Faridani, O. R., and Masucci, M. G. (2014). Epstein-Barr virus encoded microRNAs target SUMO-regulated cellular functions. *FEBS J.* 281, 4935–4950. doi: 10.1111/febs.13040

Chan, J. Y., Gao, W., Ho, W. K., Wei, W. I., and Wong, T. S. (2012). Overexpression of Epstein-Barr virus-encoded microRNA-BART7 in undifferentiated nasopharyngeal carcinoma. *Anticancer Res.* 32, 3201–3210.

Chen, H. C., Chen, G. H., Chen, Y. H., Liao, W. L., Liu, C. Y., Chang, K. P., et al. (2009). MicroRNA deregulation and pathway alterations in nasopharyngeal carcinoma. *Br. J. Cancer* 100, 1002–1011. doi: 10.1038/sj.bjc.6604948

Chen, H., Huang, J., Wu, F. Y., Liao, G., Hutt-Fletcher, L., and Hayward, S. D. (2005). Regulation of expression of the Epstein-Barr virus BamHI-A rightward transcripts. *J. Virol.* 79, 1724–1733. doi: 10.1128/JVI.79.3.1724-1733.2005

Chen, S.-J., Chen, G.-H., Chen, Y.-H., Liu, C.-Y., Chang, K.-P., Chang, Y.-S., et al. (2010). Characterization of Epstein-Barr virus miRNAome in nasopharyngeal carcinoma by deep sequencing. *PLoS ONE* 5:e12745. doi: 10.1371/journal.pone.0012745

Cohen, J. I. (2000). Epstein-Barr virus infection. *N. Engl. J. Med.* 343, 481–492. doi: 10.1056/NEJM200008173430707

Cui, C., Griffiths, A., Li, G., Silva, L. M., Kramer, M. F., Gaasterland, T., et al. (2006). Prediction and identification of herpes simplex virus 1-encoded microRNAs. *J. Virol.* 80, 5499–5508. doi: 10.1128/jvi.00200-06

Dawson, C. W., Port, R. J., and Young, L. S. (2012). The role of the EBV-encoded latent membrane proteins LMP1 and LMP2 in the pathogenesis of nasopharyngeal carcinoma (NPC). *Semin. Cancer Biol.* 22, 144–153. doi: 10.1016/j.semcancer.2012.01.004

DeBerardinis, R. J. (2011). Serine metabolism: some tumors take the road less traveled. *Cell Metab.* 14, 285–286. doi: 10.1016/j.cmet.2011.08.004

Delecluse, H. J., Feederle, R., O'Sullivan, B., and Taniere, P. (2007). Epstein Barr virus-associated tumours: an update for the attention of the working pathologist. *J. Clin. Pathol.* 60, 1358–1364. doi: 10.1136/jcp.2006.044586

Dolken, L., Malterer, G., Erhard, F., Kothe, S., Friedel, C. C., Suffert, G., et al. (2010). Systematic analysis of viral and cellular microRNA targets in cells latently infected with human gamma-herpesviruses by RISC immunoprecipitation assay. *Cell Host Microbe* 7, 324–334. doi: 10.1016/j.chom.2010.03.008

Duan, F., Liao, J., Huang, Q., Nie, Y., and Wu, K. (2012). HSV-1 miR-H6 inhibits HSV-1 replication and IL-6 expression in human corneal epithelial cells *in vitro*. *Clin. Dev. Immunol.* 2012:192791. doi: 10.1155/2012/192791

Enk, J., Levi, A., Weisblum, Y., Yamin, R., Charpak-Amikam, Y., Wolf, D. G., et al. (2016). HSV1 MicroRNA modulation of GPI anchoring and downstream immune evasion. *Cell Rep.* 17, 949–956. doi: 10.1016/j.celrep.2016.09.077

Feldman, E. R., Kara, M., Coleman, C. B., Grau, K. R., Oko, L. M., Krueger, B. J., et al. (2014). Virus-encoded microRNAs facilitate gammaherpesvirus latency and pathogenesis *in vivo*. *mBio* 5, e00981–e00914. doi: 10.1128/mBio.00981-14

Feldman, E. R., Kara, M., Oko, L. M., Grau, K. R., Krueger, B. J., Zhang, J., et al. (2016). A gammaherpesvirus noncoding RNA is essential for hematogenous dissemination and establishment of peripheral latency. *mSphere* 1, e00105–e00115 doi: 10.1128/mSphere.00105-15

Gottwein, E., Corcoran, D. L., Mukherjee, N., Skalsky, R. L., Hafner, M., Nusbaum, J. D., et al. (2011). Viral microRNA targetome of KSHV-infected primary effusion lymphoma cell lines. *Cell Host Microbe* 10, 515–526. doi: 10.1016/j.chom.2011.09.012

Grundhoff, A., Sullivan, C. S., and Ganem, D. (2006). A combined computational and microarray-based approach identifies novel microRNAs encoded by human gamma-herpesviruses. *RNA* 12, 733–750. doi: 10.1261/rna.2326106

Guido, C., Whitaker-Menezes, D., Capparelli, C., Balliet, R., Lin, Z., Pestell, R. G., et al. (2012). Metabolic reprogramming of cancer-associated fibroblasts by TGF-beta drives tumor growth: connecting TGF-beta signaling with "Warburg-like" cancer metabolism and L-lactate production. *Cell Cycle* 11, 3019–3035. doi: 10.4161/cc.21384

Hancock, M. H., Hook, L. M., Mitchell, J., and Nelson, J. A. (2017). Human cytomegalovirus MicroRNAs miR-US5-1 and miR-UL112-3p block proinflammatory cytokine production in response to nf-κb-activating factors through direct downregulation of IKKα and IKKβ. *mBio* 8, e00109–00117. doi: 10.1128/mBio.00109-17.

Haneklaus, M., Gerlic, M., Kurowska-Stolarska, M., Rainey, A. A., Pich, D., McInnes, I. B., et al. (2012). Cutting edge: miR-223 and EBV miR-BART15 regulate the NLRP3 inflammasome and IL-1beta production. *J. Immunol.* 189, 3795–3799. doi: 10.4049/jimmunol.1200312

Hook, L., Hancock, M., Landais, I., Grabski, R., Britt, W., and Nelson, J. A. (2014). Cytomegalovirus microRNAs. *Curr. Opin. Virol.* 7, 40–46. doi: 10.1016/j.coviro.2014.03.015

Hoshina, S., Sekizuka, T., Kataoka, M., Hasegawa, H., Hamada, H., Kuroda, M., et al. (2016). Profile of exosomal and intracellular microRNA in gamma-herpesvirus-infected lymphoma cell lines. *PLoS ONE* 11:e0162574. doi: 10.1371/journal.pone.0162574

Iizasa, H., Wulff, B.-E., Alla, N., Maragkakis, M., Megraw, M., Hatzigeorgiou, A., et al. (2010). Editing of Epstein-Barr virus-encoded BART6 microRNAs controls their dicer targeting and consequently affects viral latency. *J. Biol. Chem.* 285, 33358–33370. doi: 10.1074/jbc.M110.138362

Jovic, M., Naslavsky, N., Rapaport, D., Horowitz, M., and Caplan, S. (2007). EHD1 regulates beta1 integrin endosomal transport: effects on focal adhesions, cell spreading and migration. *J. Cell Sci.* 120, 802–814. doi: 10.1242/jcs.03383

Jung, Y. J., Choi, H., Kim, H., and Lee, S. K. (2014). miR-BART20-5p stabilizes Epstein-Barr virus latency by directly targeting BZLF1 and BRLF1. *J. Virol.* 88, 9027–9037. doi: 10.1128/jvi.00721-14

Jurak, I., Kramer, M. F., Mellor, J. C., van Lint, A. L., Roth, F. P., Knipe, D. M., et al. (2010). Numerous conserved and divergent microRNAs expressed by herpes simplex viruses 1 and 2. *J. Virol.* 84, 4659–4672. doi: 10.1128/jvi.02725-09

Kawauchi, K., Araki, K., Tobiume, K., and Tanaka, N. (2008). p53 regulates glucose metabolism through an IKK-NF-κB pathway and inhibits cell transformation. *Nat. Cell. Biol.* 10, 611–618. doi: 10.1038/ncb1724

Kelly, G. L., Long, H. M., Stylianou, J., Thomas, W. A., Leese, A., Bell, A. I., et al. (2009). An Epstein-Barr virus anti-apoptotic protein constitutively expressed in transformed cells and implicated in burkitt lymphomagenesis: the Wp/BHRF1 link. *PLoS Pathog.* 5:e1000341. doi: 10.1371/journal.ppat.1000341

Kenney, S. C., and Mertz, J. E. (2014). Regulation of the latent-lytic switch in Epstein-Barr virus. *Semin. Cancer Biol.* 26, 60–68. doi: 10.1016/j.semcancer.2014.01.002

Kim do, N., Song, Y. J., and Lee, S. K. (2011). The role of promoter methylation in Epstein-Barr virus (EBV) microRNA expression in EBV-infected B cell lines. *Exp. Mol. Med.* 43, 401–410. doi: 10.3858/emm.2011.43.7.044

Kim, S., Lee, S., Shin, J., Kim, Y., Evnouchidou, I., Kim, D., et al. (2011). Human cytomegalovirus microRNA miR-US4-1 inhibits $CD8^+$ T cell responses by targeting the aminopeptidase ERAP1. *Nat. Immunol.* 12, 984–991. doi: 10.1038/ni.2097

Kim, Y., Lee, S., Kim, S., Kim, D., Ahn, J. H., and Ahn, K. (2012). Human cytomegalovirus clinical strain-specific microRNA miR-UL148D targets the human chemokine RANTES during infection. *PLoS Pathog.* 8:e1002577. doi: 10.1371/journal.ppat.1002577

Landais, I., Pelton, C., Streblow, D., DeFilippis, V., McWeeney, S., and Nelson, J. A. (2015). Human cytomegalovirus miR-UL112-3p targets TLR2 and modulates the TLR2/IRAK1/NFκB signaling pathway. *PLoS Pathog.* 11:e1004881. doi: 10.1371/journal.ppat.1004881

Lei, X., Bai, Z., Ye, F., Xie, J., Kim, C. G., Huang, Y., et al. (2010). Regulation of NF-kappaB inhibitor IkappaBalpha and viral replication by a KSHV microRNA. *Nat. Cell Biol.* 12, 193–199. doi: 10.1038/ncb2019

Lo, A. K., To, K. F., Lo, K. W., Lung, R. W., Hui, J. W., Liao, G., et al. (2007). Modulation of LMP1 protein expression by EBV-encoded microRNAs. *Proc. Natl. Acad. Sci. U.S.A.* 104, 16164–16169. doi: 10.1073/pnas.0702896104

Louten, J., Beach, M., Palermino, K., Weeks, M., and Holenstein, G. (2015). MicroRNAs expressed during viral infection: biomarker potential and therapeutic considerations. *Biomark Insights* 10, 25–52. doi: 10.4137/BMI.S29512

Lung, R. W., Tong, J. H., Sung, Y. M., Leung, P. S., Ng, D. C., Chau, S. L., et al. (2009). Modulation of LMP2A expression by a newly identified Epstein-Barr virus-encoded microRNA miR-BART22. *Neoplasia* 11, 1174–1184. doi: 10.1593/neo.09888

Luo, B., Wang, Y., Wang, X.-F., Liang, H., Yan, L.-P., Huang, B.-H., et al. (2005). Expression of Epstein-Barr virus genes in EBV-associated gastric carcinomas. *World J. Gastroenterol.* 11, 629–633. doi: 10.3748/wjg.v11.i5.629

Manzano, M., Shamulailatpam, P., Raja, A. N., and Gottwein, E. (2013). Kaposi's sarcoma-associated herpesvirus encodes a mimic of cellular miR-23. *J. Virol.* 87, 11821–11830. doi: 10.1128/jvi.01692-13

Meckes, D. G. Jr., Shair, K. H., Marquitz, A. R., Kung, C. P., Edwards, R. H., and Raab-Traub, N. (2010). Human tumor virus utilizes exosomes for intercellular communication. *Proc. Natl. Acad. Sci. U.S.A.* 107, 20370–20375. doi: 10.1073/pnas.1014194107

Middeldorp, J. M., Brink, A. A., van den Brule, A. J., and Meijer, C. J. (2003). Pathogenic roles for Epstein-Barr virus (EBV) gene products in EBV-associated proliferative disorders. *Crit. Rev. Oncol. Hematol.* 45, 1–36. doi: 10.1016/S1040-8428(02)00078-1

Nachmani, D., Lankry, D., Wolf, D. G., and Mandelboim, O. (2010). The human cytomegalovirus microRNA miR-UL112 acts synergistically with a cellular microRNA to escape immune elimination. *Nat. Immunol.* 11, 806–813. doi: 10.1038/ni.1916

Nachmani, D., Stern-Ginossar, N., Sarid, R., and Mandelboim, O. (2009). Diverse herpesvirus microRNAs target the stress-induced immune ligand MICB to escape recognition by natural killer cells. *Cell Host Microbe* 5, 376–385. doi: 10.1016/j.chom.2009.03.003

Nukui, M., Mori, Y., and Murphy, E. A. (2015). A human herpesvirus 6A-encoded microRNA: role in viral lytic replication. *J. Virol.* 89, 2615–2627. doi: 10.1128/JVI.02007-14

Pattle, S., and Farrell, P. (2006). The role of Epstein-Barr virus in cancer. *Expert Opin. Biol. Ther.* 6, 1193–1205. doi: 10.1517/14712598.6.11.1193

Pegtel, D. M., Cosmopoulos, K., Thorley-Lawson, D. A., van Eijndhoven, M. A., Hopmans, E. S., Lindenberg, J. L., et al. (2010). Functional delivery of viral miRNAs via exosomes. *Proc. Natl. Acad. Sci. U.S.A.* 107, 6328–6333. doi: 10.1073/pnas.0914843107

Pfeffer, S., Sewer, A., Lagos-Quintana, M., Sheridan, R., Sander, C., Grasser, F. A., et al. (2005). Identification of microRNAs of the herpesvirus family. *Nat. Methods* 2, 269–276. doi: 10.1038/nmeth746

Pfeffer, S., Zavolan, M., Grässer, F., Chien, M., Russo, J., Ju, J., et al. (2004). Identification of virus-encoded microRNAs. *Science* 304, 734–736. doi: 10.1126/science.1096781

Plaisance-Bonstaff, K., Choi, H. S., Beals, T., Krueger, B. J., Boss, I. W., Gay, L. A., et al. (2014). KSHV miRNAs decrease expression of lytic genes in latently infected PEL and endothelial cells by targeting host transcription factors. *Viruses* 6, 4005–4023. doi: 10.3390/v6104005

Rafalski, V. A., and Brunet, A. (2011). Energy metabolism in adult neural stem cell fate. *Prog. Neurobiol.* 93, 182–203. doi: 10.1016/j.pneurobio.2010.10.007

Ramalingam, D., and Ziegelbauer, J. M. (2017). Viral microRNAs target a gene network, inhibit STAT activation, and suppress interferon responses. *Sci. Rep.* 7:40813. doi: 10.1038/srep40813

Riley, K. J., Rabinowitz, G. S., Yario, T. A., Luna, J. M., Darnell, R. B., and Steitz, J. A. (2012). EBV and human microRNAs co-target oncogenic and apoptotic viral and human genes during latency. *EMBO J.* 31, 2207–2221. doi: 10.1038/emboj.2012.63

Sadler, R. H., and Raab-Traub, N. (1995). Structural analyses of the Epstein-Barr virus BamHI A transcripts. *J. Virol.* 69, 1132–1141.

Sanchez, E. L., and Lagunoff, M. (2015). Viral activation of cellular metabolism. *Virology* 479–480, 609–618. doi: 10.1016/j.virol.2015.02.038

Sherwood, V. (2015). WNT signaling: an emerging mediator of cancer cell metabolism? *Mol. Cell Biol.* 35, 2–10. doi: 10.1128/MCB.00992-14

Skalsky, R. L., Corcoran, D. L., Gottwein, E., Frank, C. L., Kang, D., Hafner, M., et al. (2012). The viral and cellular microRNA targetome in lymphoblastoid cell lines. *PLoS Pathog.* 8:e1002484. doi: 10.1371/journal.ppat.1002484

Skalsky, R. L., Samols, M. A., Plaisance, K. B., Boss, I. W., Riva, A., Lopez, M. C., et al. (2007). Kaposi's sarcoma-associated herpesvirus encodes an ortholog of miR-155. *J. Virol.* 81, 12836–12845. doi: 10.1128/jvi.01804-07

Steer, B., Strehle, M., Sattler, C., Bund, D., Flach, B., Stoeger, T., et al. (2016). The small noncoding RNAs (sncRNAs) of murine gammaherpesvirus 68 (MHV-68) are involved in regulating the latent-to-lytic switch *in vivo*. *Sci. Rep.* 6:32128. doi: 10.1038/srep32128

Tuddenham, L., Jung, J. S., Chane-Woon-Ming, B., Dolken, L., and Pfeffer, S. (2012). Small RNA deep sequencing identifies microRNAs and other small noncoding RNAs from human herpesvirus 6B. *J. Virol.* 86, 1638–1649. doi: 10.1128/JVI.05911-11

Umbach, J. L., Kramer, M. F., Jurak, I., Karnowski, H. W., Coen, D. M., and Cullen, B. R. (2008). MicroRNAs expressed by herpes simplex virus 1 during latent infection regulate viral mRNAs. *Nature* 454, 780–783. doi: 10.1038/nature07103

Umbach, J. L., Nagel, M. A., Cohrs, R. J., Gilden, D. H., and Cullen, B. R. (2009). Analysis of human alphaherpesvirus microRNA expression in latently infected human trigeminal ganglia. *J. Virol.* 83, 10677–10683. doi: 10.1128/JVI.01185-09

Umbach, J. L., Wang, K., Tang, S., Krause, P. R., Mont, E. K., Cohen, J. I., et al. (2010). Identification of viral microRNAs expressed in human sacral ganglia latently infected with herpes simplex virus 2. *J. Virol.* 84, 1189–1192. doi: 10.1128/jvi.01712-09

Wagner, E. K., Devi-Rao, G., Feldman, L. T., Dobson, A. T., Zhang, Y. F., Flanagan, W. M., et al. (1988). Physical characterization of the herpes simplex virus latency-associated transcript in neurons. *J. Virol.* 62, 1194–1202.

Wan, X. X., Yi, H., Qu, J. Q., He, Q. Y., and Xiao, Z. Q. (2015). Integrated analysis of the differential cellular and EBV miRNA expression profiles in microdissected nasopharyngeal carcinoma and non-cancerous nasopharyngeal tissues. *Oncol. Rep.* 34, 2585–2601. doi: 10.3892/or.2015.4237

Winter, J., Jung, S., Keller, S., Gregory, R., and Diederichs, S. (2009). Many roads to maturity: microRNA biogenesis pathways and their regulation. *Nat. Cell Biol.* 11, 228–234. doi: 10.1038/ncb0309-228

Wullschleger, S., Loewith, R., and Hall, M. N. (2006). TOR signaling in growth and metabolism. *Cell* 124, 471–484. doi: 10.1016/j.cell.2006.01.016

Xia, T., O'Hara, A., Araujo, I., Barreto, J., Carvalho, E., Sapucaia, J. B., et al. (2008). EBV microRNAs in primary lymphomas and targeting of CXCL-11 by ebv-mir-BHRF1-3. *Cancer Res.* 68, 1436–1442. doi: 10.1158/0008-5472.can-07-5126

Xing, L., and Kieff, E. (2011). cis-Acting effects on RNA processing and Drosha cleavage prevent Epstein-Barr virus latency III BHRF1 expression. *J. Virol.* 85, 8929–8939. doi: 10.1128/jvi.00336-11

Yang, I. V., Wade, C. M., Kang, H. M., Alper, S., Rutledge, H., Lackford, B., et al. (2009). Identification of novel genes that mediate innate immunity using inbred mice. *Genetics* 183, 1535–1544. doi: 10.1534/genetics.109.107540

Yap, T. A., Garrett, M. D., Walton, M. I., Raynaud, F., de Bono, J. S., and Workman, P. (2008). Targeting the PI3K-AKT-mTOR pathway: progress, pitfalls, and promises. *Curr. Opin. Pharmacol.* 8, 393–412. doi: 10.1016/j.coph.2008.08.004

Ye, Y., Zhou, Y., Zhang, L., Chen, Y., Lyu, X., Cai, L., et al. (2013). EBV-miR-BART1 is involved in regulating metabolism-associated genes in nasopharyngeal carcinoma. *Biochem. Biophys. Res. Commun.* 436, 19–24. doi: 10.1016/j.bbrc.2013.05.008

Yogev, O., Lagos, D., Enver, T., and Boshoff, C. (2014). Kaposi's sarcoma herpesvirus microRNAs induce metabolic transformation of infected cells. *PLoS Pathog.* 10:e1004400. doi: 10.1371/journal.ppat.1004400

Young, L., and Murray, P. (2003). Epstein-Barr virus and oncogenesis: from latent genes to tumours. *Oncogene* 22, 5108–5121. doi: 10.1038/sj.onc.1206556

Young, L., and Rickinson, A. (2004). Epstein-Barr virus: 40 years on. *Nat. Rev. Cancer* 4, 757–768. doi: 10.1038/nrc1452

Zeng, Z. Y., Zhou, Y. H., Zhang, W. L., Xiong, W., Fan, S. Q., Li, X. L., et al. (2007). Gene expression profiling of nasopharyngeal carcinoma reveals the abnormally regulated Wnt signaling pathway. *Hum. Pathol.* 38, 120–133. doi: 10.1016/j.humpath.2006.06.023

Zhao, H., Zhang, C., Hou, G., and Song, J. (2015). MicroRNA-H4-5p encoded by HSV-1 latency-associated transcript promotes cell proliferation, invasion and cell cycle progression via p16-mediated PI3K-Akt signaling pathway in SHSY5Y cells. *Int. J. Clin. Exp. Med.* 8, 7526–7534.

Zhu, J., Pfuhl, T., Motsch, N., Barth, S., Nicholls, J., Grasser, F., et al. (2009). Identification of novel Epstein-Barr virus microRNA genes from nasopharyngeal carcinomas. *J. Virol.* 83, 3333–3341. doi: 10.1128/JVI.01689-08

8

Variation of Carbohydrate-Active Enzyme Patterns in the Gut Microbiota of Italian Healthy Subjects and Type 2 Diabetes Patients

*Matteo Soverini, Silvia Turroni, Elena Biagi, Sara Quercia, Patrizia Brigidi, Marco Candela and Simone Rampelli**

Unit of Microbial Ecology of Health, Department of Pharmacy and Biotechnology, University of Bologna, Bologna, Italy

***Correspondence:**
Simone Rampelli
simone.rampelli@unibo.it

The human gut microbiota (GM) has been associated, to date, with various complex functions, essentials for the host health. Among these, it is certainly worth noting the degradation of the so-called microbiota-accessible carbohydrates (MACs), which the GM breaks down through specific enzymes, referred to as carbohydrate-active enzymes (CAZymes). This degradation constitutes the first step in the production of short-chain fatty acids (SCFAs), key microbial small molecules having multiple health-promoting effects for the host organism. The decline in MAC dietary intake in urban Western populations forced the shrinkage of CAZyme repertoire in the GM, as shown by the literature comparing the microbiome layout between Western urban citizens and traditional rural populations. Even if this reduction in GM functional complexity has been associated with the onset of the so-called "diseases of civilization," only few information regarding the CAZyme variation within Western populations has been provided to date, and its connections with diet and health are still unexplored. In this scenario, here we explore the GM-encoded CAZyme repertoire across two Italian adult cohorts, including healthy lean subjects consuming a Mediterranean diet and obese patients affected by type 2 diabetes, consuming a high-fat diet. In order to impute the CAZyme panel, a pipeline consisting of publicly available software – QIIME, FragGeneScan and HMMER – was specifically implemented. Our study highlighted the existence of robust clusters of bacterial species sharing a common MAC degradation profile in the Italian GM, allowing the stratification of the individual GM into different steady states according to the carbohydrate degradation profile, with possible connections with diet and health.

Keywords: gut microbiota, microbiota-accessible carbohydrates, CAZymes, co-abundance groups, type 2 diabetes

INTRODUCTION

The large ensemble of bacteria that stably inhabit the distal part of our gastrointestinal tract, namely the gut microbiota (GM), is of vital importance for many physiological functions of our organism, exerting a key role in several biological processes, such as nutrition, immune function, and the regulation of the central nervous system (Neish, 2009; Hooper et al., 2012;

Nicholson et al., 2012; Honda and Littman, 2016; Sharon et al., 2016). As a strategic partner of the human holobiont, the GM expands our metabolic potential by adding degradative functions, thus enabling the metabolism of a wide range of complex polysaccharides, otherwise indigestible, including exogenous carbohydrates introduced with diet (Schnorr et al., 2014). Indeed, despite the wide distribution of complex polysaccharides in edible plants (Lattimer and Haub, 2010), our genome is astonishingly poor in genes coding for carbohydrate-active enzymes (CAZymes) (Gill et al., 2006), i.e., enzymes specifically devoted to polysaccharide degradation. Conversely, the gut microbiome (i.e., the cumulative genome of the GM) encodes for a much wider and diversified arsenal of CAZymes (El Kaoutari et al., 2013), allowing for the catabolism of the vast array of complex polysaccharides that reach the colon undigested. These molecules are converted to short-chain fatty acids (SCFAs), microbial metabolites with multiple roles in human physiology (Koh et al., 2016). This inter-kingdom cross-feeding is the basis of the mutualistic relationship we share with our intestinal microbial counterpart, which thus emerges as a key player in the co-metabolism of complex carbohydrates in our gut. In this scenario, the dietary polysaccharides that are metabolically available to gut microbes have been specifically defined as microbiota-accessible carbohydrates (MACs) (Sonnenburg and Sonnenburg, 2014) and their abundance in the host diet, and consequently their availability within the gut, has proved to be crucial for microbiota–host homeostasis.

The MAC availability in the host diet is among the aspects that have deeply changed in recent human evolutionary history, with the transition from Paleolithic hunting-gathering to Neolithic rural populations and contemporary Westernized societies (Quercia et al., 2014; Schnorr et al., 2014; Sonnenburg and Sonnenburg, 2014; Obregon-Tito et al., 2015). In particular, along with Westernization, we have witnessed a progressive reduction of the MAC content and diversity in the diet, with the transition to foods high in refined simple sugars. According to Sonnenburg et al. (2016), this reduction of dietary MACs forced the progressive impoverishment of the CAZyme repertoire in the human microbiome, compromising the overall metabolic plasticity of the human meta-organism. This was confirmed by gut metagenome studies comparing the CAZyme repertoire between traditional populations consuming high-fiber diets and Western urban citizens, which highlighted a relevant reduction of the microbial CAZyme diversity in the latter (King et al., 2012; Bhattacharya et al., 2015; Rampelli et al., 2015). Such wide GM comparative surveys provided important information on the GM-host co-evolutionary dynamics but they did not allow for a precise discrimination of the impact of individual covariates (e.g., diet, health, medication) on the GM functional repertoire. Aiming to fill this gap in knowledge, here we compared the imputed CAZyme repertoire from two cohorts of Western urban adults from Italy, overcoming the intrinsic variation of the CAZyme profiles according to geography and ethnicity (Soverini et al., 2016). In particular, we analyzed the GM structure and metadata from16 healthy subjects following a Mediterranean diet and 40 obese, type 2 diabetic (T2D) patients consuming a high-fat low-MACs diet from two previously published studies (Schnorr et al., 2014; Candela et al., 2016). Our findings highlighted the existence of a potentially limited number of well-balanced host–microbe symbiotic configurations, with a possible connection to diet and health status.

MATERIALS AND METHODS

Determination of the Pan-microbiome from Italian Healthy Subjects

The publicly available 16S rRNA sequencing data of the fecal samples of 16 Italian healthy subjects from Schnorr et al. (2014) were downloaded from the MG-RAST website[1] and taxonomically characterized to the species level using the QIIME pipeline (Caporaso et al., 2010), with blastn as an assignment method and the HMP gastrointestinal 16S rRNA dataset as reference sequences[2]. The detected species were considered part of the so-called Italian "pan-microbiome," i.e., the virtual entity gathering the vast majority of bacterial species present in the GM of the Italian population. The assembled reference genomes of these bacterial species were downloaded from the NCBI genome section[3]. Then, to characterize the CAZyme repertoire of these microorganisms, the CAZyme identification pipeline developed by Soverini et al. (2016) was applied. Briefly, ORFs were extracted from the assembled genomes using FragGeneScan 1.16 (Rho et al., 2010). From the translated ORFs, the CAZyme-coding sequences were detected using the hmmscan tool of the HMMER software package (Robert et al., 2011) and the dbCAN CAZyme database (Yin et al., 2012). The outputs were further processed by the script hmmscan-parser.sh[4], selecting only the ORFs that showed a minimum identity of 30% to the query sequences and an alignment length of at least 100 residues.

Identification of CAZyme Co-abundance Groups within the Italian Pan-microbiome

The CAZyme profiles were used to generate CAZy co-abundance groups (CCGs), which were conceived as groups of bacterial species sharing a similar CAZyme profile. In brief, the CCGs were generated by applying hierarchical Ward-linkage clustering based on Spearman correlation coefficients to the abundances of glycosyl-hydrolase (GH) and auxiliary activity (AA) families detected in the bacterial genomes. Permutational multivariate analysis of variance (function "adonis" of the vegan package in R) was used to determine whether CCGs were significantly different from each other. CAZymes were also manually classified for their ability to degrade specific substrates by consulting the publicly available CAZy database[5]. Specifically, we evaluated the ability to degrade different types of MACs: resistant starch (RS),

[1]http://metagenomics.anl.gov/linkin.cgi?project=mgp8810
[2]http://hmpdacc.org/HM16STR/healthy/
[3]https://www.ncbi.nlm.nih.gov/genome/
[4]https://github.com/carden24/Bioinformatics_scripts/blob/master/hmmscan-parser.sh
[5]http://www.cazy.org

non-digestible carbohydrates (NDC), non-starch polysaccharides (NSP), and mucins/glycoproteins (M/G). When more than one activity was found, we selected the most relevant one, i.e., the one with the highest abundance of genes involved in the degradation of a given substrate.

Assessment of Redundant Patterns of CAZymes in Italian Healthy Subjects and Type 2 Diabetes Patients

To explore CAZyme profiles in the Italian population in health and disease, we integrated the dataset used to determine the pan-microbiome with the 16S rRNA sequences of the GM from 40 patients affected by type 2 diabetes (Candela et al., 2016). The sequences were downloaded from MG-RAST[6] and analyzed using QIIME (Caporaso et al., 2010) and the HMP database, as described above for healthy subjects. The CAZyme profile of each GM was obtained by quantifying the relative abundance of each CCG, as a sum of the relative contribution of component bacterial species. We then grouped the subjects using hierarchical Ward-linkage clustering based on Spearman correlation coefficients. Separation between clusters was tested using the permutational multivariate analysis of variance (function "adonis" of vegan). All statistical analyses were computed in R version 3.1.3 using R studio version 1.0.36 with packages vegan and made4.

RESULTS

The Italian Pan-microbiome from Healthy Adults

The analysis of the publicly available 16S rRNA sequences of stool samples from 16 Italian healthy adults (aged 20–40 years, mean 32 years) consuming a standard Mediterranean diet (Schnorr et al., 2014) led to the identification of a total of 98 bacterial species, present at least once in the samples (**Supplementary Table S1**). *Faecalibacterium prausnitzii* was the most represented species, with an average relative abundance of 11 ± 0.09% (standard deviation of the mean). *Eubacterium rectale* (7 ± 0.06%), *Ruminococcus bromii* (6 ± 0.05%), and *Bifidobacterium adolescentis* (6 ± 0.06%) occurred as co-dominant species. *Subdoligranulum variabile* (3 ± 0.04%), *Ruminococcus champanellensis* (3 ± 0.02%), *Clostridium asparagiforme* (2 ± 0.01%), *Bacteroides vulgatus* (2 ± 0.03%), *Coprococcus eutactus* (2 ± 0.03%), and *Roseburia intestinalis* (1.8 ± 0.01%) were ancillary species present to a lower extent. In terms of prevalence, *F. prausnitzii, E. rectale, Butyricicoccus pullicaecorum, R. intestinalis, Ruminococcus* spp., *Flavonifractor plautii, Blautia obeum, Dorea formicigenerans* and *Anaerostipes hadrus* were present in all samples of the dataset, whereas *Methanobrevibacter smithii, Bifidobacterium catenulatum, Lactobacillus ruminis, Weissella paramesenteroides,* and *Sutterella parvirubra* were found in less than three samples, being among the least prevalent microorganisms in the analyzed Italian microbiomes.

CAZyme Repertoire in the Bacterial Species of the Italian Pan-microbiome

Reference genomes from the bacterial species included in the Italian pan-microbiome were retrieved from the NCBI database, and the respective CAZyme-coding sequences were identified. The number of these sequences varied widely between the pan-microbiome components. In particular, *Odoribacter laneus, Lactobacillus salivarius,* and *F. plautii* showed the lowest amounts of CAZyme-coding genes, while *Eubacterium biforme, Dialister succinatiphilus,* and *D. formicigenerans* the highest (see Supplementary Figure S1 for retrieving the number of CAZyme-coding sequences for each bacterial species).

To identify common patterns of MAC-degrading enzymes among the different species of the Italian pan-microbiome, we determined co-abundance associations between the bacterial CAZyme profiles and then clustered them based on similarity. Four robust CAZy Co-abundance Groups (CCGs) were identified in the Italian pan-microbiome, each one including GM species that share a similar CAZyme profile, describing the pattern of CAZyme variation within the Italian GM species (p-value < 0.001, permutation test with pseudo F ratios). CCGs were named according to the most abundant species in each group as follows: *S. variabile* (CCG1), *E. rectale* (CCG2), *R. bromii* (CCG3), and *F. prausnitzii* (CCG4) (**Figure 1**). Interestingly, *F. prausnitzii* and *R. bromii* CCGs included species with the highest amount of CAZyme-coding sequences, such as *D. succinatiphilus, D. formicigenerans,* and *E. biforme*. On the other hand, CCG1 (*S. variabile*) and CCG2 (*E. rectale*) included species with a lower amount of CAZyme genes, such as *O. laneus* and *F. plautii*. It is important to note that the bacterial genome size is not predictive of the number of encoded CAZymes (El Kaoutari et al., 2013). For example, *Bacteroides oleiciplenus, Bacterioides cellulosilyticus* and *Bacteroides ovatus*, the three species with the largest genome size in the Italian pan-microbiome (Supplementary Figure S1), were found to be included within the *S. variabile* group and show the lowest richness in the CAZyme repertoire.

Finally, we specifically evaluated the distribution of CAZyme families involved in the degradation of different types of MACs across the four CCGs (**Figure 2**). According to our findings, *E. rectale* and *F. prausnitzii* groups showed the highest number of sequences encoding for CAZymes involved in the degradation of non-digestible carbohydrates and non-starch polysaccharides, while the *R. bromii* group was the least rich in these enzymatic functions (p-value < 0.05, Wilcoxon rank sum test). Interestingly, the ability to degrade RS was evenly spread among the different CCGs.

CAZyme Distribution in the Gut Microbiome of Italian Individuals: Associations with the Diet and Health Status

We next explored the variation of CCG profiles in Italian subjects, also in association with the dietary pattern and health conditions. To this aim, the dataset of analyzed individuals was integrated

---

[6]http://metagenomics.anl.gov/mgmain.html?mgpage=project&project=mgp17675

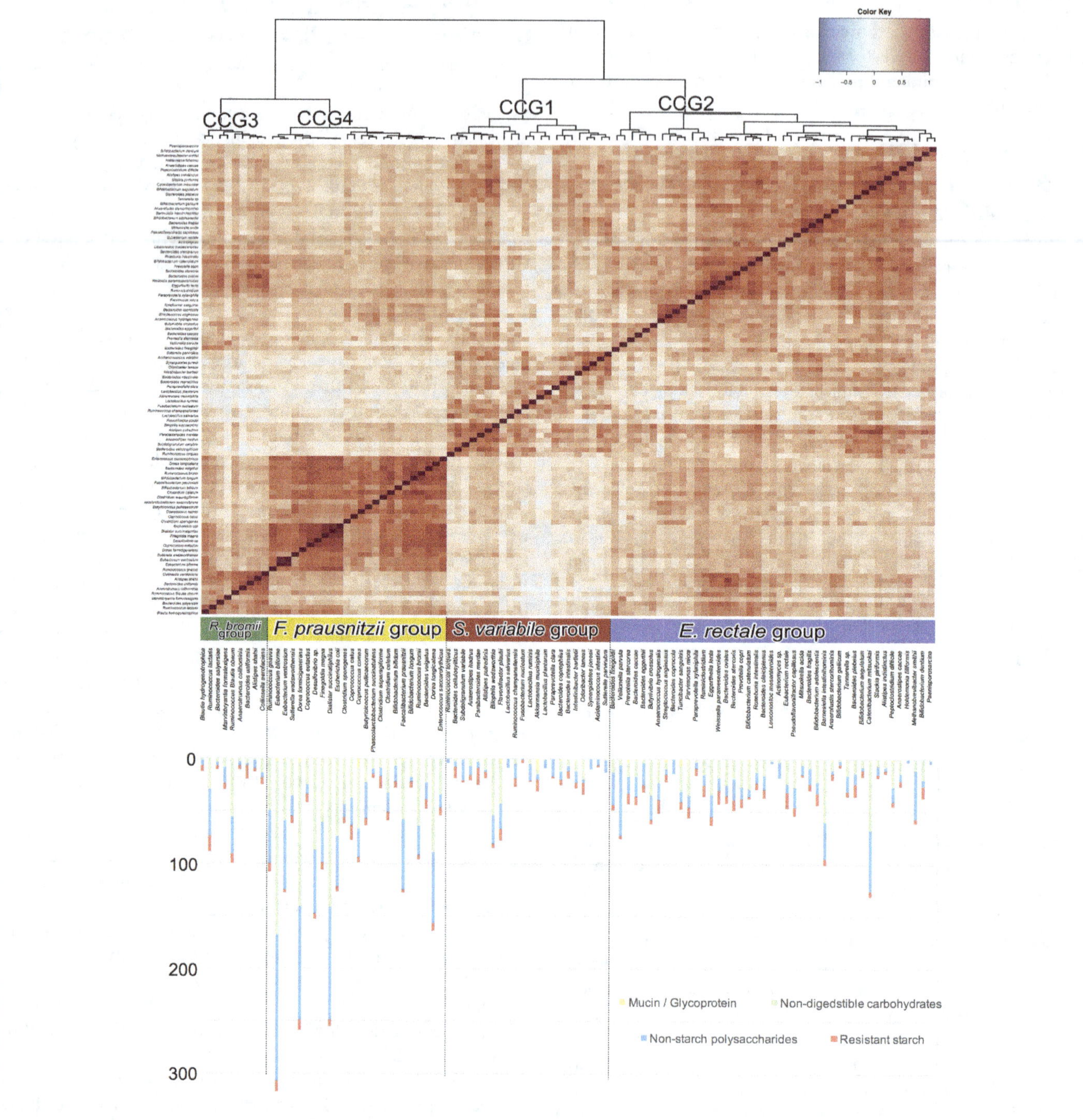

FIGURE 1 | Hierarchical clustering of the raw abundances of the CAZy glycosyl-hydrolase (GH) and auxiliary activity (AA) families in the bacterial species constituting the Italian pan-microbiome. Spearman distance and Ward's minimum variance method were used. Four CAZy Co-abundance Groups (CCGs) were identified and named according to the most abundant species in each group, as follows: CCG1 – *Subdoligranulum variabile* group (red), CCG2 – *Eubacterium rectale* group (blue), CCG3 – *Ruminococcus bromii* group (green), and CCG4 – *Faecalibacterium prausnitzii* group (yellow). Below the heatplot are reported the counts of CAZyme-coding sequences belonging to the GH and AA families, detected in the type strain reference genomes for each bacterial species, divided by class of MACs: resistant starch (RS), non-digestible carbohydrates (NDC), non-starch polysaccharides (NSP), and mucins/glycoproteins (M/G).

with publicly available16S rRNA gene sequences from 40 Italian obese patients suffering from type 2 diabetes and consuming a high-fat low-MACs diet (Candela et al., 2016). The addition of these samples did not result in an increase in the size of the Italian pan-microbiome, which still consisted of the previously identified 98 species. To compare the CCG distribution among individual gut microbiomes, for each CCG, the sum of the abundances of constituent microorganisms was calculated, and

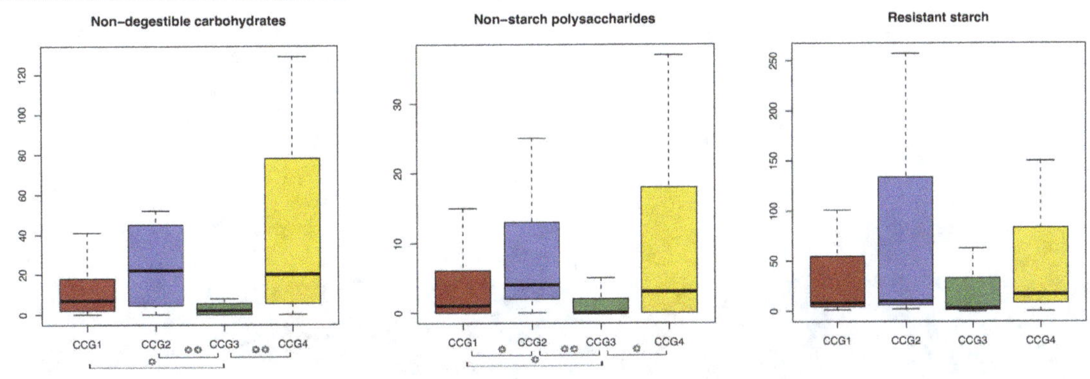

FIGURE 2 | Boxplots representing the distribution of the degradative potential of exogenous MACs in the different CAZyme Co-abundance Groups (CCGs). Square brackets at the bottom indicate a significant difference in raw abundances (single asterisk, *p*-values between 0.05 and 0.001; double asterisk, *p*-values below 0.001, Wilcoxon rank sum test).

the personal profile of CCG abundance in the GM was computed for each subject. According to a clustering analysis of the individual CCG abundance profiles, subjects could be clustered into four groups (p-value < 0.001, permutation test with pseudo F ratio), each including individuals that shared a comparable profile of the four CCGs, and therefore potentially a similar carbohydrate-degrading functional pattern. We defined these redundant patterns as CAZyTypes (CTs), i.e., clusters of different GM configurations with a similar carbohydrate-degrading profile (**Figure 3**). Interestingly, CT2 and CT4 were more represented in healthy individuals consuming a Mediterranean diet, while CT1 and CT3 occurred with higher frequency in obese T2D patients consuming a high-fat low-MACs diet. By Principal Coordinates Analysis (PCoA), we represented the CCG variation patterns in individual microbiomes in a two-dimensional space (Supplementary Figure S2), highlighting the separation of subjects based on both the CCG abundance and health status (p-value < 0.001 permutation test with pseudo F ratio).

Looking at the CCG distribution in the Italian population, we found that the most prevalent CCG was *F. prausnitzii* group, with the co-presence of *E. rectale* group as an ancillary CCG in the health-prevalent CT2 and CT4 (**Figure 3**). On the other hand, *S. variabile* group and *R. bromii* group were sporadically represented in the subjects of all CTs, but generally present in lower abundance in healthy subjects. Indeed, only three healthy subjects out of 16 showed a relative abundance of the *S. variabile* and *R. bromii* groups higher than the average contribution in the overall dataset. Conversely, a higher abundance of these two CCGs was found in T2D patients (18 out of 40).

DISCUSSION

Our work aimed at characterizing the frame of the CAZyme variation in the GM meta-community from 56 Italian subjects, of whom 16 were healthy lean adults consuming a standard Mediterranean diet (Schnorr et al., 2014) and 40 were obese T2D patients consuming a high-fat low-MACs diet (Candela et al., 2016). The pan-microbiome of the studied population included a total of 98 bacterial species and, in healthy subjects, it was dominated by *F. prausnitzii*, *E. rectale*, *R. bromii* and *B. adolescentis*, which also emerged as the most prevalent species in the GM from Italian healthy adults. When compared with previously characterized GM pan-genomes, such as that from the Chinese population (Zhang et al., 2015), the Italian one showed some peculiarities, i.e., the presence of *E. rectale* and *Bifidobacterium* and the absence of *Phascolarctobacterium* within the core community. Although both studies are based on relatively small cohorts, and a more extensive screening at the population level is needed, these data seem to suggest a certain level of country specificity in the gut microbiome structure, which may contribute to the immunological and metabolic peculiarities of the populations.

According to our findings, the bacterial species belonging to the Italian pan-microbiome showed two different types of MAC-degrading profiles, essentially characterized by a high or low content of glycosyl-hydrolase-coding sequences, respectively. As expected, the CAZyme distribution in the various species of the Italian GM was heterogeneous, and the absolute number of CAZymes was independent from the genome size. However, it should be mentioned that, for each identified species, the analysis of the CAZyme content was performed by using the type strain reference genome deposited in the NCBI database and therefore our classification was blind with respect to the possible strain-level functional variability in the CAZyme profile.

The GM species of the Italian pan-microbiome were successfully clustered into four CCGs according to the similarity of the CAZyme pattern: *S. variabile* (CCG1), *E. rectale* (CCG2), *R. bromii* (CCG3), and *F. prausnitzii* (CCG4). Interestingly, each of the identified CCGs was characterized by a peculiar structure in terms of CAZyme content. In particular, *F. prausnitzii* and *R. bromii* groups were the most enriched CCGs in terms of represented CAZyme functions, whereas *F. prausnitzii* and *E. rectale* groups were the most equipped CCGs in terms of CAZymes specifically involved in the breakdown of non-digestible carbohydrates and non-starch polysaccharides (i.e., xylans, pectins, and mannans). These observations suggest that the Italian pan-microbiome is diversified in at least

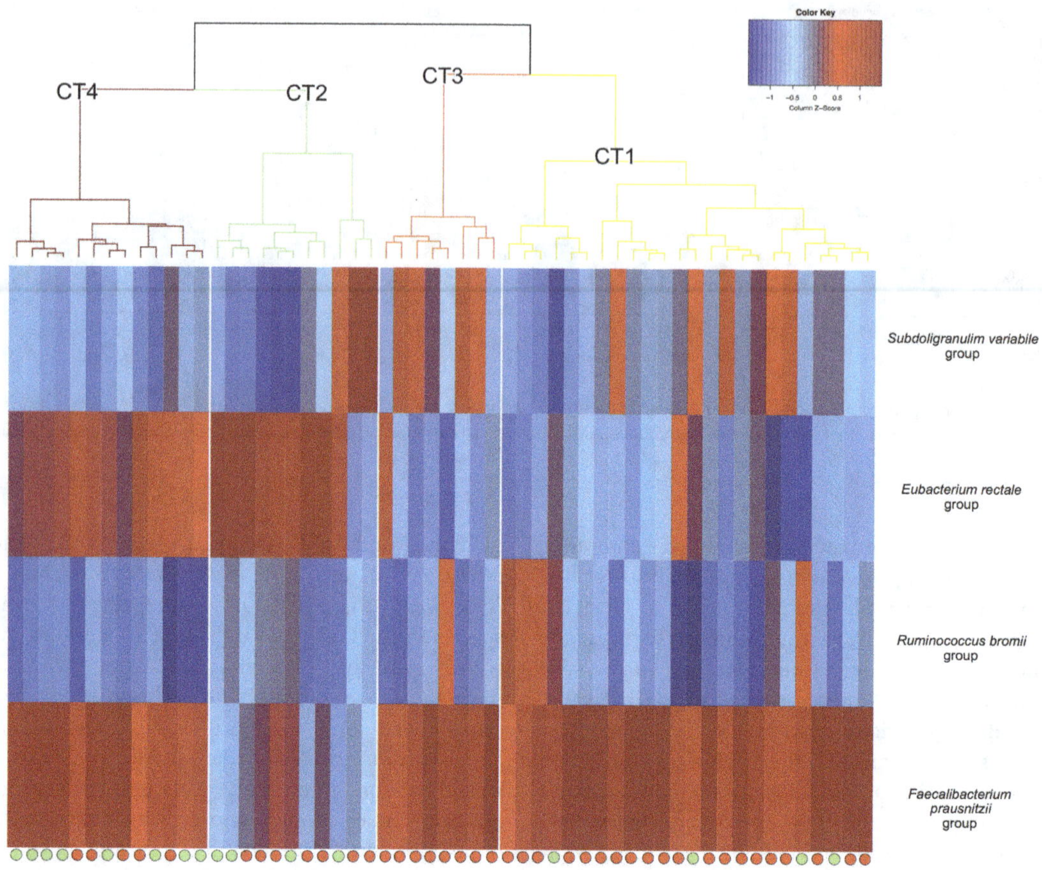

FIGURE 3 | Hierarchical clustering of the relative abundances of each CAZyme Co-abundance Group (CCG) in the gut microbiota (GM) of every subject. Bray–Curtis distance and Ward's minimum variance method were used. On the top: the four CAZyTypes (from CT1 to CT4) identified, i.e., clusters of different GM configurations with a similar carbohydrate-degrading profile. On the right: the four CCGs, named according to the most abundant species in each group (CCG1 – *Subdoligranulum variabile* group, CCG2 – *Eubacterium rectale* group, CCG3 – *Ruminococcus bromii* group, and CCG4 – *Faecalibacterium prausnitzii* group). At the bottom: green dot, healthy lean subject; red dot, obese type 2 diabetic patient.

four patterns of carbohydrate degradation, raising several open questions related to: (i) the major determinants of the co-evolutionary processes underlying this differentiation; (ii) the relative contribution of host genetics, lifestyle and diet as drivers of this functional convergence; (iii) the ultimate connections between the observed CCGs and the host metabolic phenotype.

When exploring the quantitative distribution of CCGs in the individual microbiota from all subjects analyzed, we observed four robust clusters of subjects sharing a similar CCG profile, termed from CT1 to CT4. In particular, the CT1 and CT3 clusters included CCG4 (*F. prausnitzii* group) as the most prevalent CCG, being present in all individuals, and CCG3 (*R. bromii* group) and CCG1 (*S. variabile* group) as less prevalent, ancillary, and generally mutually exclusive groups. Conversely, CT4 was dominated by both CCG4 (*F. prausnitzii* group) and CCG2 (*E. rectale* group), which equally shared the ecosystem. Finally, CT2 showed CCG2 (*E. rectale* group) as the most prevalent group and CCG4 (*F. prausnitzii* group) as ancillary and less prevalent group, except for three subjects that were dominated by CCG1 (*S. variabile* group). These observations are indicative of a different ecological behavior for the diverse CCGs. Indeed, while CCG4 (*F. prausnitzii* group) appears to co-exist with all other CCGs, CCG2 (*E. rectale* group) and the CCGs 1 (*S. variabile* group)/3 (*R. bromii* group) are mutually exclusive. Confirming this, none of the CTs showed the simultaneous presence of CCG2 and CCG1 and/or CCG3. Taken together, these data suggest that the GM-host co-evolution process has resulted in the establishment of four well-defined functional steady states, i.e., the four CTs, each determined by the CCG propensity to share the same gut environment, and each conferring to the host a specific pattern of CAZymes.

In order to explore possible associations of these CTs with the host diet and health, we explored their variation in Italian healthy adults consuming a Mediterranean diet and obese T2D patients consuming a high-fat low-MACs diet. Interestingly, according to our data, most healthy subjects belonged to the CTs 2 and 4, which were characterized by the simultaneous presence of CCG4 (*F. prausnitzii* group) and CCG2 (*E. rectale* group). Conversely, the great majority of obese T2D patients belonged to CT1 and CT3, where CCG2 (*E. rectale* group) was substituted by CCG3 (*R. bromii* group) and/or CCG1 (*S. variabile* group). Although caution is needed in interpreting results, the analysis presented here suggests that a high-fat low-MACs diet, in the context of metabolic deregulation, such as obesity and T2D, could force changes in the GM CTs, supporting the presence of CCG1 (*S. variabile* group) and/or CCG3 (*R. bromii* group) to the detriment of CCG2 (*E. rectale* group). Interestingly, compared to CCG1 and CCG3, the CCG2 showed higher levels of enzymes involved in the degradation of non-digestible carbohydrates and non-starch polysaccharides, which are indeed abundant MACs in the Mediterranean dietary regimen. Though preliminary, our data highlight a possible adaptive or maladaptive nature for each of the four CT steady states that describe the Italian pan-microbiome. Indeed, the steady states CTs 2 and 4, that were generally associated with healthy hosts, seem to be the result of an adaptive microbiome-host co-evolution process, in which the interplay between diet, gut microorganisms and the host can contribute to overall metabolic health. On the contrary, the CTs 1 and 3 that were associated with T2D and a high-fat low-MACs diet, may result from a maladaptive microbiome–host process, in which this type of diet has led to the selection of CT steady states able to contribute to metabolic and/or immunological deregulation. Supporting these hypotheses, patients suffering from Behcet's syndrome, a systemic inflammatory condition, showed a specific GM functional dysbiosis accompanied by a decreased production of SCFAs (Consolandi et al., 2015). Although the CAZyme profile has not yet been explored in patients with this disease, we can speculate that the observed reduction in SCFA biosynthesis could be the result of a maladaptive transition to CT1 or CT3, which would diminish the GM potential to provide the host with essential metabolites, such as butyrate, crucial to support immunological health.

CONCLUSION

Our findings highlighted the existence of specific and well-defined GM functional layouts (CAZyTypes, CTs) for what concerns the ecosystem capacity to metabolize MACs, and support the hypothesis that the human GM has the ability to reconfigure its own CAZyme functional layout in response to dietary changes, with possible implications for the host health and metabolic regulation.

AUTHOR CONTRIBUTIONS

SR and MS: conceived, designed and performed the analysis; SR, MS, MC, and ST: wrote the manuscript; EB, SQ, and PB: revised and edited the draft. All authors discussed the results, commented on the manuscript and approved the final version.

SUPPLEMENTARY MATERIAL

TABLE S1 | Prevalence data and average abundance of the identified 98 bacterial species in the dataset.

REFERENCES

Bhattacharya, T., Ghosh, T. S., and Mande, S. S. (2015). Global profiling of carbohydrate active enzymes in human gut microbiome. *PLOS ONE* 10:e0142038. doi: 10.1371/journal.pone.0142038

Candela, M., Biagi, E., Soverini, M., Consolandi, C., Quercia, S., Severgnini, M., et al. (2016). Modulation of gut microbiota dysbioses in type 2 diabetic patients by macrobiotic Ma-Pi 2 diet. *Br. J. Nutr.* 116, 80–93. doi: 10.1017/S0007114516001045

Caporaso, J. G., Kuczynski, J., Stombaugh, J., Bittinger, K., Bushman, F. D., Costello, E. K., et al. (2010). QIIME allows analysis of high-throughput community sequencing data. *Nat. Methods* 7, 335–336. doi: 10.1038/nmeth.f.303

Consolandi, C., Turroni, S., Emmi, G., Severgnini, M., Fiori, J., Peano, C., et al. (2015). Behçet's syndrome patients exhibit specific microbiome signature. *Autoimmun. Rev.* 14, 269–276. doi: 10.1016/j.autrev.2014.11.009

El Kaoutari, A., Armougom, F., Gordon, J. I., Raoult, D., and Henrissat, B. (2013). The abundance and variety of carbohydrate-active enzymes in the human gut microbiota. *Nat. Rev. Microbiol.* 11, 497–504. doi: 10.1038/nrmicro3050

Gill, S. R., Pop, M., Deboy, R. T., Eckburg, P. B., Turnbaugh, P. J., Samuel, B. S., et al. (2006). Metagenomic analysis of the human distal gut microbiome. *Science* 312, 1355–1359. doi: 10.1126/science.1124234

Honda, K., and Littman, D. R. (2016). The microbiota in adaptive immune homeostasis and disease. *Nature* 535, 75–84. doi: 10.1038/nature18848

Hooper, L. V., Littman, D. R., and Macpherson, A. J. (2012). Interactions between the microbiota and the immune system. *Science* 336, 1268–1273. doi: 10.1126/science.1223490

King, D. E., Mainous, A. G., and Lambourne, C. A. (2012). Trends in dietary fiber intake in the United States, 1999–2008. *J. Acad. Nutr. Diet.* 112, 642–648. doi: 10.1016/j.jand.2012.01.019

Koh, A., De Vadder, F., Kovatcheva-Datchary, P., and Bäckhed, F. (2016). From dietary fiber to host physiology: short-chain fatty acids as key bacterial metabolites. *Cell* 165, 1332–1345. doi: 10.1016/j.cell.2016.05.041

Lattimer, M. J., and Haub, M. D. (2010). Effects of dietary fiber and its components on metabolic health nutrients. *Nutrients* 2, 1266–1289. doi: 10.3390/nu2121266

Neish, A. S. (2009). Microbes in gastrointestinal health and disease. *Gastroenterology* 136, 65–80. doi: 10.1053/j.gastro.2008.10.080

Nicholson, J. K., Holmes, E., Kinross, J., Burcelin, R., Gibson, G., Jia, W., et al. (2012). Host-gut microbiota metabolic interactions. *Science* 336, 1262–1267. doi: 10.1126/science.1223813

Obregon-Tito, A. J., Tito, R. Y., Metcalf, J., Sankaranarayanan, K., Clemente, J. C., Ursell, L. K., et al. (2015). Subsistence strategies in traditional societies distinguish gut microbiomes. *Nat. Commun.* 25:6505. doi: 10.1038/ncomms7505

Quercia, S., Candela, M., Giuliani, C., Turroni, S., Luiselli, D., Rampelli, S., et al. (2014). From lifetime to evolution: timescales of human gut microbiota adaptation. *Front. Microbiol.* 5:587. doi: 10.3389/fmicb.2014.00587

Rampelli, S., Schnorr, S. L., Consolandi, C., Turroni, S., Severgnini, M., Peano, C., et al. (2015). Metagenome sequencing of the Hadza hunter-gatherer gut microbiota. *Curr. Biol.* 25, 1682–1693. doi: 10.1016/j.cub.2015.04.055

Rho, M., Tang, H., and Ye, Y. (2010). FragGeneScan: predicting genes in short and error-prone reads. *Nucleic Acids Res.* 38:e191. doi: 10.1093/nar/gkq747

Robert, D., Finn, J. C., and Sean, R. E. (2011). HMMER web server: interactive sequence similarity searching. *Nucleic Acids Res.* 39, W29–W37. doi: 10.1093/nar/gkr367

Schnorr, S. L., Candela, M., Rampelli, S., Centanni, M., Consolandi, C., Basaglia, G., et al. (2014). Gut microbiome of the Hadza hunter-gatherers. *Nat. Commun.* 15:3654. doi: 10.1038/ncomms4654

Sharon, G., Sampson, T. R., Geschwind, D. H., and Mazmanian, S. K. (2016). The central nervous system and the gut microbiome. *Cell* 167, 915–932. doi: 10.1016/j.cell.2016.10.027

Sonnenburg, E. D., Smits, S. A., Tikhonov, M., Higginbottom, S. K., Wingreen, N. S., and Sonnenburg, J. L. (2016). Diet-induced extinctions in the gut microbiota compound over generations. *Nature* 14, 212–215. doi: 10.1038/nature16504

Sonnenburg, E. D., and Sonnenburg, J. L. (2014). Starving our microbial self: the deleterious consequences of a diet deficient in microbiota-accessible carbohydrates. *Cell Metab.* 20, 779–786. doi: 10.1016/j.cmet.2014.07.003

Soverini, M., Rampelli, S., Turroni, S., Schnorr, S. L., Quercia, S., Castagnetti, A., et al. (2016). Variations in the post-weaning human gut metagenome profile as result of *Bifidobacterium* acquisition in the western microbiome. *Front. Microbiol.* 12:1058. doi: 10.3389/fmicb.2016.01058

Yin, Y., Mao, X., Yang, J. C., Chen, X., Mao, F., and Xu, Y. (2012). dbCAN: a web resource for automated carbohydrate-active enzyme annotation. *Nucleic Acids Res.* 40, 445–451. doi: 10.1093/nar/gks479

Zhang, J., Guo, Z., Xue, Z., Sun, Z., Zhang, M., Wang, L., et al. (2015). A phylo-functional core of gut microbiota in healthy young Chinese cohorts across lifestyles, geography, and ethnicities. *ISME J.* 9, 1979–1990. doi: 10.1038/ismej.2015.11

9

Role of the Human Breast Milk-Associated Microbiota on the Newborns' Immune System

Marco Toscano*[1]*, Roberta De Grandi*[1]*, Enzo Grossi*[2] *and Lorenzo Drago*[1,3]**

[1] Laboratory of Clinical Microbiology, Department of Biomedical Sciences for Health, University of Milan, Milan, Italy,
[2] Villa Santa Maria Institute, Como, Italy, [3] Clinical-Chemistry and Microbiology Lab, IRCCS Galeazzi Orthopedic Institute, University of Milan, Milan, Italy

***Correspondence:**
Lorenzo Drago
lorenzo.drago@unimi.it

The human milk is fundamental for a correct development of newborns, as it is a source not only of vitamins and nutrients, but also of commensal bacteria. The microbiota associated to the human breast milk contributes to create the "initial" intestinal microbiota of infants, having also a pivotal role in modulating and influencing the newborns' immune system. Indeed, the transient gut microbiota is responsible for the initial change from an intrauterine Th2 prevailing response to a Th1/Th2 balanced one. Bacteria located in both colostrum and mature milk can stimulate the anti-inflammatory response, by stimulating the production of specific cytokines, reducing the risk of developing a broad range of inflammatory diseases and preventing the expression of immune-mediated pathologies, such as asthma and atopic dermatitis. The aim of the present Mini Review is to elucidate the specific immunologic role of the human milk-associated microbiota and its impact on the newborn's health and life, highlighting the importance to properly study the biological interactions in a bacterial population and between the microbiota and the host. The Auto Contractive Map, for instance, is a promising analytical methodology based on artificial neural network that can elucidate the specific role of bacteria contained in the breast milk in modulating the infants' immunological response.

Keywords: human milk, milk microbiota, colostrum, immunomodulation, newborn's immune system, AutoCM

INTRODUCTION

The human milk is a rich and complete nourishment that is essential for the correct development of the infant's organism (Ballard and Morrow, 2013).

The first milk produced by mothers after the delivery is called colostrum and it is biochemically and functionally different from the mature milk (Castellote et al., 2011). Colostrum, indeed, contains high concentration of lactoferrin, Immunoglobulin A (IgA), leukocytes and specific developmental factors, and a low amount of lactose, potassium and calcium, underlying its immunological functions rather than nutritional (Kulski and Hartmann, 1981; Pang and Hartmann, 2007).

From 5 days to 2 weeks postpartum, there is the production of transitional milk which shares some characteristics of colostrum, although its main function is to support newborns at nutritional level (Henderson et al., 2008; Nommsen-Rivers et al., 2012).

Finally, 2 weeks after the delivery the milk can be considered as mature and its composition tends to be stable over the time, even if slight variations can occur during lactation (Ballard and Morrow, 2013). The main components of human milk are: (i) macronutrients, such as protein, fat and lactose, which concentration depends on the stage of lactation and maternal characteristics; (ii) micronutrients, including vitamins A, B1, B2, B12 and D that vary in human milk in relation to maternal diet and body stores; (iii) growth factor, which are strongly active on the endocrine system, nervous system, vasculature and intestinal tract; (iv) immunological factors, which are essential to defend the newborn from inflammation and infection, and for this reason, the early milk is rich in immune components that can support infants in the first delicate stages of their life; (v) the microbiota, which comprises more than 200 different bacterial species with a pivotal role in the formation of the newborn's first gut microbiota (Drago et al., 2017).

The aim of the present Mini Review is to highlight the specific and fundamental role of human milk-associated bacteria in modulating and influencing the newborns' immune system during their life.

THE MILK MICROBIOTA AND THE NEWBORN'S IMMUNE SYSTEM

The specific mechanisms that lead to the formation of the human milk microbiota are still unknown; however, there are different hypothesis that can explain the origin of milk-associated bacteria. Indeed, some microorganisms belonging to the maternal skin or infant's oral cavity may become an integral component of the milk microbiota by means of a milk flow back into mammary ducts during lactation (Rodríguez, 2014). This mechanism may justify the presence of cutaneous and oral bacteria that are recovered in the milk microbiota, such as *Streptococcus* spp. and *Staphylococcus* spp. (Gao et al., 2007; Grice et al., 2009). Interestingly, human milk contained also a great number of intestinal bacteria, which may spread from the maternal intestinal environment by a mechanism involving dendritic cells (DCs) and CD18$^+$ cells (Rodríguez, 2014); these cellular types would be able to capture intestinal microorganisms from the gut lumen and transfer them to lactating mammary glands by means of translocation, which results to be increased during late pregnancy and lactation (Rodríguez, 2014). Consequently, the milk microbiota can shape the initial intestinal microbiome of newborns, together with the maternal intestinal and vaginal microorganisms that are ingested by the neonate during the passage through the birth canal (Houghteling and Walker, 2015). Human milk can stimulate the proliferation of numerous *Bifidobacterium* and *Lactobacillus* strains, the main probiotic microorganisms present in the gut, creating an acidic environmental rich in short chain fatty acids (SCFAs) with a protective and nutritive role at intestinal level (Bode, 2012; Walker and Iyengar, 2015). The constant intake, during lactation, of bacteria contained in the human milk leads to the formation of a transient intestinal microbiota that deeply impacts on the newborn's development, acting mainly on the maturation of his immune system (Houghteling and Walker, 2015). Indeed, several studies underscored the strict link between the gut microbiota signals, the mucosal host defense and the maturation of immune system, both at intestinal and systemic level (Smith et al., 2007; Sekirov et al., 2008; Walker and Iyengar, 2015). It has been showed that an altered colonization of newborns' gut may lead to a persistent intestinal dysbiosis and, consequently, to immune-mediated and metabolic diseases during infancy and childhood (Gareau et al., 2010; Johnson and Versalovic, 2012). Moreover, breast-fed newborns have shown to possess a more stable intestinal bacterial population and a well-balanced mucosal immune response if compared to the formula-fed ones (Gronlund et al., 2000; Bezirtzoglou et al., 2011); indeed, a healthy intestinal microbiota can induce specific T cell responses and modulate substrates oxidation, decreasing the impact of autoimmune and allergic diseases not only during childhood but also in adulthood (Guaraldi and Salvatori, 2012; Palma et al., 2012). Finally, breastfeeding has been observed to have a protective role against respiratory and gastrointestinal infections between the ages of 7 and 12 months, leading to a general improvement of symptoms associated to gastrointestinal infections (Duijts et al., 2010).

Intestinal bacteria can also stimulate lymphoid elements and positively influence the maturation of both innate and adaptive immune system, as clearly demonstrated by studying germ-free animals (Cash and Hooper, 2005). It has been shown that in germ-free mice the villus capillaries develop poorly during weaning and remained in this condition also during adulthood, suggesting that the intestinal microbiota is fundamental for intestinal blood vessel to be completely developed (Martin et al., 2010). More interestingly, intestinal bacteria can promote B cell development in Peyer's Patches and increase the production of mucosal IgA, the main antibody class in secretions that acts as first line of defense (Martin et al., 2010).

Moreover, bacterial surface-expressed or secreted ligands can interact with specific receptors on mucosal immune system and enterocytes leading to a self-limited inflammatory response for preventing pathogen mucosal penetration (Round and Mazmanian, 2009; Walker and Iyengar, 2015).

As underlined by Latuga et al. (2014), all newborns have an immature immune system and the cord blood rich in anti-inflammatory T regulatory cells; furthermore, infants have a high T helper 2 (Th2) that promotes humoral immunity with the production of IL4, IL6 and IL21, thus promoting an increased B cell response and, potentially, a higher allergic sensitization (Latuga et al., 2014). The pivotal role of milk-associated microbiota in influencing the neonates' immune system is over-emphasized by the cytotoxic function promoted by microbial ligands in breast milk (Donnet-Hughes, 2008). Indeed, *in vitro* stimulation of DCs with lipopolysaccharide can lead to T-cells differentiation, supporting the hypothesis that mature milk may implement the maturation of cytotoxic Th1 cells and improve their activity against infections (M'Rabet et al., 2008). Probably, commensal colonic

TABLE 1 | Immunomodulatory activities of the human milk microbiota.

Immunological activity	Reference
Maturation of local and systemic immune system	Houghteling and Walker, 2015
Implementation of mucosal newborns' defense	Smith et al., 2007; Sekirov et al., 2008
Stimulation of specific cytokines that create a balanced microenvironment	Walker and Iyengar, 2015
Correct development of B cells	Martin et al., 2010
Stimulation of cytotoxic Th1 cells	M'Rabet et al., 2008
Correct balancing between Th1 and Th2 response	Walker and Iyengar, 2015
Development of oral tolerance	Verhasselt, 2010
Stimulation of Peyer's patches	Gross, 2007

bacteria may stimulate the release of specific cytokines that create a balanced microenvironment suitable for naive Th0 cells to ripen toward Th1 cell type (Walker and Iyengar, 2015).

Bacteroides is a bacterial genus that is very abundant in human colostrum and it may have a main role in the early stages of newborns' gut colonization, as reported by Mazmanian and Kasper (2006). In particular, the polysaccharide A located on the surface of *Bacteroides fragilis* can interact with Toll receptor 2 on intestinal DCs to stimulate cytokine production which, in turn, favor the proliferation of FOXP3 T cells in the lamina propria. FOXP3 belongs to the forhead transcription factor family bindweed in the expansion of regulatory T cells, thus having a suppressive role in the host's immune system (Kim, 2009). Therefore, it is clear that a correct stimulation of neonates' intestinal environment is fundamental for the physiological development of mucosal immune system and tolerance; the latter, in particular, is extremely important to avoid developing allergy or autoimmune diseases (Walker and Iyengar, 2015). Indeed, germ-free animals cannot develop tolerance due to the lack of intestinal bacteria and only the adequate colonization of newborns' gut can lead to a complete tolerance generation (Karlsson et al., 1999; Olszak et al., 2012).

Consequently, breastfeeding is essential for oral tolerance in newborns, as it is extremely important for the establishment of local and systemic immune tolerance to antigens ingested during lactation (Verhasselt, 2010). Infants are daily exposed to specific antigens, part of which belong directly to the human milk microbiota, and that can translocate across the intestinal barrier, being involved in the presentation by antigen-presenting cells to T lymphocytes. Furthermore, bacteria located in the human milk are fundamental to correctly stimulate the Peyer's patches, increasing the number of IgA-producing plasma cells in the intestinal environment of newborns (Gross, 2007). Consequently, IgA can trap food antigens favoring their

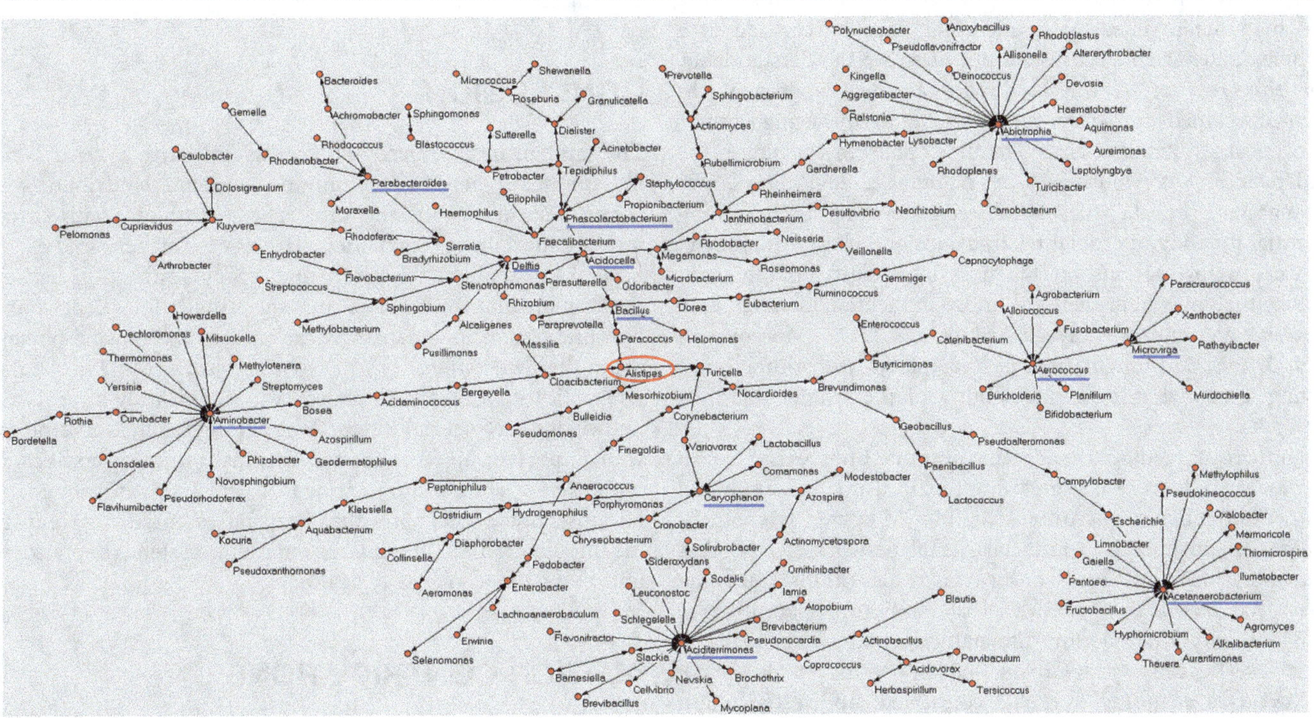

FIGURE 1 | Microbiota network of Italian mature milk. The figure shows the distribution of bacterial population contained in the Italian human mature milk. The network was obtained applying the AutoCM. The main *hubs* of the bacterial network are underlined with a blue line; red circle shows the *central node* of the network (Drago et al., 2017). As authors of the previously published manuscript, we maintain the ownership of copyright as stated in the license-to-publish we signed for the Nature Publishing Group.

elimination by specific enzymes, avoid the adherence of viruses and microorganisms to intestinal mucosa also counteracting the proliferation of pathogens and exert a direct immunomodulatory activity (Verhasselt, 2010).

Finally, the oral tolerance seems to be actively involved in the prevention of allergic diseases onset in babies, avoiding also the impact of respiratory and gastrointestinal infections during the early stages of their life (Lack, 2008).

Interestingly, some strains contained in the breast milk can stimulate immune responses in both animal and human models and their activity seems to have a moderate suppleness based on the gut environment (Fernández et al., 2013). Some *Lactobacillus* strains can enhance the production of Th1 cytokines as well as TNF-alpha even without inflammatory stimuli and activate NK cells, CD4+ and CD8+ T cells and regulatory T cells.

Table 1 summarizes the main immunomodulatory activities of human milk microbiota.

MICROBIAL NETWORK: NEW INSIGHTS INTO BACTERIAL ECOLOGY

The study of microbial interactions within a bacterial population is of extreme importance to clearly understand the specific role of microbiome. Indeed, microorganisms compete for nutrients, exchange genetic material and metabolites, being responsible of influencing the microbiota composition and the host's health (Layeghifard et al., 2017). Due to its dynamic nature and high heterogeneity, the microbiota can be considered a complex and variable ecosystem not often well understandable. For this reason, in the last years a novel approach has been developed to study the microbiota, by using graph-theoretical, systems-oriented method able to facilitate the understanding of evolutionary and complex ecological processes (Layeghifard et al., 2017). Bacterial network is becoming essential to study microbial relationships and clarify the impact of various interactions on the host by identifying the main "hubs" that may represent the most influential member in a bacterial community (Layeghifard et al., 2017). Moreover, a central node is thought to have more links with other hubs, having a pivotal role in the stability of the whole microbial network.

Numerous methods to identify network hubs exist, but in the last years there was a great interest in using and apply the Auto-Contractive map (AutoCM). AutoCM system is a fourth-generation unsupervised artificial neural network (ANN) that can outperform numerous unsupervised algorithms (Buscema and Sacco, 2016). The system uses the minimum spanning tree (MST) theory to underline the natural connections between variables (Buscema and Grossi, 2008; Buscema et al., 2008). A MST is a spanning tree of a connected, undirected graph that links all vertices together with the minimal total pondering for its edges. The concept is that as all biological and natural systems are inclined to a minimal energetic condition, the graph delineates the essential biological information of this process. The final goal of this approach is finding out all specific correlations between variables, creating a semantic map of connections in which non-linear associations are maintained. This approach allows to both highlight the relevant nodes of the system and show the network of the main relations among variables. Nodes, also defined as "hubs," are defined as variables with the highest number of relations in the map (Buscema and Grossi, 2008; Buscema et al., 2008; Buscema and Sacco, 2016).

AutoCM has already been used in the microbiological field to study the bacterial network of human colostrum and mature milk in Italian and Burundian populations, highlighting the main microbial hubs that represent the biological leading structure of the whole network (Drago et al., 2017). This mathematical approach could partially clarify the complexity of human-bacteria mutualism, and above all the role that some specific microorganisms have in the human milk.

Figure 1 shows a graphical representation of the human mature milk microbiota network obtained using AutoCM. The main bacterial hubs (blue lines) represent those microorganisms that may have a pivotal and leader role in the whole microbiota (Drago et al., 2017).

In the future, the AutoCM may be useful in understanding which microbe is directly involved in the stimulation and manipulation of newborns' immune system, maybe defining a "immunomodulatory bacterial pattern" with a pivotal role in the development of infant's immunity.

CONCLUSION

The human milk microbiota seems to have a central role in stimulate newborns' immune system, contributing to create the first transient intestinal microbiota with strong immunomodulatory activities. However, further studies are needed to highlight the direct and strong connection between the human milk microbiota and the stimulation of newborns' immune system, as to date there are no clear and specific evidence about this association.

Application of network biology will significantly improve our knowledge on bacterial interactions among the milk microbiota, with important applications for eventual targeted modification of bacterial composition, aimed to enhance the abundance of those microorganisms that may be essential not only for the modulation of the infants' immune system, but also for improving the whole host's health.

AUTHOR CONTRIBUTIONS

LD provided the general concept. LD and EG drafted part of the manuscript. MT and RDG wrote the manuscript. All authors revised and approved the manuscript.

REFERENCES

Ballard, O., and Morrow, A. L. (2013). Human milk composition: nutrients and bioactive factors. *Pediatr. Clin. North Am.* 60, 49–74. doi: 10.1016/j.pcl.2012.10.002

Bezirtzoglou, E., Tsiotsias, A., and Welling, G. W. (2011). Microbiota profile in feces of breast- and formula-fed newborns by using florescence in situ hybridization (FISH). *Anaerobe* 17, 478–482. doi: 10.1016/j.anaerobe.2011.03.009

Bode, L. (2012). Human milk oligosaccharides: every baby needs a sugar mama. *Glycobiology* 22, 1147–1162. doi: 10.1093/glycob/cws074

Buscema, M., and Grossi, E. (2008). The semantic connectivity map: an adapting self-organising knowledge discovery method in data bases. Experience in gastro-oesophageal reflux disease. *Int. J. Data Min. Bioinform.* 2, 362–404.

Buscema, M., Grossi, E., Snowdon, D., and Antuono, P. (2008). Auto-contractive maps: an artificial adaptive system for data mining. An application to Alzheimer disease. *Curr. Alzheimer Res.* 5, 481–498.

Buscema, M. B. M., and Sacco, P. L. (2016). MST Fitness Index and implicit data narratives: a comparative test on alternative unsupervised algorithms. *Phys. A* 461, 726–746.

Cash, H. L., and Hooper, L. V. (2005). Commensal bacteria shape intestinal immune system development. *ASM News* 71, 77–83.

Castellote, C., Casillas, R., Ramírez-Santana, C., Pérez-Cano, F. J., Castell, M., Moretones, M. G., et al. (2011). Premature delivery influences the immunological composition of colostrum and transitional and mature human milk. *J. Nutr.* 141, 1181–1187. doi: 10.3945/jn.110.133652

Donnet-Hughes, A. (2008). "Protective properties of human milk," in *Nutrition in Pediatrics*, 4th Edn, ed. D. Duggan (Toronto, ON: Decker Publishing), 355–362.

Drago, L., Toscano, M., De Grandi, R., Grossi, E., Padovani, E. M., and Peroni, D. G. (2017). Microbiota network and mathematic microbe mutualism in colostrum and mature milk collected in two different geographic areas: Italy versus Burundi. *ISME J.* 11, 875–884. doi: 10.1038/ismej.2016.183

Duijts, L., Jaddoe, V. W., Hofman, A., and Moll, H. A. (2010). Prolonged and exclusive breastfeeding reduces the risk of infectious diseases in infancy. *Pediatrics* 126, e18–e25. doi: 10.1542/peds.2008-3256

Fernández, L., Langa, S., Martín, V., Maldonado, A., Jiménez, E., Martín, R., et al. (2013). The human milk microbiota: origin and potential roles in health and disease. *Pharmacol. Res.* 69, 1–10. doi: 10.1016/j.phrs.2012.09.001

Gao, Z., Tseng, C., Pei, Z., and Blaser, M. J. (2007). Molecular analysis of human forearm superficial skin bacterial biota. *Proc. Natl. Acad. Sci. U.S.A.* 104, 2927–2932.

Gareau, M. G., Sherman, P. M., and Walker, W. A. (2010). Probiotics and the gut microbiota in intestinal health and disease. *Nat. Rev. Gastroenterol. Hepatol.* 7, 503–514. doi: 10.1038/nrgastro.2010.117

Grice, E. A., Kong, H. H., Conlan, S., Deming, C. B., Davis, J., Young, A. C., et al. (2009). Topographical and temporal diversity of the human skin microbiome. *Science* 324, 1190–1192. doi: 10.1126/science.1171700

Gronlund, M. M., Arvilommi, H., Kero, P., Lehtonen, O. P., and Isolauri, E. (2000). Importance of intestinal colonisation in the maturation of humoral immunity in early infancy: a prospective follow up study of healthy infants aged 0-6 months. *Arch. Dis. Child. Fetal Neonatal Ed.* 83, F186–F192.

Gross, L. (2007). Microbes colonize a baby's gut with distinction. *PLOS Biol.* 5:e191. doi: 10.1371/journal.pbio.0050191

Guaraldi, F., and Salvatori, G. (2012). Effect of breast and formula feeding on gut microbiota shaping in newborns. *Front. Cell. Infect. Microbiol.* 2:94. doi: 10.3389/fcimb.2012.00094

Henderson, J. J., Hartmann, P. E., Newnham, J. P., and Simmer, K. (2008). Effect of preterm birth and antenatal corticosteroid treatment on lactogenesis II in women. *Pediatrics* 121, e92–e100. doi: 10.1542/peds.2007-1107

Houghteling, P. D., and Walker, W. A. (2015). Why is initial bacterial colonization of the intestine important to infants' and children's health? *J. Pediatr. Gastroenterol. Nutr.* 60, 294–307. doi: 10.1097/MPG.0000000000000597

Johnson, C. L., and Versalovic, J. (2012). The human microbiome and its potential importance to pediatrics. *Pediatrics* 129, 950–960. doi: 10.1542/peds.2011-2736

Karlsson, M. R., Kahu, H., Hanson, L. A., Telemo, E., and Dahlgren, U. I. (1999). Neonatal colonization of rats induces immunological tolerance to bacterial antigens. *Eur. J. Immunol.* 29, 109–118.

Kim, C. H. (2009). FOXP3 and its role in the immune system. *Adv. Exp. Med. Biol.* 665, 17–29.

Kulski, J. K., and Hartmann, P. E. (1981). Changes in human milk composition during the initiation of lactation. *Aust. J. Exp. Biol. Med. Sci.* 59, 101–114.

Lack, G. (2008). Epidemiologic risks for food allergy. *J. Allergy Clin. Immunol.* 121, 1331–1336. doi: 10.1016/j.jaci.2008.04.032

Latuga, M. S., Stuebe, A., and Seed, P. C. (2014). A review of the source and function of microbiota in breast milk. *Semin. Reprod. Med.* 32, 68–73. doi: 10.1055/s-0033-1361824

Layeghifard, M., Hwang, D. M., and Guttman, D. S. (2017). Disentangling interactions in the microbiome: a network perspective. *Trends Microbiol.* 25, 217–228. doi: 10.1016/j.tim.2016.11.008

Martin, R., Nauta, A. J., Ben Amor, K., Knippels, L. M., Knol, J., and Garssen, J. (2010). Early life: gut microbiota and immune development in infancy. *Benef. Microbes* 1, 367–382. doi: 10.3920/BM2010.0027

Mazmanian, S. K., and Kasper, D. L. (2006). The love–hate relationship between bacterial polysaccharides and the host immune system. *Nat. Rev. Immunol.* 6, 849–858. doi: 10.1038/nri1956

M'Rabet, L., Vos, A. P., Boehm, G., and Garssen, J. (2008). Breast-feeding and its role in early development of the immune system in infants: consequences for health later in life. *J. Nutr.* 138, 1782S–1790S.

Nommsen-Rivers, L. A., Dolan, L. M., and Huang, B. (2012). Timing of stage II lactogenesis is predicted by antenatal metabolic health in a cohort of primiparas. *Breastfeed. Med.* 7, 43–49. doi: 10.1089/bfm.2011.0007

Olszak, T., An, D., Zeissig, S., Vera, M. P., Richter, J., Franke, A., et al. (2012). Microbial exposure during early life has persistent effects on natural killer T cell function. *Science* 336, 489–493. doi: 10.1126/science.1219328

Palma, G. D., Capilla, A., Nova, E., Castillejo, G., Varea, V., Pozo, T., et al. (2012). Influence of milk-feeding type and genetic risk of developing coeliac disease on intestinal microbiota of infants: the PROFICEL study. *PLOS ONE* 7:e30791. doi: 10.1371/journal.pone.0030791

Pang, W. W., and Hartmann, P. E. (2007). Initiation of human lactation: secretory differentiation and secretory activation. *J. Mammary Gland Biol. Neoplasia* 12, 211–221. doi: 10.1007/s10911-007-9054-4

Rodríguez, J. M. (2014). The origin of human milk bacteria: is there a bacterial entero-mammary pathway during late pregnancy and lactation? *Adv. Nutr.* 5, 779–784. doi: 10.3945/an.114.007229

Round, J. L., and Mazmanian, S. K. (2009). The gut microbiota shapes intestinal responses during health and disease. *Nat. Rev. Immunol.* 9, 313–323. doi: 10.1038/nri2515

Sekirov, I., Tam, N. M., Jogova, M., Robertson, M. L., Li, Y., Lupp, C., et al. (2008). Antibiotic-induced perturbations of the intestinal microbiota alter host susceptibility to enteric infection. *Infect. Immun.* 76, 4726–4736. doi: 10.1128/IAI.00319-08

Smith, K., McCoy, K. D., and Macpherson, A. J. (2007). Use of axenic animals in studying the adaptation of mammals to their commensal intestinal microbiota. *Semin. Immunol.* 19, 59–69. doi: 10.1016/j.smim.2006.10.002

Verhasselt, V. (2010). Oral tolerance in neonates: from basics to potential prevention of allergic disease. *Mucosal Immunol.* 3, 326–333. doi: 10.1038/mi.2010.25

Walker, W. A., and Iyengar, R. S. (2015). Breast milk, microbiota, and intestinal immune homeostasis. *Pediatr. Res.* 77, 220–228. doi: 10.1038/pr.2014

10

The Infectious Basis of ACPA-Positive Rheumatoid Arthritis

Lazaros I. Sakkas[1], Dimitrios Daoussis[2], Stamatis-Nick Liossis[2] and Dimitrios P. Bogdanos[1]**

[1] Department of Rheumatology and Clinical Immunology, Faculty of Medicine, School of Health Sciences, University of Thessaly, Larissa, Greece, [2] Division of Rheumatology, Department of Internal Medicine, Faculty of Medicine, University of Patras, Patras, Greece

***Correspondence:**
Lazaros I. Sakkas
lsakkas@med.uth.gr

Rheumatoid arthritis (RA) is associated with HLA-DRB1 shared epitope (HLA-DRB1SE) and anti-citrullinated protein autoantibodies (ACPAs). ACPAs precedes the onset of clinical and subclinical RA. There are strong data for three infectious agents as autoimmunity triggers in RA, namely *Porphyromonas gingivalis* and *Aggregatibacter actinomycetemcomitans* causes of periodontal disease (PD), and Epstein-Barr virus (EBV). *P. gingivalis* expresses arginine gingipains, that cleave proteins at the arginine residues, and peptidyl arginine deiminase (PPAD), which citrullinates arginine residues of proteins, thus forming neoantigens that lead to ACPA production. Peripheral blood plasmablasts from ACPA+RA patients produce ACPAs the majority of which react against *P. gingivalis*. *A. actinocycetemcomitans* produces leukotoxin A, a toxin that forms pores in the neutrophil membranes and leads to citrullination and release of citrullinated autoantigens in the gums. EBV can infect B cells and epithelial cells and resides as latent infection in resting B cells. Abs against citrullinated peptides derived from EBV nuclear antigen appear years before RA and cross-react with human citrullinated fibrin. Citrullinated proteins are potential arthritogenic autoantigens in RA. The conversion of arginine to citrulline increases the peptide binding affinity to HLA-DRB1SE. Also, citrullinated fibrinogen induces arthritis in HLA-DRB1*0401 transgenic mice, and transfer of their splenic T cells causes arthritis to recipient mice.

Keywords: anti-citrullinated protein antibodies, arthritis, Ebstein-Barr virus, HLA-DRB1 shared epitope, *Porphyromonas gingivalis*

INTRODUCTION

Rheumatoid arthritis (RA) is a systemic inflammatory disease mainly manifested with peripheral polyarthritis. The aetiopathogenesis of the disease is incompletely understood. Risk factors for RA include HLA-DR genes, periodontal disease (PD), and smoking (Bartold et al., 2005; Scher et al., 2012; Mikuls et al., 2014; Kharlamova et al., 2016). The early HLA-DR4 association of RA classified RA by many investigators as an immune-mediated disease and suggested that T cells recognized an antigen presented on HLA-DR4 molecules. The discovery of HLA-DRB1 shared epitope (SE, HLA-DRB1SE), a hypervariable DRβ chain sequence shared by all alleles associated with RA, reinforced this concept (Gregersen et al., 1987; Wordsworth et al., 1989). The discovery of autoantibodies against citrullinated antigens (ACPAs) greatly advanced our understanding of the pathogenetic mechanisms in this disease. ACPAs appear years before clinical onset of RA (Nielen et al., 2004), predict subsequent development of the disease, occur in 50–67% of RA patients, are associated with severe disease, and are highly specific for the disease (van Gaalen et al., 2004; van der Helm-van Mil et al., 2005; Alexiou et al., 2007; Barouta et al., 2017; Hensvold et al., 2017).

Citrullination is a post-translational modification of proteins in which arginine residues are converted to citrulline by the action of enzyme peptidylarginine deiminase (PAD). There are five PAD isoforms (PAD1-4, PAD6), and PAD2 and PAD4 have been implicated in RA. The production of ACPAs means break of tolerance. Tolerance is no immune response to unmodified self. Many proteins are extensively post-translationally modified that including citrullination. In this context, citrullination is a physiological process in many tissues and only in specific circumstances this leads to immune response. Thus, citrullination could create particular neoantigens that would activate T cells, which in turn will provide antigen-specific help to B cells to produce ACPA. Indeed, citrullination increases the affinity of citrullinated antigen to HLA-DRB1SE allele (Hill et al., 2003; Scally et al., 2013). ACPAs in RA recognize many citrullinated autoantigens (**Table 1**) and are associated with HLA-DRB1SE (Snir et al., 2009), and HLA-DRB1SE appears to be a risk factor for ACPA production in RA rather than an independent risk factor for RA development (van der Helm-van Mil et al., 2006). These findings and the fact that ACPAs are of IgG and IgA class suggest that T cells provide help to B cells for the subsequent ACPA production.

Although smoking is a risk factor for RA (van der Helm-van Mil et al., 2007; Lundberg et al., 2013; Hensvold et al., 2015), and increases citrullination in bronchial tissues (Makrygiannakis et al., 2008), other environmental factors, in addition to smoking, appear to play a predominant role in the development of ACPA+RA (Lee et al., 2007; Hensvold et al., 2015) and infections are likely candidates (Bogdanos and Sakkas, 2017).

INFECTIONS AS GENERATORS OF ACPA IN RA

ACPAs precede the subclinical joint inflammation in pre-RA patients (van de Sande et al., 2011) and can be detected in joints and epithelial sites, such as periodontium in PD (Nesse et al., 2012) and bronchial tissues in early RA (Reynisdottir et al., 2014). Identical citrullinated peptides were found in pulmonary bronchial tissue and synovial membrane and were found to be targets of ACPAs in RA thus providing a link between lungs and joints in ACPA+RA (Ytterberg et al., 2015). A monoclonal ACPA derived from RA patients cross-reacted with many viral, bacterial fungal and plant proteins (Tsuda et al., 2015). The most widely studied infection has been with *P. gingivalis* and Ebstein-Barr virus. The mechanisms by which these infectious agents could trigger RA are illustrated in **Figure 1**.

Porphyromonas Gingivalis

Chronic PD is very common affecting nearly 30% of adult population (Brown and Loe, 1993) and is caused by various microbes including *Porphyromonas gingivalis* (*P. gingivalis*).

P. gingivalis infection, detected by abs against *P. gingivalis* components, have been associated with ACPA in HLA-DRB1SE+RA patients. Anti-*P. gingivalis* abs, detected as abs against RgpB, potent virulent factors of *P. gingivalis* (Haffajee and Socransky, 1994; Kadowaki et al., 1998), showed stronger association with ACPA+RA (Kharlamova et al., 2016). Furthermore, there was additive interaction between these two factors. Anti-RgpB abs also showed more than additive interaction with HLA-DRB1SE in ACPA+RA (Kharlamova et al., 2016). Using anti-*P. gingivalis* lipopolysaccharide abs, one study reported association of anti-*P. gingivalis* abs with ACPA in HLA-DRB1SE+ RA patients and their relatives (Hitchon et al., 2010) whereas another study did not find an association with RA or ACPA status (Seror et al., 2015).

P. gingivalis has two unique enzymes, peptidylarginine deiminase (PPAD) and arginine ginpains (Rgps) which are expressed on the bacterial outer membrane and can also be secreted (Potempa et al., 1995; McGraw et al., 1999). Rgps are proteases that cleave proteins at arginine residues, and PPAD citrullinates both bacterial and human proteins (Wegner et al., 2010). *P. gingivalis* PAD citrullinates carboxy-terminal arginine of human proteins following proteolytic cleavage by *P. gingivalis* arginine-gingipains (Wegner et al., 2010). Crystal structure of PPAD and the use of synthetic peptides also revealed that PPAD exhibits a definitive specificity for C-terminal arginine residue created by Rgps, whereas PAD2 and PAD4 preferentially citrullinate internal arginine residues (Goulas et al., 2015; Montgomery et al., 2016). Thus *P. gingivalis* creates neoantigens, not formed by PAD2 and PAD4 and this may explain its pathogenic potential.

It is reasonable to assume that neoantigens, created by Rpgs in conjunction with PPAD in the periodontium of PD, can lead to loss of tolerance and ACPA production. In PD, increased concentrations of anti-CCP and anti-α-enolase autoAbs are detected (Lappin et al., 2013). A peptide 1 of human citrullinated α-enolase (CEP1), an immunodominant epitope, shares 92% homology with *P. gingivalis* α-enolase and cross-reacts with it (Lundberg et al., 2008). This links periodontitis with RA and suggests that periodontal infection can be the inciting agent that breaks immune tolerance in ACPA+RA, although other studies did not find association of PD with RA (Arkema et al., 2010; Eriksson et al., 2016). Using a single-cell ab cloning method, Li et al showed that peripheral blood plasmablasts in ACPA+RA patients produce ACPAs the majority of which cross-react with outer membrane antigens and/or citrullinated a-enolase from *P. gingivalis* (Li et al., 2016).

In addition, *P. gingivalis* can induce neutrophil extracellullar trap (NET) formation (Delbosc et al., 2011), another source of citrullinated autoantigens. NETs are externalized chromatin fibers containing DNA and histones, and decorated with cytoplasmic granular peptides, such as myeloperoxidase, proteinase 3, neutrophil elastase, cathepsin G, LL37, and others, in a process of programmed neutrophil death called NETosis (Yang et al., 2016). PAD4-induced citrullination is an important step in NETosis during which citrullinated histones, vimentin, α-enolase and others are externalized

TABLE 1 | Examples of citrullinated peptides which are targeted by immune responses against self and non-self immune responses in patients with rheumatoid arthritis.

Citrullinated protein/peptide	Sequence	aa	References
Fibrinogen-α chain	GPcitVVEcitHQSACKDS	36-50	Sebbag et al., 2006
Fibrinogen-α chain	VDIDIKIcitSCcitGSCS	171-185	Sebbag et al., 2006
Fibrinogen-α chain	SGIGTLDGFcitHcitHPD	501-515	Sebbag et al., 2006
Fibrinogen-α chain	citGHAKScitPVcitGIHTS	621-635	Sebbag et al., 2006
Fibrinogen-β chain	citPAPPPISGGGYcitAcit	60-74	Sebbag et al., 2006
Enolase-1	KIHAcitEIFDScitGNPTVE	5-21	Lundberg et al., 2008
Vimentin	SAVRAcitSSVPGVR	65-77	Hill et al., 2003
Vimentin	VYATcitSSAVcitLcitSSVP	60-75	Verpoort et al., 2007
Collagen II	AcitGLTGcitPGDA	359-369	Burkhardt et al., 2005
Histone 4	GAKCitHCitKVLCitDNIQGITKPAI	414-34	Corsiero et al., 2016
Histone 4	KPAICitCitLACitCitGGVKCitISGLI	431-50	Corsiero et al., 2016
P. gingivalis enolase	KIIGcitEILDScitGNPTVE	5-21	Lundberg et al., 2008
Ebstein-Barr virus EBNA1	GGDNHGCitGCitGCitGCitGCitGGGCitPGAPG	135-58	Pratesi et al., 2006
Ebstein-Barr virus EBNA2	GQSCitGQSCitGCitGCitGCitGCitGCitGKG	338-358	Pratesi et al., 2011

and recognized by ACPAs (Li et al., 2010; Pratesi et al., 2014). PAD4 is also essential for the antibacterial neutrophil immunity (Li et al., 2010). NETosis is enhanced in RA peripheral blood and synovial fluid neutrophils (Khandpur et al., 2013). A positive feedback loop between NETosis and ACPA has been proposed. ACPAs induce NETosis and NETosis provides citullinated autoantigens for ACPA production, as NET components are recognized by RA autoantibodies (Khandpur et al., 2013). Also, B cells from synovial ectopic lymphoid structures (ELS), recognize citrullinated histones of NETs. For instance, monoclonal abs generated from synovial ELS single B cell cloning from patients with ACPA+RA, recognized citrullinated histones from NETs (Corsiero et al., 2016). Neutrophils provide citrullinated autoantigens to the attention of the immune system also via immune-mediated membranolytic pathways (Romero et al., 2013), and this has led to introduction of another pathogen of PD as candidate trigger of autoimmunity in RA, namely *Aggregatibacter actinomycetemcomitans.*

Aggregatibacter Actinomycetemcomitans

Aggregatibacter actinomycetemcomitans *(A.actinomycetemcomitans)* a periodontal pathogen associated with aggressive PD (Haubek and Johansson, 2014) can cause citullination of a broad range of proteins by a completely different mechanism. *A.actinomycetemcomitans* produces leukotoxin A (LtxA), which forms pores on the cell membrane of neutrophils at the crevicular fluid of PD. This leads to neutrophil PAD activation and citrullination of a broad range of proteins, which are released from neutrophils (Konig et al., 2016a). In addition, 47% of RA patients show evidence of *A.actinimycetemcomitans* infection that is associated with ACPA presence. More interestingly, in patients with RA HLA-DRB1SE is associated with ACPA only in patients exposed to *A.actinomycetemcomitans* (Konig et al., 2016a). Thus *A.actinomycetemcomitans* is identified as a strong bacterial candidate triggering autoimmunity in RA.

Epstein-Barr Virus

Epstein-Barr virus (EBV) is a herpes virus infecting most of the adult population. EBV can infect B cells and epithelial cells and cause primary infection usually asymptomatic in childhood and then a life-long latent infection in resting memory B cells (Kalla and Hammerschmidt, 2012). High titers of anti-EBV abs are detected in RA patients (Alspaugh et al., 1981), and the EBV DNA load was found to be increased 7–10-fold in PBMCs from RA patients compared to healthy EBV carriers (Balandraud et al., 2003; Lunemann et al., 2008). Furthermore, substantial expansions of CD8+Tcells specific for EBV antigens were detected in PB (Lunemann et al., 2008) and expansions of CD8+T cells reactive against key transactivators of EBV lytic infection were also detected in RA joints (Scotet et al., 1996). Latent membrane protein (LMP) 2A through its immunoreceptor tyrosine activation motif (ITAM) phosphorylates (activates) downstream proteins of B cell receptor thus positively regulating B cell survival and activation (Swanson-Mungerson and Longnecker, 2007).

Abs against citrullinated peptide corresponding to EBV nuclear antigen (EBNA)1 (viral citrullinated peptide 1, VCP1) were detected in RA. Furthermore, affinity-purified anti-VCP1 abs reacted with citrullinated fibrinogen (Pratesi et al., 2006). More importantly, Abs against citrullinated peptides derived from EBNA2 (VCP2) along with abs against histone-4-derived citrullinated peptides appear years before the onset of clinical RA and predict subsequent development of RA (Johansson et al., 2016). These abs were associated with HLA-DRB1SE (Johansson et al., 2016). Abs against VCP1 and VCP2 cross-react with human citrullinated peptides (Pratesi et al., 2011). In particular, competition assays showed that abs to citrullinated peptide EBNA (VCP1) strongly cross-reacted with the citrullinated peptide β60-74 which bears the immunodominant epitope of citrullinated fibrin in RA (Cornillet et al., 2014, 2015). EBV latent transcripts and EBV latent and lytic proteins were detected in germinal center-like ectopic lymphoid structures (ELS) of RA synovial membrane (Croia et al.,

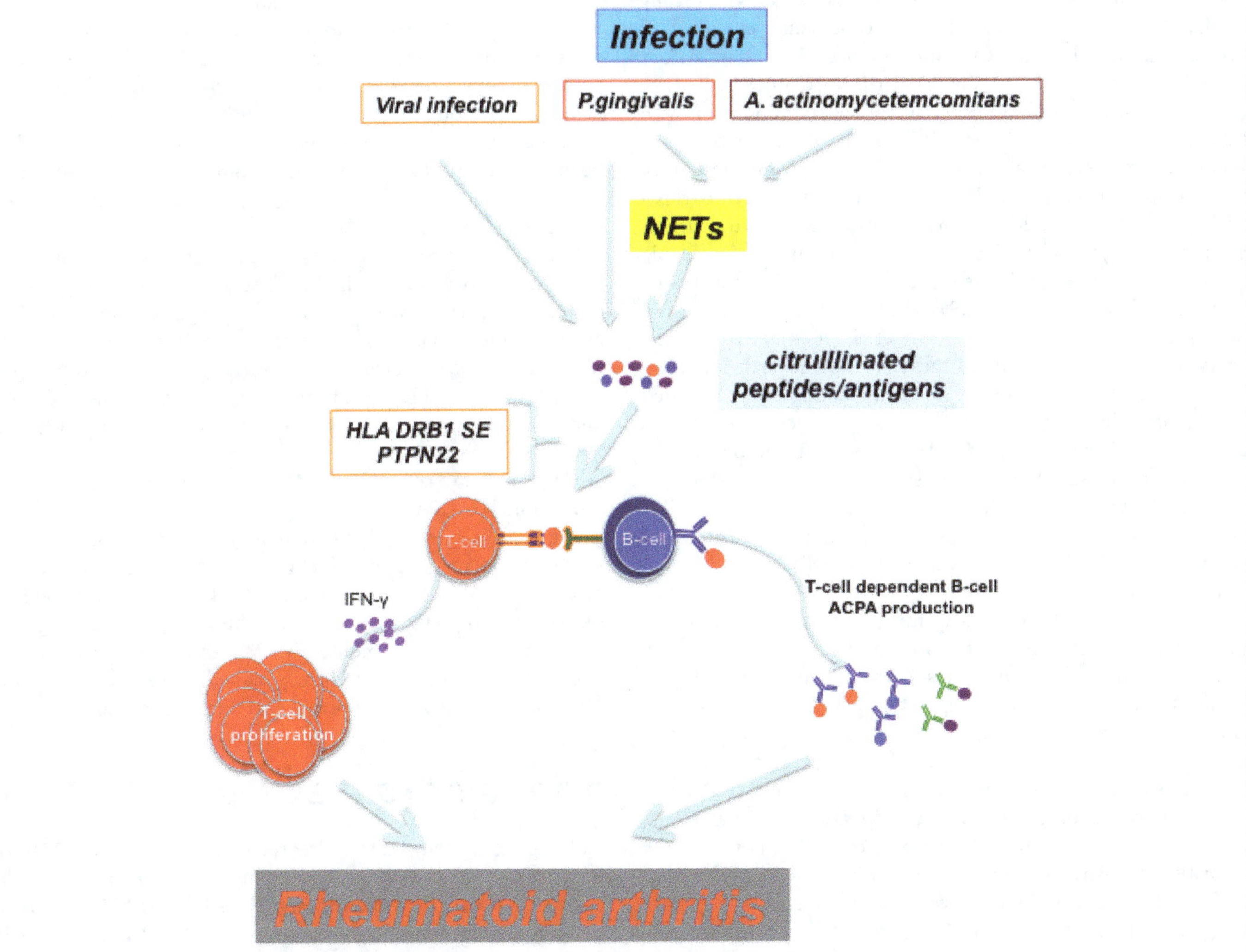

FIGURE 1 | Viral infections and periodontal disease caused by *P. gingivalis* and *A. actinocycetemcomitans* induce directly or through NETs citrullination of proteins/peptides. In an individual with proper genetic background (HLA DRB1 SE and PTPN22 risk allele R620W) T cells recognize citrullinated peptides and mount an immune response which culminates in the development of rheumatoid arthritis.

2013). Also ACPA producing plasma cells (anti-citrullinated fibrinogen abs) at the periphery of ELS were infected with EBV (expressed lytic proteins). Furthermore, ELS-containing RA synovia transplanted onto severe combined immunodeficiency (SCID) mice produced abs against citrullinated EBV proteins (VCP1 and VCP2) (Croia et al., 2013). These findings provide strong circumstantial evidence that EBV may initiate an immune response which subsequently may be re-directed against self antigens by way of cross-reactivity and epitope spreading.

CITRULLINATED PROTEINS AS ARTHRITOGENIC AUTOANTIGENS

ACPAs are associated with severe disease and are strong predictors of joint erosions in RA (Alexiou et al., 2007; Jilani and Mackworth-Young, 2015). Although association does not prove causation, several lines of evidence suggest that citrullinated proteins are likely to be arthritogenic autoantigens in RA (Sakkas et al., 2014). This means that citrullinated peptides are recognized by and activate T cells, which in turn (a) produce pro-inflammatory mediators and talk to other cells causing joint damage, and (b) provide help to B cells for ACPA production, which by themselves may be pathogenetic.

As already mentioned, the conversion of arginine to citrulline increases the affinity of citrullinated antigen binding to HLA-DRB1SE alleles (Hill et al., 2003; Scally et al., 2013). This has been confirmed in a study by Scally et al who showed that citrulline but no arginine is accommodated within the electropositive P4 pocket of RA-susceptible HLA-DRB1*0401/04 alleles (Scally et al., 2013). Furthermore, using HLA-DR4 tetramers, the authors found that citrullinated vimentin- and citrullinated aggrecan-specific T cells were present in peripheral blood of RA patients and their numbers were correlated with disease activity (Scally et al., 2013). Also, a T cell line recognizing citrullinated fibrinogen, abundant in RA joints, induced proinflammatory cytokines, and transfer of this T cell line to mice with CIA exacerbated arthritis (Cordova et al., 2013). Immunization with human fibrinogen (containing citrullinated peptides) in complete Freud adjuvant enhanced arthritis and T cells from these mice were fibrinogen-reactive and produced high levels of IL-6, IFNγ and IL-17 (Ho et al., 2010). Furthermore, adoptive transfer of plasma or T cells caused arthritis in naïve mice (Ho et al., 2010). Citrullinated fibrinogen but not unmodified fibrinogen induced arthritis in HLA-DRB1*04:01-IE transgenic mice but not in wild-type C57BL/6 mice (Hill et al., 2008). Furthermore, transfer of splenocytes from these transgenic arthritic mice caused arthritis to recipient mice, indicating that activated citrullinated fibrinogen-specific T cells are crucial for arthritis development (Yue et al., 2010). Also, a pan-PAD inhibitor (Cl-amidine) decreased the clinical severity of collagen-induced arthritis (CIA) and joint and serum protein citrullination (Willis et al., 2011). These studies show that citrullinated peptides in conjuction with HLA-DRB1SE activate T cells which become arthritogenic.

Infection with *P. ginvivalis* further contributes to joint inflammation that is dependent on citrullination. For instance, infection with *P. gingivalis* caused exacerbation of collagen-induced arthritis that was dependent on *P. gingivalis* PAD (PPAD) (Maresz et al., 2013). High levels of citrullinated proteins at the site of infection with *P. gingivalis* were detected as well as ACPAs (Maresz et al., 2013). Also, CIA was much less severe in the presence of PAD-deficient *P. gingivalis* (Gully et al., 2014). On the other hand, *P. gingivalis* components may cause arthritis through molecular mimicry. For instance, immunization of HLA-DR4-IE-transgenic mice with *P. gingivalis* α-enolase either citrullinated or noncitrullinated caused arthritis and abs reactive with human α-enolase (Kinloch et al., 2011). As already mentioned, *P. gingivalis* α-enolase shares sequence similarity with human α-enolase.

ACPAs contribute to joint inflammation and damage since they induce secretion of inflammatory cytokines and differentiation of osteoclasts. ACPA-containing immune complexes induced TNFα secretion by peripheral blood-derived macrophages (Clavel et al., 2008; Laurent et al., 2011; Sokolove et al., 2011), via toll-like receptor 4 (TLR4) and FcγR (Sokolove et al., 2011), whereas citrullinated fibrinogen stimulated TNFα production through TLR4 (England et al., 2017). Also, citrullinated histones increase macrophage TNFα production via TLR4, and immune complexes containing citrullinated histones activate macrophage production of TNFα via TLR4 and FcγR and neutrophils. Over 90% of RA patients have abs against neutrophil-derived citrullinated histones (citrullinated H2B).

P. gingivalis may also contribute to arthritis through inflammatory cytokine release. For instance, periodontal disease induced by *P. gingivalis* (Marchesan et al., 2013) or *Prevotella nigrescens* (de Aquino et al., 2014) exacerbated collagen-induced arthritis and promoted Th17 responses.

The effect of citrullinated proteins and ACPAs in wild-type animals (not transgenic animals) in the induction or exacerbation of arthritis is not certain. For instance, immunization of mice with citrullinated histone did not cause arthritis but exacerbated collagen-induced arthritis (Sohn et al., 2015). Similarly, some studies show exacerbating effect of ACPAs on collagen-induced arthritis and others suppressing effects (Kuhn et al., 2006; Shoda et al., 2011; Cantaert et al., 2013). For instance, it has been reported that co-administration of anti-citrullinated fibrinogen abs with anticollagen II abs enhanced CIA (Kuhn et al., 2006).

NETs, apart from providing targets for ACPAs, contribute to inflammatory process in RA. The nuclear and cytoplasmic molecules in NETs have antimicrobial properties, and stimulate adaptive and innate immune responses. LL37 NETs increase fibroblast-like synoviocyte IL-6 and IL-8 production (Khandpur et al., 2013). Also, LL37 can form complexes with DNA and RNA and stimulate innate TLRs (Lande et al., 2007; Ganguly et al., 2009).

ACPAs also contribute to joint erosions. ACPAs and monoclonal ACPAs derived from RA synovial fluid (SF) single B cells enhanced differentiation of osteoclasts through PAD-dependent IL-8 production. Furthermore, transfer of monoclonal ACPAs into mice induced IL-8-mediated bone loss (Krishnamurthy et al., 2016). Also, affinity-purified abs against mutated citrullinated vimentin (MCV) bind to osteoclast surface and induce osteoclastogenesis, whereas adoptive transfer of anti-MCV abs into mice causes osteopenia (Harre et al., 2012).

RELEVANCE TO TREATMENT

Although there may be few disagreements (Konig et al., 2016b), the research data outlined above imply that citrullination, in conjunction with genetic factors, such as HLA-DRB1SE, protein tyrosine phosphatase nonreceptor type 22 (PTPN22) risk allele (Joshua et al., 2016) encoding an R620W amino acid change that allows survival of autoreactive B cells (Menard et al., 2011), is the key element in breaking tolerance. Thus citrullinated peptides may offer new therapeutic strategies for RA. For instance, CTLA-4Ig blocked the development of arthritis induced by citrullinated fibrinogen in HLA-DRB1*0401 transgenic mice (Yue et al., 2010). This concept is re-enforced by the study of Gertel et al. who used citrullinate multiepitope peptide derived from prevalent citrullinated autoantigens in RA to reduce disease severity in adjuvant-induced arthritis in rats (Gertel et al., 2015). Also, citrullinated peptide autologous dendritic cells immunotherapy administered to once reduced effector T cells and increased regulatory T cells at 1 month (Benham et al., 2015).

Another strategy could be inhibition of TLR4. TLR4 is an innate immunity receptor for various ligands, including immune complexes containing ACPAs, mainly against citrullinated fibrinogen. Inhibition of TLR4 has been shown to decrease inflammatory arthritis in mouse models (Abdollahi-Roodsaz et al., 2007; Pierer et al., 2011). More importantly, the presence of ACPAs against citrullinated peptides from α-chains and β-chains of fibrinogen and histone 2A in RA patients predicts the anti-inflammatory response of TLR4 inhibition by a therapeutic ab (NI-0101) in an *ex vivo* model of RA (Hatterer et al., 2016).

Therefore, it is likely that these new therapeutic strategies will be fruitful in human RA in the near future.

AUTHOR CONTRIBUTIONS

LS, DD, SL, and DB substantially contributed on drafting the work and revising the manuscript, and approved the final version to be published. LS, DD, SL, and DB agreed to be accountable for all aspects of the work in ensuring that questions related to the accuracy or integrity of any part of the work are appropriately investigated and resolved. LS had the original idea of drafting the manuscript and overall supervision of manuscript's shaping.

FUNDING

This work was supported by the Research Committee of the University of Thessaly (Grant No. 4052).

REFERENCES

Abdollahi-Roodsaz, S., Joosten, L. A., Roelofs, M. F., Radstake, T. R., Matera, G., Popa, C., et al. (2007). Inhibition of Toll-like receptor 4 breaks the inflammatory loop in autoimmune destructive arthritis. *Arthritis Rheum.* 56, 2957–2967. doi: 10.1002/art.22848

Alexiou, I., Germenis, A., Ziogas, A., Theodoridou, K., and Sakkas, L. I. (2007). Diagnostic value of anti-cyclic citrullinated peptide antibodies in Greek patients with rheumatoid arthritis. *BMC Musculoskelet. Disord.* 8:37. doi: 10.1186/1471-2474-8-37

Alspaugh, M. A., Henle, G., Lennette, E. T., and Henle, W. (1981). Elevated levels of antibodies to Epstein-Barr virus antigens in sera and synovial fluids of patients with rheumatoid arthritis. *J. Clin. Invest.* 67, 1134–1140. doi: 10.1172/JCI110127

Arkema, E. V., Karlson, E. W., and Costenbader, K. H. (2010). A prospective study of periodontal disease and risk of rheumatoid arthritis. *J. Rheumatol.* 37, 1800–1804. doi: 10.3899/jrheum.091398

Balandraud, N., Meynard, J. B., Auger, I., Sovran, H., Mugnier, B., Reviron, D., et al. (2003). Epstein-Barr virus load in the peripheral blood of patients with rheumatoid arthritis: accurate quantification using real-time polymerase chain reaction. *Arthritis Rheum.* 48, 1223–1228. doi: 10.1002/art.10933

Barouta, G., Katsiari, C. G., Alexiou, I., Liaskos, C., Varna, A., Bogdanos, D. P., et al. (2017). Anti-MCV antibodies predict radiographic progression in Greek patients with very early (<3 months duration) rheumatoid arthritis. *Clin. Rheumatol.* 36, 885–894. doi: 10.1007/s10067-016-3494-4

Bartold, P. M., Marshall, R. I., and Haynes, D. R. (2005). Periodontitis and rheumatoid arthritis: a review. *J. Periodontol.* 76, 2066–2074. doi: 10.1902/jop.2005.76.11-S.2066

Benham, H., Nel, H. J., Law, S. C., Mehdi, A. M., Street, S., Ramnoruth, N., et al. (2015). Citrullinated peptide dendritic cell immunotherapy in HLA risk genotype-positive rheumatoid arthritis patients. *Sci. Transl. Med.* 7:290ra87. doi: 10.1126/scitranslmed.aaa9301

Bogdanos, D. P., and Sakkas, L. I. (2017). From microbiome to infectome in autoimmunity. *Curr. Opin. Rheumatol.* 29, 369–373. doi: 10.1097/BOR.0000000000000394

Brown, L. J., and Loe, H. (1993). Prevalence, extent, severity and progression of periodontal disease. *Periodontology 2000* 2, 57–71. doi: 10.1111/j.1600-0757.1993.tb00220.x

Burkhardt, H., Sehnert, B., Bockermann, R., Engstrom, A., Kalden, J. R., and Holmdahl, R. (2005). Humoral immune response to citrullinated collagen type II determinants in early rheumatoid arthritis. *Eur. J. Immunol.* 35, 1643–1652. doi: 10.1002/eji.200526000

Cantaert, T., Teitsma, C., Tak, P. P., and Baeten, D. (2013). Presence and role of anti-citrullinated protein antibodies in experimental arthritis models. *Arthritis Rheum.* 65, 939–948. doi: 10.1002/art.37839

Clavel, C., Nogueira, L., Laurent, L., Iobagiu, C., Vincent, C., Sebbag, M., et al. (2008). Induction of macrophage secretion of tumor necrosis factor alpha through Fcgamma receptor IIa engagement by rheumatoid arthritis-specific autoantibodies to citrullinated proteins complexed with fibrinogen. *Arthritis Rheum.* 58, 678–688. doi: 10.1002/art.23284

Cordova, K. N., Willis, V. C., Haskins, K., and Holers, V. M. (2013). A citrullinated fibrinogen-specific T cell line enhances autoimmune arthritis in a mouse model of rheumatoid arthritis. *J. Immunol.* 190, 1457–1465. doi: 10.4049/jimmunol.1201517

Cornillet, M., Sebbag, M., Verrouil, E., Magyar, A., Babos, F., Ruyssen-Witrand, A., et al. (2014). The fibrin-derived citrullinated peptide beta60-74Cit(6)(0),(7)(2),(7)(4) bears the major ACPA epitope recognised by the rheumatoid arthritis-specific anticitrullinated fibrinogen autoantibodies and anti-CCP2 antibodies. *Ann. Rheum. Dis.* 73, 1246–1252. doi: 10.1136/annrheumdis-2012-202868

Cornillet, M., Verrouil, E., Cantagrel, A., Serre, G., and Nogueira, L. (2015). In ACPA-positive RA patients, antibodies to EBNA35-58Cit, a citrullinated peptide from the Epstein-Barr nuclear antigen-1, strongly cross-react with the peptide beta60-74Cit which bears the immunodominant epitope of citrullinated fibrin. *Immunol. Res.* 61, 117–125. doi: 10.1007/s12026-014-8584-2

Corsiero, E., Bombardieri, M., Carlotti, E., Pratesi, F., Robinson, W., Migliorini, P., et al. (2016). Single cell cloning and recombinant monoclonal antibodies generation from RA synovial B cells reveal frequent targeting of citrullinated histones of NETs. *Ann. Rheum. Dis.* 75, 1866–1875. doi: 10.1136/annrheumdis-2015-208356

Croia, C., Serafini, B., Bombardieri, M., Kelly, S., Humby, F., Severa, M., et al. (2013). Epstein-Barr virus persistence and infection of autoreactive plasma cells in synovial lymphoid structures in rheumatoid arthritis. *Ann. Rheum. Dis.* 72, 1559–1568. doi: 10.1136/annrheumdis-2012-202352

de Aquino, S. G., Abdollahi-Roodsaz, S., Koenders, M. I., van de Loo, F. A., Pruijn, G. J., Marijnissen, R. J., et al. (2014). Periodontal pathogens directly promote autoimmune experimental arthritis by inducing a TLR2- and IL-1-driven Th17 response. *J. Immunol.* 192, 4103–4111. doi: 10.4049/jimmunol.1301970

Delbosc, S., Alsac, J. M., Journe, C., Louedec, L., Castier, Y., Bonnaure-Mallet, M., et al. (2011). *Porphyromonas gingivalis* participates in pathogenesis of human abdominal aortic aneurysm by neutrophil activation. Proof of concept in rats. *PLoS ONE* 6:e18679. doi: 10.1371/journal.pone.0018679

England, B. R., Thiele, G. M., and Mikuls, T. R. (2017). Anticitrullinated protein antibodies: origin and role in the pathogenesis of rheumatoid arthritis. *Curr. Opin. Rheumatol.* 29, 57–64. doi: 10.1097/BOR.0000000000000356

Eriksson, K., Nise, L., Kats, A., Luttropp, E., Catrina, A. I., Askling, J., et al. (2016). Prevalence of periodontitis in patients with established rheumatoid arthritis: a swedish population based case-control study. *PLoS ONE* 11:e0155956. doi: 10.1371/journal.pone.0155956

Ganguly, D., Chamilos, G., Lande, R., Gregorio, J., Meller, S., Facchinetti, V., et al. (2009). Self-RNA-antimicrobial peptide complexes activate human dendritic cells through TLR7 and TLR8. *J. Exp. Med.* 206, 1983–1994. doi: 10.1084/jem.20090480

Gertel, S., Serre, G., Shoenfeld, Y., and Amital, H. (2015). Immune tolerance induction with multiepitope peptide derived from citrullinated autoantigens attenuates arthritis manifestations in adjuvant arthritis rats. *J. Immunol.* 194, 5674–5680. doi: 10.4049/jimmunol.1402457

Goulas, T., Mizgalska, D., Garcia-Ferrer, I., Kantyka, T., Guevara, T., Szmigielski, B., et al. (2015). Structure and mechanism of a bacterial host-protein citrullinating virulence factor, *Porphyromonas gingivalis* peptidylarginine deiminase. *Sci. Rep.* 5:11969. doi: 10.1038/srep11969

Gregersen, P. K., Silver, J., and Winchester, R. J. (1987). The shared epitope hypothesis. An approach to understanding the molecular genetics of susceptibility to rheumatoid arthritis. *Arthritis Rheum.* 30, 1205–1213. doi: 10.1002/art.1780301102

Gully, N., Bright, R., Marino, V., Marchant, C., Cantley, M., Haynes, D., et al. (2014). *Porphyromonas gingivalis* peptidylarginine deiminase, a key contributor in the pathogenesis of experimental periodontal disease and experimental arthritis. *PLoS ONE* 9:e100838. doi: 10.1371/journal.pone.0100838

Haffajee, A. D., and Socransky, S. S. (1994). Microbial etiological agents of destructive periodontal diseases. *Periodontology 2000* 5, 78–111. doi: 10.1111/j.1600-0757.1994.tb00020.x

Harre, U., Georgess, D., Bang, H., Bozec, A., Axmann, R., Ossipova, E., et al. (2012). Induction of osteoclastogenesis and bone loss by human autoantibodies against citrullinated vimentin. *J. Clin. Invest.* 122, 1791–1802. doi: 10.1172/JCI60975

Hatterer, E., Shang, L., Simonet, P., Herren, S., Daubeuf, B., Teixeira, S., et al. (2016). A specific anti-citrullinated protein antibody profile identifies a group of rheumatoid arthritis patients with a toll-like receptor 4-mediated disease. *Arthritis Res. Ther.* 18:224. doi: 10.1186/s13075-016-1128-5

Haubek, D., and Johansson, A. (2014). Pathogenicity of the highly leukotoxic JP2 clone of *Aggregatibacter actinomycetemcomitans* and its geographic dissemination and role in aggressive periodontitis. *J. Oral Microbiol.* 6. doi: 10.3402/jom.v6.23980

Hensvold, A. H., Frisell, T., Magnusson, P. K., Holmdahl, R., Askling, J., and Catrina, A. I. (2017). How well do ACPA discriminate and predict RA in the general population: a study based on 12 590 population-representative Swedish twins. *Ann. Rheum. Dis.* 76, 119–125. doi: 10.1136/annrheumdis-2015-208980

Hensvold, A. H., Magnusson, P. K., Joshua, V., Hansson, M., Israelsson, L., Ferreira, R., et al. (2015). Environmental and genetic factors in the development of anticitrullinated protein antibodies (ACPAs) and ACPA-positive rheumatoid arthritis: an epidemiological investigation in twins. *Ann. Rheum. Dis.* 74, 375–380. doi: 10.1136/annrheumdis-2013-203947

Hill, J. A., Bell, D. A., Brintnell, W., Yue, D., Wehrli, B., Jevnikar, A. M., et al. (2008). Arthritis induced by posttranslationally modified (citrullinated) fibrinogen in DR4-IE transgenic mice. *J. Exp. Med.* 205, 967–979. doi: 10.1084/jem.20072051

Hill, J. A., Southwood, S., Sette, A., Jevnikar, A. M., Bell, D. A., and Cairns, E. (2003). Cutting edge: the conversion of arginine to citrulline allows for a high-affinity peptide interaction with the rheumatoid arthritis-associated HLA-DRB1*0401 MHC class II molecule. *J. Immunol.* 171, 538–541. doi: 10.4049/jimmunol.171.2.538

Hitchon, C. A., Chandad, F., Ferucci, E. D., Willemze, A., Ioan-Facsinay, A., van der Woude, D., et al. (2010). Antibodies to *porphyromonas gingivalis* are associated with anticitrullinated protein antibodies in patients with rheumatoid arthritis and their relatives. *J. Rheumatol.* 37, 1105–1112. doi: 10.3899/jrheum.091323

Ho, P. P., Lee, L. Y., Zhao, X., Tomooka, B. H., Paniagua, R. T., Sharpe, O., et al. (2010). Autoimmunity against fibrinogen mediates inflammatory arthritis in mice. *J. Immunol.* 184, 379–390. doi: 10.4049/jimmunol.0901639

Jilani, A. A., and Mackworth-Young, C. G. (2015). The role of citrullinated protein antibodies in predicting erosive disease in rheumatoid arthritis: a systematic literature review and meta-analysis. *Int. J. Rheumatol.* 2015:728610. doi: 10.1155/2015/728610

Johansson, L., Pratesi, F., Brink, M., Arlestig, L., D'Amato, C., Bartaloni, D., et al. (2016). Antibodies directed against endogenous and exogenous citrullinated antigens pre-date the onset of rheumatoid arthritis. *Arthritis Res. Ther.* 18:127. doi: 10.1186/s13075-016-1031-0

Joshua, V., Schobers, L., Titcombe, P. J., Israelsson, L., Ronnelid, J., Hansson, M., et al. (2016). Antibody responses to de novo identified citrullinated fibrinogen peptides in rheumatoid arthritis and visualization of the corresponding B cells. *Arthritis Res. Ther.* 18:284. doi: 10.1186/s13075-016-1181-0

Kadowaki, T., Nakayama, K., Yoshimura, F., Okamoto, K., Abe, N., and Yamamoto, K. (1998). Arg-gingipain acts as a major processing enzyme for various cell surface proteins in *Porphyromonas gingivalis*. *J. Biol. Chem.* 273, 29072–29076. doi: 10.1074/jbc.273.44.29072

Kalla, M., and Hammerschmidt, W. (2012). Human B cells on their route to latent infection–early but transient expression of lytic genes of Epstein-Barr virus. *Eur. J. Cell Biol.* 91, 65–69. doi: 10.1016/j.ejcb.2011.01.014

Khandpur, R., Carmona-Rivera, C., Vivekanandan-Giri, A., Gizinski, A., Yalavarthi, S., Knight, J. S., et al. (2013). NETs are a source of citrullinated autoantigens and stimulate inflammatory responses in rheumatoid arthritis. *Sci. Transl. Med.* 5:178ra40. doi: 10.1126/scitranslmed.3005580

Kharlamova, N., Jiang, X., Sherina, N., Potempa, B., Israelsson, L., Quirke, A. M., et al. (2016). Antibodies to *Porphyromonas gingivalis* indicate interaction between oral infection, smoking, and risk genes in rheumatoid arthritis etiology. *Arthritis Rheumatol.* 68, 604–613. doi: 10.1002/art.39491

Kinloch, A. J., Alzabin, S., Brintnell, W., Wilson, E., Barra, L., Wegner, N., et al. (2011). Immunization with *Porphyromonas gingivalis* enolase induces autoimmunity to mammalian alpha-enolase and arthritis in DR4-IE-transgenic mice. *Arthritis Rheum.* 63, 3818–3823. doi: 10.1002/art.30639

Konig, M. F., Abusleme, L., Reinholdt, J., Palmer, R. J., Teles, R. P., Sampson, K., et al. (2016a). *Aggregatibacter actinomycetemcomitans*-induced hypercitrullination links periodontal infection to autoimmunity in rheumatoid arthritis. *Sci. Transl. Med.* 8:369ra176. doi: 10.1126/scitranslmed.aaj1921

Konig, M. F., Giles, J. T., Nigrovic, P. A., and Andrade, F. (2016b). Antibodies to native and citrullinated RA33 (hnRNP A2/B1) challenge citrullination as the inciting principle underlying loss of tolerance in rheumatoid arthritis. *Ann. Rheum. Dis.* 75, 2022–2028. doi: 10.1136/annrheumdis-2015-208529

Krishnamurthy, A., Joshua, V., Haj Hensvold, A., Jin, T., Sun, M., Vivar, N., et al. (2016). Identification of a novel chemokine-dependent molecular mechanism underlying rheumatoid arthritis-associated autoantibody-mediated bone loss. *Ann. Rheum. Dis.* 75, 721–729. doi: 10.1136/annrheumdis-2015-208093

Kuhn, K. A., Kulik, L., Tomooka, B., Braschler, K. J., Arend, W. P., Robinson, W. H., et al. (2006). Antibodies against citrullinated proteins enhance tissue injury in experimental autoimmune arthritis. *J. Clin. Invest.* 116, 961–973. doi: 10.1172/JCI25422

Lande, R., Gregorio, J., Facchinetti, V., Chatterjee, B., Wang, Y. H., Homey, B., et al. (2007). Plasmacytoid dendritic cells sense self-DNA coupled with antimicrobial peptide. *Nature* 449, 564–569. doi: 10.1038/nature06116

Lappin, D. F., Apatzidou, D., Quirke, A. M., Oliver-Bell, J., Butcher, J. P., Kinane, D. F., et al. (2013). Influence of periodontal disease, *Porphyromonas gingivalis* and cigarette smoking on systemic anti-citrullinated peptide antibody titres. *J. Clin. Periodontol.* 40, 907–915. doi: 10.1111/jcpe.12138

Laurent, L., Clavel, C., Lemaire, O., Anquetil, F., Cornillet, M., Zabraniecki, L., et al. (2011). Fcgamma receptor profile of monocytes and macrophages from rheumatoid arthritis patients and their response to immune complexes formed with autoantibodies to citrullinated proteins. *Ann. Rheum. Dis.* 70, 1052–1059. doi: 10.1136/ard.2010.142091

Lee, H. S., Irigoyen, P., Kern, M., Lee, A., Batliwalla, F., Khalili, H., et al. (2007). Interaction between smoking, the shared epitope, and anti-cyclic citrullinated peptide: a mixed picture in three large North American rheumatoid arthritis cohorts. *Arthritis Rheum.* 56, 1745–1753. doi: 10.1002/art.22703

Li, P., Li, M., Lindberg, M. R., Kennett, M. J., Xiong, N., and Wang, Y. (2010). PAD4 is essential for antibacterial innate immunity mediated by neutrophil extracellular traps. *J. Exp. Med.* 207, 1853–1862. doi: 10.1084/jem.20100239

Li, S., Yu, Y., Yue, Y., Liao, H., Xie, W., Thai, J., et al. (2016). Autoantibodies from single circulating plasmablasts react with citrullinated antigens and *Porphyromonas gingivalis* in rheumatoid arthritis. *Arthritis Rheumatol.* 68, 614–626. doi: 10.1002/art.39455

Lundberg, K., Bengtsson, C., Kharlamova, N., Reed, E., Jiang, X., Kallberg, H., et al. (2013). Genetic and environmental determinants for disease risk in subsets of rheumatoid arthritis defined by the anticitrullinated protein/peptide antibody fine specificity profile. *Ann. Rheum. Dis.* 72, 652–658. doi: 10.1136/annrheumdis-2012-201484

Lundberg, K., Kinloch, A., Fisher, B. A., Wegner, N., Wait, R., Charles, P., et al. (2008). Antibodies to citrullinated alpha-enolase peptide 1 are specific for rheumatoid arthritis and cross-react with bacterial enolase. *Arthritis Rheum.* 58, 3009–3019. doi: 10.1002/art.23936

Lunemann, J. D., Frey, O., Eidner, T., Baier, M., Roberts, S., Sashihara, J., et al. (2008). Increased frequency of EBV-specific effector memory CD8+T cells correlates with higher viral load in rheumatoid arthritis. *J. Immunol.* 181, 991–1000. doi: 10.4049/jimmunol.181.2.991

Makrygiannakis, D., Hermansson, M., Ulfgren, A. K., Nicholas, A. P., Zendman, A. J., Eklund, A., et al. (2008). Smoking increases peptidylarginine deiminase 2 enzyme expression in human lungs and increases citrullination in BAL cells. *Ann. Rheum. Dis.* 67, 1488–1492. doi: 10.1136/ard.2007.075192

Marchesan, J. T., Gerow, E. A., Schaff, R., Taut, A. D., Shin, S. Y., Sugai, J., et al. (2013). *Porphyromonas gingivalis* oral infection exacerbates the development and severity of collagen-induced arthritis. *Arthritis Res. Ther.* 15:R186. doi: 10.1186/ar4376

Maresz, K. J., Hellvard, A., Sroka, A., Adamowicz, K., Bielecka, E., Koziel, J., et al. (2013). *Porphyromonas gingivalis* facilitates the development and progression of destructive arthritis through its unique bacterial peptidylarginine deiminase (PAD). *PLoS Pathog.* 9:e1003627. doi: 10.1371/journal.ppat.1003627

McGraw, W. T., Potempa, J., Farley, D., and Travis, J. (1999). Purification, characterization, and sequence analysis of a potential virulence factor from *Porphyromonas gingivalis*, peptidylarginine deiminase. *Infect. Immun.* 67, 3248–3256.

Menard, L., Saadoun, D., Isnardi, I., Ng, Y. S., Meyers, G., Massad, C., et al. (2011). The PTPN22 allele encoding an R620W variant interferes with the removal of developing autoreactive B cells in humans. *J. Clin. Invest.* 121, 3635–3644. doi: 10.1172/JCI45790

Mikuls, T. R., Payne, J. B., Yu, F., Thiele, G. M., Reynolds, R. J., Cannon, G. W., et al. (2014). Periodontitis and *Porphyromonas gingivalis* in patients with rheumatoid arthritis. *Arthritis Rheumatol.* 66, 1090–1100. doi: 10.1002/art.38348

Montgomery, A. B., Kopec, J., Shrestha, L., Thezenas, M. L., Burgess-Brown, N. A., Fischer, R., et al. (2016). Crystal structure of *Porphyromonas gingivalis* peptidylarginine deiminase: implications for autoimmunity in rheumatoid arthritis. *Ann. Rheum. Dis.* 75, 1255–1261. doi: 10.1136/annrheumdis-2015-207656

Nesse, W., Westra, J., van der Wal, J. E., Abbas, F., Nicholas, A. P., Vissink, A., et al. (2012). The periodontium of periodontitis patients contains citrullinated proteins which may play a role in ACPA (anti-citrullinated protein antibody) formation. *J. Clin. Periodontol.* 39, 599–607. doi: 10.1111/j.1600-051X.2012.01885.x

Nielen, M. M., van Schaardenburg, D., Reesink, H. W., van de Stadt, R. J., van der Horst-Bruinsma, I. E., de Koning, M. H., et al. (2004). Specific autoantibodies precede the symptoms of rheumatoid arthritis: a study of serial measurements in blood donors. *Arthritis Rheum.* 50, 380–386. doi: 10.1002/art.20018

Pierer, M., Wagner, U., Rossol, M., and Ibrahim, S. (2011). Toll-like receptor 4 is involved in inflammatory and joint destructive pathways in collagen-induced arthritis in DBA1J mice. *PLoS ONE* 6:e23539. doi: 10.1371/journal.pone.0023539

Potempa, J., Pike, R., and Travis, J. (1995). The multiple forms of trypsin-like activity present in various strains of *Porphyromonas gingivalis* are due to the presence of either Arg-gingipain or Lys-gingipain. *Infect. Immun.* 63, 1176–1182.

Pratesi, F., Dioni, I., Tommasi, C., Alcaro, M. C., Paolini, I., Barbetti, F., et al. (2014). Antibodies from patients with rheumatoid arthritis target citrullinated histone 4 contained in neutrophils extracellular traps. *Ann. Rheum. Dis.* 73, 1414–1422. doi: 10.1136/annrheumdis-2012-202765

Pratesi, F., Tommasi, C., Anzilotti, C., Chimenti, D., and Migliorini, P. (2006). Deiminated Epstein-Barr virus nuclear antigen 1 is a target of anti-citrullinated protein antibodies in rheumatoid arthritis. *Arthritis Rheum.* 54, 733–741. doi: 10.1002/art.21629

Pratesi, F., Tommasi, C., Anzilotti, C., Puxeddu, I., Sardano, E., Di Colo, G., et al. (2011). Antibodies to a new viral citrullinated peptide, VCP2: fine specificity and correlation with anti-cyclic citrullinated peptide (CCP) and anti-VCP1 antibodies. *Clin. Exp. Immunol.* 164, 337–345. doi: 10.1111/j.1365-2249.2011.04378.x

Reynisdottir, G., Karimi, R., Joshua, V., Olsen, H., Hensvold, A. H., Harju, A., et al. (2014). Structural changes and antibody enrichment in the lungs are early features of anti-citrullinated protein antibody-positive rheumatoid arthritis. *Arthritis Rheumatol.* 66, 31–39. doi: 10.1002/art.38201

Romero, V., Fert-Bober, J., Nigrovic, P. A., Darrah, E., Haque, U. J., Lee, D. M., et al. (2013). Immune-mediated pore-forming pathways induce cellular hypercitrullination and generate citrullinated autoantigens in rheumatoid arthritis. *Sci. Transl. Med.* 5:209ra150. doi: 10.1126/scitranslmed.3006869

Sakkas, L. I., Bogdanos, D. P., Katsiari, C., and Platsoucas, C. D. (2014). Anti-citrullinated peptides as autoantigens in rheumatoid arthritis-relevance to treatment. *Autoimmun. Rev.* 13, 1114–1120. doi: 10.1016/j.autrev.2014.08.012

Scally, S. W., Petersen, J., Law, S. C., Dudek, N. L., Nel, H. J., Loh, K. L., et al. (2013). A molecular basis for the association of the HLA-DRB1 locus, citrullination, and rheumatoid arthritis. *J. Exp. Med.* 210, 2569–2582. doi: 10.1084/jem.20131241

Scher, J. U., Ubeda, C., Equinda, M., Khanin, R., Buischi, Y., Viale, A., et al. (2012). Periodontal disease and the oral microbiota in new-onset rheumatoid arthritis. *Arthritis Rheum.* 64, 3083–3094. doi: 10.1002/art.34539

Scotet, E., David-Ameline, J., Peyrat, M. A., Moreau-Aubry, A., Pinczon, D., Lim, A., et al. (1996). T cell response to Epstein-Barr virus transactivators in chronic rheumatoid arthritis. *J. Exp. Med.* 184, 1791–1800. doi: 10.1084/jem.184.5.1791

Sebbag, M., Moinard, N., Auger, I., Clavel, C., Arnaud, J., Nogueira, L., et al. (2006). Epitopes of human fibrin recognized by the rheumatoid arthritis specific autoantibodies to citrullinated proteins. *Eur. J. Immunol.* 36, 2250–2263. doi: 10.1002/eji.200535790

Seror, R., Le Gall-David, S., Bonnaure-Mallet, M., Schaeverbeke, T., Cantagrel, A., Minet, J., et al. (2015). Association of Anti-*Porphyromonas gingivalis* antibody titers with nonsmoking status in early rheumatoid arthritis: results from the prospective French cohort of patients with early rheumatoid arthritis. *Arthritis Rheumatol.* 67, 1729–1737. doi: 10.1002/art.39118

Shoda, H., Fujio, K., Shibuya, M., Okamura, T., Sumitomo, S., Okamoto, A., et al. (2011). Detection of autoantibodies to citrullinated BiP in rheumatoid arthritis patients and pro-inflammatory role of citrullinated BiP in collagen-induced arthritis. *Arthritis Res. Ther.* 13:R191. doi: 10.1186/ar3520

Snir, O., Widhe, M., von Spee, C., Lindberg, J., Padyukov, L., Lundberg, K., et al. (2009). Multiple antibody reactivities to citrullinated antigens in sera from patients with rheumatoid arthritis: association with HLA-DRB1 alleles. *Ann. Rheum. Dis.* 68, 736–743. doi: 10.1136/ard.2008.091355

Sohn, D. H., Rhodes, C., Onuma, K., Zhao, X., Sharpe, O., Gazitt, T., et al. (2015). Local Joint inflammation and histone citrullination in a murine model of the transition from preclinical autoimmunity to inflammatory arthritis. *Arthritis Rheumatol.* 67, 2877–2887. doi: 10.1002/art.39283

Sokolove, J., Zhao, X., Chandra, P. E., and Robinson, W. H. (2011). Immune complexes containing citrullinated fibrinogen costimulate macrophages via Toll-like receptor 4 and Fcgamma receptor. *Arthritis Rheum.* 63, 53–62. doi: 10.1002/art.30081

Swanson-Mungerson, M., and Longnecker, R. (2007). Epstein-Barr virus latent membrane protein 2A and autoimmunity. *Trends Immunol.* 28, 213–218. doi: 10.1016/j.it.2007.03.002

Tsuda, R., Ozawa, T., Kobayashi, E., Hamana, H., Taki, H., Tobe, K., et al. (2015). Monoclonal antibody against citrullinated peptides obtained from rheumatoid arthritis patients reacts with numerous citrullinated microbial and food proteins. *Arthritis Rheumatol.* 67, 2020–2031. doi: 10.1002/art.39161

van der Helm-van Mil, A. H., Verpoort, K. N., Breedveld, F. C., Huizinga, T. W., Toes, R. E., and de Vries, R. R. (2006). The HLA-DRB1 shared epitope alleles are primarily a risk factor for anti-cyclic citrullinated peptide antibodies and are not an independent risk factor for development of rheumatoid arthritis. *Arthritis Rheum.* 54, 1117–1121. doi: 10.1002/art.21739

van der Helm-van Mil, A. H., Verpoort, K. N., Breedveld, F. C., Toes, R. E., and Huizinga, T. W. (2005). Antibodies to citrullinated proteins and differences in clinical progression of rheumatoid arthritis. *Arthritis Res. Ther.* 7, R949–R958. doi: 10.1186/ar1767

van der Helm-van Mil, A. H., Verpoort, K. N., le Cessie, S., Huizinga, T. W., de Vries, R. R., and Toes, R. E. (2007). The HLA-DRB1 shared epitope alleles differ in the interaction with smoking and predisposition to antibodies to cyclic citrullinated peptide. *Arthritis Rheum.* 56, 425–432. doi: 10.1002/art.22373

van de Sande, M. G., de Hair, M. J., van der Leij, C., Klarenbeek, P. L., Bos, W. H., Smith, M. D., et al. (2011). Different stages of rheumatoid arthritis: features of the synovium in the preclinical phase. *Ann. Rheum. Dis.* 70, 772–777. doi: 10.1136/ard.2010.139527

van Gaalen, F. A., Linn-Rasker, S. P., van Venrooij, W. J., de Jong, B. A., Breedveld, F. C., Verweij, C. L., et al. (2004). Autoantibodies to cyclic citrullinated peptides predict progression to rheumatoid arthritis in patients with undifferentiated arthritis: a prospective cohort study. *Arthritis Rheum.* 50, 709–715. doi: 10.1002/art.20044

Verpoort, K. N., Cheung, K., Ioan-Facsinay, A., van der Helm-van Mil, A. H., de Vries-Bouwstra, J. K., Allaart, C. F., et al. (2007). Fine specificity of the anti-citrullinated protein antibody response is influenced by the shared epitope alleles. *Arthritis Rheum.* 56, 3949–3952. doi: 10.1002/art.23127

Wegner, N., Wait, R., Sroka, A., Eick, S., Nguyen, K. A., Lundberg, K., et al. (2010). Peptidylarginine deiminase from *Porphyromonas gingivalis* citrullinates human fibrinogen and alpha-enolase: implications for autoimmunity in rheumatoid arthritis. *Arthritis Rheum.* 62, 2662–2672. doi: 10.1002/art.27552

Willis, V. C., Gizinski, A. M., Banda, N. K., Causey, C. P., Knuckley, B., Cordova, K. N., et al. (2011). N-alpha-benzoyl-N5-(2-chloro-1-iminoethyl)-L-ornithine amide, a protein arginine deiminase inhibitor, reduces the severity of murine collagen-induced arthritis. *J. Immunol.* 186, 4396–4404. doi: 10.4049/jimmunol.1001620

Wordsworth, B. P., Lanchbury, J. S., Sakkas, L. I., Welsh, K. I., Panayi, G. S., and Bell, J. I. (1989). HLA-DR4 subtype frequencies in rheumatoid arthritis indicate that DRB1 is the major susceptibility locus within the HLA class II region. *Proc. Natl. Acad. Sci. U.S.A.* 86, 10049–10053. doi: 10.1073/pnas.86.24.10049

Yang, H., Biermann, M. H., Brauner, J. M., Liu, Y., Zhao, Y., and Herrmann, M. (2016). New insights into neutrophil extracellular traps: mechanisms of formation and role in inflammation. *Front. Immunol.* 7:302. doi: 10.3389/fimmu.2016.00302

Ytterberg, A. J., Joshua, V., Reynisdottir, G., Tarasova, N. K., Rutishauser, D., Ossipova, E., et al. (2015). Shared immunological targets in the lungs and joints of patients with rheumatoid arthritis: identification and validation. *Ann. Rheum. Dis.* 74, 1772–1777. doi: 10.1136/annrheumdis-2013-204912

Yue, D., Brintnell, W., Mannik, L. A., Christie, D. A., Haeryfar, S. M., Madrenas, J., et al. (2010). CTLA-4Ig blocks the development and progression of citrullinated fibrinogen-induced arthritis in DR4-transgenic mice. *Arthritis Rheum.* 62, 2941–2952. doi: 10.1002/art.27597

11

Dietary and Microbial Metabolites in the Regulation of Host Immunity

Naoko Shibata[1,2,3]*, Jun Kunisawa*[1,3,4,5]** and Hiroshi Kiyono*[1,6]

[1] *Division of Mucosal Immunology, Department of Microbiology and Immunology and International Research and Development Center for Mucosal Vaccines, The Institute of Medical Science, The University of Tokyo, Tokyo, Japan,* [2] *Department of Mucosal Immunology, School of Medicine, Chiba University, Chiba, Japan,* [3] *Laboratory of Vaccine Materials and Laboratory of Gut Environmental System, National Institutes of Biomedical Innovation, Health and Nutrition, Osaka, Japan,* [4] *Graduate School of Medicine, Graduate School of Pharmaceutical Sciences, Graduate School of Dentistry, Osaka University, Osaka, Japan,* [5] *Department of Microbiology and Infectious Diseases, Kobe University Graduate School of Medicine, Kobe, Japan,* [6] *Department of Immunology, Graduate School of Medicine, Chiba University, Chiba, Japan*

Correspondence:
Jun Kunisawa
kunisawa@nibiohn.go.jp

Mucosal surfaces in the body, especially the intestine, are constantly exposed to trillions of microbiomes. Accumulating evidence has revealed that changes in the composition of the gut microbiome, especially that of the commensal bacteria population, are frequently associated with immunologic disorders. These changes coincide with changes in the production of certain dietary metabolites. Recent studies have uncovered the molecular and cellular mechanisms underlying the relationships among diet, commensal bacteria, and the host immune system. In this review, we describe how dietary and microbial metabolites modulate host immunity.

Keywords: microbiome, metabolite, fatty acid, vitamin

INTRODUCTION

Mucosal surfaces, especially that of the gastrointestinal tract, are constantly exposed to a wide variety of antigens including trillions of bacteria and fungi, as well as dietary components and their metabolites. The host immune system discriminates between harmful and beneficial antigens, simultaneously inducing immune responses to exclude harmful antigens while tolerating beneficial antigens to establish appropriate homeostatic conditions in the gut.

It has long been recognized that commensal bacteria regulate host responses, including immunity, but, due to the difficulty of culturing the intestinal microbiome, it has been challenging to obtain information. In addition, because dietary and microbial metabolites are generated in a complex network that includes the diet, host, and intestinal microbiome, it is difficult to analyze such metabolites. However, recent advances in genome-based analysis of bacteria has enabled direct analysis of the intestinal microbiome without culturing; this analysis has revealed that changes in the composition of the gut microbiome are associated with immunologic disorders and diseases (Browne et al., 2017). In addition, advances in high throughput metabolomics have allowed immunologists to investigate metabolites generated in the intestine and to discover that these changes in the microbiome composition coincide with changes in either useful or harmful metabolites involved in the regulation of immune responses. For example, commensal bacteria are

---

Abbreviations: AA, arachidonic acid; DC, dendritic cell; DHA, docosahexaenoic acid; EPA, eicosapentaenoic acid; FAO, fatty acid oxidation; FP, formylpterin; GPR, G-protein-coupled receptor; IEC, intestinal epithelial cell; IL, interleukin; LCFA, long-chain fatty acid; MAIT, mucosal-associated invariant T cell; MR1, MHC-like protein 1; PD1, Protectin D1; PPAR, peroxisome proliferator-activated receptor; Rv, resolving; SCFA, short-chain fatty acid; TCA, tricarboxylic acid; TLR, toll-like receptor; TNF, tumor necrosis factor; TX, Thromboxane.

involved in the extraction, synthesis, and absorption of many nutrients and metabolites including short- and LCFAs, and vitamins (Hirata and Kunisawa, 2017).

In this review, we describe recent findings regarding the role of the gut microbiome–diet interaction in the generation of immunologically active metabolites.

LONG-CHAIN FATTY ACIDS IN THE CONTROL OF IMMUNE RESPONSES

Fatty acids are an essential nutrient that is mainly obtained from the diet. Generally, dietary oils are composed of various LCFAs. LCFAs primarily serve as a source of energy and membrane components, but they are also actively involved in the regulation of immune responses by being metabolized into lipid metabolites (**Figure 1**) (Hirata and Kunisawa, 2017).

Studies to date have mainly focused on the lipid metabolites generated after absorption into the body. Among LCFAs, ω3 and ω6 LCFAs are essential FAs, meaning that they are not generated by mammals, including humans (Hirata and Kunisawa, 2017). These essential FAs are metabolized into bioactive lipid mediators through reactions that are mediated by several series of oxidative enzymes, such as cyclooxygenases, lipoxygenases, and cytochrome P450 monooxygenases (Arita, 2012). It is thought that ω3 LCFAs have anti-allergic and anti-inflammatory properties, whereas ω6 LCFAs have pro-inflammatory properties (Arita, 2012; Serhan, 2017). AA and linoleic acid are the major ω6 LCFA, whereas α-linolenic acid abundantly present in linseed or perilla oil, EPA and DHA abundantly present in fish oils are typical ω3 LCFAs. TX B_2, an AA derivative, is a potent vasoconstrictor and platelet activator, whereas TXB_3, an EPA derivative, has barely any physiological effects. Dietary supplementation with EPA has been shown to reduce TXB_2 levels in plasma and cellular fatty acid and to induce a shift to less reactive platelets and to reduce blood pressure in response to pressor hormones (Weber et al., 1986). In another study, dietary supplementation with ω3 LCFAs suppressed the ability of monocytes to synthesize inflammatory cytokines, such as interleukin-1 (IL-1) and TNF, which was accompanied by a decreased ratio of AA to EPA in the membrane phospholipids of the monocytes (Endres et al., 1989). Since the conversion of ω3 and ω6 LCFAs to bioactive lipid mediators shares the same series of enzymes, competition exists between AA and EPA/DHA for metabolism. This competition is one of the mechanisms through which EPA inhibits the inflammatory properties of AA.

In addition to the competition between ω3 and ω6 LCFAs, some lipid metabolites of ω3 LCFAs exhibit anti-inflammatory or anti-allergy effects (Arita, 2012; Kunisawa et al., 2015a). E-series Rv are derived from EPA, whereas D-series Rv and Protectin D1 (PD1) are derived from DHA. RvD1, RvD2, RvE1, and PD1 activate inflammation resolution programs by reducing levels of pro-inflammatory cytokines, including IL-6, IL-1β, IL-23, and TNFα, and neutrophil influx, and by promoting macrophage phagocytosis of apoptotic cells and inflammatory debris (Schwab et al., 2007; Spite et al., 2009; Chiang et al., 2012).

In addition to these studies, we previously reported that allergic diarrhea was ameliorated when mice were maintained on linseed oil rich in ω3 α-linolenic acid (Kunisawa et al., 2015a). The α-linolenic acid is metabolized to eicosapentaenoic acid, levels of which also increased in the intestine of mice maintained on linseed oil. When we performed lipidomics analysis, we identified 17,18-epoxy-eicosatetraenoic acid as an anti-allergic lipid metabolite derived from eicosapentaenoic acid (Kunisawa et al., 2015a). Given that synthetic 17,18-epoxy-eicosatetraenoic acid administration is sufficient to inhibit allergic diarrhea, this lipid metabolite appears to be effective in the control of intestinal allergy.

Although these lipid metabolites seem to be generated in the body, several lines of evidence indicate that commensal bacteria also express enzymes that participate in LCFA metabolism (**Figure 1**). Indeed, germ-free animals exhibit alterations of composition in their lipid metabolites (Claus et al., 2008; Martin et al., 2009; Chiang et al., 2012). In this regard, we identified conjugated linoleic acids, oxo FAs, and hydroxy FAs as microbial lipid metabolites (Kishino et al., 2013). These metabolites are formed in the intestine through the action of commensal bacteria, especially *Lactobacillus plantarum* (Kishino et al., 2013). Indeed, these lipid metabolites are abundant in the intestinal lumen of specific pathogen-free mice but are scarce in germ-free mice (Kishino et al., 2013). Of note, these lipid metabolites are detected not only in the intestinal lumen but also in the serum, suggesting that these microbial lipid metabolites act both in the intestinal lumen and elsewhere in the body.

Administration of 10-hydroxy-cis-12-octadecenoic acid, one of the microbial lipid metabolites, has been reported to ameliorate experimental colitis by enhancing tight junctions on epithelial cells. Signaling though LCFA receptors is mediated by GPR40, which suppresses TNFR2 gene expression and NF-κB via the MEK-ERK pathway (Miyamoto et al., 2015). LCFAs are also recognized by PPARs, which also modulate immune reactions and allergic diseases (Ricote et al., 1998; Fukui et al., 2009). For example, it was reported that probiotic bacteria in the intestine produce conjugated linoleic acids, which target PPAR-γ in macrophages to suppress the inflammatory response (Bassaganya-Riera et al., 2012). In other studies, *Bacteroides thetaiotaomicron* activated PPAR-γ, which decreased NF-κB–dependent IL-8 production (Kelly et al., 2004), and *Enterococcus faecalis* activated PPAR-γ1 in IECs thereby increasing the production of IL-10 in human newborn babies (Are et al., 2008). Although it remains unclear which types of lipids act as ligands for these PPRA receptors, these microbial lipids and lipid metabolites may prevent allergy and inflammation.

As mentioned before, RvD1, RvD2, RvE1, and PD1 participate in the activation of inflammation resolution programs (Schwab et al., 2007; Spite et al., 2009; Chiang et al., 2012). It is important to note that commensal bacteria are also involved in this process (Chiang et al., 2012). Given that germ-free mice have increased levels of endogenous RvD1 and PD1 in their colon (Chiang et al., 2012), these reports suggest that microbial suppression of RvD1 and PD1 production may be involved in the regulation of the host immune defense against invading pathogens.

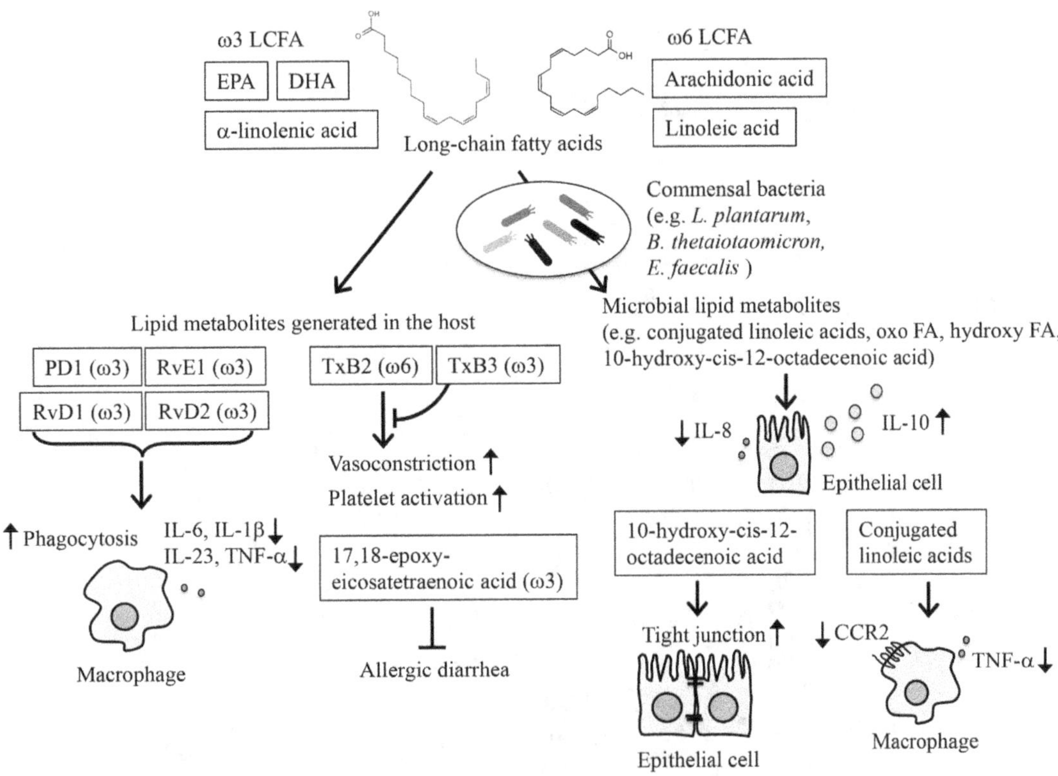

FIGURE 1 | Modification of immune responses by lipid metabolites. LCFAs are converted to bioactive lipid metabolites by host enzymes and commensal bacteria (e.g., *L. plantarum*, *B. thetaiotaomicron*, *E. faecalis*), and participate in the regulation of immune responses. Among LCFAs, ω3 LCFAs, such as EPA, DHA, and α-linolenic acid, and ω6 LCFA, such as AA and linoleic acid, are essential FAs. PD1, RvE1, RvD1, and RvD2, which are derived from EPA/DHA, activate inflammation resolution programs by modifying monocyte functions, such as inhibiting the production of inflammatory cytokines while enhancing phagocytosis. TxB3, derived from EPA, competitively inhibits the vasoconstriction and platelet activation induced by TxB2, which is derived from AA. 17,18-epoxy-eicosatetraenoic acid is derived from ω3 LCFA and participates in the amelioration of allergic diarrhea. Microbial lipid metabolites inhibit IL-8 production and activate IL-10 production from IECs. Conjugated linoleic acids inhibit the inflammatory responses of macrophages. 10-hydroxy-cis-12-octadecenoic acid, generated by commensal bacteria, enhances the tight junctions on IECs.

SHORT-CHAIN FATTY ACIDS IN THE CONTROL OF IMMUNE RESPONSES

Short-chain fatty acids are present at high concentrations in the intestine as bacterial fermentation products of dietary indigestible polysaccharides such as cellulose (**Figure 2**) (Wong et al., 2006). Because mammals lack the enzymes to degrade polysaccharides, germ-free mice exhibit remarkably decreased amounts of SCFAs and increased amounts of indigestible oligosaccharide, a bacterial fermentation substrate (Hoverstad and Midtvedt, 1986).

Among SCFAs, acetate, propionate, and butyrate have been well studied. Accumulated evidence indicated that these SCFAs modify several cellular processes including gene expression, chemotaxis, differentiation, proliferation, and apoptosis, which affect various biological responses including the immune response (**Figure 2**) (Correa et al., 2016). Generally, SCFAs are recognized on the cell surface by G-protein coupled receptors (GPRs) such as GPR41, GPR43, GPR109A, and Olfr78 (Bolognini et al., 2016). SCFAs are also transported by monocarboxylate transporter-1 and the sodium-dependent monocarboxylate transporter-1 and by passive diffusion across the plasma membrane into the cytoplasm (Thwaites and Anderson, 2007).

Because SCFAs are found at high concentrations in the intestine, they are in direct contact with the IECs. IECs take up SCFAs through both passive and active mechanisms into their cytosol, where the SCFAs, especially butyrate, are used as a source of ATP for energy metabolism (den Besten et al., 2013). In addition to their role in energy metabolism, SCFAs enhance some immune surveillance functions of IECs by increasing the expression of certain antimicrobial peptides; for example, butyrate increases the expression of LL-37 and CAP-18 (Raqib et al., 2006), and modulating cytokine (CCL20 and IL-8) production (Iraporda et al., 2015). In addition, the activation of GPR43 and GPR109a by SCFAs in IECs reportedly resulted in an increase in the production of IL-18, a cytokine involved in the maintenance of epithelial integrity (Singh et al., 2014; Macia et al., 2015).

Short-chain fatty acids are also known to enhance the induction of Treg cells in the intestine. A key molecule involved in this event is the butyrate receptor GPR109a expressed on DCs. Indeed, in one study, GPR109a-deficient mice were found

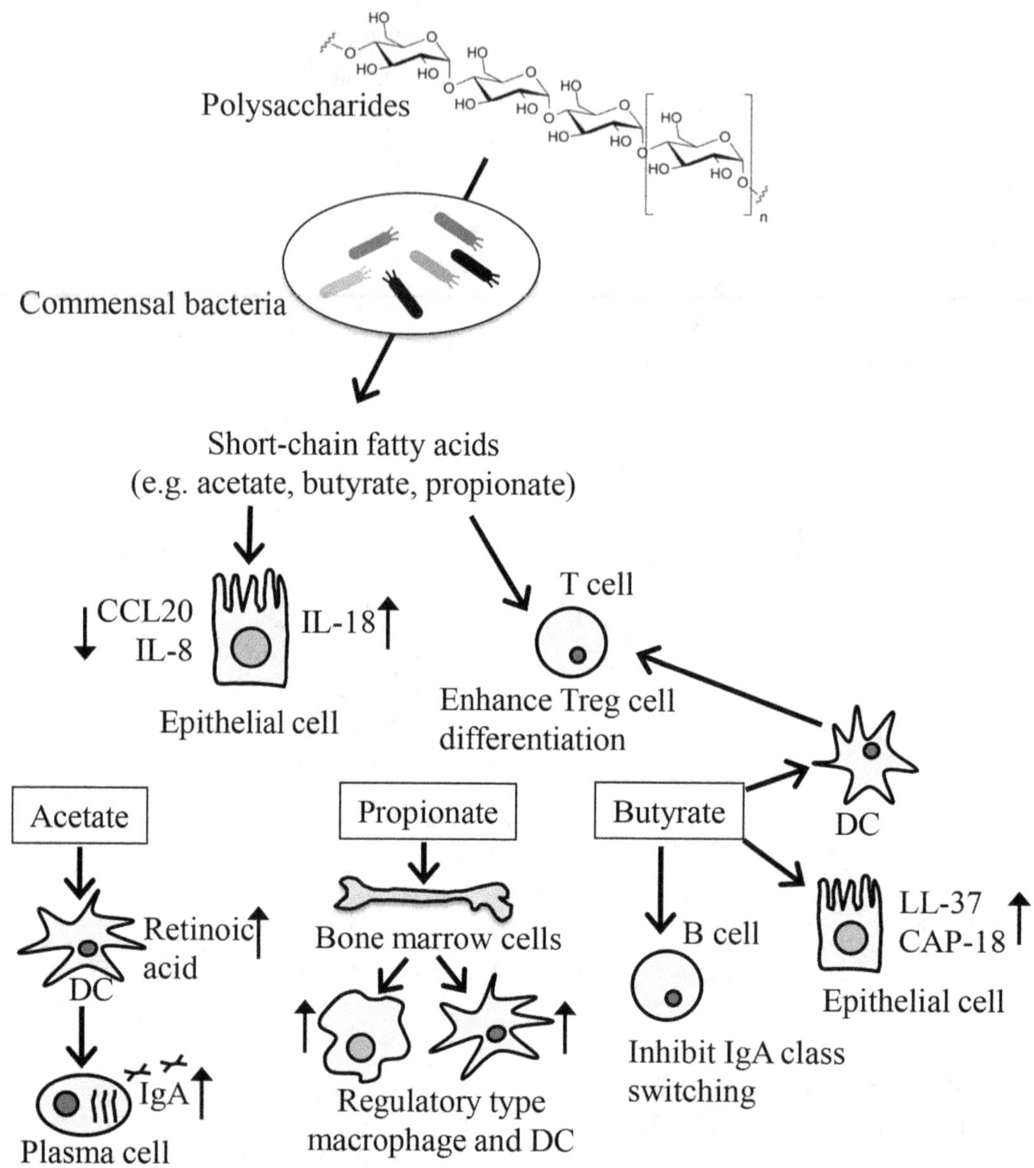

FIGURE 2 | Modification of immune responses by SCFAs produced by microbial fermentation. SCFAs are produced by bacterial fermentation of dietary indigestible polysaccharides and participate in the regulation of energy metabolism, cellular function, and differentiation. SCFAs, such as acetate, butyrate, and propionate, are taken up by IECs, where they inhibit the production of inflammatory cytokines such as CCL20 and IL-8 and enhance the production of IL-18, which is involved in IEC integrity. Butyrate participates in the production of antimicrobial peptides such as LL-37 and CAP-18. SCFAs also directly enhance the differentiation of Treg cells. Butyrate acts on DCs to enhance DC-induced Treg cell differentiation. Acetate enhances the production of retinoic acids from DCs, which promote IgA production, whereas butyrate inhibits the IgA class switching of B cells. Propionate enhances the generation of regulatory type of macrophages and DCs from bone marrow cells.

to have reduced numbers of Treg cells (Singh et al., 2014). In another study, SCFAs were found to directly affect the preferential differentiation of T cells to Treg cells with concurrent enhancement of histone H3 acetylation in the Foxp3 locus by butyrate, or the GPR43-mediated pathway (Furusawa et al., 2013; Smith et al., 2013). Consistent with these findings, mice lacking either GPR43 or GPR109a show exacerbated symptoms in food-allergy models (Tan et al., 2016). In addition to GPR43 and GPR109a, Slc5a8, a Na^+-coupled high-affinity transporter for SCFAs such as butyrate, plays an important role in the increased expression of indoleamine 2,3-dioxygenase 1 and aldehyde dehydrogenase in DCs, which results in the preferential induction of $FoxP3^+$ Treg cells (Gurav et al., 2015).

Besides their effects in the intestine, SCFAs exhibit several anti-allergic properties after absorption into the body. For example, mice fed a high-fiber, but not mice fed a low-fiber, showed increased levels of SCFAs in the blood and were protected against allergic inflammation in the lung (Trompette et al., 2014). In this case, propionate enhanced the generation of macrophage and DC precursors from bone marrow cells, which is dependent on GPR41 but not GPR43. DCs and macrophages generated in this process are highly phagocytic but impaired in their ability to promote the effector function of Th2 cells, thereby blocking allergic responses (Trompette et al., 2014).

Short-chain fatty acid are also involved in the production of intestinal IgA. The acetate-GPR43 axis positively regulates this process. Indeed, supplementation of acetate promotes intestinal IgA production in a GPR43-dependent manner (Wu et al., 2017). As an underlying mechanism, it was demonstrated that acetate induces the expression of aldehyde dehydrogenase in DCs, which converts vitamin A to retinoic acid for the promotion of IgA production (Wu et al., 2017). In contrast to the positive effects of acetate on intestinal IgA production, butyrate has been reported to suppress class switching to IgA through the upregulation of miR-155, -181b, -361, -23b, -30a, and -125b in B cells, which silence AID and Blimp-1 (White et al., 2014). These findings collectively suggest that a balance among SCFAs controls the immunologic status quo in both humoral and cellular immunity.

Short-chain fatty acids regulate IEC functions controlled by TLRs. IECs express several TLRs, including TLR2/1, TLR4, TLR5, and TLR9, which mainly recognize bacterial lipoproteins, lipopolysaccharides, flagellin, and DNA, respectively (de Kivit et al., 2014). SCFAs have been reported to modify immune responses by altering TLR-induced inflammatory gene expression through the inhibition of histone deacetylases (Lin et al., 2015). For example, when IECs were incubated with butyrate or propionate and then stimulated with flagellin, a ligand for TLR5 (Oh et al., 2014), the expression levels of pro-inflammatory cytokines such as TNF-α were upregulated, whereas those of chemotactic chemokines, such as IL-8 and monocyte chemotactic protein-1, were downregulated (Lin et al., 2015). A similar regulation pathway, mediated by TLR ligands and SCFAs, has been observed in hematopoietic cells (Mirmonsef et al., 2012). Given that many TLR ligands are present in not only pathogenic but also commensal bacteria and that SCFAs are produced by these bacteria via fermentation, the combination of TLR ligands and SCFAs seems to be an essential component of one of the commensal-mediated immune regulation pathways. Of note, flagellin-initiated TLR5 stimulation plays essential roles in the induction of immune responses against trivalent inactivated influenza vaccine-induced antibody responses (Oh et al., 2014). These reports indicate that the effectiveness of vaccination varies depending on the balance between commensal bacteria carrying flagellins and commensal bacteria contributing to the synthesis of SCFAs.

VITAMIN B FAMILY IN THE CONTROL OF IMMUNE RESPONSES

Mammals do not have biosynthetic pathways for vitamins and therefore must obtain vitamins externally. Of course, diets are a general source of vitamins, but commensal bacteria also produce vitamins and simultaneously consume dietary vitamins. Therefore, both diet and commensal bacteria determine the vitamin contents in the intestine (**Figure 3**).

Vitamins are required for the maintenance of many biological responses by acting as antioxidants, transcription factors, and cofactors for metabolic enzymes in the generation, conversion, and digestion of fatty acids, nucleotides, carbohydrate, and amino acids. Immune cells require all of these processes for their development, differentiation, and activation and therefore vitamin deficiency is frequently associated with increased risk of infectious, allergic, and inflammatory diseases (**Figure 3**) (Kunisawa and Kiyono, 2015; Suzuki and Kunisawa, 2015).

Vitamin B3 (nicotinic acid) supplementation acts on monocytes to dampen TLR2- and TLR4-induced release of inflammatory mediators such as TNF-α, IL-6, and monocyte chemotactic protein-1 (Digby et al., 2012). These effects are mediated by GPR109a, a vitamin B3 receptor expressed on monocytes (Digby et al., 2012). Vitamin B3 also reduces macrophage production of pro-inflammatory cytokines, including IL-1, IL-6, and TNF-α, in a murine model of atherosclerosis (Lipszyc et al., 2013). Collectively, these findings suggest that vitamin B3 exerts its anti-inflammatory properties by modulating immune cells.

The vitamin B complex also contributes to energy metabolism. Currently, the metabolic processes in immune cells are recognized as the emerging field of immunometabolism (Buck et al., 2017; Mills et al., 2017). The core function of metabolic pathways is the synthesis or degradation of sugars, fatty acids, nucleic acids, or proteins, coupled to the consumption or generation of ATP by oxidative phosphorylation or glycolysis. Changes in these metabolic pathways are frequently associated with immune cell functions such as cell proliferation and the production of cytokines, chemokines, and antibodies (Buck et al., 2017; Mills et al., 2017). Recent advances in our understanding of immunometabolism have revealed that quiescent or regulatory-type cells such as naïve T and B cells, Treg cells, and M2 macrophages use anabolic pathways for energy generation from the TCA cycle, such as FAO, whereas activated or inflammatory cells (e.g., Th1, Th2, Th17, IgA-producing plasma cells, M1 macrophages) use catabolic pathways and shift to glycolysis for energy generation (Buck et al., 2017; Kunisawa, 2017; Mills et al., 2017).

In metabolic energy pathways, vitamin B2 and its active forms (e.g., flavin adenine dinucleotide) function as cofactors for various enzymatic reactions such as the TCA cycle and FAO (Huskisson et al., 2007). FAO is necessary for the generation of acetyl-CoA, which enters the TCA cycle in mitochondria to produce energy. Studies using rodent models have shown that vitamin B2 deficiency reduces the activity of acyl-CoA dehydrogenases, which participate in the dehydrogenation step of FAO, and that vitamin B2 supplementation rescues the activity of these enzymes (Sakurai et al., 1982). As with vitamin B2, vitamin B1 (also known as thiamine) and its derivatives (e.g., thiamine pyrophosphate) acts as a cofactor for several enzymes such as pyruvate dehydrogenase and α-ketoglutarate dehydrogenase that are involved in TCA cycle (Frank et al., 2007). In agreement with the importance of energy metabolism in immune system, mice maintained on diets lacking the vitamin B complex show impaired immunity (Kunisawa et al.,

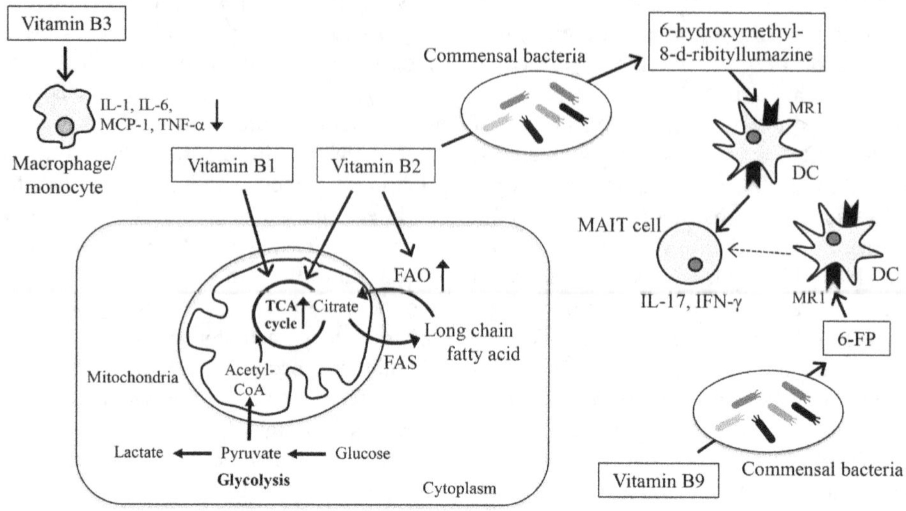

FIGURE 3 | Modification of energy metabolism and immune responses by vitamins. Vitamins are involved in the maintenance of immunological homeostasis in the gut through the regulation of energy metabolism, cellular function, and differentiation. Glucose enters the cell and is metabolized to pyruvate, which is then converted to lactate (glycolysis) or enters the TCA cycle for energy generation. In the TCA cycle, citrate can be transferred out of the mitochondria into the cytoplasm, where it is used for fatty acid synthesis (FAS). Fatty acids can be degraded in the mitochondria and enter the TCA cycle to produce energy (FAO). Vitamins B1 and B2 act as cofactors for enzymes involved in the TCA cycle. Vitamin B2 also acts as a cofactor for enzymes involved in FAO. Vitamin B3 inhibits the production of inflammatory cytokines such as TNF-α, IL-6, IL-1, MCP-1 from macrophages and monocytes. Vitamins B2 and B9 are metabolized by commensal bacteria and converted to 6-hydroxymethyl-8-D-ribityllumazine and 6-FP, respectively. 6-hydroxymethyl-8-D-ribityllumazine activates MAIT cells, whereas 6-FP binds to MR1 without activating MAIT cells.

2015b; Suzuki and Kunisawa, 2015; Hosomi and Kunisawa, 2017).

In addition to their direct effects on immune cells and energy metabolism, microbial metabolites of some B vitamins act as ligands for immune cells, especially mucosal-associated invariant T (MAIT) cells. Activated MAIT cells produce IL-17 and IFN-γ and help exclude infectious bacteria (Bourhis et al., 2013). Because MAIT cells are found in several inflammatory tissues in brain and kidney cancer patients, accompanied by reduced numbers of MAIT cells in the circulating blood, it is thought that MAIT cells infiltrate the inflammatory tissues and contribute to inflammatory disease (Bourhis et al., 2013). MAIT cells are innate-like T cells that recognize MHC-like protein 1 (MR1)-restricted presentation. Intriguingly, the microbial metabolite of vitamin B2 (riboflavin) 6-hydroxymethyl-8-D-ribityllumazine has been shown to activate MAIT cells (Kjer-Nielsen et al., 2012; Patel et al., 2013). Similarly, a microbial vitamin B9 metabolite, 6-formyl pterin (6-FP), has been shown to bind to MR1; however; unlike 6-hydroxymethyl-8-D-ribityllumazine, 6-FP cannot activate MAIT cells (Kjer-Nielsen et al., 2012; Patel et al., 2013). In line with these findings, a previous study suggests that acetyl-6-FP, an analog of 6-FP, acts as antagonist of MR1 in the inhibition of MR1-dependent MAIT cell activation (Eckle et al., 2014). Taking into account that the kinds and levels of biosynthesized B vitamins differ among bacteria (Magnusdottir et al., 2015), these findings collectively suggest that the balance between the amount of vitamin B2 and B9 as well as the type of bacteria and its metabolism are critical factors in determining MAIT cell activation.

CONCLUSION

There are many immune cells in the intestine, where biological communication between dietary components and microorganisms produces numerous kinds of metabolites. These dietary or microbial metabolites affect cell composition and function and alter energy metabolism. Accumulating evidence has revealed the importance of these changes in cell composition, function, and energy metabolism in the control of host immune responses and the subsequent incidence of inflammatory, allergic, and infectious diseases. It should be noted that not all of the results obtained in the rodent models can be directly translated to humans, because their diets and commensal bacteria differ greatly. In this context, it is important to utilize cohort studies and clinical data that include the effects of antibiotic treatment. In addition, it will be important to apply novel and/or improved technologies such as single-cell omics, whole-genome sequencing, non-target metabolomics, and bioinformatics in future research. Understanding the integrated mechanisms by which diet, microbiota, and metabolites influence the function of the immune system would be an interesting topic for future study that could provide new strategies for the control of immune and infectious diseases.

AUTHOR CONTRIBUTIONS

All authors listed have made a substantial, direct and intellectual contribution to the work, and approved it for publication.

ACKNOWLEDGMENTS

This review article contains results obtained from our studies that were supported at least in part by grants from the Core Research for Evolutional Science and Technology Program of the Japan Agency for Medical Research and Development (HK); by the Ministry of Education, Culture, Sports, Science, and Technology of Japan (Grants-in-Aid for Scientific Research S [HK; 23229004], for Scientific Research B [JK; 26293111], for Scientific Research on Innovative Areas [JK; 16H01373], for Young Scientists B [NS; 17K17686], and for a JSPS Research Fellow [NS; 17J07480]); by the Practical Research Project for Allergic Diseases and Immunology (Research on Allergic Diseases and Immunology) and for the Research on Development of New Drugs (Adjuvant Database Project) from the Japan Agency for Medical Research and Development (AMED; JK, and HK) and by the Ministry of Health, Labour and Welfare (MHLW) (JK); by the Science and Technology Research Promotion Program for Agriculture, Forestry, Fisheries, and Food Industry (JK); and by the Astellas Foundation for Research on Metabolic Disorders (JK), the Public Health Research Foundation for Public Health Science (NS), the Terumo Foundation for Life Science and Arts (JK), and the Suzuken Memorial Foundation (JK).

REFERENCES

Are, A., Aronsson, L., Wang, S., Greicius, G., Lee, Y. K., Gustafsson, J. A., et al. (2008). Enterococcus faecalis from newborn babies regulate endogenous PPARgamma activity and IL-10 levels in colonic epithelial cells. *Proc. Natl. Acad. Sci. U.S.A.* 105, 1943–1948. doi: 10.1073/pnas.0711734105

Arita, M. (2012). Mediator lipidomics in acute inflammation and resolution. *J. Biochem.* 152, 313–319. doi: 10.1093/jb/mvs092

Bassaganya-Riera, J., Viladomiu, M., Pedragosa, M., De Simone, C., Shaykhutdinov, R., Carbo, A., et al. (2012). Probiotic bacteria produce conjugated linoleic acid locally in the gut that targets macrophage PPAR gamma to suppress colitis. *PLOS ONE* 7:e31238. doi: 10.1371/journal.pone.0031238

Bolognini, D., Tobin, A. B., Milligan, G., and Moss, C. E. (2016). The pharmacology and function of receptors for short-chain fatty acids. *Mol. Pharmacol.* 89, 388–398. doi: 10.1124/mol.115.102301

Bourhis, L. L., Mburu, Y. K., and Lantz, O. (2013). MAIT cells, surveyors of a new class of antigen: development and functions. *Curr. Opin. Immunol.* 25, 174–180. doi: 10.1016/j.coi.2013.01.005

Browne, H. P., Neville, B. A., Forster, S. C., and Lawley, T. D. (2017). Transmission of the gut microbiota: spreading of health. *Nat. Rev. Microbiol.* 15, 531–543. doi: 10.1038/nrmicro.2017.50

Buck, M. D., Sowell, R. T., Kaech, S. M., and Pearce, E. L. (2017). Metabolic instruction of immunity. *Cell* 169, 570–586. doi: 10.1016/j.cell.2017.04.004

Chiang, N., Fredman, G., Backhed, F., Oh, S. F., Vickery, T., Schmidt, B. A., et al. (2012). Infection regulates pro-resolving mediators that lower antibiotic requirements. *Nature* 484, 524–528. doi: 10.1038/nature11042

Claus, S. P., Tsang, T. M., Wang, Y., Cloarec, O., Skordi, E., Martin, F. P., et al. (2008). Systemic multicompartmental effects of the gut microbiome on mouse metabolic phenotypes. *Mol. Syst. Biol.* 4:219. doi: 10.1038/msb.2008.56

Correa, R. O., Fachi, J. L., Vieira, A., Sato, F. T., and Vinolo, M. A. R. (2016). Regulation of immune cell function by short-chain fatty acids. *Clin. Exp. Immunol.* 5:e73. doi: 10.1038/cti.2016.17

de Kivit, S., Tobin, M. C., Forsyth, C. B., Keshavarzian, A., and Landay, A. L. (2014). Regulation of intestinal immune responses through TLR activation: implications for pro- and prebiotics. *Front. Immunol.* 5:60. doi: 10.3389/fimmu.2014.00060

den Besten, G., van Eunen, K., Groen, A. K., Venema, K., Reijngoud, D. J., and Bakker, B. M. (2013). The role of short-chain fatty acids in the interplay between diet, gut microbiota, and host energy metabolism. *J. Lipid Res.* 54, 2325–2340. doi: 10.1194/jlr.R036012

Digby, J. E., Martinez, F., Jefferson, A., Ruparelia, N., Chai, J., Wamil, M., et al. (2012). Anti-inflammatory effects of nicotinic acid in human monocytes are mediated by GPR109A dependent mechanisms. *Arterioscler. Thromb. Vasc. Biol.* 32, 669–676. doi: 10.1161/ATVBAHA.111.241836

Eckle, S. B., Birkinshaw, R. W., Kostenko, L., Corbett, A. J., McWilliam, H. E., Reantragoon, R., et al. (2014). A molecular basis underpinning the T cell receptor heterogeneity of mucosal-associated invariant T cells. *J. Exp. Med.* 211, 1585–1600. doi: 10.1084/jem.20140484

Endres, S., Ghorbani, R., Kelley, V. E., Georgilis, K., Lonnemann, G., Van Der Meer, J. W. M., et al. (1989). The effect of dietary supplementation with n-3 polyunsaturated fatty acids on the synthesis of interleukin-1 and tumor necrosis factor by mononuclear cells. *N. Engl. J. Med.* 320, 265–271. doi: 10.1056/NEJM198902023200501

Frank, R. A., Leeper, F. J., and Luisi, B. F. (2007). Structure, mechanism and catalytic duality of thiamine-dependent enzymes. *Cell Mol. Life Sci* 64, 892–905. doi: 10.1007/s00018-007-6423-5

Fukui, N., Honda, K., Ito, E., and Ishikawa, K. (2009). Peroxisome proliferator-activated receptor γ negatively regulates allergic rhinitis in mice. *Allergol. Int. Off. J. Jpn. Soc. Allergol.* 58, 247–253. doi: 10.2332/allergolint.08-OA-0047

Furusawa, Y., Obata, Y., Fukuda, S., Endo, T. A., Nakato, G., Takahashi, D., et al. (2013). Commensal microbe-derived butyrate induces the differentiation of colonic regulatory T cells. *Nature* 504, 446–450. doi: 10.1038/nature12721

Gurav, A., Sivaprakasam, S., Bhutia, Y. D., Boettger, T., Singh, N., and Ganapathy, V. (2015). Slc5a8, a Na+-coupled high-affinity transporter for short-chain fatty acids, is a conditional tumour suppressor in colon that protects against colitis and colon cancer under low-fibre dietary conditions. *Biochem. J.* 469, 267–278. doi: 10.1042/BJ20150242

Hirata, S. I., and Kunisawa, J. (2017). Gut microbiome, metabolome, and allergic diseases. *Allergol. Int.* 66, 523–528. doi: 10.1016/j.alit.2017.06.008

Hosomi, K., and Kunisawa, J. (2017). The specific roles of vitamins in the regulation of immunosurveillance and maintenance of immunologic homeostasis in the gut. *Immune Netw.* 17, 13–19. doi: 10.4110/in.2017.17.1.13

Hoverstad, T., and Midtvedt, T. (1986). Short-chain fatty acids in germfree mice and rats. *J. Nutr.* 116, 1772–1776.

Huskisson, E., Maggini, S., and Ruf, M. (2007). The role of vitamins and minerals in energy metabolism and well-being. *J. Int. Med. Res.* 35, 277–289. doi: 10.1177/147323000703500301

Iraporda, C., Errea, A., Romanin, D. E., Cayet, D., Pereyra, E., Pignataro, O., et al. (2015). Lactate and short chain fatty acids produced by microbial fermentation downregulate proinflammatory responses in intestinal epithelial cells and myeloid cells. *Immunobiology* 220, 1161–1169. doi: 10.1016/j.imbio.2015.06.004

Kelly, D., Campbell, J. I., King, T. P., Grant, G., Jansson, E. A., Coutts, A. G., et al. (2004). Commensal anaerobic gut bacteria attenuate inflammation by regulating nuclear-cytoplasmic shuttling of PPAR-gamma and RelA. *Nat. Immunol.* 5, 104–112. doi: 10.1038/ni1018

Kishino, S., Takeuchi, M., Park, S. B., Hirata, A., Kitamura, N., Kunisawa, J., et al. (2013). Polyunsaturated fatty acid saturation by gut lactic acid bacteria affecting host lipid composition. *Proc. Natl. Acad. Sci. U.S.A.* 110, 17808–17813. doi: 10.1073/pnas.1312937110

Kjer-Nielsen, L., Patel, O., Corbett, A. J., Le Nours, J., Meehan, B., Liu, L., et al. (2012). MR1 presents microbial vitamin B metabolites to MAIT cells. *Nature* 491, 717–723. doi: 10.1038/nature11605

Kunisawa, J. (2017). Metabolic changes during B cell differentiation for the production of intestinal IgA antibody. *Cell Mol. Life Sci.* 74, 1503–1509. doi: 10.1007/s00018-016-2414-8

Kunisawa, J., Arita, M., Hayasaka, T., Harada, T., Iwamoto, R., Nagasawa, R., et al. (2015a). Dietary omega3 fatty acid exerts anti-allergic effect through the conversion to 17,18-epoxyeicosatetraenoic acid in the gut. *Sci. Rep.* 5:9750. doi: 10.1038/srep09750

Kunisawa, J., and Kiyono, H. (2015). Vitamins mediate immunological homeostasis and diseases at the surface of the body. *Endocr. Metab. Immune Disord. Drug Targets* 15, 25–30. doi: 10.2174/1871530314666141021114651

Kunisawa, J., Sugiura, Y., Wake, T., Nagatake, T., Suzuki, H., Nagasawa, R., et al. (2015b). Mode of bioenergetic metabolism during B cell differentiation in the intestine determines the distinct requirement for vitamin B1. *Cell Rep.* 13, 122–131. doi: 10.1016/j.celrep.2015.08.063

Lin, M. Y., de Zoete, M. R., van Putten, J. P. M., and Striijbis, K. (2015). Redirection of epithelial immune responses by short-chain fatty acids through inhibition of histone deacetylases. *Front. Immunol.* 6:554. doi: 10.3389/fimmu.2015.00554

Lipszyc, P. S., Cremaschi, G. A., Zubilete, M. Z., Bertolino, M. L., Capani, F., Genaro, A. M., et al. (2013). Niacin modulates pro-inflammatory cytokine secretion. A potential mechanism involved in its anti-atherosclerotic effect. *Open Cardiovasc. Med. J.* 7, 90–98. doi: 10.2174/1874192401307010090

Macia, L., Tan, J., Vieira, A. T., Leach, K., Stanley, D., Luong, S., et al. (2015). Metabolite-sensing receptors GPR43 and GPR109A facilitate dietary fibre-induced gut homeostasis through regulation of the inflammasome. *Nat. Commun.* 6:6734. doi: 10.1038/ncomms7734

Magnusdottir, S., Ravcheev, D., de Crécy-Lagard, V., and Thiele, I. (2015). Systematic genome assessment of B-vitamin biosynthesis suggests co-operation among gut microbes. *Front. Genet.* 6:148. doi: 10.3389/fgene.2015.00148

Martin, F. P., Sprenger, N., Yap, I. K., Wang, Y., Bibiloni, R., Rochat, F., et al. (2009). Panorganismal gut microbiome-host metabolic crosstalk. *J. Proteome Res.* 8, 2090–2105. doi: 10.1021/pr801068x

Mills, E. L., Kelly, B., and O'Neill, L. A. J. (2017). Mitochondria are the powerhouses of immunity. *Nat. Immunol.* 18, 488–498. doi: 10.1038/ni.3704

Mirmonsef, P., Zariffard, M. R., Gilbert, D., Makinde, H., Landay, A. L., and Spear, G. T. (2012). Short-chain fatty acids induce pro-inflammatory cytokine production alone and in combination with toll-like receptor ligands. *Am. J. Reprod. Immunol.* 67, 391–340.

Miyamoto, J., Mizukure, T., Park, S. B., Kishino, S., Kimura, I., Hirano, K., et al. (2015). A gut microbial metabolite of linoleic acid, 10-hydroxy-cis-12-octadecenoic acid, ameliorates intestinal epithelial barrier impairment partially via GPR40-MEK-ERK pathway. *J. Biol. Chem.* 290, 2902–2918. doi: 10.1074/jbc.M114.610733

Oh, J. Z., Ravindran, R., Chassaing, B., Carvalho, F. A., Maddur, M. S., Bower, M., et al. (2014). TLR5-mediated sensing of gut microbiota is necessary for antibody responses to seasonal influenza vaccination. *Immunity* 41, 478–492. doi: 10.1016/j.immuni.2014.08.009

Patel, O., Kjer-Nielsen, L., Le Nours, J., Eckle, S. B., Birkinshaw, R., Beddoe, T., et al. (2013). Recognition of vitamin B metabolites by mucosal-associated invariant T cells. *Nat. Commun.* 4:2142. doi: 10.1038/ncomms3142

Raqib, R., Sarker, P., Bergman, P., Ara, G., Lindh, M., Sack, D. A., et al. (2006). Improved outcome in shigellosis associated with butyrate induction of an endogenous peptide antibiotic. *Proc. Natl. Acad. Sci. U.S.A.* 103, 9178–9183. doi: 10.1073/pnas.0602888103

Ricote, M., Li, A. C., Willson, T. M., Kelly, C. J., and Glass, C. K. (1998). The peroxisome proliferator-activated receptor-γ is a negative regulator of macrophage activation. *Nature* 391, 79–82. doi: 10.1038/34178

Sakurai, T., Miyazawa, S., Furuta, S., and Hashimoto, T. (1982). Riboflavin deficiency and beta-oxidation systems in rat liver. *Lipids* 17, 598–604. doi: 10.1007/BF02535365

Schwab, J. M., Chiang, N., Arita, M., and Serhan, C. N. (2007). Resolvin E1 and protectin D1 activate inflammation-resolution programmes. *Nature* 447, 869–874. doi: 10.1038/nature05877

Serhan, C. N. (2017). Treating inflammation and infection in the 21st century: new hints from decoding resolution mediators and mechanisms. *FASEB J.* 31, 1273–1288. doi: 10.1096/fj.201601222R

Singh, N., Gurav, A., Sivaprakasam, S., Brady, E., Padia, R., Shi, H., et al. (2014). Activation of Gpr109a, receptor for niacin and the commensal metabolite butyrate, suppresses colonic inflammation and carcinogenesis. *Immunity* 40, 128–139. doi: 10.1016/j.immuni.2013.12.007

Smith, P. M., Howitt, M. R., Panikov, N., Michaud, M., Gallini, C. A., Bohlooly, Y. M., et al. (2013). The microbial metabolites, short-chain fatty acids, regulate colonic Treg cell homeostasis. *Science* 341, 569–573. doi: 10.1126/science.1241165

Spite, M., Norling, L. V., Summers, L., Yang, R., Cooper, D., Petasis, N. A., et al. (2009). Resolvin D2 is a potent regulator of leukocytes and controls microbial sepsis. *Nature* 461, 1287–1291. doi: 10.1038/nature08541

Suzuki, H., and Kunisawa, J. (2015). Vitamin-mediated immune regulation in the development of inflammatory diseases. *Endocr. Metab. Immune Disord. Drug Targets* 15, 212–215. doi: 10.2174/18715303156661503161 22128

Tan, J., McKenzie, C., Vuillermin, P. J., Goverse, G., Vinuesa, C. G., Mebius, R. E., et al. (2016). Dietary fiber and bacterial SCFA enhance oral tolerance and protect against food allergy through diverse cellular pathways. *Cell Rep.* 15, 2809–2824. doi: 10.1016/j.celrep.2016.05.047

Thwaites, D. T., and Anderson, C. M. (2007). H+-coupled nutrient, micronutrient and drug transporters in the mammalian small intestine. *Exp. Physiol.* 92, 603–619. doi: 10.1113/expphysiol.2005.029959

Trompette, A., Gollwitzer, E. S., Yadava, K., Sichelstiel, A. K., Sprenger, N., Ngom-Bru, C., et al. (2014). Gut microbiota metabolism of dietary fiber influences allergic airway disease and hematopoiesis. *Nat. Med.* 20, 159–166. doi: 10.1038/nm.3444

Weber, P. C., Fischer, S., Schacky, C. V., Lorenz, R., and Strasser, T. (1986). The conversion of dietary eicosapentaenoic acid to prostanoids and leukotrienes in man. *Prog. Lipid Res.* 25, 273–276. doi: 10.1016/0163-7827(86)90056-1

White, C. A., Pone, E. J., Lam, T., Tat, C., Hayama, K. L., Li, G., et al. (2014). Histone deacetylase inhibitors upregulate B cell microRNAs that silence AID and Blimp-1 expression for epigenetic modulation of antibody and autoantibody responses. *J. Immunol.* 193, 5933–5950. doi: 10.4049/jimmunol.1401702

Wong, J. M., de Souza, R., Kendall, C. W., Emam, A., and Jenkins, D. J. (2006). Colonic health: fermentation and short chain fatty acids. *J. Clin. Gastroenterol.* 40, 235–243. doi: 10.1097/00004836-200603000-00015

Wu, W., Sun, M., Chen, F., Cao, A. T., Liu, H., Zhao, Y., et al. (2017). Microbiota metabolite short-chain fatty acid acetate promotes intestinal IgA response to microbiota which is mediated by GPR43. *Mucosal Immunol.* 10, 946–956. doi: 10.1038/mi.2016.114

12

Fecal Microbiota Transplantation, Commensal *Escherichia coli* and *Lactobacillus johnsonii* Strains Differentially Restore Intestinal and Systemic Adaptive Immune Cell Populations Following Broad-Spectrum Antibiotic Treatment

*Ira Ekmekciu[1], Eliane von Klitzing[1], Christian Neumann[2,3], Petra Bacher[2], Alexander Scheffold[2,3], Stefan Bereswill[1] and Markus M. Heimesaat[1]**

[1] Intestinal Microbiology Research Group, Institute of Microbiology, Charité – Universitätsmedizin Berlin, corporate member of Freie Universität Berlin, Humboldt-Universität zu Berlin, and Berlin Institute of Health, Berlin, Germany, [2] Department of Cellular Immunology, Clinic for Rheumatology and Clinical Immunology, Charité – Universitätsmedizin Berlin, corporate member of Freie Universität Berlin, Humboldt-Universität zu Berlin, and Berlin Institute of Health, Berlin, Germany, [3] German Rheumatism Research Center, Leibniz Association, Berlin, Germany

***Correspondence:**
Markus M. Heimesaat
markus.heimesaat@charite.de

The essential role of the intestinal microbiota in the well-functioning of host immunity necessitates the investigation of species-specific impacts on this interplay. Aim of this study was to examine the ability of defined Gram-positive and Gram-negative intestinal commensal bacterial species, namely *Escherichia coli* and *Lactobacillus johnsonii*, respectively, to restore immune functions in mice that were immunosuppressed by antibiotics-induced microbiota depletion. Conventional mice were subjected to broad-spectrum antibiotic treatment for 8 weeks and perorally reassociated with *E. coli*, *L. johnsonii* or with a complex murine microbiota by fecal microbiota transplantation (FMT). Analyses at days (d) 7 and 28 revealed that immune cell populations in the small and large intestines, mesenteric lymph nodes and spleens of mice were decreased after antibiotic treatment but were completely or at least partially restored upon FMT or by recolonization with the respective bacterial species. Remarkably, *L. johnsonii* recolonization resulted in the highest CD4+ and CD8+ cell numbers in the small intestine and spleen, whereas neither of the commensal species could stably restore those cell populations in the colon until d28. Meanwhile less efficient than FMT, both species increased the frequencies of regulatory T cells and activated dendritic cells and completely restored intestinal memory/effector T cell populations at d28. Furthermore, recolonization with either single species maintained pro- and anti-inflammatory immune functions in parallel. However, FMT could most effectively recover the decreased frequencies of cytokine producing CD4+ lymphocytes in mucosal and systemic compartments. *E. coli* recolonization increased the production of cytokines such as TNF, IFN-γ, IL-17, and IL-22, particularly in the small intestine. Conversely, only *L. johnsonii* recolonization maintained colonic IL-10 production. In summary,

FMT appears to be most efficient in the restoration of antibiotics-induced collateral damages to the immune system. However, defined intestinal commensals such as *E. coli* and *L. johnsonii* have the potential to restore individual functions of intestinal and systemic immunity. In conclusion, our data provide novel insights into the distinct role of individual commensal bacteria in maintaining immune functions during/following dysbiosis induced by antibiotic therapy thereby shaping host immunity and might thus open novel therapeutical avenues in conditions of perturbed microbiota composition.

Keywords: commensal intestinal microbiota, *Escherichia coli*, *Lactobacillus johnsonii*, fecal microbiota transplantation, secondary abiotic (gnotobiotic) mice, intestinal mucosal and peripheral and central immunity, immune-modulating effects, immune restoration

INTRODUCTION

Approximately 10^{13} microorganisms, collectively known as microbiota, reside in the human gastrointestinal tract (Sender et al., 2016) and have increasingly received well-deserved attention regarding their deep impact on the physiology and well-being of the mammalian host. The microbiota composition is characterized by vast inter-individual variations and is furthermore influenced by numerous factors, including genetics (Org et al., 2015), mode of delivery (Biasucci et al., 2010), age (Palmer et al., 2007), diet (Ericsson and Franklin, 2015), hospitalization (Penders et al., 2006), exposure to pathogens and/or antibiotics (Buffie et al., 2012; Carding et al., 2015). It has been shown that bacteria belonging to the phyla *Firmicutes*, *Bacteroidetes*, *Proteobacteria*, *Actinobacteria*, and *Fusobacteria* comprise the vast majority of the mammalian intestinal microbiota (Eckburg et al., 2005; Palmer et al., 2007; Hill et al., 2012) and both bacterial density and diversity increase from the proximal to the distal gut (Sommer and Backhed, 2013). *Firmicutes* are Gram-positive bacteria, which include the large class of *Clostridia* and the lactic acid bacteria (Zhang et al., 2015), while *Escherichia coli* (Gram-negative, rod-shaped bacteria belonging to the family *Enterobacteriaceae* and phylum *Proteobacteria*) represent the predominant facultative anaerobe member of the mammalian gastrointestinal tract (Finegold et al., 1983; Tenaillon et al., 2010). The small intestinal microbiota is dominated by the families *Lactobacillaceae* and *Enterobacteriaceae*, whereas species from the families *Bacteroidaceae*, *Prevotellaceae*, *Rikenellaceae*, *Lachnospiraceae*, and *Ruminococcaceae* can be detected in the colon (Donaldson et al., 2016). While the microbiota is of paramount importance for numerous metabolic processes, including vitamin synthesis (LeBlanc et al., 2013) and digestion of dietary compounds (Backhed et al., 2005), compelling evidence points toward its impact on the maturation, development and function of the innate and adaptive immune system of the host (Macpherson and Harris, 2004; Sommer and Backhed, 2013).

Lactic acid bacteria exert important functions in the modulation of immune responses and have successfully been used as probiotics in inflammatory conditions of mice and men. For instance, *Lactobacillus rhamnosus* GG has been shown to exert preventive and therapeutic effects in atopic eczema and dermatitis (Isolauri et al., 2000; Kalliomaki et al., 2001, 2003; Viljanen et al., 2005). Moreover, treating IL-10 deficient mice with *L. plantarum* attenuated the severity of colonic inflammation by reducing mucosal IL-12p40 and IFN-γ levels (Schultz et al., 2002). In our own previous work, we could further demonstrate that a single commensal *L. johnsonii* strain was able to attenuate both intestinal mucosal and systemic pro-inflammatory immune responses upon murine infection with the enteropathogen *Campylobacter jejuni* (Bereswill et al., 2017). Kwon et al. (2010) have proposed that the observed beneficial anti-inflammatory properties may be elicited due to induction of regulatory DCs and regulatory T cells (Treg).

Gram-negative commensals, such as members of the family *Enterobacteriaceae*, tend to be neglected, but may, nevertheless, be potent immune-modulators (Zeuthen et al., 2006). This is best corroborated by the probiotic strain *E. coli* Nissle 1917, which has conclusively been shown efficient in the treatment of ulcerative colitis and is considered as an effective alternative to the standard maintenance therapy, i.e., mesalazine (Kruis et al., 2004; Henker et al., 2008; Schultz, 2008).

Importantly, Hessle et al. (2000, 2005) and Skovbjerg et al. (2010) have shown the differing impact of Gram-positive and Gram-negative bacteria on the modulation of cytokine production patterns, given that *in vitro* co-culturing of human PBMC with Gram-positive bacteria leads to elevated levels of IL-12, IL-1β, IFN-γ, and TNF, while Gram-negative bacteria rather induce IL-6, IL-8, and IL-10. In contrast, from monocytes derived human DC have been shown to produce comparable levels of IL-12 and TNF in response to commensal Gram-positive and Gram-negative bacteria (Karlsson et al., 2004; Zeuthen et al., 2006).

Murine studies have further underlined the impact of individual bacterial species on distinct immune cell populations. For instance, segmented filamentous bacteria (SFB) have been identified to induce the expansion of IL-17 producing Th17 cells (Ivanov et al., 2008), while *Clostridium* species of clusters IV and XIVa promoted accumulation of Treg in the colonic lamina propria (LP) of mice (Atarashi et al., 2011). The differentiation of CD4+ T cells into Treg locally in the LP as well as in the

Abbreviations: ABx, secondary abiotic; BSA, bovine serum albumin; CFU, colony forming units; DC, dendritic cells; FMT, fecal microbiota transplantation; IFN-γ, interferon-γ; IL, interleukin; LPL, lamina propria lymphocytes; LPS, lipopolysaccharide; MLN, mesenteric lymph nodes; PBS, phosphate buffered saline; PBMC, peripheral blood mononuclear cells; PP, Peyer's patches; PSA, polysaccharide A; SFB, segmented filamentous bacteria; SPF, special pathogen free; Th, T helper cell; TLR, toll-like receptor; TNF, tumor necrosis factor; Treg, regulatory T cells.

circulation is also supported by TLR-2 mediated sensing of the Gram-negative bacterium *Bacteroides fragilis* (Round et al., 2011). Moreover, treatment of IL-$10^{-/-}$ mice with *L. plantarum* has been shown to attenuate the severity of colonic inflammation by reducing mucosal IL-12p40 and IFN-γ levels (Schultz et al., 2002). However, elucidating the differential impact of Gram-positive and Gram-negative commensals on the immune cell homeostasis in *in vivo* models, and identifying the species specific mechanisms of immunomodulation remains difficult and challenging, yet of utmost interest.

In our previous works, we have shown that normally developed mice rendered void of intestinal microbiota through a quintuple antibiotic therapy (i.e., secondary abiotic mice, ABx mice), display numerous changes of intestinal mucosal and systemic immune cell subsets, which can, however, almost completely be restored through reintroduction of intestinal antigens via fecal microbiota transplantation (FMT) (Ekmekciu et al., 2017a,b). Furthermore we were able to demonstrate that recolonization of ABx mice with VSL#3, a probiotic mixture consisting of eight bacterial species (namely *Streptococcus thermophilus, Bifidobacterium breve, B. longum, B. infantis, Lactobacillus acidophilus, L. plantarum, L. paracasei,* and *L. delbrueckii* subsp. *bulgaricus*), elicits IL-10 production by lymphocytes in the small and large intestinal LP, MLN and spleen, but does not influence the production of pro-inflammatory cytokines (Ekmekciu et al., 2017a,b). The impact of probiotics on cytokine production has been extensively investigated, and it has been proposed, that some strains might promote mainly IL-12 production, thus inducing Th1 type immune responses, which are known to protect from pathogens. Other strains, however, more effectively impacted the production of the anti-inflammatory IL-10, thereby limiting excessive immune responses as observed in autoimmune and allergic diseases, for instance (Fujiwara et al., 2004; Foligne et al., 2007; Shida et al., 2011).

Niess et al. (2008) have previously further addressed the role of commensal organisms in the recruitment of pro-inflammatory cytokine producing CD4+ cells in the colonic lamina propria and proposed that these cell types might contribute to the immunopathogenesis of colitis. However, a fine-tuned balance between pro- and anti-inflammatory immune responses at mucosal and systemic sites is of utmost importance for the vertebrate host. For instance, a reduction of the IL-17 producing Th17 cell compartment playing a pivotal role in protection against bacterial and fungal pathogens (Aujla et al., 2007) may explain the increased susceptibility of microbiota depleted mice to pathogens (Croswell et al., 2009; Stiemsma et al., 2014).

In the present study, we investigated the role of two important representatives of Gram-negative (namely *E. coli*) and Gram-positive (namely *L. johnsonii*) commensals, both derived from the gut microbiota of healthy mice, in restoring numbers of distinct immune cell subsets following antibiotic treatment as compared to FMT in C57Bl/6j ABx mice. To address this, we analyzed the immune responses exerted by lymphocytes within the small and large intestinal LP, MLN and spleen of microbiota-depleted mice upon reassociation with *E. coli* or *L. johnsonii* and upon FMT at day (d) 7 and d28 post recolonization. We furthermore surveyed the cytokine production patterns assessing TNF, IFN-γ, IL-17, IL-22, and IL-10 secretion by CD4+ lymphocytes in respective compartments.

MATERIALS AND METHODS

Ethics Statement

All animal experiments were conducted according to the European Guideline for animal welfare (2010/63/EU) with approval from the commission for animal experiments headed by the "Landesamt für Gesundheit und Soziales" (LaGeSo, Berlin, Germany, registration numbers G0097/12 and G0184/12). Animal welfare was examined twice daily by assessment of clinical conditions including weight loss.

Generation of Secondary Abiotic (Gnotobiotic) Mice

All animals were bred, raised and housed in the facilities of the "Forschungseinrichtungen für Experimentelle Medizin" (FEM, Charité – University Medicine Berlin, Germany) under specific pathogen-free (SPF) conditions. Secondary abiotic mice were generated through quintuple antibiotic treatment for 8 weeks via the drinking water as previously described (Heimesaat et al., 2006; Bereswill et al., 2011; Fiebiger et al., 2016; Ekmekciu et al., 2017a,b).

Bacterial Recolonization

Three days prior bacterial recolonization experiments, the antibiotic cocktail was withdrawn and replaced by sterile drinking water (*ad libitum*). Successful depletion of the intestinal microbiota was confirmed and FMT performed as described previously (Ekmekciu et al., 2017a,b). Furthermore, secondary abiotic mice were recolonized with 10^9 CFU of either *E. coli* or *L. johnsonii* in 0.3 ml PBS (Gibco Life Technologies, Paisley, United Kingdom) by gavage on day 0. The applied *E. coli* strain constitutes a commensal isolate derived from a naive conventionally colonized C57BL/6j wildtype mouse and did not express known virulence factors such as stx 1 and 2, hlyA, cspA, catA, katA, and astA as confirmed in a reference laboratory (Heimesaat et al., 2007; Haag et al., 2012). The *L. johnsonii* strain had initially been isolated from the feces of a healthy female 3 months old C57BL/6j wildtype mouse as previously described (Bereswill et al., 2017). For FMT fresh murine fecal samples were collected from 10 age and sex matched SPF control mice, pooled, dissolved in 10 ml sterile PBS and the supernatant perorally applied by gavage (in 0.3 ml PBS) in order to reconstitute secondary abiotic (i.e., gnotobiotic) mice with a complex intestinal microbiota as shown previously (Heimesaat et al., 2006; Ekmekciu et al., 2017a,b).

Sampling Procedures

Mice were sacrificed by isoflurane treatment (Abbott, Greifswald, Germany) at d7 or d28 following bacterial recolonization. Luminal large intestinal samples as well as *ex vivo* biopsies from spleen, MLN, ileum, and colon were taken under sterile conditions. Intestinal samples were collected in parallel for microbiological and immunological analyses.

Quantitative Analysis of Bacterial Colonization

Total intestinal loads of *E. coli* and *L. johnsonii* were quantitated in fecal and colonic samples over time post recolonization or upon necropsy. Respective samples were dissolved in PBS and serial dilutions streaked onto appropriate solid culture media: *E. coli* was detected on Columbia agar supplemented with 5% sheep blood and MacConkey agar (Oxoid, Wesel, Germany) following aerobic incubation at 37°C for 48 h. *L. johnsonii* loads were determined on Columbia agar supplemented with 5% sheep blood, Columbia-CNA agar supplemented with colistin and nalidixic acid and MRS agar (all from Oxoid) in parallel and incubated under microaerobic and obligate anaerobic conditions (in jars using CampyGen and AnaeroGen gas packs, respectively; both from Oxoid) at 37°C for at least 2 days. Bacterial species were identified according to their typical morphological appearances and biochemical properties. The detection limit of viable bacteria was ≈100 CFU/g.

Lymphocyte Isolation from Spleen and Mesenteric Lymph Nodes

Single cell suspensions were generated from spleens and MLN, and erythrocytes were removed from splenic samples by 1.66% ammonium chloride. All samples were resuspended in volumes of 5 ml (spleen) and 2 ml (MLN) PBS/0.5% BSA (Sigma–Aldrich, St. Louis, MO, United States) and subjected to further processing (Cording et al., 2013).

Lamina Propria Lymphocyte Isolation

Lamina propria lymphocyte isolation followed a standard protocol with minor modifications as described previously (Sheridan and Lefrancois, 2012; Ekmekciu et al., 2017b). Briefly, the intestines were cut into 0.5 cm pieces and incubated twice in 25 ml 1 mM dithioerythritol (DTE; Carl Roth) in Hanks balanced salt solution (HBSS; Gibco) for 20 min at 37°C at 220 rpm. Afterward the intestines were introduced to 1.3 mM ethylenediaminetetraacetic acid (EDTA; life technologies, Eugene, OR, United States) solution in HBSS and were shaken again twice herein for 30 min at 37°C at 220 rpm. After each incubation, the epithelial cell layer containing the intraepithelial lymphocytes was removed by intensive vortexing and passing through a 70 μm cell strainer, and new solution (DTE or EDTA) was added. After the second EDTA incubation the cells were washed with RPMI 1640 (Gibco) containing 5% fetal calf serum (FCS; Biochrom, Berlin, Germany) and were subsequently placed in 35 ml digestion solution containing 0.5 mg/ml collagenase A (Roche, Mannheim, Germany), 0.5 mg/ml DNAse I (Roche), 10% FCS, 1 mM of each $CaCl_2$ and $MgCl_2$ (both Carl Roth) in RPMI 1640 (Gibco). Digestion was performed through incubation for 45 min at 37°C and 220 rpm. After incubation the digested tissues were washed in RPMI supplemented with 5% FCS and centrifuged for 6 min at 4°C and 350 × *g*. The pellets were resuspended in 5 ml 44% Percoll (GE Healthcare, Uppsala, Sweden) and overlaid on 5 ml 67% Percoll in a 15 ml Falcon tube. Percoll gradient separation was performed by centrifugation at 600 × *g* for 20 min at room temperature. LPL were collected from the interphase, washed once and suspended in 1 ml of PBS/0.5% BSA.

Surface and Intracellular Stainings and Flow Cytometry

Surface staining was performed using a mix of the following antibodies: FITC-anti-CD4 (Clone RM4-5; 1:200), PerCP-anti-CD8 (Clone 53-6.7; 1:100), PacBlue-anti-B220 (Clone RA3-6B2, 1:200), APC-Cy7-anti-CD25 (Clone PC61, 1:200), PE-anti-CD44 (Clone IM7, 1:200), APC-anti-CD86 (Clone B7-2, 1:200) (all from BD Biosciences, San Jose, CA, United States).

For intracellular staining cells from spleen, MLN and intestinal LP were restimulated for 5 h with 10 ng/ml phorbol myristate acetate (PMA) and 1 μg/ml ionomycin, in a tissue culture incubator at 37°C (both Sigma–Aldrich). The 10 μg/ml brefeldin A (Sigma–Aldrich) were added to the cell suspensions after 1 h of polyclonal restimulation. Then cells were treated with LIVE/DEAD Fixable Aqua Dead Cell Stain kit (life technologies) and hereafter fixed with 2% paraformaldehyde (PFA; Sigma–Aldrich) for 20 min at room temperature. Cells were stained in 0.5% saponin (Sigma–Aldrich) using a mix of the following antibodies: PacBlue-Anti-CD4 (Clone RM4-5; 1:400), PE-Cy7-anti-IFN-γ (Clone XMG 1.2; 1:400), APC-Cy7-anti-TNF-α (Clone MP6-XT22; 1:400) (all three from BD Biosciences), FITC-anti-IL17A (Clone TC11-18H10.1; 1:200, BioLegend, San Diego, CA, United States), PE-anti-IL10 (Clone JESS-16E3; 1:100), APC-anti-IL22 (Clone IL22JOP; 1:100) (both from eBioscience). After gating for lymphocytes and excluding doublets only living cells were included in further analyses. CD4 and CD8 cells were gated on living cells, whereas CD86+ (activated dendritic) cells were identified in the CD4-CD8- compartment. All data were acquired on a MACSQuant analyzer (Miltenyi Biotec, Bergisch Gladbach, Germany) and were analyzed with FlowJo Software v10.1 (Tree star, Ashland, OR, United States).

Statistical Analysis

Medians, means, standard deviations (SD) and significance levels were determined using Mann–Whitney *U* test or one-way analysis of variance (ANOVA) with Tukey's *post hoc* test for multiple comparisons (GraphPad Prism Software v6, La Jolla, CA, United States) as indicated. Two-sided probability (p) values ≤ 0.05 were considered significant. Experiments were reproduced twice and pooled data are shown ($n = 8$–15 per group).

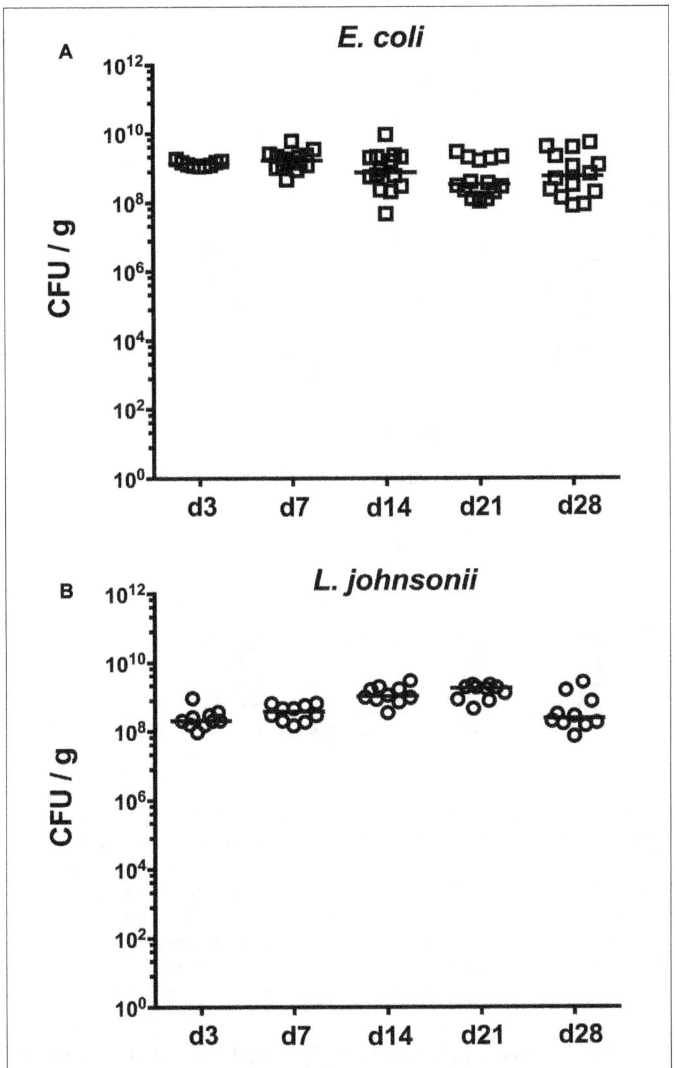

FIGURE 1 | Kinetics of intestinal bacterial colonization densities following bacterial recolonization of secondary abiotic mice. Secondary abiotic mice were generated by broad-spectrum antibiotic treatment and perorally recolonized with **(A)** *E. coli* (open squares) or **(B)** *L. johnsonii* (open circles) on day (d) 0 as described in "Materials and Methods." Bacterial colonization densities were assessed in fecal samples (colony forming units per gram, CFU/g) over time upon recolonization as indicated by culture. Medians (black bars) are indicated. Data were pooled from three independent experiments.

RESULTS

Kinetics of Intestinal Colonization Densities Following Recolonization of Secondary Abiotic Mice with *E. coli* or *L. johnsonii*

In the present study, we investigated the immunomodulatory properties of representative Gram-negative or Gram-positive intestinal bacterial species (namely, *E. coli* and *L. johnsonii*, respectively) in comparison to a complex gut microbiota in mice that had been treated with broad-spectrum antibiotic compounds. To address this, conventionally reared mice were subjected to a quintuple antibiotic cocktail rendering them secondary abiotic (Ekmekciu et al., 2017a,b), and after a sufficient wash-out period ABx mice were perorally recolonized with respective bacterial species or the complex intestinal microbiota by FMT. Importantly, the intestinal microbiota composition of ABx mice that had been subjected to FMT was comparable to naive conventionally colonized counterparts as confirmed previously (Ekmekciu et al., 2017a,b). As early as 3 days upon initial recolonization we assessed intestinal colonization efficiencies of respective species over time (**Figure 1**). Cultural analyses of fecal samples revealed that *E. coli* (**Figure 1A**) and *L. johnsonii* (**Figure 1B**) stably colonized the murine intestinal tract, both with high median loads of $>10^8$ CFU per gram feces until necropsy at d28. Of note, none of the interventions carried out in this study (i.e., antibiotic treatment, recolonization with *E. coli*/*L. johnsonii*, FMT) led to any adverse clinical effects in mice such as wasting, diarrhea, occurrence of blood in feces or microscopic signs of intestinal inflammation including epithelial apoptosis (data not shown).

T Cell Populations in Murine Intestinal and Systemic Compartments Following FMT or Recolonization of Secondary Abiotic Mice with *E. coli* or *L. johnsonii*

To examine the impact of *E. coli* and *L. johnsonii* versus complex gut microbiota on distinct immune cell populations after antibiotic microbiota depletion, we isolated lymphocytes from small and large intestinal LP, MLN and spleen and analyzed defined immune cell populations by flow cytometry on d7 and d28 post recolonization. Firstly, we analyzed the CD4+ (**Figures 2**, **3**) and CD8+ lymphocytes (**Supplementary Figures S1**, **S2**) and assessed both the relative abundances (i.e., percentages) and the absolute cell numbers of respective immune cell populations. After the antibiotic treatment the abundance of CD4+ T helper lymphocytes declined in both the small and large intestines, but could be fully restored upon FMT ($p < 0.05$–0.001; **Figures 2A,B**). Mice harboring *E. coli* or *L. johnsonii* displayed slightly higher percentages of CD4+ cells in their small intestine without reaching significant levels (n.s. vs ABx; **Figure 2A**). In the colon, however, *E. coli* recolonization resulted in higher frequencies of CD4+ cells at d7, but decreased again until d28 (**Figure 2A**). Interestingly, in the MLN the percentage of the CD4+ lymphocytes was at its lowest at d7 post FMT ($p < 0.05$ vs. N; **Figure 2C**), but reached naive levels thereafter. In the spleens of *L. johnsonii* colonized mice we detected higher frequencies of CD4+ lymphocytes than in their with *E. coli* colonized counterparts at d28 ($p < 0.05$–0.01; **Figure 2D**). Furthermore, *L. johnsonii* recolonization led to the highest absolute CD4+ cell numbers in the murine small intestine ($p < 0.05$–0.001; **Figure 3A**). At d7 following either recolonization higher numbers of CD4+ lymphocytes could be observed in the colonic LP as compared to ABx mice ($p < 0.05$–0.01; **Figure 3B**), but declined until d28. Notably, at d28 after *L. johnsonii* colonization mice also displayed the highest numbers of CD4+ cells in the

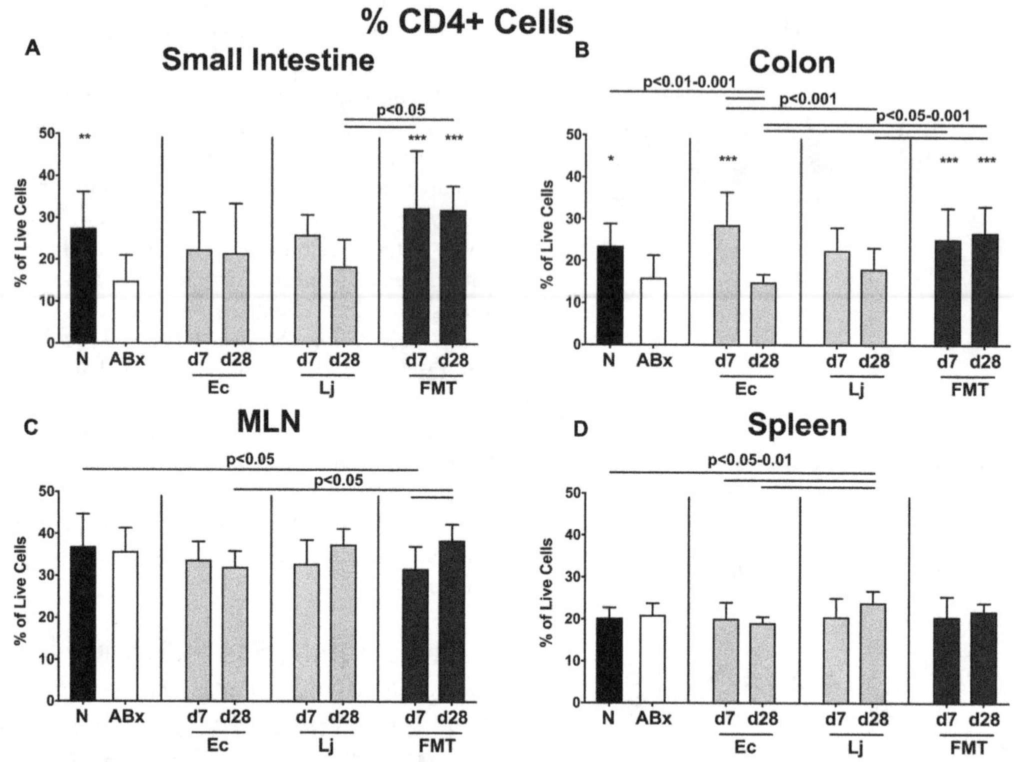

FIGURE 2 | Percentages of CD4+ cells in intestinal and systemic compartments of secondary abiotic and recolonized mice. Secondary abiotic mice were generated by broad-spectrum antibiotic treatment and perorally recolonized by gavage. Subsequently, lymphocytes from small intestinal and colonic lamina propria, MLN and spleen were isolated, and analyzed by flow cytometry as described in "Materials and Methods." The percentages of the CD4+ lymphocyte population within the **(A)** small intestine, **(B)** colon, **(C)** MLN, and **(D)** spleen of naive conventional mice (N), secondary abiotic mice (ABx) and mice re-associated with either *E. coli* (Ec), *L. johnsonii* (Lj) or complex intestinal microbiota by FMT on d7 and d28 post-recolonization are depicted. Columns represent means +SD. Significance levels (*p*-values) determined with one-way ANOVA test followed by Tukey post-correction test for multiple comparisons are indicated. Significant differences as compared to secondary abiotic mice are indicated by asterisks (*$p < 0.05$; **$p < 0.01$; ***$p < 0.001$). Data were pooled from three independent experiments.

splenic (and hence systemic) compartment ($p < 0.05$–0.001; **Figure 3D**).

Interestingly, the microbiota depletion-induced decreases of the CD8+ cell abundances within the small and large intestinal LP were accompanied by increases of these cells in the spleen ($p < 0.01$–0.001 ABx vs. naive; **Supplementary Figures S1A,B,D**). Single strain mono-colonization could restore this cell population in the small intestine rather late, i.e., until d28 post recolonization with either *E. coli* or *L. johnsonii* ($p < 0.05$–0.001; **Supplementary Figure S1**). Remarkably, neither *E. coli* nor *L. johnsonii* colonization impacted the decline of colonic CD8+ cell numbers, which could only be restored upon FMT at d28 (**Supplementary Figure S1B**). At d7 post FMT, mice displayed the lowest frequencies of CD8+ cells in their MLN, which, however, increased until d28 (**Supplementary Figure S1C**). Moreover, at d7 following either recolonization, mice exerted lower percentages of splenic CD8+ cells than their ABx counterparts ($p < 0.05$–0.001; **Supplementary Figure S1D**). This effect, however, could be preserved over time in *E. coli* recolonized mice only. Remarkably, mice harboring single commensal species in their gut displayed higher CD8+ lymphocyte numbers in the small intestinal LP at d28 as compared to mice that had been subjected to FMT ($p < 0.05$–0.001; **Supplementary Figure S2A**). Until d7, however, only *L. johnsonii* but not *E. coli* could sufficiently restore the antibiotics-induced decreased colonic CD8+ lymphocytes ($p < 0.01$ vs. ABx; **Supplementary Figure S2B**). In line with the splenic CD4+ lymphocytes, the highest splenic CD8+ lymphocyte numbers could be detected in *L. johnsonii* colonized mice at d28 post recolonization ($p < 0.001$; **Supplementary Figure S2D**).

Activated T Cells (Including Treg), Memory/Effector T Cells and Activated Dendritic Cells in Murine Intestinal and Systemic Compartments Following FMT or Recolonization of Secondary Abiotic Mice with *E. coli* or *L. johnsonii*

We further expanded our investigations by analyzing the activation status of defined immune cell populations. Therefore we stained for surface markers CD25 (**Figure 4**), CD44 (**Figure 5** and **Supplementary Figure S3**) and CD86 (**Supplementary Figure S4**) characteristic for activated T cells (including Treg), memory/effector T cells and activated DCs, respectively (Sprent and Surh, 2002; Wallet et al., 2005;

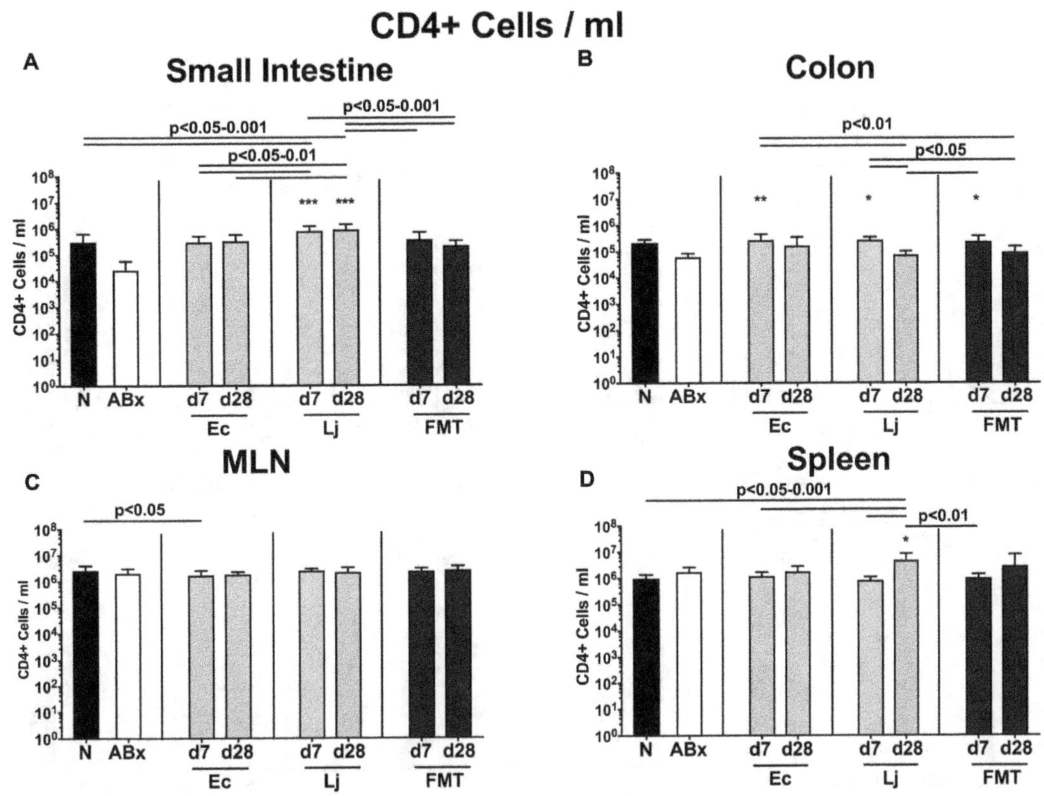

FIGURE 3 | Absolute cell numbers of CD4+ cells in intestinal and systemic compartments of secondary abiotic and recolonized mice. Secondary abiotic mice were generated by broad-spectrum antibiotic treatment and perorally recolonized by gavage. Subsequently, lymphocytes from small intestinal and colonic lamina propria, MLN and spleen were isolated, and analyzed by flow cytometry as described in "Materials and Methods." Concentrations of CD4+ lymphocytes in the **(A)** small intestine, **(B)** colon, **(C)** MLN, and **(D)** spleen of naive conventional mice (N), secondary abiotic mice (ABx) and mice re-associated with either *E. coli* (Ec), *L. johnsonii* (Lj) or complex intestinal microbiota by FMT on d7 and d28 post-recolonization are depicted. Columns represent means +SD. Significance levels (*p*-values) determined with one-way ANOVA test followed by Tukey post-correction test for multiple comparisons are indicated. Significant differences as compared to secondary abiotic mice are indicated by asterisks (*$p < 0.05$; **$p < 0.01$; ***$p < 0.001$). Data were pooled from three independent experiments.

Ostman et al., 2006). Broad-spectrum antibiotic treatment led to a significant reduction of the CD4+CD25+ abundances in all analyzed immunological compartments (**Figures 4A–D**). At d7 post FMT, mice displayed the highest percentages of CD4+CD25+ cells, which were even higher than in naive untreated SPF controls. However, both *E. coli* and *L. johnsonii* induced a significant increase of CD25 expression in lymphocytes derived from the small intestine, colon and spleen as early as d7 post recolonization ($p < 0.05$–0.001 vs. ABx; **Figures 4A,B,D**), whereas notably, *L. johnsonii* exerted a more pronounced effect than *E. coli* in the colon at d7 ($p < 0.05$–0.001 vs. Ec; **Figure 4B**). Moreover, only *L. johnsonii* was able to restore CD4+CD25+ cells in the MLN ($p < 0.001$ vs. ABx; **Figure 4C**).

Similarly, microbiota-depleted mice exhibited an overall reduction of the CD4+CD44+ memory/effector cell subset ($p < 0.001$ vs. N; **Figures 5A–D**). In the small and large intestine *E. coli, L. johnsonii* and FMT were equally capable of restoring this cell population as early as d7 post recolonization ($p < 0.01$–0.001 vs. ABx; **Figures 5A,B**). This also held true for the MLN, albeit in this compartment *L. johnsonii* could restore the abundances of CD4+CD44+ cells only rather late in the course, i.e., until d28 post recolonization. In contrast, *E. coli*, but not *L. johnsonii* colonization resulted in restored frequencies of splenic memory CD4+ cells at d28 post recolonization ($p < 0.001$ vs. ABx; **Figure 5D**).

Moreover, reduced abundances of CD8+CD44+ cells could be observed in the small intestine, colon, MLN and spleen of with antibiotics treated mice ($p < 0.001$ vs. N; **Supplementary Figures S3A–D**). Already at d7 following recolonization (regardless of the regimen) frequencies of CD8+ memory cells were elevated in the small intestine and spleen, whereas, in contrast to FMT, either single species colonization could normalize colonic CD8+ memory cells only until d28. In the MLN, *E. coli* was able to restore the CD8+ memory/effector cells more effectively than *L. johnsonii*, considering that abundances of CD8+CD44+ cells were comparable in *E. coli* mono-associated and naive mice (**Supplementary Figure S3C**).

The expression of the surface molecule CD86, a co-stimulatory protein marking activated DC, showed a strong intestinal

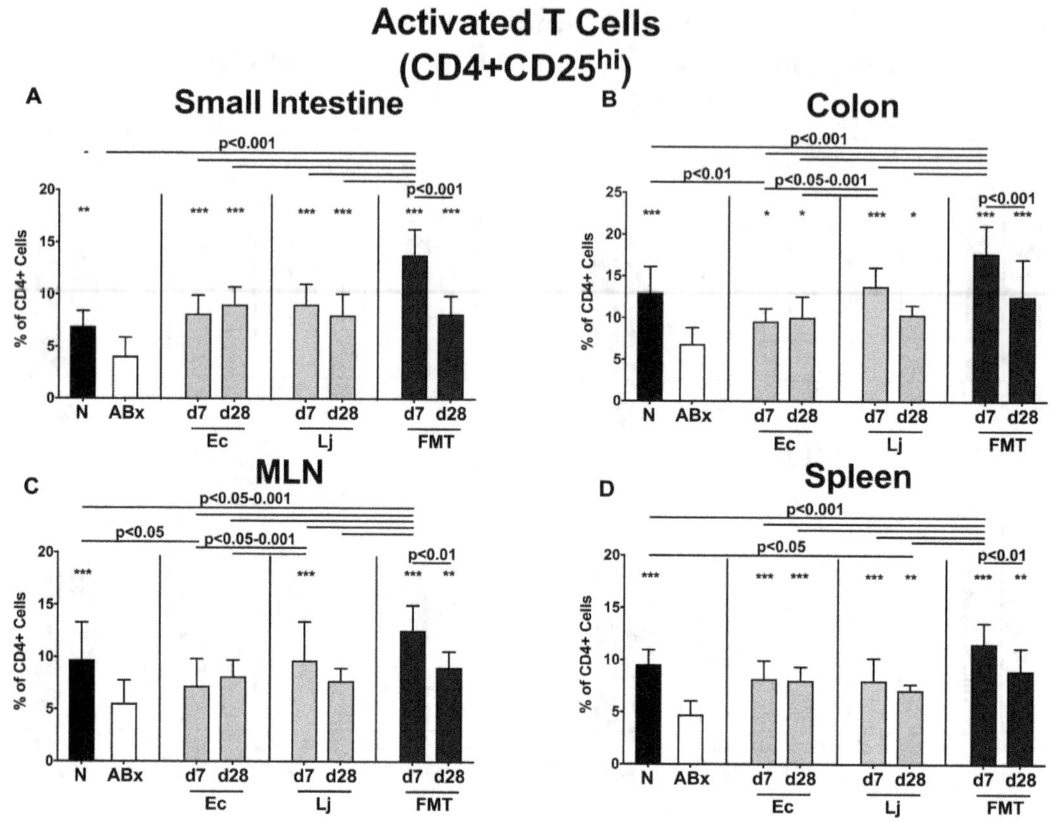

FIGURE 4 | Activated T cells (including Treg) in intestinal and systemic compartments of secondary abiotic and recolonized mice. Secondary abiotic mice were generated by broad-spectrum antibiotic treatment and perorally recolonized by gavage. Subsequently, lymphocytes from small intestinal and colonic lamina propria, MLN and spleen were isolated, and analyzed by flow cytometry as described in "Materials and Methods." The frequencies of activated T cells (including Treg, CD4+CD25+, gated on CD4+ cells) in the **(A)** small intestine, **(B)** colon, **(C)** MLN and **(D)** spleen of naive conventional mice (N), secondary abiotic mice (ABx) and mice re-associated with either *E. coli* (Ec), *L. johnsonii* (Lj) or complex intestinal microbiota by FMT on d7 and d28 post-recolonization are depicted. Columns represent means +SD. Significance levels (*p*-values) determined with one-way ANOVA test followed by Tukey post-correction test for multiple comparisons are indicated. Significant differences as compared to secondary abiotic mice are indicated by asterisks ($^*p < 0.05$; $^{**}p < 0.01$; $^{***}p < 0.001$). Data were pooled from three independent experiments.

microbiota dependence, as indicated by a strong reduction of CD86+ cells in mucosal and systemic compartments of secondary abiotic mice ($p < 0.001$ vs. N; **Supplementary Figures S4A–D**). Small intestinal CD86+ cells in mice harboring single bacterial species were more abundant than in ABx mice, however, lower than in their naive or with FMT treated counterparts (**Supplementary Figure S4A**). Moreover, only FMT, but neither *E. coli* nor *L. johnsonii*, could recover this antibiotics-induced reduction of CD86+ cell frequencies in the MLN until d28 (**Supplementary Figure S4C**). Splenic CD86+ cells displayed the highest abundance at d7 post FMT, but could also be restored to basal naive levels by either *E. coli* or *L. johnsonii* recolonization alone ($p < 0.001$ vs. ABx; **Supplementary Figure S4C**).

Taken together, our data indicate that depending on the respective immunological compartment and immune cell subset, single bacterial commensal species may be as effective as complex microbiota in reversing antibiotics induced collateral damages on intestinal mucosal and systemic immunity.

Production of Pro- and Anti-inflammatory Cytokines by CD4+ Cells in Murine Intestinal and Systemic Compartments Following FMT or Recolonization of Secondary Abiotic Mice with *E. coli* or *L. johnsonii*

We further addressed the impact of *E. coli* and *L. johnsonii* recolonization on the cytokine production pattern of CD4+ lymphocytes in intestinal mucosal, peripheral and systemic immunological sites and therefore determined the frequencies of TNF (**Figure 6**), IFN-γ (**Figure 7**), IL-17 (**Figure 8**), IL-22 (**Figure 9**), and IL-10 (**Figure 10**) producing CD4+ lymphocytes in the small and large intestines, MLN and spleens of recolonized mice.

The antibiotics-induced decreases of TNF producing CD4+ cells in the small and large intestines were accompanied by increased abundances in the MLN and spleen ($p < 0.01$–0.001 ABx vs. N; **Figures 6A–D**). Small intestinal TNF production was at it highest at d7 following *E. coli* recolonization,

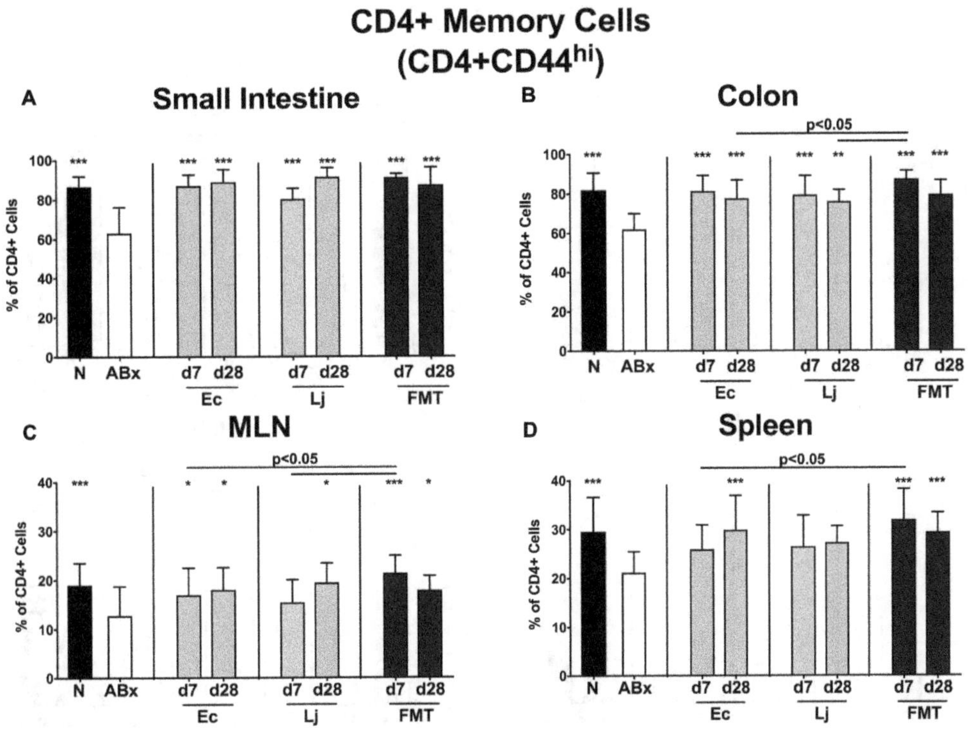

FIGURE 5 | CD4+ memory/effector T cells in intestinal and systemic compartments of secondary abiotic and recolonized mice. Secondary abiotic mice were generated by broad-spectrum antibiotic treatment and perorally recolonized by gavage. Subsequently, lymphocytes from small intestinal and colonic lamina propria, MLN and spleen were isolated, and analyzed by flow cytometry as described in "Materials and Methods." The proportions of CD4+ memory/effector cells ($CD4+CD44^{hi}$, gated on CD4+ cells) in the **(A)** small intestine, **(B)** colon, **(C)** MLN and **(D)** spleen of naive conventional mice (N), secondary abiotic mice (ABx) and mice re-associated with either *E. coli* (Ec), *L. johnsonii* (Lj) or complex intestinal microbiota by FMT on d7 and d28 post-recolonization are depicted. Columns represent means +SD. Significance levels (*p*-values) determined with one-way ANOVA test followed by Tukey post-correction test for multiple comparisons are indicated. Significant differences as compared to secondary abiotic mice are indicated by asterisks ($^{*}p < 0.05$; $^{**}p < 0.01$; $^{***}p < 0.001$). Data were pooled from three independent experiments.

but further declined thereafter, while it remained unaffected by *L. johnsonii* during the entire observation period. In addition, either recolonization regimen resulted in higher abundances of TNF producing CD4+ cells in the colonic LP at d7, whereas none of them could sustain this effect until d28. Of note, microbial reassociation of ABx mice dampened TNF production in the MLN ($p < 0.05$–0.01 vs. ABx; **Figure 6C**), except for FMT at d28. *E. coli* and complex microbiota could additionally reduce the TNF production in the spleen at d7 ($p < 0.01$–0.001 vs. ABx, n.s. vs. N; **Figure 6D**).

Furthermore, a significant reduction of IFN-γ producing CD4+ cells could be detected in the small and large intestines of secondary abiotic mice ($p < 0.001$ vs. N; **Figures 7A,B**). *E. coli* at d7 and d28, as well as *L. johnsonii* and FMT at d7 could completely restore the IFN-γ production in the small intestine. Colonic IFN-γ expressing CD4+ cells also increased upon either recolonization regimen at d7 ($p < 0.001$; **Figure 7B**). In contrast, IFN-γ production remained largely unaffected by antibiotic treatment and subsequent bacterial reassociation in the MLN and spleen of mice (**Figures 7C,D**).

Furthermore, IL-17 expressing CD4+ cells were strongly diminished in all analyzed immunological compartments upon microbial depletion, but could be fully restored by FMT ($p < 0.05$–0.001; **Figures 8A–D**). Mono-association with *E. coli* resulted in elevated IL-17 production in the small intestine and colon at both d7 and d28, as well as in the MLN at d7 and spleen at d28 (**Figures 8A–D**). Mice harboring *L. johnsonii* alone displayed higher abundances of CD4+IL17+ cells than ABx mice in the colon and spleen at d7 post recolonization. In addition, decreased percentages of IL-22 producing CD4+ cells following broad-spectrum antibiotic treatment were detected in either compartment ($p < 0.01$–0.001; **Figures 9A–D**). Small intestinal IL-22 expression was most distinctly induced by *E. coli* as early as d7 and by FMT at d7 only (**Figure 9A**). Mono-associated mice further displayed slightly higher abundances of colonic IL-22 producing CD4+ cells than their ABx counterparts, which were, however, only significantly higher in the case of *E. coli* at d7 ($p < 0.05$ vs. ABx; **Figure 9B**). Either recolonization regimen could restore the CD4+IL22+ immune cell subset in the MLN at d7, but only *E. coli* was able to sustain this effect until d28. Moreover, recolonized mice showed similar frequencies of IL-22 producing CD4+ lymphocytes in the systemic compartment as their naive, untreated counterparts, regardless of the intervention or time point ($p < 0.05$–0.001; **Figures 9C,D**).

Overall, the IL-10 expressing CD4+ lymphocytes were down-regulated in the absence of the intestinal microbiota

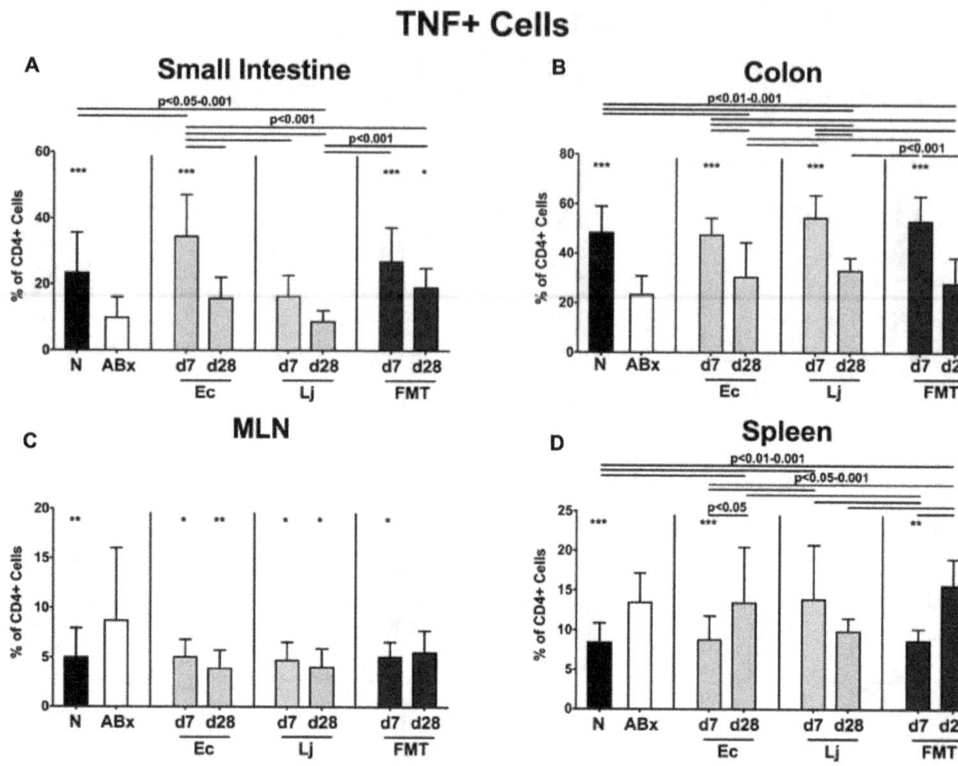

FIGURE 6 | TNF producing CD4+ cells in intestinal and systemic compartments of secondary abiotic and recolonized mice. Secondary abiotic mice were generated by broad-spectrum antibiotic treatment and perorally recolonized by gavage. Subsequently, lymphocytes were isolated from small intestinal and colonic lamina propria, MLN, and spleen and stimulated with PMA/ionomycin in presence of brefeldin A and subsequently analyzed by flow cytometry. The percentages of IFN-γ producing CD4+ cells in the **(A)** small intestine, **(B)** colon, **(C)** MLN and **(D)** spleen of naive conventional mice (N), secondary abiotic mice (ABx) and mice re-associated with either *E. coli* (Ec), *L. johnsonii* (Lj) or complex intestinal microbiota by FMT on d7 and d28 post-recolonization are depicted. Columns represent means +SD. Significance levels (p-values) determined with one-way ANOVA test followed by Tukey post-correction test for multiple comparisons are indicated. Significant differences as compared to secondary abiotic mice are indicated by asterisks (*$p < 0.05$; **$p < 0.01$; ***$p < 0.001$). Data were pooled from three independent experiments.

($p < 0.05$–0.001; **Figures 10A–D**). Both *E. coli* and *L. johnsonii* mono-colonization, however, could sufficiently restore the CD4+IL10+ cells in the small intestines, whereas only *L. johnsonii* could achieve this effect in the colon (**Figures 10A,B**). Increased abundances of IL-10 producing CD4+ cells were also detected upon *E. coli* recolonization at d7 in the MLN and d28 in both MLN and spleen. The IL-10 production in the MLN and spleen could also be restored at d7 following *L. johnsonii* recolonization, but this effect could not be sustained until d28 post recolonization.

DISCUSSION

In the present study, we aimed at comparing the short- and long-term effects of a single representative Gram-negative and Gram-positive intestinal commensal species, namely of *E. coli* and *L. johnsonii*, respectively, versus the complex gut microbiota in shaping host immunity following antibiotics-induced microbiota depletion. These species were chosen for the following reasons. Firstly, both commensals are common inhabitants of the intestinal ecosystem, and although lactobacilli are quantitatively more abundant than *E. coli* (Castillo et al., 2006), the latter represents the predominant facultative anaerobe Gram-negative strain within the mammalian gastrointestinal tract (Finegold et al., 1983; Tenaillon et al., 2010). Furthermore, in our previous works we could confirm differential immunomodulatory properties of either strain under defined immunopathological conditions. For instance, *E. coli*, but not *L. johnsonii*, aggravated Th1-driven pro-inflammatory immune responses in murine ileitis (Heimesaat et al., 2006, 2007). Furthermore, *L. johnsonii* was able to attenuate intestinal and systemic pro-inflammatory and to augment anti-inflammatory immune responses upon *C. jejuni* infection of secondary abiotic mice (Bereswill et al., 2017), and has further been shown to be effective against enteric including infectious morbidities (Lievin-Le Moal and Servin, 2014), hence resulting in its commercial probiotic application (e.g., Nestlé LC1).

Here, we unraveled immunomodulatory properties of respective commensals at two different time points following recolonization of antibiotics-treated mice, but in the absence of immunopathological conditions. Performing kinetic analysis in this context is important, given that intestinal responses are

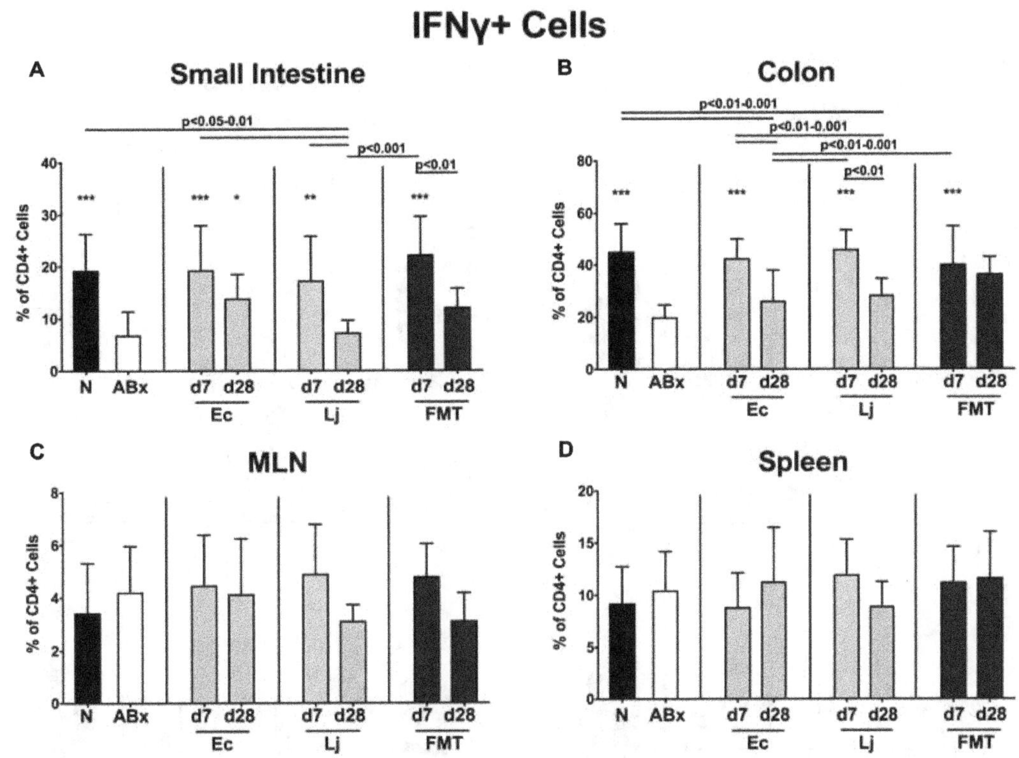

FIGURE 7 | IFN-γ producing CD4+ cells in intestinal and systemic compartments of secondary abiotic and recolonized mice. Secondary abiotic mice were generated by broad-spectrum antibiotic treatment and perorally recolonized by gavage. Subsequently, lymphocytes were isolated from small intestinal and colonic lamina propria, MLN, and spleen and stimulated with PMA/ionomycin in presence of brefeldin A and subsequently analyzed by flow cytometry. The percentages of TNF producing CD4+ cells in the **(A)** small intestine, **(B)** colon, **(C)** MLN and **(D)** spleen of naive conventional mice (N), secondary abiotic mice (ABx) and mice re-associated with either *E. coli* (Ec), *L. johnsonii* (Lj) or complex intestinal microbiota by FMT on d7 and d28 post-recolonization are depicted. Columns represent means +SD. Significance levels (*p*-values) determined with one-way ANOVA test followed by Tukey post-correction test for multiple comparisons are indicated. Significant differences as compared to secondary abiotic mice are indicated by asterisks (* $p < 0.05$; ** $p < 0.01$; *** $p < 0.001$). Data were pooled from three independent experiments.

highly dynamic over time after the transfer of microbiota into germ-free animals (El Aidy et al., 2012; Tomas et al., 2015).

Cultural analysis of fecal samples revealed that either commensal strain was able to stably colonize the murine intestinal tract at high intestinal loads throughout the observation period. Our previous work revealed that upon cessation of antibiotic therapy neither regrowth of intestinal bacterial commensals nor changes in the immune cell populations could be observed, further supporting that the observed immune responses of the mucosal and systemic sites can be exclusively attributed to defined bacterial commensal recolonization (Ekmekciu et al., 2017a,b).

Overall, single-strain recolonization appeared to be, to some extent, less effective in restoring immune cell populations after broad-spectrum antibiotic treatment than the complex microbiota upon FMT, given that mono-colonized mice displayed a lack of full recovery of affected cell populations. Following mono-colonization of mice both common and strict strain-specific immune responses could be observed over time. For instance, *E. coli* and *L. johnsonii* had a minor impact on the relative abundances of intestinal CD4+ and CD8+ cells when compared to antibiotics-treated mice, while FMT resulted in cell percentages comparable to naive conventionally colonized counterparts. Furthermore, *E. coli*, but not *L. johnsonii* recolonization could increase colonic CD4+ abundances at d7, but not later on. Whereas small intestinal CD8+ cells could be reestablished only rather late upon mono-colonization, colonic CD8+ cells were virtually unaffected. In the systemic compartment, however, the observed increases in percentages of splenic CD8+ cells in microbiota-depleted mice could be reversed by both *E. coli* and *L. johnsonii* until d7, and remained lower in *E. coli* recolonized mice later on. These results underline the importance of examining immunological sequelae of gut microbiota-interventive strategies, not only at mucosal surfaces, but also on the systemic level of the immune system, given that the presence/absence and distinct composition of the gut microbiota might also affect splenic lymphocytes. This rationale is supported by the former findings that the *Bacteroides fragilis* driven differentiation of Treg was not limited to the LP, but could also be detected in the circulation (Round et al., 2011).

Interestingly, recolonization with *L. johnsonii* resulted in highest CD4+ lymphocyte numbers in the small intestinal LP, supporting former evidence from a clinical investigation, where the application of another *Lactobacillus* strain, namely *L. reuteri*,

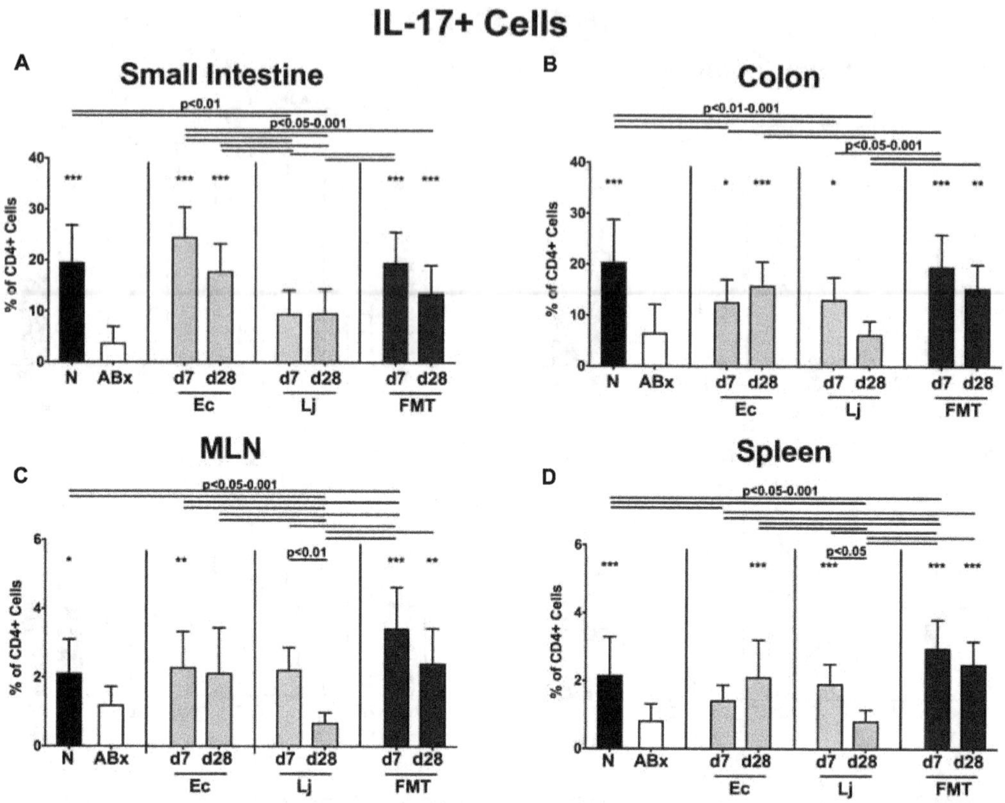

FIGURE 8 | IL-17 producing CD4+ cells in intestinal and systemic compartments of secondary abiotic and recolonized mice. Secondary abiotic mice were generated by broad-spectrum antibiotic treatment and perorally recolonized by gavage. Subsequently, lymphocytes were isolated from small intestinal and colonic lamina propria, MLN, and spleen and stimulated with PMA/ionomycin in presence of brefeldin A and subsequently analyzed by flow cytometry. The percentages of IL-17 producing CD4+ cells in the **(A)** small intestine, **(B)** colon, **(C)** MLN and **(D)** spleen of naive conventional mice (N), secondary abiotic mice (ABx) and mice re-associated with either *E. coli* (Ec), *L. johnsonii* (Lj) or complex intestinal microbiota by FMT on d7 and d28 post-recolonization are depicted. Columns represent means +SD. Significance levels (*p*-values) determined with one-way ANOVA test followed by Tukey post-correction test for multiple comparisons are indicated. Significant differences as compared to secondary abiotic mice are indicated by asterisks (**p* < 0.05; ***p* < 0.01; ****p* < 0.001). Data were pooled from three independent experiments.

led to a significant increase in ileal CD4+ cells (Valeur et al., 2004). In our study, either commensal strain was able to promote CD25 expression on CD4+ lymphocytes in the small and large intestines as well as in the spleen, but only *L. johnsonii* was able to achieve the same effect in MLN. Of note, at d7 following recolonization, *L. johnsonii* was a stronger inducer of the colonic activated T cells (including Treg) than *E. coli*. The dependence of Treg on intestinal bacterial antigens has been demonstrated before. Atarashi et al. (2011) showed that treatment of mice with vancomycin, an antibiotic compound directed mainly against Gram-positive bacteria, resulted in reduced numbers of colonic Treg (Zarkan et al., 2016). A study conducted with germ-free rats revealed that colonic CD25+ cells were higher in animals co-colonized with *E. coli* and *L. plantarum* 299v, than in those harboring *E. coli* alone (Herías et al., 1999). This indicates that increased microbiota diversity and synergistic effects between species may elicit a stronger immunomodulatory effect on activated T cells and the Treg population, which is supported by our findings that FMT induced the most prominent expression of CD25 in all analyzed immunological compartments.

Unlike FMT, single-strain recolonization resulted in an only partial restoration of the intestinal activated DC (CD86+) cells, which remained, however, lower than in untreated SPF mice. Former evidence suggests, that the activation, maturation and cytokine production of DC upon bacterial stimulation is highly dose dependent (Evrard et al., 2011). Our data indicate that the activation of DC may furthermore be dependent on the diversity of presented microbial antigens.

In vitro studies applying PBMC revealed that Gram-positive and Gram-negative bacteria differentially induced cytokine expression patterns (Hessle et al., 2000, 2005; Skovbjerg et al., 2010). Therefore we analyzed the production of pro- and anti-inflammatory cytokines, including TNF, IFN-γ, IL-17, IL-22, and IL-10 in mice following recolonization with either *E. coli* or *L. johnsonii*. Intestinal *E. coli* colonization had a more prominent effect on TNF production by lymphocytes than *L. johnsonii*. At d7 following *E. coli* application, TNF levels measured in intestinal, peripheral and systemic immune compartments were comparable to those in naive mice. However, this effect could

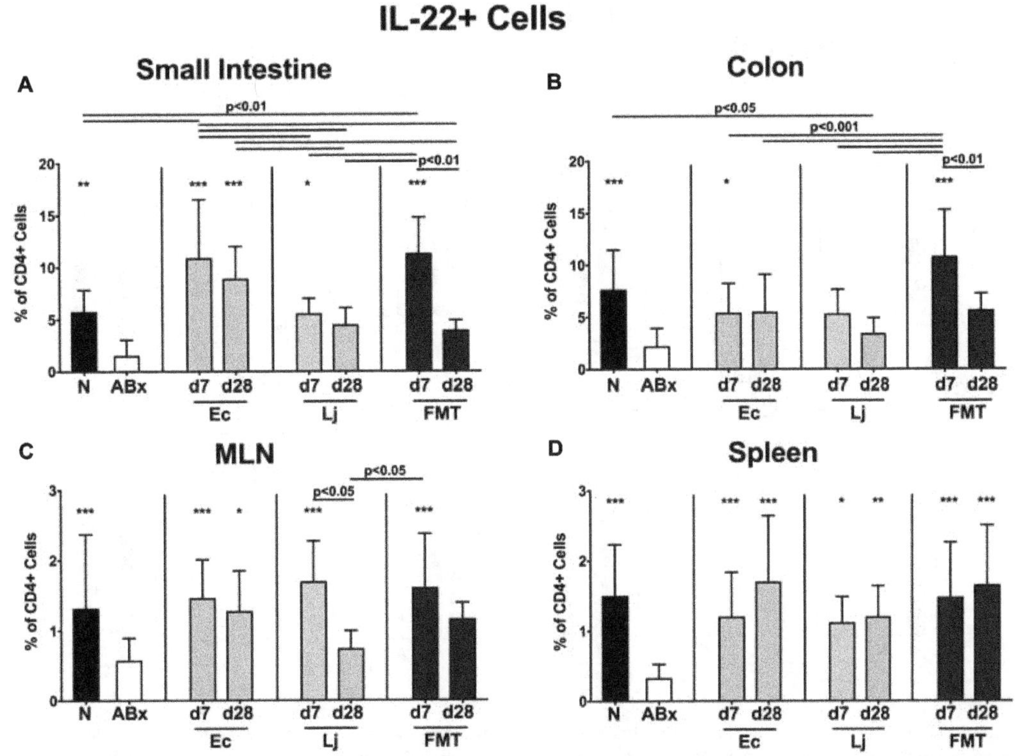

FIGURE 9 | IL-22 producing CD4+ cells in intestinal and systemic compartments of secondary abiotic and recolonized mice. Secondary abiotic mice were generated by broad-spectrum antibiotic treatment and perorally recolonized by gavage. Subsequently, lymphocytes were isolated from small intestinal and colonic lamina propria, MLN, and spleen and stimulated with PMA/ionomycin in presence of brefeldin A and subsequently analyzed by flow cytometry. The percentages of IL-22 producing CD4+ cells in the **(A)** small intestine, **(B)** colon, **(C)** MLN and **(D)** spleen of naive conventional mice (N), secondary abiotic mice (ABx) and mice re-associated with either *E. coli* (Ec), *L. johnsonii* (Lj) or complex intestinal microbiota by FMT on d7 and d28 post-recolonization are depicted. Columns represent means +SD. Significance levels (*p*-values) determined with one-way ANOVA test followed by Tukey post-correction test for multiple comparisons are indicated. Significant differences as compared to secondary abiotic mice are indicated by asterisks ($^*p < 0.05$; $^{**}p < 0.01$; $^{***}p < 0.001$). Data were pooled from three independent experiments.

be preserved until d28 in MLN only. While excessive TNF production has conclusively been linked to chronic inflammation in numerous organs including the gastrointestinal tract (Kollias et al., 1999; Popa et al., 2007), it is important to recognize the protective roles of TNF against epithelial injury and disease susceptibility. In a murine ileitis model increased TNF levels resulted in improved epithelial barrier functions and prevention from disease onset (Pagnini et al., 2009). Moreover, TNF deficient mice were more prone to acute colitis, thus leading to the conclusion that TNF might have protective functions in normal gut homeostasis and intestinal epithelial integrity (Naito et al., 2003). Rakoff-Nahoum et al. (2004) suggested that the production of intestinal epithelial tissue-protective factors, including TNF, is regulated via TLR-mediated recognition of commensal bacteria, while we here provide further evidence that the adaptive immune system may also contribute to this effect.

Furthermore, both *E. coli* and *L. johnsonii* were able to promote the small intestinal and colonic production of IFN-γ by CD4+ cells as early as d7 post recolonization, whereas this cytokine remained highly expressed until d28 only in the small intestines of *E. coli* recolonized mice. The abundance of IFN-γ expressing CD4+ lymphocytes in the MLN and spleen remained unaffected by any of the interventions. These data seem to contradict *in vitro* findings, which suggest that Gram-positive bacteria tend to be stronger inducers of IFN-γ and TNF than Gram-negative species (Hessle et al., 2000, 2005; Skovbjerg et al., 2010). Apart from the general difficulty of directly applying *in vitro* results to vertebrates exhibiting a complex intestinal microbiota and distinct intra-luminal milieu interacting with the fine-tuned immune system in health and disease, it is also highly likely that human PBMC and murine CD4+ cells differently respond to bacterial stimuli, given former evidence regarding the differences in cytokine patterns between human monocytes and human DC upon bacterial stimulation (Karlsson et al., 2004).

Moreover, *E. coli* recolonization seemed to favor a Th17 immune cell differentiation, particularly in the small intestine, given that the production of the two key cytokines of this cell population, i.e., IL-17 and IL-22, was significantly higher in CD4+ cells isolated from with *E. coli* recolonized mice as compared to mice harboring *L. johnsonii* only. Th17 polarization

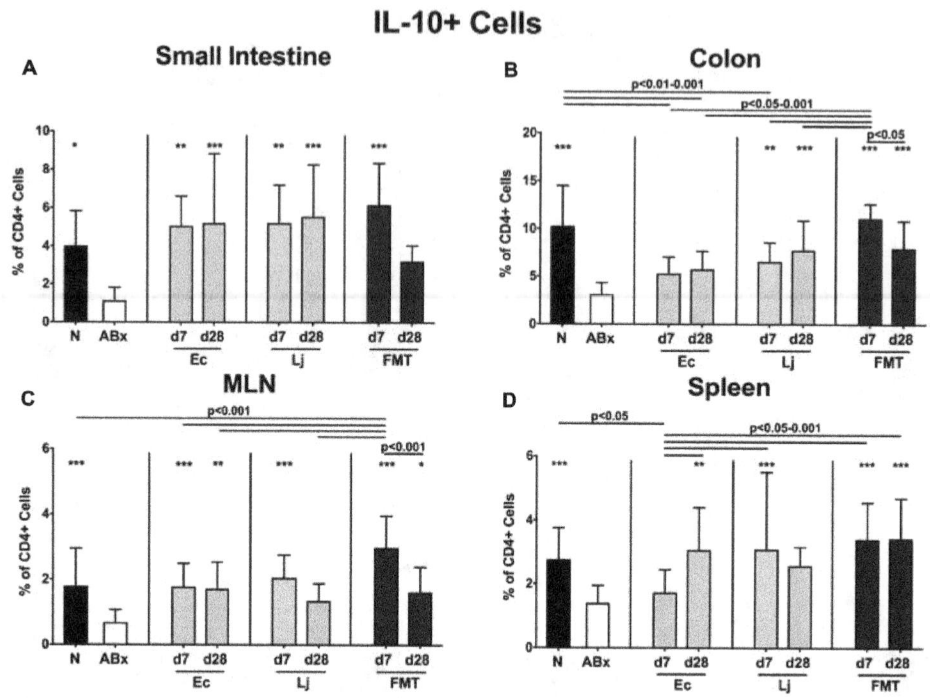

FIGURE 10 | IL-10 producing CD4+ cells in intestinal and systemic compartments of secondary abiotic and recolonized mice. Secondary abiotic mice were generated by broad-spectrum antibiotic treatment and perorally recolonized by gavage. Subsequently, lymphocytes were isolated from small intestinal and colonic lamina propria, MLN, and spleen and stimulated with PMA/ionomycin in presence of brefeldin A and subsequently analyzed by flow cytometry. The percentages of IL-10 producing CD4+ cells in the **(A)** small intestine, **(B)** colon, **(C)** MLN and **(D)** spleen of naive conventional mice (N), secondary abiotic mice (ABx) and mice re-associated with either *E. coli* (Ec), *L. johnsonii* (Lj) or complex intestinal microbiota by FMT on d7 and d28 post-recolonization are depicted. Columns represent means +SD. Significance levels (*p*-values) determined with one-way ANOVA test followed by Tukey post-correction test for multiple comparisons are indicated. Significant differences as compared to secondary abiotic mice are indicated by asterisks (*$p < 0.05$; **$p < 0.01$; ***$p < 0.001$). Data were pooled from three independent experiments.

is determined by the co-stimulation and cytokine provision from the DC (Perona-Wright et al., 2009), whereby IL-23 plays a particularly important role in the sustenance of Th17 cell responses *in vivo* (Mangan et al., 2006; McGeachy et al., 2009). It is tempting to speculate that commensal *E. coli* more strongly induce IL-23 production of DC, thus leading to a Th17 cell differentiation. Interestingly, a study conducted with human PBMC revealed that myeloid DC do indeed produce higher levels of IL-23 when stimulated with *E. coli* (Manuzak et al., 2012). Furthermore, *E. coli* heat-labile enterotoxin (synergizing with LPS) has been shown to induce IL-1β and IL-23 secretion by DC, which in turn promoted IL-17 and IFN-γ production by CD4+ T cells (Brereton et al., 2011).

Lactobacillus johnsonii recolonized mice, however, displayed higher abundances of CD4+IL-17+ cells in the colon and spleen and of CD4+IL22+ cells in the small intestinal LP and MLN as compared to their secondary abiotic counterparts at d7 post recolonization. Nonetheless, all the aforementioned immune cell populations declined back to the levels observed in secondary abiotic mice until 4 weeks after *L. johnsonii* recolonization. It has been known for a while now, that specific bacterial species such as SFB are required for the differentiation of small intestinal Th17 cells in germ-free mice (Ivanov et al., 2008; Gaboriau-Routhiau et al., 2009). A more recent investigation revealed that extracellular pathogens, such as *Citrobacter rodentium* and *E. coli* O157:H7 can also induce Th17 differentiation following adhesion to intestinal epithelial cells (Atarashi et al., 2015). Importantly, a common pilus adherence factor, which mediates adhesion to epithelial cells, has been reported for both pathogenic and commensal *E. coli* species (Rendón et al., 2007), indicating that the observed effects on the Th17 cells may be mediated through adherence of this commensal *E. coli*.

Furthermore, both *E. coli* and *L. johnsonii* could restore the antibiotics-induced reduction of IL-10 producing CD4+ cells in the small intestines, but only the latter could achieve the same effect in the colon, indicating commensal species-specific anti-inflammatory properties. Our results are well in line with a comprehensive analysis of numerous *Lactobacillus* species suggesting that species derived from healthy mice can be largely classified as potentially anti-inflammatory (Gorska et al., 2016). Notably, these data support the already proposed concept and evidence, that probiotic bacteria including *L. johnsonii* exert health-promoting effects through induction of regulatory/anti-inflammatory host immune responses (Di Giacinto et al., 2005; Kwon et al., 2010). However, it is highly likely that *L. johnsonii* and other probiotic species exert additional beneficial functions through

IL-10 independent mechanisms, given their capability to attenuate the severity of colonic inflammation in IL-10 deficient mice.

The reintroduction of complex microbiota into the host via FMT is a well-known therapy dating back to the Chinese Dong-jin dynasty in the fourth century (Zhang et al., 2012) and has undergone a renaissance recently as a therapeutic option for the treatment of recurrent and refractory *Clostridium difficile* toxin induced acute necrotizing pseudo-membranous enterocolitis (van Nood et al., 2009; Rohlke et al., 2010; Brandt et al., 2012; Fischer et al., 2016; Scaldaferri et al., 2016).

In summary, the restoration of immune cell populations following broad-spectrum antibiotic treatment by commensal bacterial mono-colonization appears to be less effective than by complex intestinal microbiota association upon FMT, but depends both on the respective immune cell subtypes and analyzed compartments and does hence not follow a clear cut pattern. Nevertheless, mono-colonization of secondary abiotic mice with defined Gram-negative or Gram-positive species has a deep impact on shaping the host immune system and drives both pro- as well as anti-inflammatory immune responses on the mucosal, peripheral and systemic level in parallel. However, *E. coli* appears to favor pro-inflammatory immune responses, while *L. johnsonii* has a stronger impact on anti-inflammatory immune cell subsets.

CONCLUSION

Future studies should further unravel the fine-tuned interplay between the well-orchestrated concert within the complex intestinal microbiota intestinal on one side and the different members of the immune system on the other in health and disease subsequently providing potential novel treatment options for immunopathological intestinal and extra-intestinal morbidities.

AUTHOR CONTRIBUTIONS

IE: Performed experiments, analyzed data, and wrote paper. EvK: Performed experiments. CN: Suggested critical parameters in design of experiments, supplied antibodies. PB: Suggested critical parameters in design of experiments, supplied antibodies. AS: Provided advice in design and performance of experiments. SB: Provided advice in design and performance of experiments, co-edited paper. MH: Designed and performed experiments, analyzed data, and co-wrote paper.

FUNDING

This work was supported by grants from the German Research Foundation (DFG) to SB (SFB633, TP A7), MH (SFB633, TP B6), AS (SFB633, TP A1), IE and EvK (SFB633; Immuco) and by the German Federal Ministries of Education and Research (BMBF) to SB and MH (PAC-Campy 01KI1725D).

ACKNOWLEDGMENTS

The authors thank Michaela Wattrodt, Ursula Rüschendorf, Alexandra Bittroff-Leben, Ulrike Fiebiger, Ines Puschendorf, Gernot Reifenberger, and the staff of the animal research facility of the Charité - University Medicine Berlin for excellent technical assistance and animal breeding.

SUPPLEMENTARY MATERIAL

FIGURE S1 | Percentages of CD8+ cells in intestinal and systemic compartments of secondary abiotic and recolonized mice. Secondary abiotic mice were generated by broad-spectrum antibiotic treatment and perorally recolonized by gavage. Subsequently, lymphocytes from small intestinal and colonic lamina propria, MLN and spleen were isolated, and analyzed by flow cytometry as described in "Materials and Methods." The percentages of the CD8+ lymphocyte population within the **(A)** small intestine, **(B)** colon, **(C)** MLN and **(D)** spleen of naive conventional mice (N), secondary abiotic mice (ABx) and mice re-associated with either *E. coli* (Ec), *L. johnsonii* (Lj) or complex intestinal microbiota by FMT on d7 and d28 post-recolonization are depicted. Columns represent means +SD. Significance levels (p-values) determined with one-way ANOVA test followed by Tukey post-correction test for multiple comparisons are indicated. Significant differences as compared to secondary abiotic mice are indicated by asterisks (*$p < 0.05$; **$p < 0.01$; ***$p < 0.001$). Data were pooled from three independent experiments.

FIGURE S2 | Absolute cell numbers of CD8+ cells in intestinal and systemic compartments of secondary abiotic and recolonized mice. Secondary abiotic mice were generated by broad-spectrum antibiotic treatment and perorally recolonized by gavage. Subsequently, lymphocytes from small intestinal and colonic lamina propria, MLN and spleen were isolated, and analyzed by flow cytometry as described in "Materials and Methods." The concentrations of CD8+ lymphocytes in the **(A)** small intestine, **(B)** colon, **(C)** MLN and **(D)** spleen of naive conventional mice (N), secondary abiotic mice (ABx) and mice re-associated with either *E. coli* (Ec), *L. johnsonii* (Lj) or complex intestinal microbiota by FMT on d7 and d28 post-recolonization are depicted. Columns represent means +SD. Significance levels (p-values) determined with one-way ANOVA test followed by Tukey post-correction test for multiple comparisons are indicated. Significant differences as compared to secondary abiotic mice are indicated by asterisks (*$p < 0.05$; **$p < 0.01$; ***$p < 0.001$). Data were pooled from three independent experiments.

FIGURE S3 | CD8+ memory/effector T cells in intestinal and systemic compartments of secondary abiotic and recolonized mice. Secondary abiotic mice were generated by broad-spectrum antibiotic treatment and perorally recolonized by gavage. Subsequently, lymphocytes from small intestinal and colonic lamina propria, MLN and spleen were isolated, and analyzed by flow cytometry as described in "Materials and Methods." The proportions of CD8+ memory/effector cells (CD8+CD44^{hi}, gated on CD8+ cells) in the **(A)** small intestine, **(B)** colon, **(C)** MLN and **(D)** spleen of naive conventional mice (N), secondary abiotic mice (ABx) and mice re-associated with either *E. coli* (Ec), *L. johnsonii* (Lj) or complex intestinal microbiota by FMT on d7 and d28 post-recolonization are depicted. Columns represent means +SD. Significance levels (p-values) determined with one-way ANOVA test followed by Tukey post-correction test for multiple comparisons are indicated. Significant differences as compared to secondary abiotic mice are indicated by asterisks (*$p < 0.05$; **$p < 0.01$; ***$p < 0.001$). Data were pooled from three independent experiments.

FIGURE S4 | Activated DCs in intestinal and systemic compartments of secondary abiotic and recolonized mice. Secondary abiotic mice were generated by broad-spectrum antibiotic treatment and perorally recolonized by gavage.

Subsequently, lymphocytes from small intestinal and colonic lamina propria, MLN and spleen were isolated, and analyzed by flow cytometry as described in "Materials and Methods." The frequencies of activated DCs (CD86+, gated on CD4-CD8- live cells) in the **(A)** small intestine, **(B)** colon, **(C)** MLN and **(D)** spleen of naive conventional mice (N), secondary abiotic mice (ABx) and mice re-associated with either *E. coli* (Ec), *L. johnsonii* (Lj) or complex intestinal microbiota by FMT on d7 and d28 post-recolonization are depicted. Columns represent means +SD. Significance levels (*p*-values) determined with one-way ANOVA test followed by Tukey post-correction test for multiple comparisons are indicated. Significant differences as compared to secondary abiotic mice are indicated by asterisks (*$p < 0.05$; **$p < 0.01$; ***$p < 0.001$). Data were pooled from three independent experiments.

REFERENCES

Atarashi, K., Tanoue, T., Ando, M., Kamada, N., Nagano, Y., Narushima, S., et al. (2015). Th17 cell induction by adhesion of microbes to intestinal epithelial cells. *Cell* 163, 367–380. doi: 10.1016/j.cell.2015.08.058

Atarashi, K., Tanoue, T., Shima, T., Imaoka, A., Kuwahara, T., Momose, Y., et al. (2011). Induction of colonic regulatory T cells by indigenous *Clostridium* species. *Science* 331, 337–341. doi: 10.1126/science.1198469

Aujla, S. J., Dubin, P. J., and Kolls, J. K. (2007). Th17 cells and mucosal host defense. *Semin. Immunol.* 19, 377–382. doi: 10.1016/j.smim.2007.10.009

Backhed, F., Ley, R. E., Sonnenburg, J. L., Peterson, D. A., and Gordon, J. I. (2005). Host-bacterial mutualism in the human intestine. *Science* 307, 1915–1920. doi: 10.1126/science.1104816

Bereswill, S., Ekmekciu, I., Escher, U., Fiebiger, U., Stingl, K., and Heimesaat, M. M. (2017). *Lactobacillus johnsonii* ameliorates intestinal, extra-intestinal and systemic pro-inflammatory immune responses following murine *Campylobacter jejuni* infection. *Sci. Rep.* 7:2138. doi: 10.1038/s41598-017-02436-2

Bereswill, S., Fischer, A., Plickert, R., Haag, L. M., Otto, B., Kuhl, A. A., et al. (2011). Novel murine infection models provide deep insights into the "menage a trois" of *Campylobacter jejuni*, microbiota and host innate immunity. *PLOS ONE* 6:e20953. doi: 10.1371/journal.pone.0020953

Biasucci, G., Rubini, M., Riboni, S., Morelli, L., Bessi, E., and Retetangos, C. (2010). Mode of delivery affects the bacterial community in the newborn gut. *Early Hum. Dev.* 86(Suppl. 1), 13–15. doi: 10.1016/j.earlhumdev.2010.01.004

Brandt, L. J., Aroniadis, O. C., and Mellow, M. (2012). Long-term follow-up of colonoscopic fecal microbiota transplant for recurrent *Clostridium difficile* infection. *Am. J. Gastroenterol.* 107, 1079–1087. doi: 10.1038/ajg.2012.60

Brereton, C. F., Sutton, C. E., Ross, P. J., Iwakura, Y., Pizza, M., Rappuoli, R., et al. (2011). *Escherichia coli* heat-labile enterotoxin promotes protective Th17 responses against infection by driving innate IL-1 and IL-23 production. *J. Immunol.* 186, 5896–5906. doi: 10.4049/jiimunol.1003789

Buffie, C. G., Jarchum, I., Equinda, M., Lipuma, L., Gobourne, A., Viale, A., et al. (2012). Profound alterations of intestinal microbiota following a single dose of clindamycin results in sustained susceptibility to *Clostridium difficile*-induced colitis. *Infect. Immun.* 80, 62–73. doi: 10.1128/IAI.05496-11

Carding, S., Verbeke, K., Vipond, D. T., Corfe, B. M., and Owen, L. J. (2015). Dysbiosis of the gut microbiota in disease. *Microb. Ecol. Health Dis.* 26:26191. doi: 10.3402/mehd.v26.26191

Castillo, M., Martin-Orue, S. M., Manzanilla, E. G., Badiola, I., Martin, M., and Gasa, J. (2006). Quantification of total bacteria, enterobacteria and lactobacilli populations in pig digesta by real-time PCR. *Vet. Microbiol.* 114, 165–170. doi: 10.1016/j.vetmic.2005.11.055

Cording, S., Fleissner, D., Heimesaat, M. M., Bereswill, S., Loddenkemper, C., Uematsu, S., et al. (2013). Commensal microbiota drive proliferation of conventional and Foxp3(+) regulatory CD4(+) T cells in mesenteric lymph nodes and Peyer's patches. *Eur. J. Microbiol. Immunol. (Bp)* 3, 1–10. doi: 10.1556/EuJMI.3.2013.1.1

Croswell, A., Amir, E., Teggatz, P., Barman, M., and Salzman, N. H. (2009). Prolonged impact of antibiotics on intestinal microbial ecology and susceptibility to enteric *Salmonella* infection. *Infect. Immun.* 77, 2741–2753. doi: 10.1128/IAI.00006-09

Di Giacinto, C., Marinaro, M., Sanchez, M., Strober, W., and Boirivant, M. (2005). Probiotics ameliorate recurrent Th1-mediated murine colitis by inducing IL-10 and IL-10-dependent TGF-β-bearing regulatory cells. *J. Immunol.* 174, 3237–3246. doi: 10.4049/jimmunol.174.6.3237

Donaldson, G. P., Lee, S. M., and Mazmanian, S. K. (2016). Gut biogeography of the bacterial microbiota. *Nat. Rev. Microbiol.* 14, 20–32. doi: 10.1038/nrmicro3552

Eckburg, P. B., Bik, E. M., Bernstein, C. N., Purdom, E., Dethlefsen, L., Sargent, M., et al. (2005). Diversity of the human intestinal microbial flora. *Science* 308, 1635–1638. doi: 10.1126/science.1110591

Ekmekciu, I., von Klitzing, E., Fiebiger, U., Escher, U., Neumann, C., Bacher, P., et al. (2017a). Immune responses to broad-spectrum antibiotic treatment and fecal microbiota transplantation in mice. *Front. Immunol.* 8:397. doi: 10.3389/fimmu.2017.00397

Ekmekciu, I., von Klitzing, E., Fiebiger, U., Neumann, C., Bacher, P., Scheffold, A., et al. (2017b). The probiotic compound VSL#3 modulates mucosal, peripheral, and systemic immunity following murine broad-spectrum antibiotic treatment. *Front. Cell Infect. Microbiol.* 7:167. doi: 10.3389/fcimb.2017.00167

El Aidy, S., van Baarlen, P., Derrien, M., Lindenbergh-Kortleve, D. J., Hooiveld, G., Levenez, F., et al. (2012). Temporal and spatial interplay of microbiota and intestinal mucosa drive establishment of immune homeostasis in conventionalized mice. *Mucosal Immunol.* 5, 567–579. doi: 10.1038/mi.2012.32

Ericsson, A. C., and Franklin, C. L. (2015). Manipulating the gut microbiota: methods and challenges. *ILAR J.* 56, 205–217. doi: 10.1093/ilar/ilv021

Evrard, B., Coudeyras, S., Dosgilbert, A., Charbonnel, N., Alame, J., Tridon, A., et al. (2011). Dose-dependent immunomodulation of human dendritic cells by the probiotic *Lactobacillus rhamnosus* Lcr35. *PLOS ONE* 6:e18735. doi: 10.1371/journal.pone.0018735

Fiebiger, U., Bereswill, S., and Heimesaat, M. M. (2016). Dissecting the interplay between intestinal microbiota and host immunity in health and disease: lessons learned from germfree and gnotobiotic animal models. *Eur. J. Microbiol. Immunol. (Bp)* 6, 253–271. doi: 10.1556/1886.2016.00036

Finegold, S., Sutter, V., and Mathisen, G. (1983). *Human Intestinal Microflora in Health and Disease*, ed. D. J. Hentges (Cambridge, MA: Academic Press, Inc.), 3–31.

Fischer, M., Kao, D., Kelly, C., Kuchipudi, A., Jafri, S. M., Blumenkehl, M., et al. (2016). Fecal microbiota transplantation is safe and efficacious for recurrent or refractory *Clostridium difficile* infection in patients with inflammatory Bowel disease. *Inflamm. Bowel Dis.* 22, 2402–2409. doi: 10.1097/mib.0000000000000908

Foligne, B., Nutten, S., Grangette, C., Dennin, V., Goudercourt, D., Poiret, S., et al. (2007). Correlation between in vitro and in vivo immunomodulatory properties of lactic acid bacteria. *World J. Gastroenterol.* 13, 236–243. doi: 10.3748/wjg.v13.i2.236

Fujiwara, D., Inoue, S., Wakabayashi, H., and Fujii, T. (2004). The anti-allergic effects of lactic acid bacteria are strain dependent and mediated by effects on both Th1/Th2 cytokine expression and balance. *Int. Arch. Allergy Immunol.* 135, 205–215. doi: 10.1159/000081305

Gaboriau-Routhiau, V., Rakotobe, S., Lecuyer, E., Mulder, I., Lan, A., Bridonneau, C., et al. (2009). The key role of segmented filamentous bacteria in the coordinated maturation of gut helper T cell responses. *Immunity* 31, 677–689. doi: 10.1016/j.immuni.2009.08.020

Gorska, S., Sandstrom, C., Wojas-Turek, J., Rossowska, J., Pajtasz-Piasecka, E., Brzozowska, E., et al. (2016). Structural and immunomodulatory differences among lactobacilli exopolysaccharides isolated from intestines of mice with experimentally induced inflammatory bowel disease. *Sci. Rep.* 6:37613. doi: 10.1038/srep37613

Haag, L. M., Fischer, A., Otto, B., Plickert, R., Kuhl, A. A., Gobel, U. B., et al. (2012). *Campylobacter jejuni* induces acute enterocolitis in gnotobiotic IL-$10^{-/-}$ mice via Toll-like-receptor-2 and -4 signaling. *PLOS ONE* 7:e40761. doi: 10.1371/journal.pone.0040761

Heimesaat, M. M., Bereswill, S., Fischer, A., Fuchs, D., Struck, D., Niebergall, J., et al. (2006). Gram-negative bacteria aggravate murine small intestinal Th1-type immunopathology following oral infection with *Toxoplasma gondii*. *J. Immunol.* 177, 8785–8795. doi: 10.4049/jimmunol.177.12.8785

Heimesaat, M. M., Fischer, A., Jahn, H. K., Niebergall, J., Freudenberg, M., Blaut, M., et al. (2007). Exacerbation of murine ileitis by Toll-like receptor 4 mediated sensing of lipopolysaccharide from commensal *Escherichia coli*. *Gut* 56, 941–948. doi: 10.1136/gut.2006.104497

Henker, J., Muller, S., Laass, M. W., Schreiner, A., and Schulze, J. (2008). Probiotic *Escherichia coli* Nissle 1917 (EcN) for successful remission maintenance of ulcerative colitis in children and adolescents: an open-label pilot study. *Z. Gastroenterol.* 46, 874–875. doi: 10.1055/s-2008-1027463

Herías, M. V., Hessle, C., Telemo, E., Midtvedt, T., Hanson, L., and Wold, A. E. (1999). Immunomodulatory effects of *Lactobacillus plantarum* colonizing the intestine of gnotobiotic rats. *Clin. Exp. Immunol.* 116, 283–290. doi: 10.1046/j.1365-2249.1999.00891.x

Hessle, C., Andersson, B., and Wold, A. E. (2000). Gram-positive bacteria are potent inducers of monocytic interleukin-12 (IL-12) while Gram-negative bacteria preferentially stimulate IL-10 production. *Infect. Immun.* 68, 3581–3586. doi: 10.1128/IAI.68.6.3581-3586.2000

Hessle, C. C., Andersson, B., and Wold, A. E. (2005). Gram-positive and Gram-negative bacteria elicit different patterns of pro-inflammatory cytokines in human monocytes. *Cytokine* 30, 311–318. doi: 10.1016/j.cyto.2004.05.008

Hill, D. A., Siracusa, M. C., Abt, M. C., Kim, B. S., Kobuley, D., Kubo, M., et al. (2012). Commensal bacteria-derived signals regulate basophil hematopoiesis and allergic inflammation. *Nat. Med.* 18, 538–546. doi: 10.1038/nm.2657

Isolauri, E., Arvola, T., Sutas, Y., Moilanen, E., and Salminen, S. (2000). Probiotics in the management of atopic eczema. *Clin. Exp. Allergy* 30, 1604–1610. doi: 10.1046/j.1365-2222.2000.00943.x

Ivanov, I., Frutos Rde, L., Manel, N., Yoshinaga, K., Rifkin, D. B., Sartor, R. B., et al. (2008). Specific microbiota direct the differentiation of IL-17-producing T-helper cells in the mucosa of the small intestine. *Cell Host Microbe* 4, 337–349. doi: 10.1016/j.chom.2008.09.009

Kalliomaki, M., Salminen, S., Arvilommi, H., Kero, P., Koskinen, P., and Isolauri, E. (2001). Probiotics in primary prevention of atopic disease: a randomised placebo-controlled trial. *Lancet* 357, 1076–1079. doi: 10.1016/s0140-6736(00)04259-8

Kalliomaki, M., Salminen, S., Poussa, T., Arvilommi, H., and Isolauri, E. (2003). Probiotics and prevention of atopic disease: 4-year follow-up of a randomised placebo-controlled trial. *Lancet* 361, 1869–1871. doi: 10.1016/s0140-6736(03)13490-3

Karlsson, H., Larsson, P., Wold, A. E., and Rudin, A. (2004). Pattern of cytokine responses to gram-positive and gram-negative commensal bacteria is profoundly changed when monocytes differentiate into dendritic cells. *Infect. Immun.* 72, 2671–2678. doi: 10.1128/IAI.72.5.2671-2678.2004

Kollias, G., Douni, E., Kassiotis, G., and Kontoyiannis, D. (1999). The function of tumour necrosis factor and receptors in models of multi-organ inflammation, rheumatoid arthritis, multiple sclerosis and inflammatory bowel disease. *Ann. Rheum. Dis.* 58(Suppl. 1), I32–I39. doi: 10.1136/ard.58.2008.i32

Kruis, W., Fric, P., Pokrotnieks, J., Lukas, M., Fixa, B., Kascak, M., et al. (2004). Maintaining remission of ulcerative colitis with the probiotic *Escherichia coli* Nissle 1917 is as effective as with standard mesalazine. *Gut* 53, 1617–1623. doi: 10.1136/gut.2003.037747

Kwon, H. K., Lee, C. G., So, J. S., Chae, C. S., Hwang, J. S., Sahoo, A., et al. (2010). Generation of regulatory dendritic cells and CD4+Foxp3+ T cells by probiotics administration suppresses immune disorders. *Proc. Natl. Acad. Sci. U.S.A.* 107, 2159–2164. doi: 10.1073/pnas.0904055107

LeBlanc, J. G., Milani, C., de Giori, G. S., Sesma, F., van Sinderen, D., and Ventura, M. (2013). Bacteria as vitamin suppliers to their host: a gut microbiota perspective. *Curr. Opin. Biotechnol.* 24, 160–168. doi: 10.1016/j.copbio.2012.8.005

Lievin-Le Moal, V., and Servin, A. L. (2014). Anti-infective activities of lactobacillus strains in the human intestinal microbiota: from probiotics to gastrointestinal anti-infectious biotherapeutic agents. *Clin. Microbiol. Rev.* 27, 167–199. doi: 10.1128/cmr.00080-13

Macpherson, A. J., and Harris, N. L. (2004). Interactions between commensal intestinal bacteria and the immune system. *Nat. Rev. Immunol.* 4, 478–485. doi: 10.1038/nri1373

Mangan, P. R., Harrington, L. E., O'Quinn, D. B., Helms, W. S., Bullard, D. C., Elson, C. O., et al. (2006). Transforming growth factor-beta induces development of the T(H)17 lineage. *Nature* 441, 231–234. doi: 10.1038/nature04754

Manuzak, J., Dillon, S., and Wilson, C. (2012). Differential interleukin-10 (IL-10) and IL-23 production by human blood monocytes and dendritic cells in response to commensal enteric bacteria. *Clin. Vaccine Immunol.* 19, 1207–1217. doi: 10.1128/CVI.00282.12

McGeachy, M. J., Chen, Y., Tato, C. M., Laurence, A., Joyce-Shaikh, B., Blumenschein, W. M., et al. (2009). The interleukin 23 receptor is essential for the terminal differentiation of interleukin 17-producing effector T helper cells *in vivo*. *Nat. Immunol.* 10, 314–324. doi: 10.1038/ni.1698

Naito, Y., Takagi, T., Handa, O., Ishikawa, T., Nakagawa, S., Yamaguchi, T., et al. (2003). Enhanced intestinal inflammation induced by dextran sulfate sodium in tumor necrosis factor-alpha deficient mice. *J. Gastroenterol. Hepatol.* 18, 560–569. doi: 10.1046/j.1440-1746.2003.03034.x

Niess, J. H., Leithauser, F., Adler, G., and Reimann, J. (2008). Commensal gut flora drives the expansion of proinflammatory CD4 T cells in the colonic lamina propria under normal and inflammatory conditions. *J. Immunol.* 180, 559–568. doi: 10.4049/jimmunol.180.1.559

Org, E., Parks, B. W., Joo, J. W., Emert, B., Schwartzman, W., Kang, E. Y., et al. (2015). Genetic and environmental control of host-gut microbiota interactions. *Genome Res.* 25, 1558–1569. doi: 10.1101/gr.194118.115

Ostman, S., Rask, C., Wold, A. E., Hultkrantz, S., and Telemo, E. (2006). Impaired regulatory T cell function in germ-free mice. *Eur. J. Immunol.* 36, 2336–2346. doi: 10.1002/eji.200535244

Pagnini, C., Saeed, R., Bamias, G., Arseneau, K. O., Pizarro, T. T., and Cominelli, F. (2009). Probiotics promote gut health through stimulation of epithelial innate immunity. *Proc. Natl. Acad. Sci. U.S.A.* 107, 454–459. doi: 10.1073/pnas.0910307107

Palmer, C., Bik, E. M., DiGiulio, D. B., Relman, D. A., and Brown, P. O. (2007). Development of the human infant intestinal microbiota. *PLOS Biol.* 5:e177. doi: 10.1371/journal.pbio.0050177

Penders, J., Thijs, C., Vink, C., Stelma, F. F., Snijders, B., Kummeling, I., et al. (2006). Factors influencing the composition of the intestinal microbiota in early infancy. *Pediatrics* 118, 511–521. doi: 10.1542/peds.2005-2824

Perona-Wright, G., Jenkins, S. J., O'Connor, R. A., Zienkiewicz, D., McSorley, H. J., Maizels, R. M., et al. (2009). A pivotal role for CD40-mediated IL-6 production by dendritic cells during IL-17 induction *in vivo*. *J. Immunol.* 182, 2809–2815. doi: 10.4049/jimmunol.0803553

Popa, C., Netea, M. G., van Riel, P. L., van der Meer, J. W., and Stalenhoef, A. F. (2007). The role of TNF-alpha in chronic inflammatory conditions, intermediary metabolism, and cardiovascular risk. *J. Lipid Res.* 48, 751–762. doi: 10.1194/jlr.R600021-JLR200

Rakoff-Nahoum, S., Paglino, J., Eslami-Varzaneh, F., Edberg, S., and Medzhitov, R. (2004). Recognition of commensal microflora by toll-like receptors is required for intestinal homeostasis. *Cell* 118, 229–241. doi: 10.1016/j.cell.2004.07.002

Rendón, M. A., Saldaña, Z., Erdem, A. L., Monteiro-Neto, V., Vázquez, A., Kaper, J. B., et al. (2007). Commensal and pathogenic *Escherichia coli* use a common pilus adherence factor for epithelial cell colonization. *Proc. Natl. Acad. Sci. U.S.A.* 104, 10637–10642. doi: 10.1073/pnas.0704104104

Rohlke, F., Surawicz, C. M., and Stollman, N. (2010). Fecal flora reconstitution for recurrent *Clostridium difficile* infection: results and methodology. *J. Clin. Gastroenterol.* 44, 567–570. doi: 10.1097/MCG.0b013e3181dadb10

Round, J. L., Lee, S. M., Li, J., Tran, G., Jabri, B., Chatila, T. A., et al. (2011). The Toll-like receptor 2 pathway establishes colonization by a commensal of the human microbiota. *Science* 332, 974–977. doi: 10.1126/science.1206095

Scaldaferri, F., Pecere, S., Petito, V., Zambrano, D., Fiore, L., Lopetuso, L. R., et al. (2016). Efficacy and mechanisms of action of fecal microbiota transplantation in ulcerative colitis: pitfalls and promises from a first meta-analysis. *Transplant. Proc.* 48, 402–407. doi: 10.1016/j.transproceed.2015.12.040

Schultz, M. (2008). Clinical use of *E. coli* Nissle 1917 in inflammatory bowel disease. *Inflamm. Bowel. Dis.* 14, 1012–1018. doi: 10.1002/ibd.20377

Schultz, M., Veltkamp, C., Dieleman, L. A., Grenther, W. B., Wyrick, P. B., Tonkonogy, S. L., et al. (2002). *Lactobacillus plantarum* 299V in the treatment and prevention of spontaneous colitis in interleukin-10-deficient mice. *Inflamm. Bowel Dis.* 8, 71–80. doi: 10.1097/00054725-200203000-00001

Sender, R., Fuchs, S., and Milo, R. (2016). Are we really vastly outnumbered? revisiting the ratio of bacterial to host cells in humans. *Cell* 164, 337–340. doi: 10.1016/j.cell.2016.01.013

Sheridan, B. S., and Lefrancois, L. (2012). Isolation of mouse lymphocytes from small intestine tissues. *Curr. Protoc. Immunol.* 3, 3.19.1–3.19.11. doi: 10.1002/0471142735.im0319s99

Shida, K., Nanno, M., and Nagata, S. (2011). Flexible cytokine production by macrophages and T cells in response to probiotic bacteria: a possible mechanism by which probiotics exert multifunctional immune regulatory activities. *Gut Microbes* 2, 109–114. doi: 10.4161/gmic.2.2.15661

Skovbjerg, S., Martner, A., Hynsjo, L., Hessle, C., Olsen, I., Dewhirst, F. E., et al. (2010). Gram-positive and gram-negative bacteria induce different patterns of cytokine production in human mononuclear cells irrespective of taxonomic relatedness. *J. Interferon Cytokine Res.* 30, 23–32. doi: 10.1089/jir.2009.0033

Sommer, F., and Backhed, F. (2013). The gut microbiota–masters of host development and physiology. *Nat. Rev. Microbiol.* 11, 227–238. doi: 10.1038/nrmicro2974

Sprent, J., and Surh, C. D. (2002). T cell memory. *Annu. Rev. Immunol.* 20, 551–579. doi: 10.1146/annurev.immunol.20.100101.151926

Stiemsma, L. T., Turvey, S. E., and Finlay, B. B. (2014). An antibiotic-altered microbiota provides fuel for the enteric foe. *Cell Res.* 24, 5–6. doi: 10.1038/cr.2013.142

Tenaillon, O., Skurnik, D., Picard, B., and Denamur, E. (2010). The population genetics of commensal *Escherichia coli*. *Nat. Rev. Microbiol.* 8, 207–217. doi: 10.1038/nrmicro2298

Tomas, J., Reygner, J., Mayeur, C., Ducroc, R., Bouet, S., Bridonneau, C., et al. (2015). Early colonizing *Escherichia coli* elicits remodeling of rat colonic epithelium shifting toward a new homeostatic state. *ISME J.* 9, 46–58. doi: 10.1038/ismej.2014.111

Valeur, N., Engel, P., Carbajal, N., Connolly, E., and Ladefoged, K. (2004). Colonization and immunomodulation by *Lactobacillus reuteri* ATCC 55730 in the human gastrointestinal tract. *Appl. Environ. Microbiol.* 70, 1176–1181. doi: 10.1128/AEM.70.2.1176-1181.2004

van Nood, E., Speelman, P., Kuijper, E. J., and Keller, J. J. (2009). Struggling with recurrent *Clostridium difficile* infections: is donor faeces the solution? *Euro Surveill.* 14:19316.

Viljanen, M., Savilahti, E., Haahtela, T., Juntunen-Backman, K., Korpela, R., Poussa, T., et al. (2005). Probiotics in the treatment of atopic eczema/dermatitis syndrome in infants: a double-blind placebo-controlled trial. *Allergy* 60, 494–500. doi: 10.1111/j.1398-9995.2004.00514.x

Wallet, M. A., Sen, P., and Tisch, R. (2005). Immunoregulation of dendritic cells. *Clin. Med. Res.* 3, 166–175. doi: 10.3121/cmr.3.3.166

Zarkan, A., Macklyne, H.-R., Truman, A. W., Hesketh, A. R., and Hong, H.-J. (2016). The frontline antibiotic vancomycin induces a zinc starvation response in bacteria by binding to Zn(II). *Sci. Rep.* 6:19602. doi: 10.1038/srep19602

Zeuthen, L. H., Christensen, H. R., and Frokiaer, H. (2006). Lactic acid bacteria inducing a weak interleukin-12 and tumor necrosis factor alpha response in human dendritic cells inhibit strongly stimulating lactic acid bacteria but act synergistically with gram-negative bacteria. *Clin. Vaccine Immunol.* 13, 365–375. doi: 10.1128/cvi.13.3.365-375.2006

Zhang, F., Luo, W., Shi, Y., Fan, Z., and Ji, G. (2012). Should we standardize the 1,700-year-old fecal microbiota transplantation?. *Am. J. Gastroenterol.* 107, 1755–1755. doi: 10.1038/ajg.2012.251

Zhang, Y. J., Li, S., Gan, R. Y., Zhou, T., Xu, D. P., and Li, H. B. (2015). Impacts of gut bacteria on human health and diseases. *Int. J. Mol. Sci.* 16, 7493–7519. doi: 10.3390/ijms16047493

13

Bifidobacteria and their Molecular Communication with the Immune System

Lorena Ruiz, Susana Delgado, Patricia Ruas-Madiedo, Borja Sánchez* and Abelardo Margolles

Dairy Research Institute, Spanish National Research Council (Instituto de Productos Lácteos de Asturias – CSIC), Villaviciosa, Spain

****Correspondence:***
Borja Sánchez
borja.sanchez@csic.es

Bifidobacterium represents a genus within the phylum Actinobacteria which is one of the major phyla in the healthy intestinal tract of humans. *Bifidobacterium* is one of the most abundant genera in adults, but its predominance is even more pronounced in infants, especially during lactation, when they can constitute the majority of the total bacterial population. They are one of the pioneering colonizers of the early gut microbiota, and they are known to play important roles in the metabolism of dietary components, otherwise indigestible in the upper parts of the intestine, and in the maturation of the immune system. Bifidobacteria have been shown to interact with human immune cells and to modulate specific pathways, involving innate and adaptive immune processes. In this mini-review, we provide an overview of the current knowledge on the immunomodulatory properties of bifidobacteria and the mechanisms and molecular players underlying these processes, focusing on the corresponding implications for human health. We deal with *in vitro* models suitable for studying strain-specific immunomodulatory activities. These include peripheral blood mononuclear cells and T cell-mediated immune responses, both effector and regulatory cell responses, as well as the modulation of the phenotype of dendritic cells, among others. Furthermore, preclinical studies, mainly germ-free, gnotobiotic, and conventional murine models, and human clinical trials, are also discussed. Finally, we highlight evidence supporting the immunomodulatory effects of bifidobacterial molecules (proteins and peptides, exopolysaccharides, metabolites, and DNA), as well as the role of bifidobacterial metabolism in maintaining immune homeostasis through cross-feeding mechanisms.

Keywords: bifidobacteria, *Bifidobacterium*, microbiota, immunomodulation, T cell response, PRRs, MAMPs

EARLY COLONIZATION OF BIFIDOBACTERIA AND PROPER IMMUNE DEVELOPMENT

Microbiota establishment in newborns involves the assembly of a novel microbial community, a process that is dependent on several factors, including the mother's physiology (age, metabolic state, lifestyle, or even the potential transfer of microorganisms from mother to child before birth), mode of delivery, genetic background, environmental factors, type of feeding and early antibiotic use, among others (Hill et al., 2017). Similar results were found for preterm neonates, which are less abundantly colonized by bifidobacteria (Arboleya et al., 2012). Infant feeding is also a critical factor for bifidobacterial establishment in the gut, and breast-fed infants have been shown to possess higher levels of bifidobacteria than formula-fed infants (Yatsunenko et al., 2012); these high bifidobacterial levels decrease after breast milk cessation (Davis et al., 2016).

Pioneering studies revealed reduced levels of bifidobacteria in the gut microbiota composition of infants at high risk of atopic disease at 3 weeks and 3 months of age, and a higher incidence of atopic disease was found in this group of infants by the age of 1 year (Kalliomaki et al., 2001). Similarly, lower bifidobacterial levels were found in 3-month-old infants who later developed atopy at 2 years of age, or asthma at 4 years of age (Fujimura et al., 2016). All these data point to a critical role for bifidobacteria in the maturation of our immune system from gestation to childhood, suggesting that the low abundance of these early colonizers is associated with a deviated physiological state in infancy. Indeed, current evidence suggests a role of early life bifidobacteria establishment in programming future health. Therefore, it is of great importance to know the specific strains (and species) able to regulate immune responses, either directly or indirectly through the modulation of the gut microbiota, and the underlying mechanisms, in order to design dietary strategies focused on preventing immune-related disorders.

STRAIN-SPECIFIC IMMUNOMODULATORY ACTIVITIES/*IN VITRO* AND *IN VIVO* MODELS OF STUDY

In Vitro Models

In vitro models have important limitations but they enable the preliminary screening of the effects that bacterial cells or fractions might have on different components of the immune response (Kobayashi et al., 2017). Most *in vitro* models based on immune cells employ peripheral blood mononuclear cells (PBMCs). In this way, whole cells of *B. longum*, *B. breve*, *B. bifidum*, and *B. animalis* subsp. *lactis* strains demonstrated capacity to induce dendritic cell (DC) maturation, and a species/strain-dependent T cell polarization response (Medina et al., 2007; López et al., 2010; Nicola et al., 2016). These studies revealed that, while *B. animalis* and many *B. longum* strains induced the production of the modulatory cytokine IL10 to varying degrees, the greatest strain-dependent differences were displayed in TNFα and INFγ production (**Figure 1**). Stimulation of PBMCs with subcellular fractions of bifidobacteria, including cytoplasmic, surface extracts, and supernatants, has also allowed the identification of molecular determinants of the elicited effects. For instance, a trypsin-labile cytoplasmic fraction of a *B. bifidum* strain was identified as the effector of $CD8^+$ T cell activation; and supernatants of *B. breve* BB99 and *B. longum* 1941 exerted a regulatory T cell induction (Mouni et al., 2009). PBMC models are thus useful to identify desirable immune profiles in probiotic strain screenings (Liu et al., 2016).

Other *in vitro* models differentiate DCs, a specialized type of antigen presenting cells, from monocytes. DCs are regarded as the main guardians of the intestinal mucosa and are important in initiating the microbiota–immune system cross-talk. Their pattern recognition receptors (PRRs) interact with specific microbial-associated molecular patterns (MAMPs), which orchestrated molecular cascades that will determine the nature of the immune response (Hoarau et al., 2008; Wittmann et al., 2013). *In vitro* differentiated DCs allowed the identification of specific domains of a *B. bifidum* surface protein and the exopolysaccharide (EPS) of *B. longum* 35624, as the effectors of the immune responses elicited by the strains (Guglielmetti et al., 2014; Schiavi et al., 2016). DC models have also been used to predict the anti-inflammatory potential of bifidobacterial strains/molecules in specific population groups; for instance, bifidobacteria improved antigen uptake and processing by DC from Crohn's disease patients (Strisciuglio et al., 2015).

Other *in vitro* models using immune cells employ murine splenocytes (Tanabe et al., 2008; Srutkova et al., 2015), macrophage-like cell lines (He et al., 2002; Lee et al., 2012; Mokrozub et al., 2015), or cells isolated from the gut-associated lymphoid tissues (GALT) (Hidalgo-Cantabrana et al., 2014), although they have not been widely used to examine the immunomodulation potential of bifidobacteria and thus their utility to predict immune responses is yet to be confirmed.

The immunomodulation potential of bifidobacteria has also been studied on enterocytes including Caco-2 or HT29 cell models (Bahrami et al., 2011; Chichlowski et al., 2012; Khokhlova et al., 2012; Arboleya et al., 2015; Sánchez et al., 2015; Luongo et al., 2017). Although the immune response of epithelial cells is much more limited than the one exerted by specialized immune cells, enterocytes are more directly exposed to the intestinal milieu and are considered to play a key role in initiating the bifidobacteria–host interactions.

Beyond that, co-culture systems employing both immune and intestinal cells have also been implemented to study microbial–host interactions and promise to overcome some of the limitations of single cell type models (Duell et al., 2011). However, few studies have used them on bifidobacteria (Pozo-Rubio et al., 2011). The application of organized multicellular systems like intestinal organoids for these kinds of studies is envisaged (Noel et al., 2017).

In Vivo Models

Germ-free (GF) and conventional *in vivo* models, including healthy and disease-induced models, have shed light on the immune modulation capability of bifidobacterial strains including live and heat-killed cells (Sugahara et al., 2017). Screening of a large collection of gut symbionts on GF mice identified a *B. adolescentis* strain which induces a robust Th17 response, albeit not inducing intestinal inflammation (Tan et al., 2016). However, immune responses may vary strongly depending on the health status of the host, as the human sera of *Clostridium difficile* patients were shown to be more reactive against *B. longum* extracts than that of healthy individuals (Górska et al., 2016).

In vivo models of intestinal diseases have demonstrated the potential of *B. bifidum* and *B. animalis* strains to restore immune markers and intestinal barrier in low chronic inflammation models (Philippe et al., 2011). Similarly, *B. longum* CECT

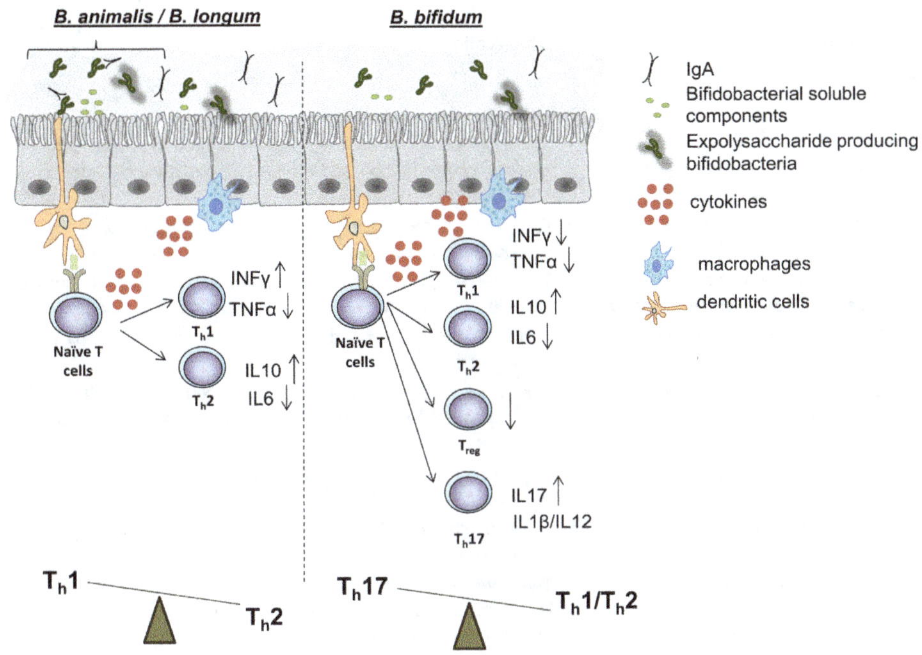

FIGURE 1 | Schematic representation of the effects on immune functions that certain strains of *B. animalis*, *B. longum* **(Left)**, and *B. bifidum* **(Right)** have demonstrated in *in vitro* and *in vivo* experiments. Many *B. animalis* and *B. longum* strains have demonstrated capacity to promote a Th1 response, while, on the contrary, some *B. bifidum* strains have been revealed capable to induce a Th17 polarization. Treg responses can also be regulated by certain strains of other species. Immunomodulatory properties are strain-dependent, and further evidence is needed in order to give to each bifidobacteria species a specific immune response in the intestinal mucosa.

7347 attenuated the production of inflammatory cytokines and the $CD4^+$ T cell-mediated immune response in a gliadin-induced enteropathy model (Laparra et al., 2012). Other disease models, described below, have been tested in literature. In food-allergy models, a vesicle-derived protein from *B. longum* (Kim et al., 2016) and a *B. animalis* (Ezendam et al., 2008) strain, administered during lactation, exerted immunomodulatory effects. In a gut model, *B. longum* strain 51-A reduced inflammation (Vieira et al., 2015). Finally, in obesity models, *B. pseudocatenulatum* restored the lymphocyte–macrophage balance and *B. adolescentis* IM38 improved high-fat-diet induced colitis inhibiting NF-κB activation (Moya-Pérez et al., 2015; Lim and Kim, 2017). Furthermore, the role of bifidobacteria in responsiveness to immunotherapy has recently been suggested. Accordingly, using tumor models in mice, *Bifidobacterium* administration was shown to improve tumor-specific immunity and response to therapy through augmented DC function, opening new avenues to exploit the bifidobacterial-immune dialog in the context of this disease (Sivan et al., 2015).

Finally, non-murine *in vivo* models, like pig models, are very attractive for the study of microbe–host interactions due to the similarities in the gastrointestinal function and development between pigs and humans. In this context, bifidobacterial administration in neonatal piglets has been shown to increase the production of intestinal IL-10 (Herfel et al., 2013), and to improve B and T cell responses following rotavirus vaccination (Vlasova et al., 2013; Kandasamy et al., 2014; Ishizuka et al., 2016). In addition, colonization with a combination of lactobacilli and bifidobacteria in non-vaccinated gnotobiotic piglets reduced the severity of rotavirus infection, while in vaccinated animals enhanced Th1 (Chattha et al., 2013). Thus, *in vivo* models closer to humans are valuable to study the immunomodulatory potential of certain strains, should be "particularly in the context of pig models in order to study pre-term birth and necrotizing enterocolitis (NEC)" (Oosterloo et al., 2014).

Humans

Different immunoreactive proteins from two *B. longum* strains have been identified in mono-colonized mice, rabbit, and human sera, revealing that the effects are strain and host specific (Górska et al., 2016) and emphasizing the need to further support *in vitro* immunomodulatory effects in clinical trials. A summary of human studies that focus on the immunomodulatory effects of bifidobacterial consumption in multiple disorders, in some of which gut microbial ecology dysbiosis and altered immune profiles coexist, is presented in **Table 1**.

MOLECULAR STRUCTURES DRIVING SPECIFIC IMMUNOMODULATORY EFFECTS

Findings from the last 10 years support the idea that bifidobacteria exert their beneficial effects on host health through the immunomodulatory action of some of their surface-associated molecules (Hoarau et al., 2006; Ewaschuk et al., 2008).

TABLE 1 | *Bifidobacterium* role on diseases with an immunological component.

Species/strains tested	Population	Observations	Reference
Intervention studies			
B. lactis BB12	Healthy adults	Four weeks administration of yogurt with the strain resulted in lower expression of TLR-2 on $CD14^{+}HLA\text{-}DR^{+}$ cells and reduction in TNF-α secretion	Meng et al., 2017
B. lactis Bi-07	Healthy elderly adults	Four weeks administration improved phagocytic activity of monocytes and granulocytes	Maneerat et al., 2014
B. animalis ssp. *lactis* HN019	Systematic meta-analysis on four clinical trials/healthy elderly subjects	The strain supplementation resulted in increased PMN phagocytic capacity and moderately increased NK cell tumoricidal activity	Miller et al., 2017
B. animalis LKM512	Atopic dermatitis adult patients	Administration into a yogurt daily for 4 weeks induced a Th1-type cytokine profile	Matsumoto et al., 2007
B. lactis NCC2818	Seasonal allergic rhinitis to grass pollen/adults	Eight weeks probiotic administration reduced Th2-cytokines secretion and CD63 expressing basophiles correlating to improved symptoms	Singh et al., 2013
B. lactis HN019	Metabolic syndrome patients	Decrease in TNFα and IL6 correlated to improvement in cardiovascular risk markers	Bernini et al., 2016
B. breve BR03 and *B. breve* B632	Cystic fibrosis/children	Three months administration of the two strains combination reduced proinflammatory markers	Klemenak et al., 2015
Lb. gasseri KS-13, *B. bifidum G9-1*, and *B. longum MM-2*	Healthy elderly population	Three weeks administration of probiotic mix maintained CD4+ lymphocytes and resulted in a more anti-inflammatory cytokines profile with increased IL-10	Spaiser et al., 2015
B. breve M-16V and *B. longum* BB536	Prenatal administration to pregnant mothers 1 month prior delivery and to the infants during 6 months	Reduced risk of developing eczema in the probiotic group	Enomoto et al., 2014
B. longum BB536, *B. infantis* M-63, *B. breve* M-16V mixture	Seasonal allergic rhinitis and intermittent asthma/children	Improvement of symptoms following 4 weeks of probiotic administration	Miraglia Del Giudice et al., 2017
B. longum BB536	Healthy newborns	The number of IFN-γ secretion cells and the ratio of IFN-γ/IL-4 secretion cells was increased, suggesting improvement of Th1 function	Wu et al., 2016
B. longum BB536	Elderly subjects receiving enteral tube feeding	Twelve weeks administration resulted in increased serum IgA and maintenance of NC cell activity	Akatsu et al., 2013
B. longum 35624	Patients of ulcerative colitis (UC), chronic fatigue syndrome (CFS), and psoriasis, as compared to healthy controls	Six to eight weeks of probiotic administration reduced CRP, TNFα, and IL6 in UC, CFS, and psoriasis patients	Groeger et al., 2013
B. infantis NLS	Celiac adults	Six weeks probiotic administration reduced Paneth cells numbers and expression of α-defensine-5, as compared to patients under a gluten-free diet without probiotic supplementation	Pinto-Sánchez et al., 2017
B. longum CECT 7347	Children with newly diagnosed coeliac disease	Three months administration resulted in reduced peripheral CD3+ lymphocytes, TNFα, and sIgA in stools	Olivares et al., 2014
Observational studies			
B. breve	Eczema risk in children at high risk of allergic disease	Early *B. breve* colonization was associated to reduced risk of eczema	Ismail et al., 2016
Bifidobacterium spp. and *B. adolescentis*	Allergic asthma in adults	Reduction in gut bifidobacterial representation and *B. adolescentis* prevalence within the bifidobacterial group in the studied population	Hevia et al., 2016
B. pseudocatenulatum	Gout patients	*B. pseudocatenulatum* depletion in gout patients	Guo et al., 2016

Summary of observational and intervention studies in humans.

This is based on the interaction of a specific bifidobacteria molecule, a MAMP, with a PRR presents on the membrane of epithelial/immune cells, which mostly configures the cellular structure of the intestinal mucosa (Sutterwala and Flavell, 2009). Although mucosa itself is differently organized, depending on the gut section considered, bifidobacteria are thought to exert their immunomodulatory activity mainly in the colon and in the distal part of the ileum, where up to 46% of the Peyer's patches are located (Van Kruiningen et al., 2002). Scientific evidence has shown the presence of immunomodulatory compounds in bifidobacteria spent medium which are released during bacterial growth (**Figure 1**).

Proteins and Peptides

Bifidobacterial proteins are one of the targets of human immunoglobulins, notably IgA, which is secreted into the gut lumen in order to control the commensal microbiota populations. Up to six different extracellular proteins from the strains *B. longum* subsp. *longum* NCIMB 8809, *B. bifidum* LMG 11041^{T}, and *B. animalis* subsp. *lactis* IPLA 4549 were recognized by pooled sera from healthy individuals, or Inflammatory Bowel Disease (IBD) patients (Hevia et al., 2014). Perhaps the best known example of an immunomodulatory protein is the extracellular serpin secreted by *B. longum* subsp. *longum*. Serpin stands for serine protease inhibitor and includes different families that share the ability to bind and irreversibly inactivate proteases. The gene coding for serpin is not widely distributed among the genus *Bifidobacterium*, being present in up to nine species so far (Turroni et al., 2010a). More precisely, the targets of serpin secreted by *B. longum* are two important pro-inflammatory proteases: human neutrophil and pancreatic elastases (Ivanov et al., 2006), proteases that have been shown to induce the serpin gene through a two-component regulatory system (Alvarez-Martin et al., 2012). Limiting the local action of these proteases suggests a role of bifidobacteria in the maintenance of gut homeostasis.

Other well-known protein structures with an immunomodulatory action are pili, which self-assemble on the bifidobacteria surface in the form of filaments and have a primary function of adherence to the intestinal surface (Turroni et al., 2014). Lower levels of IL10 and higher levels of TNFα were detected in the murine cecum mucosa as a response to the presence of a *Lactococcus lactis* strain, genetically modified for producing *B. bifidum* pili. This response was not observed in the wild-type strain, suggesting a specific interaction of these structures with the gastrointestinal mucosa (Turroni et al., 2013). Another protein with an immunomodulatory effect is the peptidoglycan hydrolase TgaA, a surface-associated protein in *B. bifidum*, which was shown to induce IL2 production in monocyte-derived dendritic cell (MoDC), the key cytokine in T_{reg} cell expansion (Zelante et al., 2012; Guglielmetti et al., 2014). Finally, our own work has revealed the presence of immunomodulatory peptides encrypted in the sequences of bifidobacteria proteins. In this sense, a peptide contained within the sequence of the protein translocase subunit SecA of *B. longum* DJ010A triggered a marked Th17 response when incubated with human PBMCs (Hidalgo-Cantabrana et al., 2017b).

EPSs

EPSs are carbohydrate polymers that are synthesized and exhibited in the bifidobacterial surface (Hidalgo-Cantabrana et al., 2014). Although the exact molecular mechanisms have not been described so far, EPSs have a great impact on the host immune function (Hidalgo-cantabrana et al., 2012). In a murine model, the EPS-producing strain *B. breve* UCC2003 was associated with increases in the mucosal levels of the pro-inflammatory IL12, INFγ, and TNFα which turned out to protect against *Citrobacter* infection (Fanning et al., 2012). Murine J77A.1 macrophages challenged with the EPS produced by strain *B. longum* BCRC 14634 increased the production of the anti-inflammatory cytokine IL10 when compared to basal conditions, and when challenged with lipopolysaccharide, the presence of the EPS was linked to lower levels of the pro-inflammatory cytokine TNFα (Wu et al., 2010). It is noteworthy that the rhamnose-rich, high-molecular weight EPS isolated from the strain *B. animalis* subsp. *lactis* IPLA-R1 was able to increase IL10 production in a PBMC model and to decrease the TNFα production in human colonic biopsies (Hidalgo-Cantabrana et al., 2015). Moreover, the administration of strain IPLA-R1 to Wistar rats was associated with higher serum levels of TGFβ and lower serum levels of the pro-inflammatory interleukin IL6 (Salazar et al., 2014).

EPS produced by specific bifidobacteria strains have been shown as molecules able to prevent exacerbated pro-inflammatory responses. *B. longum* subsp. *longum* 35624 is a strain which has shown clinical efficacy in Irritable Bowel Syndrome, a human condition cursing with chronic mucosal inflammation (Altmann et al., 2016). The anti-inflammatory effects elicited by this strain were shown to rely in its surface-associated EPS, which prevented expansion of the pro-inflammatory Th17 response compared to an exopolysaccharide-negative mutant derivative (Schiavi et al., 2016).

Finally, recent data on a mouse model of pathological cell shedding, EPS from *B. breve* UCC2003 appeared to confer protective effect through MyD88-dependent signaling (Hughes et al., 2017). Diversity of gene clusters responsible for EPS biosynthesis is high among bifidobacterial species/strains (not to mention variations in the level of EPS production) and this diversity may hold tremendous potential for strain-specific immune responses.

DNA

Bifidobacteria possess genomes with high G+C proportions, and un-methylated CpG motifs derived from them can interact with the TLR 9 present on immune cells. Several publications have reported on the immunomodulatory activity of bifidobacterial DNA. CpG motifs have in one case been linked to a promotion of the T_h1 response, dedicated to fight intracellular pathogens such as viruses (Ménard et al., 2010). Another work described an oligodeoxynucleotide derived from the *B. longum* BB536 strain able to inhibit anti-ovalbumin–IgE titres in a murine model of type-I allergic response after ovalbumin injection (Takahashi et al., 2006).

BIFIDOBACTERIAL METABOLISM TRIGGERS CROSS-FEEDING MECHANISMS THAT MAINTAIN IMMUNE HOMEOSTASIS IN THE GUT

Many efforts are currently being pursued to understand the metabolic fluxes within the gut ecosystem among bifidobacteria, other members of the gut microbiota and the human host (Hidalgo-Cantabrana et al., 2017a). A major metabolic contribution elicited by bifidobacteria from their host is represented by the breakdown of non-digestible, diet-derived glycans, and carbohydrates provided by the host known as host-derived glycans [mucins and human milk oligosaccharides (HMOs)] (Milani et al., 2015). Mucin is a host-produced glycan that constitutes one of the main barriers covering the gastrointestinal mucosa (Tailford et al., 2015). Among bifidobacteria, only members of *B. bifidum* species have been shown to efficiently metabolize mucin

(Ruas-Madiedo et al., 2008; Turroni et al., 2010b; Ruiz et al., 2011). HMOs are present in high concentrations in human colostrum and breast milk. Bifidobacteria, which dominate during early life, are among the best described gut bacteria with the ability to utilize HMOs. Several species possess glycosyl hydrolases that cleave specific linkages within the HMO molecules, the best characterized being those synthesized by *B. bifidum* (Ruiz et al., 2016). HMOs are preferentially fermented by *B. bifidum* and *B. longum* species which, together with *B. breve*, are the most abundant in breast-fed infant gut microbiota (Sela and Mills, 2010). Thus, the ability of these species to utilize these otherwise indigestible carbohydrates explains their abundance in breast-fed neonates (Zivkovic et al., 2011).

Metabolic cross-feeding mechanisms in the gut are commonly exploited by primary microbial degraders like bifidobacteria which, thanks to partial extracellular hydrolysis of specific complex carbohydrates (e.g., host-produced glycans), provide monosaccharides, oligosaccharides, or metabolites for other microbial gut inhabitants (De Vuyst and Leroy, 2011). As an example, *B. bifidum* PRL2010 is a strain specialized in the extracellular breakdown of host-glycans and, thus, in the release of simple sugars that can be utilized by other members of the (bifido)bacterial community (Turroni et al., 2016). The subsequent fermentative metabolism of these carbohydrates generates end-metabolites, such as acetate and lactate, which are the main end-products of the bifidobacteria catabolism. Acetate released in the gut by bifidobacteria is used as substrates for other microbial gut fermenters, mainly butyrate and propionate producers (Flint et al., 2015). The production of these two major short-chain fatty acid metabolites have been shown to have anti-inflammatory effects, and promotes and regulates the pool of colonic T_{reg} cells (Arpaia et al., 2013; Smith et al., 2013). By inhibiting histone deacetylase activity in DC and T cells, butyrate acts in the differentiation of T_{reg} cells, increasing the expression of the T_{reg} marker FoxP3 (Furusawa et al., 2013). Signalization has been proposed to be mediated by the butyrate receptors in epithelial and immune cells named FFAR3 (free fatty acid receptor 3) and GPR109A (Ahmed et al., 2009; Remely et al., 2014).

CONCLUDING REMARKS

Bifidobacterial cells, their subcellular fractions, or specific molecules produced by these microorganisms, hold an important potential to trigger immunomodulatory responses involved in the maintenance of our healthy physiological state. However, these responses are poorly understood and need for more research on how this molecular communication between bifidobacteria and host cells is performed. Additionally, the increasing knowledge on the role played by different gut microbiota members, and the understanding of the cross-talk and cross-feeding interaction processes between bifidobacteria, the host, and the surrounding network of intestinal microbes, should facilitate the synergistic use of different intestinal microorganisms to modulate the immunological and inflammatory processes in a microbial dependent way.

AUTHOR CONTRIBUTIONS

AM and BS designed the structure of the mini-review. LR, SD, PR-M, BS, and AM wrote the manuscript and drafted the first version of the manuscript. All authors reviewed the final version of the manuscript.

ACKNOWLEDGMENTS

LR is a postdoctoral researcher supported by the *Juan de la Cierva* Postdoctoral Trainee Program of the Spanish Ministry of Economy and Competitiveness (MINECO; IJCI-2015-23196). BS and AM thanks MINECO for the funding of the project AGL2016-78311-R and PR-M for the project AGL2015-64901-R. SD is supported by a research contract associated to the project BIO2014-55019-JIN from the Spanish "Plan Estatal de I+D+i".

REFERENCES

Ahmed, K., Tunaru, S., and Offermanns, S. (2009). GPR109A, GPR109B and GPR81, a family of hydroxy-carboxylic acid receptors. *Trends. Pharmacol. Sci.* 30, 557–562. doi: 10.1016/j.tips.2009.09.001

Akatsu, H., Iwabuchi, N., Xiao, J., Matsuyama, Z., Kurihara, R., Okuda, K., et al. (2013). Clinical effects of probiotic *Bifidobacterium longum* BB536 on immune function and intestinal microbiota in elderly patients receiving enteral tube feeding. *J. Parenter Enteral Nutr.* 37, 631–640. doi: 10.1177/0148607112467819

Altmann, F., Kosma, P., O'Callaghan, A., Leahy, S., Bottacini, F., Molloy, E., et al. (2016). Genome analysis and characterisation of the exopolysaccharide produced by *Bifidobacterium longum* subsp. *longum* 35624™. *PLOS ONE* 11:e0162983. doi: 10.1371/journal.pone.0162983

Alvarez-Martin, P., O'Connell Motherway, M., Turroni, F., Foroni, E., Ventura, M., and van Sinderen, D. (2012). A two-component regulatory system controls autoregulated serpin expression in *Bifidobacterium breve* UCC2003. *Appl. Environ. Microbiol.* 78, 7032–7041. doi: 10.1128/AEM.01776-12

Arboleya, S., Bahrami, B., Macfarlane, S., Gueimonde, M., Macfarlane, G. T., and de los Reyes-Gavilán, C. G. (2015). Production of immune response mediators by HT-29 intestinal cell-lines in the presence of *Bifidobacterium*-treated infant microbiota. *Benef. Microbes* 6, 543–552. doi: 10.3920/BM2014.0111

Arboleya, S., Binetti, A., Salazar, N., Fernandez, N., Solis, G., Hernandez-Barranco, A., et al. (2012). Establishment and development of intestinal microbiota in preterm neonates. *FEMS Microbiol. Ecol.* 79, 763–772. doi: 10.1111/j.1574-6941.2011.01261.x [Epub. 2011 Dec. 15].

Arpaia, N., Campbell, C., Fan, X., Dikiy, S., van der Veeken, J., deRoos, P., et al. (2013). Metabolites produced by commensal bacteria promote peripheral regulatory T-cell generation. *Nature* 504, 451–455. doi: 10.1038/nature12726

Bahrami, B., Macfarlane, S., and Macfarlane, G. T. (2011). Induction of cytokine formation by human intestinal bacteria in gut epithelial cell lines. *J. Appl. Microbiol.* 110, 353–363. doi: 10.1111/j.1365-2672.2010.04889.x

Bernini, L. J., Simão, A. N. C., Alfieri, D. F., Lozovoy, M. A. B., Mari, N. L., de Souza, C. H., et al. (2016). Beneficial effects of *Bifidobacterium lactis* on lipid profile and cytokines in patients with metabolic syndrome: a randomized trial. Effects of probiotics on metabolic syndrome. *Nutrition* 32, 716–719. doi: 10.1016/j.nut.2015.11.001

Chattha, K. S., Vlasova, A. N., Kandasamy, S., Rajashekara, G., and Saif, L. J. (2013). Divergent immunomodulating effects of probiotics on T cell responses to oral attenuated human rotavirus vaccine and virulent human rotavirus infection in a neonatal gnotobiotic piglet disease model. *J. Immunol.* 191, 2446–2456. doi: 10.4049/jimmunol.1300678

Chichlowski, M., De Lartigue, G., German, J. B., Raybould, H. E., and Mills, D. A. (2012). Bifidobacteria isolated from infants and cultured on human milk oligosaccharides affect intestinal epithelial function. *J. Pediatr. Gastroenterol. Nutr.* 55, 321–327. doi: 10.1097/MPG.0b013e31824fb899

Davis, M. Y., Zhang, H., Brannan, L. E., Carman, R. J., and Boone, J. H. (2016). Rapid change of fecal microbiome and disappearance of *Clostridium difficile* in a colonized infant after transition from breast milk to cow milk. *Microbiome* 4:53. doi: 10.1186/s40168-016-0198-6

De Vuyst, L., and Leroy, F. (2011). Cross-feeding between bifidobacteria and butyrate-producing colon bacteria explains bifidobacterial competitiveness, butyrate production, and gas production. *Int. J. Food Microbiol.* 149, 73–80. doi: 10.1016/j.ijfoodmicro.2011.03.003

Duell, B. J., Cripps, A. W., Mark, A., Schembri, M. A., and Ulett, G. C. (2011). Epithelial cell coculture models for studying infectious diseases: benefits and limitations. *J. Biomed. Biotechnol.* 2011:852419. doi: 10.1155/2011/852419

Enomoto, T., Sowa, M., Nishimori, K., Shimazu, S., Yoshida, A., Yamada, K., et al. (2014). Effects of bifidobacterial supplementation to pregnant women and infants in the prevention of allergy development in infants and on fecal microbiota. *Allergol. Int.* 63, 575–585. doi: 10.2332/allergolint.13-OA-0683

Ewaschuk, J. B., Diaz, H., Meddings, L., Diederichs, B., Dmytrash, A., Backer, J., et al. (2008). Secreted bioactive factors from *Bifidobacterium infantis* enhance epithelial cell barrier function. *Am. J. Physiol. Gastrointest. Liver Physiol.* 295, G1025–G1034. doi: 10.1152/ajpgi.90227.2008

Ezendam, J., de Klerk, A., Gremmer, E. R., and van Loveren, H. (2008). Effects of Bifidobacterium animalis administered during lactation on allergic and autoimmune responses in rodents. *Clin. Exp. Immunol.* 154, 424–431. doi: 10.1111/j.1365-2249.2008.03788.x

Fanning, S., Hall, L. J., Cronin, M., Zomer, A., MacSharry, J., Goulding, D., et al. (2012). Bifidobacterial surface-exopolysaccharide facilitates commensal-host interaction through immune modulation and pathogen protection. *Proc. Natl. Acad. Sci. U.S.A.* 109, 2108–2113. doi: 10.1073/pnas.1115621109

Flint, H. J., Duncan, S. H., Scott, K. P., and Louis, P. (2015). Links between diet, gut microbiota composition and gut metabolism. *Proc. Nutr. Soc.* 74, 13–22. doi: 10.1017/S0029665114001463

Fujimura, K. E., Sitarik, A. R., Havstad, S., Lin, D. L., Levan, S., Fadrosh, D., et al. (2016). Neonatal gut microbiota associates with childhood multisensitized atopy and T cell differentiation. *Nature Med.* 22, 1187–1191. doi: 10.1038/nm.4176

Furusawa, Y., Obata, Y., Fukuda, S., Endo, T., Nakato, G., Takahashi, D., et al. (2013). Commensal microbe-derived butyrate induces the differentiation of colonic regulatory T cells. *Nature* 504, 446–450. doi: 10.1038/nature12721

Górska, S., Dylus, E., Rudawska, A., Brzozowska, E., Srutkova, D., Schwarzer, M., et al. (2016). Immunoreactive Proteins of *Bifidobacterium longum* ssp. *longum CCM* 7952 and *Bifidobacterium longum* ssp. longum CCDM 372 Identified by Gnotobiotic Mono-Colonized Mice Sera, Immune Rabbit Sera and Non-immune Human Sera. *Front. Microbiol.* 7:1537. doi: 10.3389/fmicb.2016.01537

Groeger, D., O'Mahony, L., Murphy, E. F., Bourke, J. F., Dinan, T. G., Kiely, B., et al. (2013). Bifidobacterium infantis 35624 modulates host inflammatory processes beyond the gut. *Gut Microbes* 4, 325–339. doi: 10.4161/gmic.25487

Guglielmetti, S., Zanoni, I., Balzaretti, S., Miriani, M., Taverniti, V., De Noni, I., et al. (2014). Murein lytic enzyme TgaA of Bifidobacterium bifidum MIMBb75 modulates dendritic cell maturation through its cysteine- and histidine-dependent amidohydrolase/peptidase (CHAP) amidase domain. *Appl. Environ. Microbiol.* 80, 5170–5177. doi: 10.1128/AEM.00761-14

Guo, Z., Zhang, J., Wang, Z., Ang, K. Y., Huang, S., Hou, Q., et al. (2016). Intestinal microbiota distinguish gout patients from healthy humans. *Sci. Rep.* 6:20602. doi: 10.1038/srep20602

He, F., Morita, H., Ouwehand, A. C., Hosoda, M., Hiramatsu, M., Kurisaki, J., et al. (2002). Stimulation of the secretion of pro-inflammatory cytokines by bifidobacterium strains. *Microbiol. Immunol.* 46, 781–785. doi: 10.1111/j.1348-0421.2002.tb02765.x

Herfel, T. M., Jacobi, S. K., Lin, X., Jouni, Z. E., Chichlowski, M., Stahl, C. H., et al. (2013). Dietary supplementation of *Bifidobacterium longum* strain AH1206 increases its cecal abundance and elevates intestinal interleukin-10 expression in the neonatal piglet. *Food Chem. Toxicol.* 60, 116–122. doi: 10.1016/j.fct.2013.07.020

Hevia, A., López, P., Suárez, A., Jacquot, C., Urdaci, M. C., Margolles, A., et al. (2014). Association of levels of antibodies from patients with inflammatory bowel disease with extracellular proteins of food and probiotic bacteria. *Biomed Res. Int.* 2014:351204. doi: 10.1155/2014/351204

Hevia, A., Milani, C., López, P., Donado, C. D., Cuervo, A., González, S., et al. (2016). Allergic patients with long-term asthma display low levels of *Bifidobacterium adolescentis*. *PLOS ONE* 11:e0147809. doi: 10.1371/journal.pone.0147809

Hidalgo-cantabrana, C., Arboleya, S., Sánchez, B., Gueimonde, M., de los Reyes-Gavilán, C. G., Margolles, A., et al. (2012). "Intestinal Microbiota as a source of probiotic *Bifidobacterium* strains: challenges and opportunities for the development of functional foods," in *Beneficial Microbes in Fermented and Functional Foods*, eds R. Rai and J. A. Bai (Boca Raton, FL: CRC Press).

Hidalgo-Cantabrana, C., Delgado, S., Ruiz, L., Ruas-Madiedo, P., Sánchez, B., and Margolles, A. (2017a). Bifidobacteria and their health-promoting effects. *Microbiol. Spectr.* 5:BAD-0010-2016. doi: 10.1128/microbiolspec.BAD-0010-2016

Hidalgo-Cantabrana, C., Moro-García, M. A., Blanco-Míguez, A., Fernández-Riverola, F., Lourenço, A., Alonso-Arias, R., et al. (2017b). *In silico* screening of the human gut metaproteome identifies Th17-promoting peptides encrypted in proteins of commensal bacteria. *Front. Microbiol.* 8:1726. doi: 10.3389/fmicb.2017.01726

Hidalgo-Cantabrana, C., Sánchez, B., Álvarez-Martín, P., López, P., Martínez-Álvarez, N., Delley, M., et al. (2015). A single mutation in the gene responsible for the mucoid phenotype of *Bifidobacterium animalis* subsp. *lactis* confers surface and functional characteristics. *Appl. Environ. Microbiol.* 81, 7960–7968. doi: 10.1128/AEM.02095-15

Hidalgo-Cantabrana, C., Sánchez, B., Milani, C., Ventura, M., Margolles, A., and Ruas-Madiedo, P. (2014). Genomic overview and biological functions of exopolysaccharide biosynthesis in *Bifidobacterium* spp. *Appl. Environ. Microbiol.* 80, 9–18. doi: 10.1128/AEM.02977-13

Hill, C. J., Lynch, D. B., Murphy, K., Ulaszewska, M., Jeffery, I. B., O'Shea, C., et al. (2017). Evolution of gut microbiota composition from birth to 24 weeks in the INFANTMET cohort. *Microbiome* 5:4. doi: 10.1186/s40168-016-0213-y

Hoarau, C., Lagaraine, C., Martin, L., Velge-Roussel, F., and Lebranchu, Y. (2006). Supernatant of *Bifidobacterium breve* induces dendritic cell maturation, activation, and survival through a Toll-like receptor 2 pathway. *J. Allergy Clin. Immunol.* 117, 696–702. doi: 10.1016/j.jaci.2005.10.043

Hoarau, C., Martin, L., Faugaret, D., Baron, C., Dauba, A., Aubert-Jacquin, C., et al. (2008). Supernatant from *Bifidobacterium* differentially modulates transduction signaling pathways for biological functions of human dendritic cells. *PLOS ONE* 3:e2753. doi: 10.1371/journal.pone.0002753

Hughes, K. R., Harnisch, L. C., Alcon-Giner, C., Mitra, S., Wright, C. J., Ketskemety, J., et al. (2017). *Bifidobacterium breve* reduces apoptotic epithelial cell shedding in an exopolysaccharide and MyD88-dependent manner. *Open Biol.* 7:160155. doi: 10.1098/rsob.160155

Ishizuka, T., Kanmani, P., Kobayashi, H., Miyazaki, A., Soma, J., Suda, Y., et al. (2016). Immunobiotic bifidobacteria strains modulate rotavirus immune response in porcine intestinal epitheliocytes via pattern recognition receptor signaling. *PLOS ONE* 11:e0152416. doi: 10.1371/journal.pone.0152416

Ismail, I. H., Boyle, R. J., Licciardi, P. V., Oppedisano, F., Lahtinen, S., Robins-Browne, R. M., et al. (2016). Early gut colonization by *Bifidobacterium breve* and *B. catenulatum* differentially modulates eczema risk in children at high risk of developing allergic disease. *Pediatr. Allergy Immunol.* 27, 838–846. doi: 10.1111/pai.12646

Ivanov, D., Emonet, C., Foata, F., Affolter, M., Delley, M., Fisseha, M., et al. (2006). A serpin from the gut bacterium *Bifidobacterium longum* inhibits eukaryotic elastase-like serine proteases. *J. Biol. Chem.* 281, 17246–17252. doi: 10.1074/jbc.M601678200

Kalliomaki, M., Kirjavainen, P., Eerola, E., Kero, P., Salminen, S., and Isolauri, E. (2001). Distinct patterns of neonatal gut microflora in infants in whom atopy was and was not developing. *J. Allergy Clin. Immunol.* 107, 129–134. doi: 10.1067/mai.2001.111237

Kandasamy, S., Chattha, K. S., Vlasova, A. N., Rajashekara, G., and Saif, L. J. (2014). Lactobacilli and Bifidobacteria enhance mucosal B cell responses and differentially modulate systemic antibody responses to an oral human rotavirus vaccine in a neonatal gnotobiotic pig disease model. *Gut Microbes* 5, 639–651. doi: 10.4161/19490976.2014.969972

Khokhlova, E. V., Smeianov, V. V., Efimov, B. A., Kafarskaia, L. I., Pavlova, S. I., and Shkoporov, A. N. (2012). Anti-inflammatory properties of intestinal *Bifidobacterium* strains isolated from healthy infants. *Microbiol. Immunol.* 56, 27–39. doi: 10.1111/j.1348-0421.2011.00398.x

Kim, J.-H., Jeun, E.-J., Hong, C.-P., Kim, S.-H., Jang, M. S., Lee, E.-J., et al. (2016). Extracellular vesicle derived protein from *Bifidobacterium longum* alleviates food allergy through mast cell suppression. *J. Allergy Clin. Immunol.* 137, 507–516. doi: 10.1016/j.jaci.2015.08.016

Klemenak, M., Dolinšek, J., Langerholc, T., Di Gioia, D., and Mičetić-Turk, D. (2015). Administration of *Bifidobacterium breve* decreases the production of TNF-α in children with celiac disease. *Dig. Dis. Sci.* 60, 3386–3392. doi: 10.1007/s10620-015-3769-7

Kobayashi, H., Kanmani, P., Ishizuka, T., Miyazaki, A., Soma, J., Albarracin, L., et al. (2017). Development of an *in vitro* immunobiotic evaluation system against rotavirus infection in bovine intestinal epitheliocytes. *Benef. Microbes* 8, 309–321. doi: 10.3920/BM2016.0155

Laparra, J. M., Olivares, M., Gallina, O., and Sanz, Y. (2012). *Bifidobacterium longum* CECT 7347 modulates immune responses in a gliadin-induced enteropathy animal model. *PLOS ONE* 7:e30744. doi: 10.1371/journal.pone.0030744

Lee, D.-K., Kim, M.-J., Ham, J.-W., An, H.-M., Cha, M.-K., Lee, S.-W., et al. (2012). *In Vitro* evaluation of antibacterial activities and anti-inflammatory effects of *Bifidobacterium* spp. addressing acne vulgaris. *Arch. Pharm. Res.* 35, 1065–1071. doi: 10.1007/s12272-012-0614-9

Lim, S.-M., and Kim, D.-H. (2017). *Bifidobacterium adolescentis* IM38 ameliorates high-fat diet–induced colitis in mice by inhibiting NF-κB activation and lipopolysaccharide production by gut microbiota. *Nutr. Res.* 41, 86–96. doi: 10.1016/j.nutres.2017.04.003

Liu, Y., Gibson, G. R., and Walton, G. E. (2016). An *in vitro* approach to study effects of prebiotics and probiotics on the faecal microbiota and selected immune parameters relevant to the elderly. *PLOS ONE* 11:e0162604. doi: 10.1371/journal.pone.0162604

López, P., Gueimonde, M., Margolles, A., and Suárez, A. (2010). Distinct *Bifidobacterium* strains drive different immune responses in vitro. *Int. J. Food Microbiol.* 138, 157–165. doi: 10.1016/j.ijfoodmicro.2009.12.023

Luongo, D., Treppiccione, L., Sorrentino, A., Ferrocino, I., Turroni, S., Gatti, M., et al. (2017). Immune-modulating effects in mouse dendritic cells of lactobacilli and bifidobacteria isolated from individuals following omnivorous, vegetarian and vegan diets. *Cytokine* 97, 141–148. doi: 10.1016/j.cyto.2017.06.007

Maneerat, S., Lehtinen, M. J., Childs, C. E., Forssten, S. D., Alhoniemi, E., Tiphaine, M., et al. (2014). Consumption of *Bifidobacterium lactis* Bi-07 by healthy elderly adults enhances phagocytic activity of monocytes and granulocytes. *J. Nutr. Sci.* 2, e44. doi: 10.1017/jns.2013.31

Matsumoto, M., Aranami, A., Ishige, A., Watanabe, K., and Benno, Y. (2007). LKM512 yogurt consumption improves the intestinal environment and induces the T-helper type 1 cytokine in adult patients with intractable atopic dermatitis. *Clin. Exp. Allergy* 37, 358–370. doi: 10.1111/j.1365-2222.2007.02642.x

Medina, M., Izquierdo, E., Ennahar, S., and Sanz, Y. (2007). Differential immunomodulatory properties of *Bifidobacterium logum* strains: relevance to probiotic selection and clinical applications. *Clin. Exp. Immunol.* 150, 531–538. doi: 10.1111/j.1365-2249.2007.03522.x

Ménard, O., Gafa, V., Kapel, N., Rodriguez, B., Butel, M. J., and Waligora-Dupriet, A. J. (2010). Characterization of immunostimulatory CpG-rich sequences from different *Bifidobacterium* species. *Appl. Environ. Microbiol.* 76, 2846–2855. doi: 10.1128/AEM.01714-09

Meng, H., Ba, Z., Lee, Y., Peng, J., Lin, J., Fleming, J. A., et al. (2017). Consumption of *Bifidobacterium animalis* subsp. *lactis* BB-12 in yogurt reduced expression of TLR-2 on peripheral blood-derived monocytes and pro-inflammatory cytokine secretion in young adults. *Eur. J. Nutr.* 56, 649–661. doi: 10.1007/s00394-015-1109-5

Milani, C., Lugli, G. A., Duranti, S., Turroni, F., Mancabelli, L., Ferrario, C., et al. (2015). Bifidobacteria exhibit social behavior through carbohydrate resource sharing in the gut. *Sci. Rep.* 5:15782. doi: 10.1038/srep15782

Miller, L. E., Lehtoranta, L., and Lehtinen, M. J. (2017). The Effect of *Bifidobacterium animalis* ssp. *lactis* HN019 on cellular immune function in healthy elderly subjects: systematic review and meta-analysis. *Nutrients* 9:E191. doi: 10.3390/nu9030191

Miraglia Del Giudice, M., Indolfi, C., Capasso, M., Maiello, N., Decimo, F., and Ciprandi, G. (2017). *Bifidobacterium* mixture (B longum BB536, B infantis M-63, B breve M-16V) treatment in children with seasonal allergic rhinitis and intermittent asthma. *Ital. J. Pediatr.* 43:25. doi: 10.1186/s13052-017-0340-5

Mokrozub, V. V., Lazarenko, L. M., Sichel, L. M., Babenko, L. P., Lytvyn, P. M., Demchenko, O. M., et al. (2015). The role of beneficial bacteria wall elasticity in regulating innate immune response. *EPMA J.* 6, 13. doi: 10.1186/s13167-015-0035-1

Mouni, F., Aissi, E., Hernández, J., Gorocica, P., Bouquelet, S., Zenteno, E., et al. (2009). Effect of *Bifidobacterium bifidum* DSM 20082 cytoplasmic fraction on human immune cells. *Immunol. Invest.* 38, 104–115. doi: 10.1080/08820130802608303

Moya-Pérez, A., Neef, A., and Sanz, Y. (2015). *Bifidobacterium pseudocatenulatum* CECT 7765 reduces obesity-associated inflammation by restoring the lymphocyte-macrophage balance and gut microbiota structure in high-fat diet-fed mice. *PLOS ONE* 10:e0126976. doi: 10.1371/journal.pone.0126976

Nicola, S., Amoruso, A., Deidda, F., Pane, M., Allesina, S., Mogna, L., et al. (2016). Searching for the perfect homeostasis: five strains of *Bifidobacterium longum* from centenarians have a similar behavior in the production of cytokines. *J. Clin. Gastroenterol.* 50, S126–S130. doi: 10.1097/MCG.0000000000000678

Noel, G., Baetz, N. W., Staab, J. F., Donowitz, M., Kovbasnjuk, O., Pasetti, M. P., et al. (2017). A primary human macrophage-enteroid co-culture model to investigate mucosal gut physiology and host-pathogen interactions. *Sci. Rep.* 7:45270. doi: 10.1038/srep45270

Olivares, M., Castillejo, G., Varea, V., and Sanz, Y. (2014). Double-blind, randomised, placebo-controlled intervention trial to evaluate the effects of *Bifidobacterium longum* CECT 7347 in children with newly diagnosed coeliac disease. *Br. J. Nutr.* 112, 30–40. doi: 10.1017/S0007114514000609

Oosterloo, B. C., Premkumar, M., Stoll, B., Olutoye, O., Thymann, T., Sangild, P. T., et al. (2014). Dual purpose use of preterm piglets as a model of pediatric GI disease. *Vet. Immunol. Immunopathol.* 159, 156–165. doi: 10.1016/j.vetimm.2014.02.012

Philippe, D., Heupel, E., Blum-Sperisen, S., and Riedel, C. U. (2011). Treatment with Bifidobacterium bifidum 17 partially protects mice from Th1-driven inflammation in a chemically induced model of colitis. *Int. J. Food Microbiol.* 149, 45–49. doi: 10.1016/j.ijfoodmicro.2010.12.020

Pinto-Sánchez, M. I., Smecuol, E. C., Temprano, M. P., Sugai, E., González, A., Moreno, M. L., et al. (2017). *Bifidobacterium infantis* NLS super strain reduces the expression of α-defensin-5, a marker of innate immunity, in the mucosa of active celiac disease patients. *J. Clin. Gastroenterol.* 51, 814–817. doi: 10.1097/MCG.0000000000000687

Pozo-Rubio, T., Mujico, J. R., Marcos, A., Puertollano, E., Nadal, I., Sanz, Y., et al. (2011). Immunostimulatory effect of faecal *Bifidobacterium* species of breast-fed and formula-fed infants in a peripheral blood mononuclear cell/Caco-2 co-culture system. *Br. J. Nutr.* 106, 1216–1223. doi: 10.1017/S0007114511001656

Remely, M., Aumueller, E., Merold, C., Dworzak, S., Hippe, B., Zanner, J., et al. (2014). Effects of short chain fatty acid producing bacteria on epigenetic regulation of FFAR3 in type 2 diabetes and obesity. *Gene* 537, 85–92. doi: 10.1016/j.gene.2013.11.081

Ruas-Madiedo, P., Gueimonde, M., Fernández-García, M., de los Reyes-Gavilán, C. G., and Margolles, A. (2008). Mucin degradation by *Bifidobacterium* strains isolated from the human intestinal microbiota. *Appl. Environ. Microbiol.* 74, 1936–1940. doi: 10.1128/AEM.02509-07

Ruiz, L., Delgado, S., Ruas-Madiedo, P., Margolles, A., and Sánchez, B. (2016). Proteinaceous molecules mediating *Bifidobacterium*-host interactions. *Front. Microbiol.* 7:1193. doi: 10.3389/fmicb.2016.01193

Ruiz, L., Gueimonde, M., Coute, Y., Salminen, S., Sánchez, J. C., de los Reyes-Gavilán, C. G., et al. (2011). Evaluation of the ability of *Bifidobacterium longum* to metabolize human intestinal mucus. *FEMS Microbiol. Lett.* 314, 125–130. doi: 10.1111/j.1574-6968.2010.02159.x

Salazar, N., López, P., Garrido, P., Moran, J., Cabello, E., Gueimonde, M., et al. (2014). Immune modulating capability of two exopolysaccharide-producing *Bifidobacterium* strains in a wistar rat model. *Biomed Res. Int.* 2014:106290. doi: 10.1155/2014/106290

Sánchez, B., González-Rodriguez, I., Arboleya, S., López, P., Suárez, A., Ruas-Madiedo, P., et al. (2015). The effects of *Bifidobacterium breve* on immune mediators and proteome of HT29 cells monolayers. *Biomed. Res. Int.* 2015:479140. doi: 10.1155/2015/479140

Schiavi, E., Gleinser, M., Molloy, E., Groeger, D., Frei, R., Ferstl, R., et al. (2016). The surface-associated exopolysaccharide of *Bifidobacterium longum* 35624 plays an essential role in dampening host proinflammatory responses and repressing local TH17 responses. *Appl. Environ. Microbiol.* 82, 7185–7196. doi: 10.1128/AEM.02238-16

Sela, D. A., and Mills, D. A. (2010). Nursing our microbiota: molecular linkages between bifidobacteria and milk oligosaccharides. *Trends Microbiol.* 18, 298–307. doi: 10.1016/j.tim.2010.03.008

Singh, A., Hacini-Rachinel, F., Gosoniu, M. L., Bourdeau, T., Holvoet, S., Doucet-Ladeveze, R., et al. (2013). Immune-modulatory effect of probiotic *Bifidobacterium lactis* NCC2818 in individuals suffering from seasonal allergic rhinitis to grass pollen: an exploratory, randomized, placebo-controlled clinical trial. *Eur. J. Clin. Nutr.* 67, 161–167. doi: 10.1038/ejcn.2012.197

Sivan, A., Corrales, L., Hubert, N., Williams, J. B., Aquino-Michaels, K., Earley, Z. M., et al. (2015). Commensal *Bifidobacterium* promotes antitumor immunity and facilitates anti-PD-L1 efficacy. *Science* 350, 1084–1089. doi: 10.1126/science.aac4255

Smith, P. M., Howitt, M. R., Panikov, N., Michaud, M., Gallini, C. A., Bohlooly, Y. M., et al. (2013). The microbial metabolites, short-chain fatty acids, regulate colonic Treg cell homeostasis. *Science* 341, 569–573. doi: 10.1126/science.1241165

Spaiser, S. J., Culpepper, T., Nieves, C., Ukhanova, M., Mai, V., Percival, S. S., et al. (2015). Lactobacillus gasseri KS-13, *Bifidobacterium bifidum* G9-1, and *Bifidobacterium longum* MM-2 ingestion induces a less inflammatory cytokine profile and a potentially beneficial shift in gut microbiota in older adults: a randomized, double-blind, placebo-controlled, crossover study. *J. Am. Coll. Nutr.* 34, 459–469. doi: 10.1080/07315724.2014.983249

Srutkova, D., Schwarzer, M., Hudcovic, T., Zakostelska, Z., Drab, V., Spanova, A., et al. (2015). *Bifidobacterium longum* CCM 7952 promotes epithelial barrier function and prevents acute DSS-induced colitis in strictly strain-specific manner. *PLOS ONE* 10:e0134050. doi: 10.1371/journal.pone.0134050

Strisciuglio, C., Miele, E., Giugliano, F. P., Vitale, S., Andreozzi, M., Vitale, A., et al. (2015). Bifidobacteria enhance antigen sampling and processing by dendritic cells in pediatric inflammatory bowel disease. *Inflamm. Bowel Dis.* 21, 1491–1498. doi: 10.1097/MIB.0000000000000389

Sugahara, H., Yao, R., Odamaki, T., and Xiao, J. Z. (2017). Differences between live and heat-killed bifidobacteria in the regulation of immune function and the intestinal environment. *Benef. Microbes* 8, 463–472. doi: 10.3920/BM2016.0158

Sutterwala, F. S., and Flavell, R. A. (2009). NLRC4/IPAF: a CARD carrying member of the NLR family. *Clin. Immunol.* 130, 2–6. doi: 10.1016/j.clim.2008.08.011

Tailford, L. E., Crost, E. H., Kavanaugh, D., and Juge, N. (2015). Mucin glycan foraging in the human gut microbiome. *Front. Genet.* 6:81. doi: 10.3389/fgene.2015.00081

Takahashi, N., Kitazawa, H., Iwabuchi, N., Xiao, J. Z., Miyaji, K., Iwatsuki, K., et al. (2006). Immunostimulatory oligodeoxynucleotide from *Bifidobacterium longum* suppresses Th2 immune responses in a murine model. *Clin. Exp. Immunol.* 145, 130–138. doi: 10.1111/j.1365-2249.2006.03111.x

Tan, T. G., Sefik, E., Geva-Zatorsky, N., Kua, L., Naskar, D., Teng, F., et al. (2016). Identifying species of symbiont bacteria from the human gut that, alone, can induce intestinal Th17 cells in mice. *Proc. Natl. Acad. Sci. U.S.A.* 113, E8141–E8150. doi: 10.1073/pnas.1617460113

Tanabe, S., Kinuta, Y., and Saito, Y. (2008). Bifidobacterium infantis suppresses proinflammatory interleukin-17 production in murine splenocytes and dextran sodium sulfate-induced intestinal inflammation. *Int. J. Mol. Med.* 22, 181–185. doi: 10.3892/ijmm_00000006

Turroni, F., Bottacini, F., Foroni, E., Mulder, I., Kim, J. H., Zomer, A., et al. (2010b). Genome analysis of *Bifidobacterium bifidum* PRL2010 reveals metabolic pathways for host-derived glycan foraging. *Proc. Natl. Acad. Sci. U.S.A.* 107, 19514–19519. doi: 10.1073/pnas.1011100107

Turroni, F., Foroni, E., O'Connell Motherway, M., Bottacini, F., Giubellini, V., Zomer, A., et al. (2010a). Characterization of the serpin-encoding gene of *Bifidobacterium breve* 210B. *Appl. Environ. Microbiol.* 76, 3206–3219. doi: 10.1128/AEM.02938-09

Turroni, F., Milani, C., Duranti, S., Mancabelli, L., Mangifesta, M., Viappiani, A., et al. (2016). Deciphering bifidobacterial-mediated metabolic interactions and their impact on gut microbiota by a multi-omics approach. *ISME J.* 10, 1656–1668. doi: 10.1038/ismej.2015.236

Turroni, F., Serafini, F., Foroni, E., Duranti, S., O'Connell Motherway, M., Taverniti, V., et al. (2013). Role of sortase-dependent pili of *Bifidobacterium bifidum* PRL2010 in modulating bacterium-host interactions. *Proc. Natl. Acad. Sci. U.S.A.* 110, 11151–11156. doi: 10.1073/pnas.1303897110

Turroni, F., Serafini, F., Mangifesta, M., Arioli, S., Mora, D., van Sinderen, D., et al. (2014). Expression of sortase-dependent pili of *Bifidobacterium bifidum* PRL2010 in response to environmental gut conditions. *FEMS Microbiol. Lett.* 357, 23–33. doi: 10.1111/1574-6968.12509

Van Kruiningen, H. J., West, A. B., Freda, B. J., and Holmes, K. A. (2002). Distribution of Peyer's patches in the distal ileum. *Inflamm. Bowel Dis.* 8, 180–185. doi: 10.1097/00054725-200205000-00004

Vieira, A. T., Galvão, I., Amaral, F. A., Teixeira, M. M., Nicoli, J. R., and Martins, F. S. (2015). Oral treatment with *Bifidobacterium longum* 5 1A reduced inflammation in a murine experimental model of gout. *Benef. Microbes* 6, 799–806. doi: 10.3920/BM2015.0015

Vlasova, A. N., Chattha, K. S., Kandasamy, S., Liu, Z., Esseili, M., Shao, L., et al. (2013). Lactobacilli and bifidobacteria promote immune homeostasis by modulating innate immune responses to human rotavirus in neonatal gnotobiotic pigs. *PLOS ONE* 8:e76962. doi: 10.1371/journal.pone.0076962

Wittmann, A., Autenrieth, I. B., and Frick, J.-S. (2013). Plasmacytoid dendritic cells are crucial in *Bifidobacterium adolescentis*-mediated inhibition of *Yersinia enterocolitica* infection. *PLOS ONE* 8:e71338. doi: 10.1371/journal.pone.0071338

Wu, B.-B., Yang, Y., Xu, X., and Wang, W.-P. (2016). Effects of *Bifidobacterium* supplementation on intestinal microbiota composition and the immune response in healthy infants. *World J. Pediatr.* 12, 177–182. doi: 10.1007/s12519-015-0025-3

Wu, M. H., Pan, T. M., Wu, Y. J., Chang, S. J., Chang, M. S., and Hu, C. Y. (2010). Exopolysaccharide activities from probiotic *Bifidobacterium*: immunomodulatory effects (on J774A.1 macrophages) and antimicrobial properties. *Int. J. Food Microbiol.* 144, 104–110. doi: 10.1016/j.ijfoodmicro.2010.09.003

Yatsunenko, T., Rey, F. E., Manary, M. J., Trehan, I., Dominguez-Bello, M. G., Contreras, M., et al. (2012). Human gut microbiome viewed across age and geography. *Nature* 486, 222–227. doi: 10.1038/nature11053

Zelante, T., Fric, J., Wong, A. Y. W., and Ricciardi-Castagnoli, P. (2012). Interleukin-2 production by dendritic cells and its immuno-regulatory functions. *Front. Immunol.* 3:161. doi: 10.3389/fimmu.2012.00161

Zivkovic, A. M., German, J. B., Lebrilla, C. B., and Mills, D. A. (2011). Human milk glycobiome and its impact on the infant gastrointestinal microbiota. *Proc. Natl. Acad. Sci. U.S.A.* 108, 4653–4658. doi: 10.1073/pnas.1000083107

14

Modulatory Influence of Segmented Filamentous Bacteria on Transcriptomic Response of Gnotobiotic Mice Exposed to TCDD

Robert D. Stedtfeld[1]*, Benli Chai[2], Robert B. Crawford[3,4], Tiffany M. Stedtfeld[1], Maggie R. Williams[1], Shao Xiangwen[1], Tomomi Kuwahara[5], James R. Cole[2], Norbert E. Kaminski[3,4], James M. Tiedje[2] and Syed A. Hashsham[1,2]*

[1] Department of Civil and Environmental Engineering, East Lansing, MI, United States, [2] Center for Microbial Ecology, Michigan State University, East Lansing, MI, United States, [3] Institute for Integrative Toxicology, Michigan State University, East Lansing, MI, United States, [4] Department of Pharmacology and Toxicology, Michigan State University, East Lansing, MI, United States, [5] Department of Molecular Bacteriology, Institute of Health Biosciences, University of Tokushima Graduate School, Tokushima, Japan

***Correspondence:**
Syed A. Hashsham
hashsham@egr.msu.edu
Robert D. Stedtfeld
stedtfel@msu.edu

Environmental toxicants such as 2,3,7,8-tetrachlorodibenzo-*p*-dioxin (TCDD), an aryl hydrocarbon receptor (AhR), are known to induce host toxicity and structural shifts in the gut microbiota. Key bacterial populations with similar or opposing functional responses to AhR ligand exposure may potentially help regulate expression of genes associated with immune dysfunction. To examine this question and the mechanisms for AhR ligand-induced bacterial shifts, C57BL/6 gnotobiotic mice were colonized with and without segmented filamentous bacteria (SFB) – an immune activator. Mice were also colonized with polysaccharide A producing *Bacteroides fragilis* – an immune suppressor to serve as a commensal background. Following colonization, mice were administered TCDD (30 μg/kg) every 4 days for 28 days by oral gavage. Quantified with the nCounter® mouse immunology panel, opposing responses in ileal gene expression (e.g., genes associated with T-cell differentiation via the class II major histocompatibility complex) as a result of TCDD dosing and SFB colonization were observed. Genes that responded to TCDD in the presence of SFB did not show a significant response in the absence of SFB, and vice versa. Regulatory T-cells examined in the mesenteric lymph-nodes, spleen, and blood were also less impacted by TCDD in mice colonized with SFB. TCDD-induced shifts in abundance of SFB and *B. fragilis* compared with previous studies in mice with a traditional gut microbiome. With regard to the mouse model colonized with individual populations, results indicate that TCDD-induced host response was significantly modulated by the presence of SFB in the gut microbiome, providing insight into therapeutic potential between AhR ligands and key commensals.

Keywords: TCDD, segmented filamentous bacteria, gnotobiotic mice, regulatory T-cells, gut dysbiosis, host microbe response, *B. fragilis*

INTRODUCTION

Dysbiosis of certain key immune modulating commensals can influence host disposition to disease and environmental exposure (Snedeker and Hay, 2012). Specific individual bacterial groups can also revive or influence differentiation of T-cells observed in germ free or antibiotic-treated mice (Faith et al., 2014; Sefik et al., 2015; Honda and Littman, 2016). For example, multiple immune activating strains isolated from mice and human stool including segmented filamentous bacteria (SFB) induce Th_{17} cells in animal studies (Gaboriau-Routhiau et al., 2009; Ivanov et al., 2009; Atarashi et al., 2015; Tan et al., 2016). Alternatively, bacteria such as *Bacteroides fragilis* promote the expression of T_{reg} cells through polysaccharide A (PSA) production (Troy and Kasper, 2010). Dysregulation of T_{reg}/Th_{17} cells can lead to various disease outcomes (Hand and Belkaid, 2010; Ivanov and Littman, 2010). For example, *Helicobacter pylori* succeeds in colonizing the gut by causing changes in both T_{reg} and Th_{17} cells (Kao et al., 2010). Thus imbalanced levels of T-cells can influence protection against pathogens or autoimmune diseases (Fantini et al., 2007; Peck and Mellins, 2010).

Attention to environmental exposure such as dioxins and other persistent organic pollutants has increased due to possible contributions to autoimmune diseases (Hertz-Picciotto et al., 2008), among others such as developmental disorders (Lee et al., 2007), obesity (Ibrahim et al., 2011), and diabetes (Taylor et al., 2013). Mediated in part through the aryl hydrocarbon receptor (AhR), 2,3,7,8-tetrachlorodibenzo-*p*-dioxin (TCDD, a porotype for studying the bioactivity for AhR) and other dioxins promote multiple toxic health effects including immune suppression (Kerkvliet et al., 2002, 2009). Thus, AhR ligands are also critically linked to the balance of T_{reg}/Th_{17} cells (Ho and Steinman, 2008; Mustafa et al., 2008; Quintana et al., 2008; Veldhoen et al., 2008; Chmill et al., 2010; Marshall and Kerkvliet, 2010; Veldhoen and Duarte, 2010; Zhang et al., 2010). For example, AhR ligands have been shown to abrogate inflammation caused by Crohn's disease (Benson and Shepherd, 2011), which may in part be initially caused by commensal dysbiosis. While not completely understood, the pleiotropy type relationship between AhR modulating environmental toxicants, host, and gut commensals may potentially be employed to therapeutically modulate health.

Emerging studies also suggest that environmental toxicants such as TCDD (Lefever et al., 2016; Stedtfeld et al., 2017b) and other AhR ligands interact with gut commensals (Hubbard et al., 2015; Zhang et al., 2015; Murray et al., 2016). Previous murine studies with a traditional gut microbiome found that TCDD induced structural shifts in key bacterial populations; with increasing abundance of SFB (Bhaduri, 2015; Stedtfeld et al., 2017a) and decreasing abundance of *Bacteroidetes* in response to TCDD (Lefever et al., 2016). Known opposing T-cell host responses to SFB and exposure to TCDD suggest that expansion of SFB could potentially abrogate or lessen TCDD-induced toxicity and differentiation of regulatory T-cells (Marshall et al., 2008; Ivanov et al., 2009). It was also unknown if SFB response was due to structural shifts in other bacterial populations (e.g., decreased abundance in *Bacteroidetes*), or due to TCDD-induced shifts in the host.

To answer these questions and examine the modulatory potential of an immune activating bacteria in animals exposed to TCDD, gnotobiotic mice were colonized with and without SFB. Mice were also colonized with immune suppressing (Round and Mazmanian, 2010; Troy and Kasper, 2010; Atarashi et al., 2011) PSA producing *B. fragilis* to serve as a commensal background. A separate group of mice was also mono-colonized with SFB or non-colonized to further verify the modulatory potential.

MATERIALS AND METHODS

Animal Models and Bacterial Cocktails

Germ-free female C57BL/6 mice were bred and maintained at the Germ-Free Mouse Facility housed in the Unit for Laboratory Animal Medicine at the University of Michigan (Ann Arbor, MI, United States) and maintained in germ-free isolators. Mice were orally colonized with bacteria 4–6 weeks after birth (Supplementary Figure S1). TCDD dosing started 4 weeks after colonization. A previously described TCDD dosing regimen of 30 μg/kg (AccuStandard, New Haven, CT, United States) by oral gavage once every 4 days for 28 days (Fader et al., 2015; Nault et al., 2015) was used. Mice were dosed by oral gavage with 0.1 ml of sesame oil vehicle control (Sigma–Aldrich, St. Louis, MO, United States) or TCDD in sesame oil vehicle.

Results shown in this study are based on the following two experiments and animal numbers: Experiment 1 consisted of untreated (vehicle) with *B. fragilis* mono-colonization ($n = 4$), TCDD treated with *B. fragilis* mono-colonization ($n = 4$), an untreated (vehicle) with co-colonization of SFB and *B. fragilis* groups ($n = 4$), and TCDD-treated with co-colonization of both groups ($n = 4$).

To further verify modulation potential of SFB, experiments were replicated in the absence of *B. fragilis* including untreated (vehicle) uncolonized (UC; $n = 4$), TCDD-treated UC ($n = 4$), untreated (vehicle) with SFB mono-colonization ($n = 4$), and TCDD-treated with SFB mono-colonization ($n = 4$). One untreated mouse mono-colonized with SFB and one co-colonized treated mouse died prior to sacrifice. Mice had access to sterile water and food *ad libitum*. All animals received humane care in compliance with the animal use protocol approved by the University of Michigan, U of M Animal Welfare Assurance (A3114-01). Handling of blood and tissue exposed to TCDD was carried out as per MSU's Environmental Health and Safety approved protocols under AUF numbers 02/14-030-00.

Bacteroides fragilis (DSM 2151) used for colonization was grown in Brucella broth (AS-105, Anaerobe Systems, Morgan Hill, CA, United States). *Candidatus* Savagella SFB-mouse-Japan, isolated as described previously (Kuwahara et al., 2011), was used for SFB groups. SFB was provided through an MTA between MSU and Kagawa University, Japan (No. AGR2015-00006 Kagawa University) and used as per approved protocols for handling BSL2 organisms. Prior to the association of bacteria into germ-free mice, qPCR was used to estimate abundance of bacteria and confirmed by Sanger sequencing of the 16S rRNA gene to ensure correct bacterial species. qPCR reactions included 1 ng of DNA extracted from fecal pellets, 18 μl Master Mix, and 1 μl of 10 mM primer mix in a 20 μl reaction. PCR conditions were as previously described (Bouskra et al., 2008). Briefly, cycling consisted of an initial 95°C for 5 min, 40 cycles of 95°C for 55 s, 60°C for 55 s, and 72°C for 1.5 min. Amplicons from three biological replicates (used for oral gavage) were purified using the Qiagen PCR purification kit and sequenced using the 96-capillary electrophoretic ABI 3730xl platform. Sequenced samples showed 99% identity with published mouse SFB sequences in the NCBI database (Accession Numbers: CP008713.1, AP012209.1, and AP012202.1). *B. fragilis* colonized groups were also inoculated with additional commensals including *Faecalibacterium prausnitzii* DSM 17677, *Ruminococcus bromii* Strain VPI 6883, *R. obeum* DSM 25238, *Butyrivibrio fibrisolvens* DSM 3071, and *Eubacterium rectale* DSM 17629 to serve as a background; however, only *B. fragilis* and SFB colonized to detectable levels in matrices tested.

Collection of Fecal Pellets and Isolation of Tissue

Fresh fecal pellets were collected and analyzed every 8 days to ensure colonization, no contamination of unwanted bacterial groups, and examine the influence of TCDD on bacterial abundance. Fecal pellets were placed in RNA/DNA stabilizer (Zymo Research Corp, Irvine, CA, United States) and stored in a −20°C freezer. Whole blood, spleen, mesenteric lymph nodes, and intestinal tissues were collected at the time of sacrifice. Mice were weighed prior to sacrifice. Two intestinal sections were removed and used for subsequent analysis, including the cecum and the ileum. For the ileum, a 0.25 cm segment proximal to the cecum was removed and stored for all animals. For the cecum, sections of content and tissue were both removed and placed in the same vial. Intestinal tissue samples were immediately placed on RNA stabilizer and stored at −80°C.

Transcriptomic Response Analysis with qPCR and nCounter®

RNA was extracted from ileum and cecum of all mice to evaluate the transcriptome response of SFB and *B. fragilis* in response to TCDD and the response of host immune cells. In detail, the PureLink RNA Mini Kit with Trizol (12183018A, Ambion/Thermo Fisher Scientific, Waltham, MA, United States) was used to extract RNA from mouse tissue and content. Two additional steps were used to digest DNA including the DNase 1 (Invitrogen/Thermo Fisher Scientific, Waltham, MA, United States) and Turbo DNase I Kit (Life Technologies/Thermo Fisher Scientific, Waltham, MA, United States). After each step, isolated RNA was quantified using a Qubit (Life Technologies), and assessed for purity using the Nanodrop ND-1000 UV-Vis spectrophotometer (Nanodrop Products, Wilmington, DE, United States).

2,3,7,8-Tetrachlorodibenzo-*p*-dioxin-induced expression of both bacterial members was monitored in the ileum and cecum using qPCR. For mRNA analysis of bacteria, qPCR primers were designed from sequences available for the colonized organisms. Genes targeting SFB functions were selected based on potential interaction with host immunity (Pamp et al., 2012) including the putative hemolysin A producing gene (BAK56433.1), and the putative rubrerythrin producing gene (BAK56170.1). Primers targeting *B. fragilis* gene clusters *wcfQ* (CAH07088.1) responsible for biosynthesis of PSA (Troutman et al., 2014) were selected due to known influence in signaling naïve T-cells differentiation into T_{reg} cells (Troy and Kasper, 2010). Primers were designed as previously described (Stedtfeld et al., 2008). Briefly, qPCR primers were designed from sequences downloaded from NCBI using Primer Express (Applied Biosystems) default settings; with a maximum length of 150 bases, and a theoretical melting temperature of 59°C. NCBI BLAST analysis (Altschul et al., 1997) was used to check theoretical specificity of designed primers against the GenBank database (Supplementary Table S1). cDNA was synthesized via random primers as instructed in the High Capacity cDNA Reverse Transcription Kit (Thermo Fisher Scientific, Waltham, MA, United States). qPCR was performed using a custom SmartChip^{TM} (Wafergen Biosystems, Fremont, CA, United States) with species-specific 16S rRNA gene and functional gene primers (Supplementary Table S1). Briefly, Wafergen's Custom SmartChip^{TM} array allows for 5,184 qPCR reactions with 100 nl volumes to be run in parallel. Sample/primers were dispensed into the SmartChip^{TM} using a Multi-sample Nano-dispenser (Wafergen Biosystems, Fremont, CA, United States). PCR cycling conditions and initial data processing were performed as previously described (Wang et al., 2014; Stedtfeld et al., 2016). Amplification reactions on the SmartChip^{TM} consisted of 1× LightCycler 480 SYBR® Green I Master Mix (Roche Inc., United States), nuclease-free PCR-grade water, 50 ng/μl cDNA template per sample, and 0.5 μM of each forward and reverse primer. Thermal cycling included an initial denaturation at 95°C for 3 min, followed by 40 cycles of denaturation at 95°C for 30 s, and annealing at 60°C for 1 min. Each primer/sample combination was tested in triplicate. Genetic copies were estimated as previously described (Looft et al., 2012). Negative controls with no templates were also included on the array.

2,3,7,8-Tetrachlorodibenzo-*p*-dioxin-induced ileal expression of host maker genes related to immune function was quantified using the nCounter® mouse immunology panel. In detail, 200 ng of digested RNA was submitted per sample using the nCounter® (NanoString Technologies, Seattle, WA, United States). NanoString's nCounter® mouse immunology panel contains probes targeting 547 immunology-related mouse genes (Reis et al., 2011).

qPCR of gDNA from Fecal Pellets

Genomic DNA was also extracted from fecal pellets 18–20 days after colonization and 21 days after initial treatment (following the sixth dose of TCDD) using the PowerSoil Extraction Kit (MoBio). qPCR was performed using species-specific 16S rRNA gene primers (Supplementary Table S1). Assays were performed in parallel using the Wafergen SmartChip^{TM} with the same reaction conditions described above for cDNA; however, only 0.1 ng/μl of gDNA was used per sample. Results showed colonization of SFB and *B. fragilis* in the groups expected to contain these populations.

Flow Cytometry of Whole Blood, Splenocytes, and Mesenteric Lymph Nodes

Regulatory T-cell responses were measured in mesenteric lymph nodes, blood, and spleen. Trunk blood was collected into heparin-treated tubes followed by red blood cell lysis using a standard ACK lysing protocol (BD Biosciences, San Jose, CA, United States). Whole blood leukocytes were washed and counted, 1–2 $\times$ 10^6 leukocytes were stained with antibodies for analysis by flow cytometry. Spleens and mesenteric lymph nodes were isolated and made into single-cell suspensions by removing the capsule and connective tissue via mechanical disruption. Cells were then washed and 1–2 $\times$ 10^6 lymphocytes stained with antibodies for analysis by flow cytometry. Subsequently, Fc receptors on peripheral blood, lymph node, and spleen-derived leukocytes were blocked with an anti-mouse CD16/CD32 (BD Biosciences, San Jose, CA, United States), and the cells were stained for extracellular proteins using the following antibodies (Biolegend, San Diego, CA, United States) CD3, CD4, CD25, and NK1.1. Samples were incubated for 20 min at 4°C, and washed twice with FACS buffer (1$\times$ HBSS containing 1% BSA and 0.1% sodium azide). Next, cells were fixed with Cytofix (BD Biosciences, San Jose, CA, United States) and resuspended in FACS buffer. For intercellular protein staining, cells that were previously fixed after surface staining were permeabilized with FoxP3 Perm Buffer (Biolegend, San Diego, CA, United States) by incubating the cells in the perm buffer for 10 min, followed by the addition of the antibodies (FoxP3 and IL-17F (Biolegend, San Diego, CA, United States) directly to the cells and incubated for an additional 30 min at room temperature. Cells were washed four times in the Perm Buffer and after the last wash cells were re-suspended in FACs buffer. Cells were analyzed using a FACSCanto II Flow Cytometer (BD Biosciences, San Jose, CA, United States) and the data analyzed with Flowjo software (ver. 8.8.7 Treestar Software, Ashland, OR, United States), with a gating strategy as shown in Supplementary Figure S2. The percentage of Th_{17} cells was near the detection limit in measured matrices, as the background ranged from 0.001 to 0.08% in whole blood samples for IL17 staining.

Statistical Analysis and Host/Bacterial Functional Gene Annotation

qPCR was analyzed for absolute abundance based on mass of tissue used to extract DNA and extraction yield, or normalized for relative expression of 16S rRNA gene specific to SFB or *B. fragilis*.

For data obtained using the nCounter®, expression counts were normalized to the geometric mean of multiple housekeeping genes including Rpl19, Ppia, G6pdx, Tubb5, Alas1, Tbp Gusb, Hprt, Gapdh (all had %CV <50) with an algorithm developed by NanoString Technologies. Genes with a maximum normalized expression count of 10 or less among all colonized groups were removed. The Shapiro–Wilk test was used to evaluate normality of data. If necessary, the variance between compared groups was corrected with the Geisser–Greenhouse method. For comparison of more than two groups, one-way ANOVA followed by a multiple comparison Sidak test was performed. When normal distribution was satisfied, a Student's *t*-test was used for comparing differences between two groups. Otherwise, the non-parametric Mann–Whitney test was used. Statistical analysis and some plots were generated using Prism (version 7 for Windows; GraphPad Software, San Diego, CA, United States), additional plots were rendered using Excel or Cytoscape v. 3.3.0 (Institute for Systems Biology, Seattle, WA, United States). Genes were deemed significantly different if $p < 0.05$.

Genes that responded to TCDD and colonization were analyzed for enriched functions using the database for annotation, visualization, and integrated discovery (DAVID) v6.8 (Huang et al., 2009a,b). Gene ontology-biological processes (GO-BPs) were used for clustering the enrichment analysis. Functional groups with an enrichment score (ES)$\geq$1.3 were considered significantly enriched, representing the $-$log scale geometric mean $p < 0.05$.

RESULTS

Transcriptomic Response of Ileal Immune Cells

The influence of SFB on TCDD-induced transcriptomic response was measured using the nCounter® mouse immunology panel (**Figure 1** and Supplementary Table S2). Comparisons were made between groups of mice (Supplementary Figure S1) that remained uncolonized (UC), mice mono-colonized with *B. fragilis* (B), mice mono-colonized with SFB (SFB), and mice co-colonized with both bacteria (SFB+B) to examine: (i) influence of TCDD in presence of SFB (SFB+B, **Figure 1A**) and (ii) influence of TCDD in absence of SFB (UC and *B. fragilis* groups, **Figure 1B**). The influence of SFB colonization was determined by comparing vehicle dosed SFB+B vs B groups; and the influence of *B. fragilis* was determined by comparing vehicle dosed UC vs B groups. Results showed that 11 genes were significantly influenced by TCDD in the presence of SFB (**Figure 1A**). Nine out of 11 of these genes had an opposing response between TCDD and SFB colonization, in terms of transcript regulation. The two genes with similar responses between SFB colonization and TCDD (*cfd*, *Il2rb*) had a conflicting response between TCDD and colonization of *B. fragilis*. The influence of SFB on TCDD-induced host response was further verified in comparing UC with SFB mono-colonized groups (Supplementary Figure S3).

Nine genes were influenced by TCDD in the absence of SFB (**Figure 1B**), all of which were no longer significantly up/down regulated in the presence of SFB. All nine of the genes influenced by TCDD in the absence of SFB were up/down regulated in the same direction as SFB colonization. Influence of SFB colonization in **Figure 1B** was measured by comparing SFB vs UC groups. TCDD-induced responses in groups with and without SFB exhibited opposing modulation of genes associated with immune cell function.

A majority of genes that responded to TCDD in presence/absence of SFB are related to T-cell differentiation

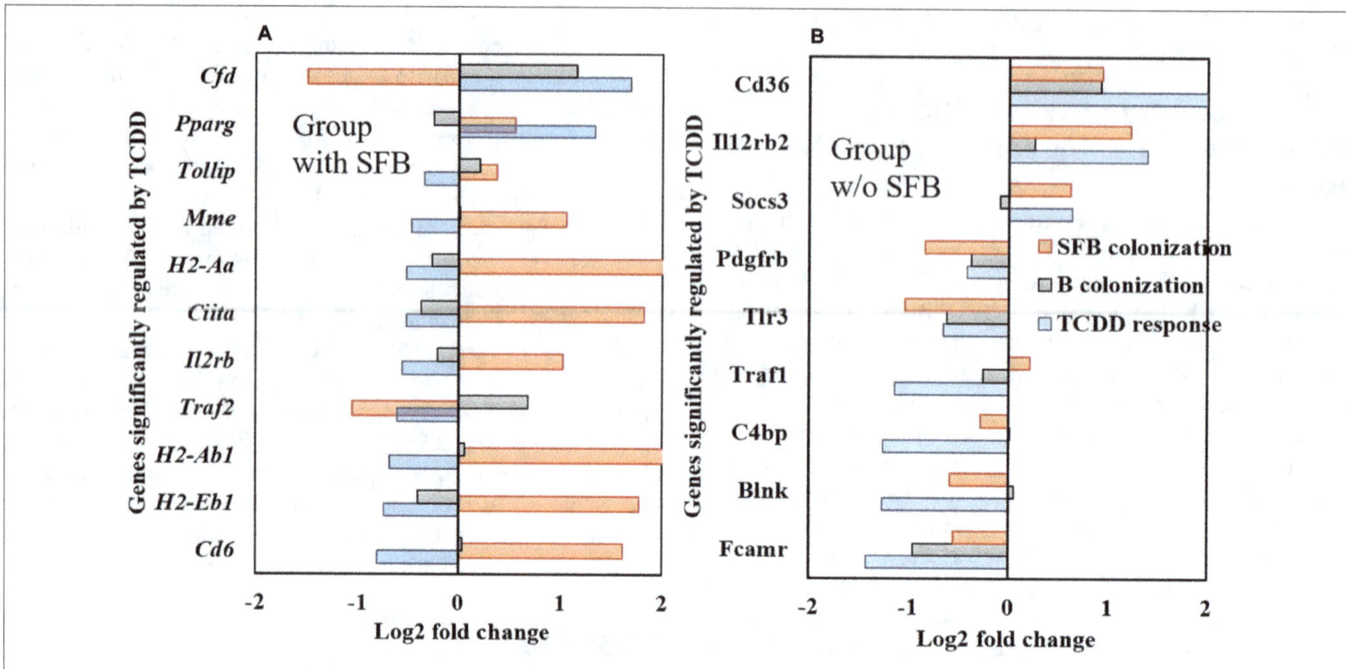

FIGURE 1 | nCounter® mouse immunology panel analysis of genes in ileal tissue that were significantly influenced in response to TCDD in mice **(A)** with SFB, and **(B)** without SFB. Line color indicates gene regulation due to TCDD (blue). For comparative analysis of genes significantly influenced by TCDD, fold change expression due to SFB and *B. fragilis* colonization is also shown regardless of significance. For comparative analysis of SFB colonization (red), the vehicle dosed group colonized with *B. fragilis* was compared with the vehicle dosed group co-colonized with SFB and *B. fragilis*. For comparative analysis of *B. fragilis* colonization (gray), the vehicle dosed group colonized with *B. fragilis* was compared with the uncolonized vehicle dosed group.

including: *Il1β*, *Ciita*, *H2-Eb1*, and *H2-Aa* which were significantly upregulated in response to SFB, and were downregulated in response to TCDD. These genes encode the class II, major histocompatibility complex (MHC II), transactivator, which is required for SFB induction of Th_{17} cells (Lecuyer et al., 2012; Goto et al., 2014). The *Il1β* gene, which has also been shown to substitute TGFβ in differentiation of T-cells (Ghoreschi et al., 2010), was also upregulated with SFB and downregulated with TCDD (Supplementary Figure S3). In the group without SFB, TCDD induced downregulation of genes related to T-cells (*Traf1*) and activation of NF-κB (*Tlr3*) and genes related to regulation of IgA and IgM (*Fcamr, Pdcd1*) homeostasis (Kawamoto et al., 2012; Ouchida et al., 2012).

Colonization with SFB had a greater overall influence on immune gene expression compared to TCDD (**Figures 1A,B, 2A**). In total, 93 genes were influenced by SFB colonization; and 83 of these were up-regulated. To identify the function of genes that responded to colonization and TCDD, the DAVID v6.8 (Huang et al., 2009a,b) was used. Seven and zero significant clusters were observed in response to SFB and *B. fragilis* colonization, respectively (**Figure 2B**). Three enriched clusters functionally associated with T-cell differentiation and inflammatory response (**Figure 2C**) were identified from the genes that responded to TCDD in one or more groups.

Response of Regulatory T Cells

2,3,7,8-Tetrachlorodibenzo-*p*-dioxin-induced responses to T_{reg} cells in the mesenteric lymph node, blood, and spleen were less impacted in the presence of SFB, which is known to promote differentiation of cytokines toward Th_{17} cells (**Figure 3**). TCDD-induced differentiation of T_{reg} was greater in the group mono-colonized with PSA producing *B. fragilis*. The percent of $CD3^+$ and $CD4^+$ in the spleen and mesenteric lymph nodes of groups with SFB was also less influenced by TCDD (**Table 1**). Colonization and TCDD also tended to influence Th_{17} cells in an expected manner; however, Th_{17} measurements were near the limit of detection (Supplementary Figure S4).

Response of Colonized Bacteria

qPCR analysis showed that TCDD significantly influenced the abundance of SFB and *B. fragilis* in the absence of other gut commensals (**Figure 4**). In detail, the absolute abundance of SFB was significantly higher in response to TCDD (**Figure 4B**). Increased SFB abundance was also verified with gDNA extracted from fecal pellets, and using assays targeting the SFB *fliC* functional gene (Supplementary Table S3). Overall, a 2.8-fold higher level of SFB ($p = 0.038$) was observed in response to TCDD. In contrast, the absolute abundance of *B. fragilis*, measured using species-specific *rplB* gene primers, significantly ($p = 0.029$) decreased 2.1-fold in mice dosed with TCDD (**Figure 4A**). The cecal and ileal abundance of *B. fragilis* and SFB did not differ among co-colonized or mono-colonization groups (Supplementary Table S3). Thus, bacterial abundances in both groups of mice were plotted and analyzed concurrently.

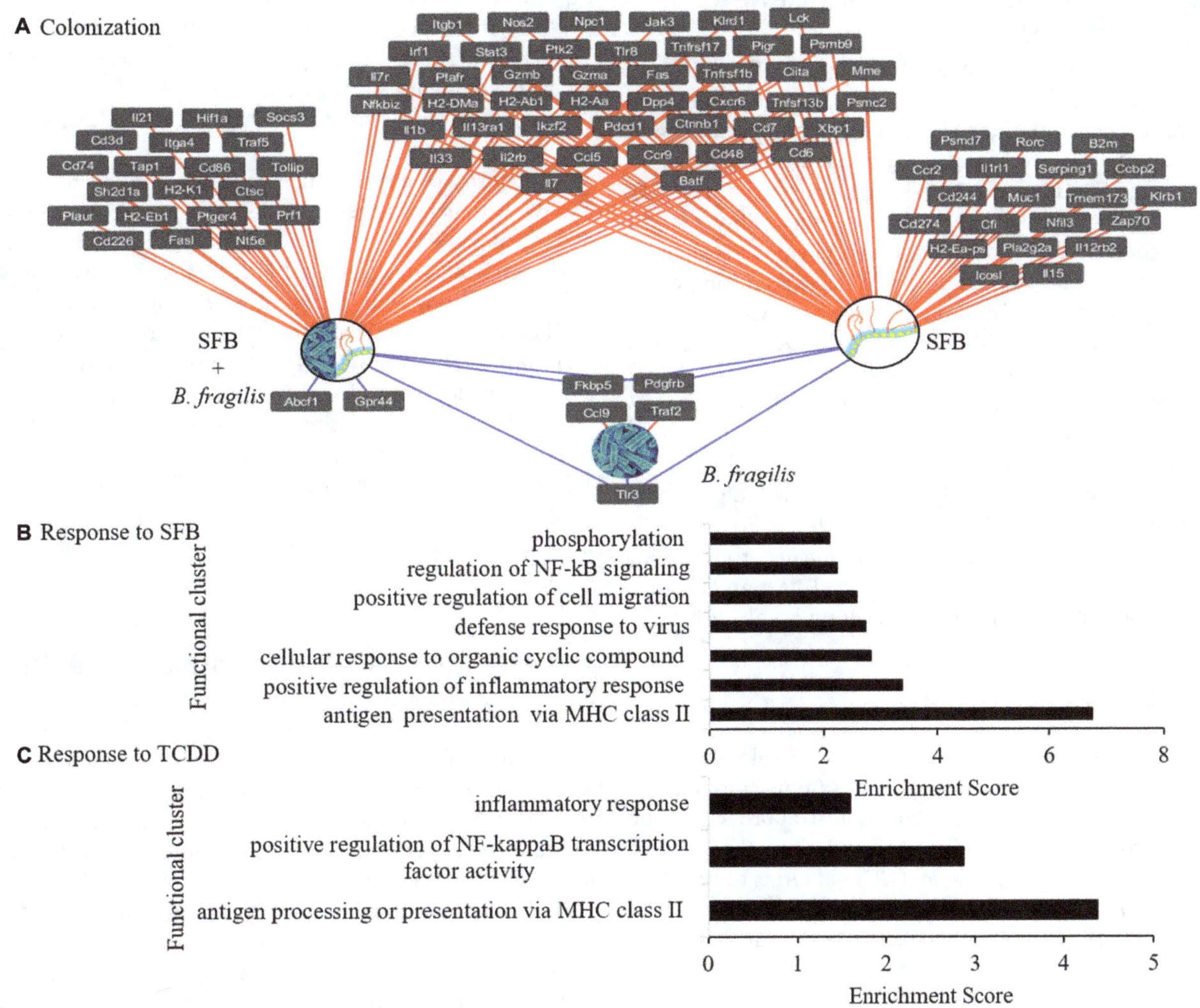

FIGURE 2 | nCounter® mouse immunology panel analysis and functional response. **(A)** Genes in ileal tissue that responded to SFB colonization. Line color and direction indicate upregulated (red) and downregulated (blue) genes. Abbreviations include mice that were mono-colonized with SFB (SFB), mono-colonized with *B. fragilis* (B) and co-colonized (SFB+B). **(B,C)** Functional clusters identified using the DAVID using nCounter® mouse immunology panel analysis with gene expression of ileal tissue showing **(B)** clusters of genes that responded to colonization with SFB, and **(C)** clusters of genes that responded to TCDD in presence and absence of SFB. Functional clusters with scores =1.3 were included as significantly enriched.

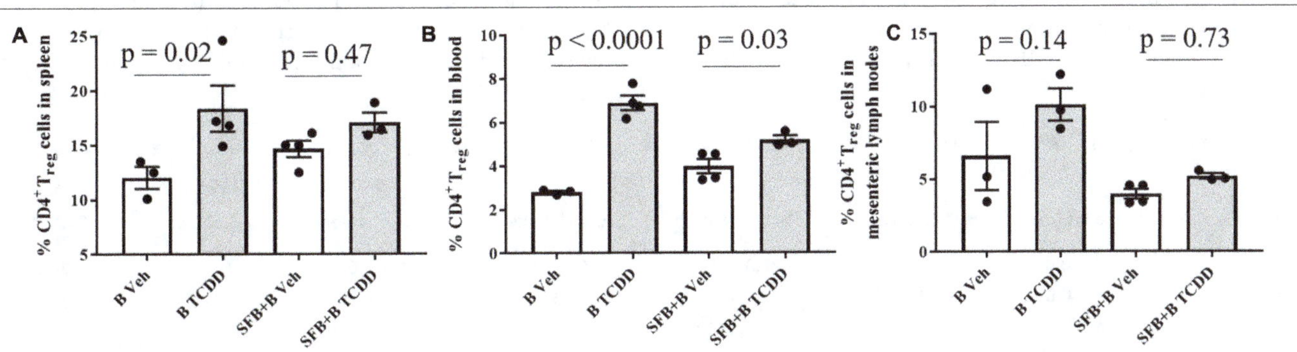

FIGURE 3 | Percent CD4$^+$ T_{reg} measured in **(A)** spleen, **(B)** whole blood, and **(C)** mesenteric lymph nodes in C57BL/6 female mice after TCDD (30 μg/kg) or vehicle (sesame oil) treatment by oral gavage once every 4 days for 28 days. Gray bars are TCDD dosed and white bars are vehicle dosed mice. Values represent mean percent and error bars represent standard error in presence/absence of SFB. *P*-values are shown between vehicle- (Veh) and TCDD-treated groups.

Response of Select Functional Genes from Colonized Bacteria

The expression of select functional SFB and *B. fragilis* genes was also quantified via qPCR to examine responses putative to host interaction. In the ileum of the SFB colonized group, expression of the hemolysin A producing genes was downregulated in response to TCDD (**Figure 4D** and Supplementary Table S3). Hemolysin A has been shown to decrease the ability of host cells to phagocytize bacteria and undergo chemotaxis *in vitro* (Cavalieri and Snyder, 1982). Host macrophage recruiting genes were downregulated in the jejunum of mice dosed with TCDD in previously described studies (Fader et al., 2015). Down-regulation of this gene was only observed in the SFB mono-colonized group, as the expression was below the limit of detection in the group that also had *B. fragilis*.

Expression of the *wcf* gene involved in PSA production by *B. fragilis* was also measured. In detail, the *wcfQ* gene was significantly upregulated in the cecum of the *B. fragilis* colonized mice (**Figure 4C**) in response to TCDD. *B. fragilis* produce PSA as a control mechanism to induce regulatory T-cells and create a more self-tolerable growth environment (Round et al., 2011).

DISCUSSION

Comparative analysis between gnotobiotic mice colonized with and without SFB was performed to examine modulatory responses to TCDD. Noting the reductionist approach of the mouse model colonized with individual populations, the presence of SFB had an opposing response to TCDD in terms of host ileal immune gene expression, and helped modulate levels of TCDD-induced regulatory T-cells in blood, spleen, and mesenteric lymph nodes.

Opposing Influence of SFB Colonization and TCDD on Host

Transcriptomic response fell into two categories including: (i) only responding to TCDD in opposition to SFB colonization and (ii) only responding to TCDD in the group without SFB. In the first category, genes influenced by TCDD would not have differed if had they not been expressed via colonization of SFB. This is evident in that none of the MHC II genes were differentially expressed in response to TCDD in groups without SFB. Within the second category, SFB reduced impact of TCDD on host immune gene expression. Verification of SFB influence in groups without *B. fragilis* further verifies opposing responses with TCDD (Supplementary Figure S3).

A majority of ileal immune genes were down-regulated with TCDD, with gene expression corresponding with differentiation of regulatory T-cells. In the presence of SFB, only two genes were significantly upregulated in response to TCDD (*Pparg* and *cfd*) in the group with background *B. fragilis*. The peroxisome proliferator-activated receptor-γ (*Pparg*) is a nuclear acceptor that inhibits NFκB activity. The downregulation of this gene has been associated with ulcerative colitis (Dubuquoy et al., 2003), and its increased expression correlates with anti-inflammatory responses, which is akin to what has been observed with TCDD (Benson and Shepherd, 2011). The genes that responded to TCDD in the absence of SFB (e.g., *Il12rb2*, *Cd36*) also regulate the number of regulatory T-cells and suppression of an inflammatory response (Zhao et al., 2008; Cecil et al., 2009).

Influence of T-Cell Response in Health

2,3,7,8-Tetrachlorodibenzo-*p*-dioxin-induced response of regulatory T-cells in the mesenteric lymph nodes was less impacted in groups colonized with SFB, extending to blood and spleen matrices beyond the gut (**Figure 3**). Differences in regulatory T-cell responses among the colonized groups further indicate the influence of gut commensals on host disposition to TCDD. The impact of TCDD on regulatory T-cells has been shown to influence susceptibility to infection in the gut (Thigpen et al., 1975). However, the modulatory influence of SFB or Th_{17} inducers isolated from human stool (Tan et al., 2016) may help modulate susceptibility to bacterial infection and abrogate TCDD-induced response.

TCDD-Induced Host Response Favors SFB

2,3,7,8-Tetrachlorodibenzo-*p*-dioxin-induced down-regulation of host immune genes that were activated with SFB colonization may provide a more favorable environment for SFB proliferation. This is evident in opposing functional inflammatory responses. Previous studies have found that mice deficient in mucosal

TABLE 1 | Body weight and T-cell number ($CD3^+$ and $CD4^+$) in spleen, blood, and mesenteric lymph nodes (lymph) after TCDD (30 μg/kg) or vehicle (sesame oil) treatment of mice by oral gavage once every 4 days for 28 days.

Group	Mouse wt (mg)	%$CD3^+$ lymph	%$CD4^+$ lymph	%$CD3^+$ spleen	%$CD4^+$ spleen	%$CD3^+$ blood	%$CD4^+$ blood
UC Veh	28.3 ± 0.8	48.2 ± 3.2	27.3 ± 1.4	27.8 ± 1.3	14.8 ± 0.9	18.0 ± 1.7	10.5 ± 0.6
B Veh	27.1 ± 0.6	45.2 ± 9.5	18.7 ± 4.6	29.2 ± 1.0	17.0 ± 0.6	22.9 ± 5.6	11.5 ± 2.9
SFB+B Veh	28.5 ± 0.6	48.8 ± 3.9	25.7 ± 2.2	25.0 ± 2.3	12.5 ± 1.4	20.7 ± 1.8	9.6 ± 1.0
UC TCDD	25.3 ± 0.6*	43.1 ± 3.6	20.4 + 2.1	19.9 ± 2.5*	10.3 ± 1.2*	20.8 ± 2.3	9.8 ± 1.0
B TCDD	24.5 ± 1.0*	72.9 ± 1.5*	34.6 ± 1.1*	23.9 ± 1.2*	13.7 ± 1.0*	20.7 ± 0.9	10.0 ± 1.0
SFB+B TCDD	26.1 ± 0.8*	49.1 ± 4.0	25.6 ± 1.9	24.3 ± 2.3	12.8 ± 1.2	25.0 ± 2.0	12.0 ± 1.0

*Numbers indicate mean and standard error. Abbreviations identify mice that remained uncolonized (UC) or were mono-colonized with B. fragilis (B) and co-colonized (SFB+B). Vehicle dosed mice (Veh) and TCDD dosed mice (TCDD). *Significant difference between TCDD and vehicle-dosed groups ($p < 0.05$).*

immunity maintainers displayed a 10-fold increase in SFB abundance in fecal pellets (Upadhyay et al., 2012). Studies have also shown that mice lacking an enzyme critical to the production of IgA had an overgrowth of SFB despite the presence of other commensal organisms (Suzuki et al., 2004). TCDD also tended to reduce expression of the flagella receptor Toll-like receptor 5 gene *TLR5* gene 2.0-fold ($p = 0.06$) in the ileum of UC mice. Increased levels of flagella producing bacterial members have previously been observed in mice lacking the *TLR5* gene (Cullender et al., 2013). As such, TCDD appears to repress host immune cell gene expression in the gut, permitting proliferation of SFB. Downregulation of mRNA from measured SFB functional genes putative to evasion from host defense has similar implications.

A similar shift in SFB abundance was also observed in mice with a traditional gut microbiome; however, it was unknown if this was due to the expansion of other bacterial populations or changes in nutrients caused by commensal fluctuations. In detail, previous studies described an increased ratio of *Firmicutes* to *Bacteroidetes* in response to TCDD (Lefever et al., 2016; Stedtfeld et al., 2017a), and higher levels of *Proteobacteria* (Stedtfeld et al., 2017b). The expansion in these predominantly flagella producing groups (Lozupone et al., 2012) may in part influence the relative levels of *Bacteroidetes* and SFB. However, similar shifts in both bacteria in the gnotobiotic mice indicate this response can occur solely via TCDD-induced modulation of the host.

TCDD-Induced Host Response Influences *B. fragilis*

The abundance of *B. fragilis* decreased in response to TCDD in the gnotobiotic mice. While the reduced abundance of *Bacteroidetes* was previously observed in TCDD-dosed mice with a traditional gut microbiome (Bhaduri, 2015; Lefever et al., 2016), the causation for this dysregulation is unclear. Previous studies performed by Round et al. (2011) suggest that *B. fragilis* favors an immunosuppressed environment, and that expression of *B. fragilis* PSA is a defense or colonization mechanism to increase differentiations of T_{reg} cells. In accordance, it would seem that PSA-producing genes should be downregulated to balance the levels of T_{reg} cells induced by TCDD. However, the upregulation of mRNA genes clusters related to the production of PSA indicates that *B. fragilis* are in a state of distress in response to TCDD. In addition, TCDD did not significantly influence the abundance of *Bacteroidetes* or other key commensals when tested *in vitro* in this (Supplementary Figure S5) or previously

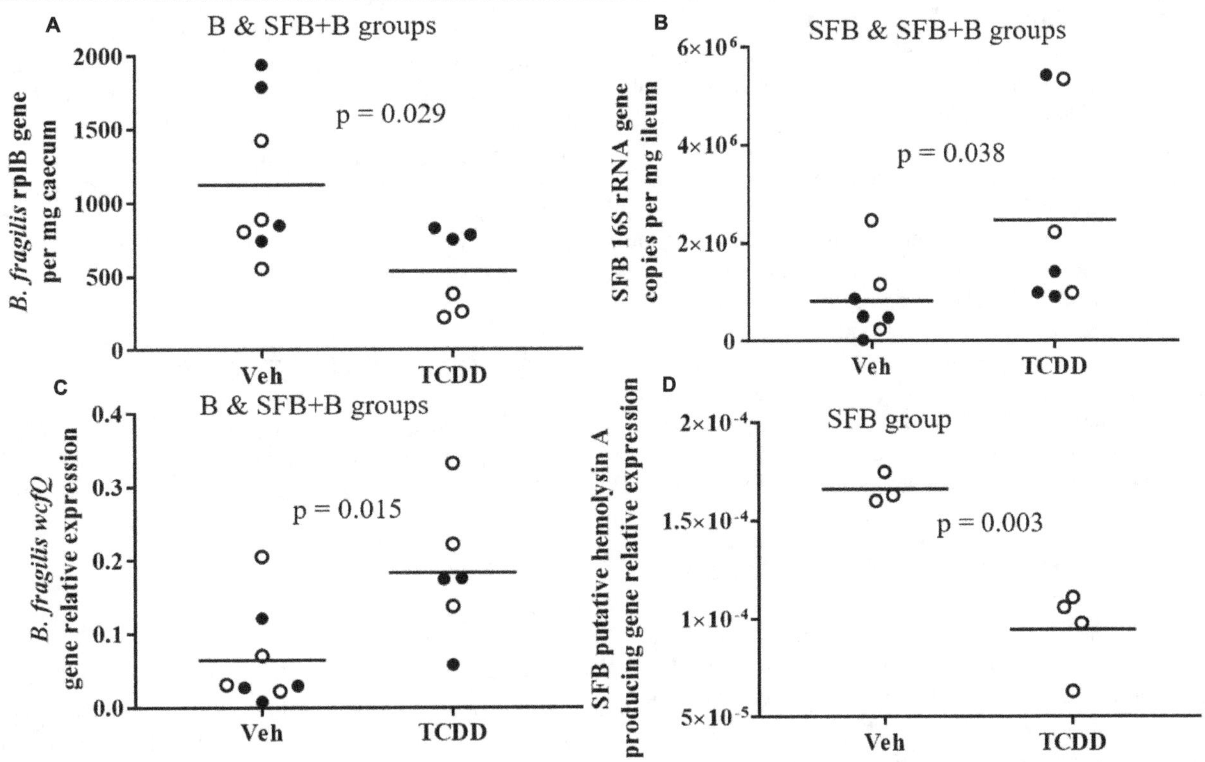

FIGURE 4 | *Bacteroides fragilis* and SFB abundance and selected functional gene expression based on isolated RNA. **(A)** Absolute abundance of *B. fragilis* expression measured with specific *rplB* gene primers in cecum content from respective groups. **(B)** Absolute abundance of SFB expression using species-specific 16S rRNA gene primers from ileum of respective groups. **(C)** PSA biosynthesizing *wcfQ* gene normalized expression, measured with cecum content from respective groups. **(D)** SFB functional genes putative to interaction with host immunity (hemolysin A producing gene) normalized expression, measured with ileal RNA from SFB mono-colonized mice. SFB functional genes in co-colonized group are not included as the genes were expressed below detection limit in two or more biological replicates. Bars represent mean normalized abundance. Open dots indicate mono-colonized groups, closed dots indicate co-colonized groups. Abbreviations include vehicle dosed (Veh) and TCDD treated (TCDD).

described studies (Lefever et al., 2016). Collectively, shifts in *B. fragilis* function and abundance also appear to be the result of TCDD-elicited changes in host.

Relevance of TCDD Dose

Considering a half-life of 7–11 days for TCDD (Gasiewicz et al., 1983; Birnbaum, 1986), mice in this study had an estimated concentration of 60.5–90.7 μg/kg TCDD at sacrifice. One previously measured human exposure event resulted in comparable levels; with lipid-adjusted blood levels of 56 μg/kg TCDD in children near a 1976 plant accident in Seveso, Italy (Bertazzi et al., 1993). In addition, the lowest observable effect level of TCDD on inhibiting an immune response (IgM secretion) was lower in human (0.3 nM) than mice (3 nM) in lymphocytes tissue tested *in vitro* (Wood et al., 1993). We have also observed significantly higher levels of SFB at doses $\geq$1.0 μg/kg TCDD in other studies (Bhaduri, 2015). Thus, similar responses to those described here may occur with 10- to 100-fold less TCDD, warranting additional experiments. While environmental levels of TCDD are typically lower than that used in this study and are thought to be decreasing in the environment, cumulative exposure to other AhR ligands such as polyaromatic hydrocarbons and flame retardants is increasing (Lim et al., 2008; Wiseman et al., 2011).

TCDD versus Other AhR Ligands

The AhR ligand response demonstrated in this study differs from those published by Zhang et al. (2015). In detail, their study with wild-type mice orally dosed with 2,3,7,8-tetrachlorodibenzofuran (TCDF), a less potent AhR activator, heightened host inflammation, reduced levels of SFB, and increased abundance of *Bacteroidetes* over *Firmicutes*. However, our results showed reduced levels of host immune gene expression, which has also been previously described in the jejunum in response to TCDD (Fader et al., 2015) and AhR activation (Monteleone et al., 2013). Dissimilar responses may be due to differences in AhR ligand potency, which has been reported in a study comparing TCDD and 6-formylindolo[3,2-b]carbazole (Farmahin et al., 2016). Future studies addressing AhR activity and influence to host and gut microbes in response to different ligands throughout the gut are necessary (Zhang et al., 2017).

Differences in Murine and Human Models

Before inferring if TCDD and presence/absence of SFB would have a similar influence on humans compared to the murine model, both the host and microbial phenotype must be considered. Differences in host phenotype have been described previously (Kreisman and Cobb, 2011), with varied gene expression in response to TCDD depending on the measured tissue and host species (Kovalova et al., 2017). In regards to microbiota, recent meta-analysis has shown that 90 and 89% of bacterial phyla and genera, respectively, are shared between mice and the human gut microbiota (Krych et al., 2013), with the most abundant bacterial species being common in both. Studies examining the presence of SFB in human microbiome have conflicting results (Klaasen et al., 1993; Qin et al., 2010; Caselli et al., 2013; Yin et al., 2013; Shukla et al., 2015), which may be due to variability in the methods or matrices used for measuring SFB. However, immune-activating bacterial groups isolated from human gut microbiome appear to have a similar response to SFB in the capacity to differentiate T-cells in mice (Tan et al., 2016). Commercially available probiotic consortia have also been shown to contain Th_{17} cell inducers in mice (Tan et al., 2016), highlighting the therapeutic potential of immune-activating bacteria to modulate host response to TCDD.

Collectively, the presence of SFB significantly influenced host response to TCDD in the matrices measured. TCDD exposure also appeared to provide a more favorable environment for SFB. *B. fragilis* also responded to TCDD-induced shifts in the host, expressing higher levels of the *wcfQ* gene, a PSA-producing gene cluster. TCDD did not appear to influence abundance of these bacterial groups *in vitro* in TCDD-dosed batch reactors (Supplementary Figure S5), further suggesting that the bacterial response of SFB and *B. fragilis* is in part due to TCDD induced influences on the host.

Follow-up studies are underway to further elucidate causation of functional dysbiosis with *B. fragilis*. This will include the analysis of additional genes related to host interaction and immune tolerance. Further identification of key bacterial species and functional genes may facilitate attempts to manipulate the intestinal microbiome toward a protective and healthy state. Future studies will also examine the ability of other human bacterial commensals to influence TCDD-induced response in the absence of SFB. These studies may lead to new therapeutic approaches to treat intestinal pathogens and resulting autoimmune diseases.

AUTHOR CONTRIBUTIONS

RS, TS, and SH wrote the manuscript; RS, SH, JT, NK, RC, JC, and TK contributed to experimental design; and SH, BC, RC, TS, RS, SX, and MW aided in collection of tissue, measurements, and data analysis.

FUNDING

This work was supported by the National Institute of Environmental Health Sciences Superfund Basic Research Program (NIEHS SBRP P42ES04911) with contributions from Project 1, 4, 5, and Core-B.

ACKNOWLEDGMENT

We would like to thank Kathryn Eaton and her laboratory team at the University of Michigan Germ Free Facility.

REFERENCES

Altschul, S. F., Madden, T. L., Schäffer, A. A., Zhang, J., Zhang, Z., Miller, W., et al. (1997). Gapped BLAST and PSI-BLAST: a new generation of protein database search programs. *Nucleic Acids Res.* 25, 3389–3402. doi: 10.1093/nar/25.17.3389

Atarashi, K., Tanoue, T., Ando, M., Kamada, N., Nagano, Y., Narushima, S., et al. (2015). Th17 cell induction by adhesion of microbes to intestinal epithelial cells. *Cell* 163, 367–380. doi: 10.1016/j.cell.2015.08.058

Atarashi, K., Tanoue, T., Shima, T., Imaoka, A., Kuwahara, T., Momose, Y., et al. (2011). Induction of colonic regulatory T Cells by indigenous Clostridium species. *Science* 331, 337–341. doi: 10.1126/science.1198469

Benson, J. M., and Shepherd, D. M. (2011). Aryl hydrocarbon receptor activation by TCDD reduces inflammation associated with Crohn's Disease. *Toxicol. Sci.* 120, 68–78. doi: 10.1093/toxsci/kfq360

Bertazzi, P. A., Pesatori, A. C., Consonni, D., Tironi, A., Landi, M. T., and Zocchetti, C. (1993). Cancer incidence in a population accidentally exposed to 2,3,7,8-tetrachlorodibenzo-para-dioxin. *Epidemiology* 4, 398–406. doi: 10.1097/00001648-199309000-00004

Bhaduri, P. (2015). *Exposure to 2, 3, 7, 8-Tetrachlorodibenzo-p-Dioxin Differentially Impacts Key Members of Mice Gut Microbiome.* East Lansing, MI: Michigan State University.

Birnbaum, L. S. (1986). Distribution and excretion of 2,3,7,8-tetrachlorodibenzo-p-dioxin in congenic strains of mice which differ at the Ah locus. *Drug Metab. Dispos.* 14, 34–40.

Bouskra, D., Brézillon, C., Bérard, M., Werts, C., Varona, R., Boneca, I. G., et al. (2008). Lymphoid tissue genesis induced by commensals through NOD1 regulates intestinal homeostasis. *Nature* 456, 507–510. doi: 10.1038/nature07450

Caselli, M., Tosini, D., GafÃ, R., Gasbarrini, A., and Lanza, G. (2013). Segmented filamentous bacteria-like organisms in histological slides of ileo-cecal valves in patients with ulcerative colitis. *Am. J. Gastroenterol.* 108, 860–861. doi: 10.1038/ajg.2013.61

Cavalieri, S., and Snyder, I. (1982). Effect of *Escherichia coli* alpha-hemolysin on human peripheral leukocyte function in vitro. *Infect. Immun.* 37, 966–974.

Cecil, D., Appleton, C., Polewski, M., Mort, J., Schmidt, A., Bendele, A., et al. (2009). The pattern recognition receptor CD36 is a chondrocyte hypertrophy marker associated with suppression of catabolic responses and promotion of repair responses to inflammatory stimuli. *J. Immunol.* 182, 5024–5031. doi: 10.4049/jimmunol.0803603

Chmill, S., Kadow, S., Winter, M., Weighardt, H., and Esser, C. (2010). 2,3,7,8-Tetrachlorodibenzo-p-dioxin impairs stable establishment of oral tolerance in mice. *Toxicol. Sci.* 118, 98–107. doi: 10.1093/toxsci/kfq232

Cullender, T. C., Chassaing, B., Janzon, A., Kumar, K., Muller, C. E., Werner, J. J., et al. (2013). Innate and adaptive immunity interact to quench microbiome flagellar motility in the gut. *Cell Host Microbe* 14, 571–581. doi: 10.1016/j.chom.2013.10.009

Dubuquoy, L., Jansson, E. A., Deeb, S., Rakotobe, S., Karoui, M., Colombel, J. F., et al. (2003). Impaired expression of peroxisome proliferator-activated receptor gamma in ulcerative colitis. *Gastroenterology* 124, 1265–1276. doi: 10.1016/S0016-5085(03)00271-3

Fader, K. A., Nault, R., Ammendolia, D. A., Harkema, J. R., Williams, K. J., Crawford, R. B., et al. (2015). 2, 3, 7, 8-Tetrachlorodibenzo-p-Dioxin (TCDD) alters lipid metabolism and depletes immune cell populations in the jejunum of C57BL/6 mice. *Toxicol. Sci.* 148, 567–580. doi: 10.1093/toxsci/kfv206

Faith, J., Ahern, P., Ridaura, V., Cheng, J., and Gordon, J. (2014). Identifying gut microbe-host phenotype relationships using combinatorial communities in gnotobiotic mice. *Sci. Transl. Med.* 6, 220ra11. doi: 10.1126/scitranslmed.3008051

Fantini, M., Rizzo, A., Fina, D., Caruso, R., Becker, C., Neurath, M., et al. (2007). IL-21 regulates experimental colitis by modulating the balance between Treg and Th17 cells. *Eur. J. Immunol.* 37, 3155–3163. doi: 10.1002/eji.200737766

Farmahin, R., Crump, D., O'Brien, J. M., Jones, S. P., and Kennedy, S. W. (2016). Time-dependent transcriptomic and biochemical responses of 6-Formylindolo [3, 2-b] carbazole (FICZ) and 2, 3, 7, 8-tetrachlorodibenzo-p-dioxin (TCDD) are explained by AHR activation time. *Biochem. Pharmacol.* 115, 134–143. doi: 10.1016/j.bcp.2016.06.005

Gaboriau-Routhiau, V., Rakotobe, S., Lecuyer, E., Mulder, I., Lan, A., Bridonneau, C., et al. (2009). The key role of segmented filamentous bacteria in the coordinated maturation of gut helper T cell responses. *Immunity* 31, 677–689. doi: 10.1016/j.immuni.2009.08.020

Gasiewicz, T., Geiger, L., Rucc, G., and Neal, R. (1983). Distribution, excretion, and metabolism of 2, 3, 7, 8-tetrachlorodibenzo-p-dioxin in C57BL/6J, DBA/2J, and B6D2F1/J mice. *Drug Metab. Dispos.* 11, 397–403.

Ghoreschi, K., Laurence, A., Yang, X., Tato, C. M., Mcgeachy, M. J., Konkel, J. E., et al. (2010). Generation of pathogenic TH17 cells in the absence of TGF-β signalling. *Nature* 467, 967–971. doi: 10.1038/nature09447

Goto, Y., Panea, C., Nakato, G., Cebula, A., Lee, C., Diez, M. G., et al. (2014). Segmented filamentous bacteria antigens presented by intestinal dendritic cells drive mucosal Th17 cell differentiation. *Immunity* 40, 594–607. doi: 10.1016/j.immuni.2014.03.005

Hand, T., and Belkaid, Y. (2010). Microbial control of regulatory and effector T cell responses in the gut. *Curr. Opin. Immunol.* 22, 63–72. doi: 10.1016/j.coi.2010.01.008

Hertz-Picciotto, I., Park, H., Dostal, M., Kocan, A., Trnovec, T., and Sram, R. (2008). Prenatal exposures to persistent and non-persistent organic compounds and effects on immune system development. *Basic Clin. Pharmacol. Toxicol.* 102, 146–154. doi: 10.1111/j.1742-7843.2007.00190.x

Ho, P. P., and Steinman, L. (2008). The aryl hydrocarbon receptor: a regulator of Th17 and Treg cell development in disease. *Cell Res.* 18, 605–608. doi: 10.1038/cr.2008.63

Honda, K., and Littman, D. R. (2016). The microbiota in adaptive immune homeostasis and disease. *Nature* 535, 75–84. doi: 10.1038/nature18848

Huang, D. W., Sherman, B. T., and Lempicki, R. A. (2009a). Bioinformatics enrichment tools: paths toward the comprehensive functional analysis of large gene lists. *Nucleic Acids Res.* 37, 1–13. doi: 10.1093/nar/gkn923

Huang, D. W., Sherman, B. T., and Lempicki, R. A. (2009b). Systematic and integrative analysis of large gene lists using DAVID bioinformatics resources. *Nat. Protoc.* 4, 44–57. doi: 10.1038/nprot.2008.211

Hubbard, T., Murray, I., Bisson, W., Lahoti, T., Gowda, K., Amin, S., et al. (2015). Adaptation of the human aryl hydrocarbon receptor to sense microbiota-derived indoles. *Sci. Rep.* 5:12689. doi: 10.1038/srep12689

Ibrahim, M., Fjære, E., Lock, E., Naville, D., Amlund, H., Meugnier, E., et al. (2011). Chronic consumption of farmed salmon containing persistent organic pollutants causes insulin resistance and obesity in mice. *PLoS ONE* 6:e25170. doi: 10.1371/journal.pone.0025170

Ivanov, I., and Littman, D. (2010). Segmented filamentous bacteria take the stage. *Mucosal Immunol.* 3, 209–212. doi: 10.1038/mi.2010.3

Ivanov, I. I., Atarashi, K., Manel, N., Brodie, E. L., Shima, T., Karaoz, U., et al. (2009). Induction of intestinal Th17 cells by segmented filamentous bacteria. *Cell* 139, 485–498. doi: 10.1016/j.cell.2009.09.033

Kao, J., Zhang, M., Miller, M., Mills, J., Wang, B., Liu, M., et al. (2010). *Helicobacter pylori* immune escape is mediated by dendritic cell-induced Treg skewing and Th17 suppression in mice. *Gastroenterology* 138, 1046–1054. doi: 10.1053/j.gastro.2009.11.043

Kawamoto, S., Tran, T., Maruya, M., Suzuki, K., Doi, Y., Tsutsui, Y., et al. (2012). The inhibitory receptor PD-1 regulates IgA selection and bacterial composition in the gut. *Science* 336, 485–489. doi: 10.1126/science.1217718

Kerkvliet, N. I., Shepherd, D. M., and Baecher-Steppan, L. (2002). T lymphocytes are direct, aryl hydrocarbon receptor (AhR)-dependent targets of 2, 3, 7, 8-tetrachlorodibenzo-p-dioxin (TCDD): AhR expression in both CD4+ and CD8+ T cells is necessary for full suppression of a cytotoxic T lymphocyte response by TCDD. *Toxicol. Appl. Pharmacol.* 185, 146–152. doi: 10.1006/taap.2002.9537

Kerkvliet, N. I., Steppan, L. B., Vorachek, W., Oda, S., Farrer, D., Wong, C. P., et al. (2009). Activation of aryl hydrocarbon receptor by TCDD prevents diabetes in NOD mice and increases Foxp3+ T cells in pancreatic lymph nodes. *Immunotherapy* 1, 539–547. doi: 10.2217/imt.09.24

Klaasen, H., Koopman, J. P., Van den Brink, M. E., Bakker, M. H., Poelma, F. G. J., and Beynen, A. C. (1993). Intestinal, segmented, filamentous bacteria in a wide range of vertebrate species. *Lab. Anim.* 27, 141–150. doi: 10.1258/002367793780810441

Kovalova, N., Nault, R., Crawford, R., Zacharewski, T., and Kaminski, N. (2017). Comparative analysis of TCDD-induced AhR-mediated gene expression in human, mouse and rat primary B cells. *Toxicol. Appl. Pharmacol.* 316, 95–106. doi: 10.1016/j.taap.2016.11.009

Kreisman, L. S. C., and Cobb, B. A. (2011). Glycoantigens induce human peripheral Tr1 cell differentiation with gut-homing specialization. *J. Biol. Chem.* 286, 8810–8818. doi: 10.1074/jbc.M110.206011

Krych, L., Hansen, C. H. F., Hansen, A. K., van den Berg, F. W. J., and Nielsen, D. S. (2013). Quantitatively different, yet qualitatively alike: a meta-analysis of the mouse core gut microbiome with a view towards the human gut microbiome. *PLoS ONE* 8:e62578. doi: 10.1371/journal.pone.0062578

Kuwahara, T., Ogura, Y., Oshima, K., Kurokawa, K., Ooka, T., Hirakawa, H., et al. (2011). The lifestyle of the segmented filamentous bacterium: a non-culturable gut-associated immunostimulating microbe inferred by whole-genome sequencing. *DNA Res.* 18, 291–303. doi: 10.1093/dnares/dsr022

Lecuyer, E., Rakotobe, S., Lebreton, C., Picard, M., Mccoy, K. D., Macpherson, A. J., et al. (2012). Segmented filamentous bacterium uses secondary and tertiary lymphoid tissues to induce Gut IgA and specific T helper 17 cell responses. *Immunity* 17, 457–459. doi: 10.1016/j.immuni.2014.03.009

Lee, D., Jacobs, D., and Porta, M. (2007). Association of serum concentrations of persistent organic pollutants with the prevalence of learning disability and attention deficit disorder. *J. Epidemiol. Community Health* 61, 591–596. doi: 10.1136/jech.2006.054700

Lefever, D. E., Xu, J., Chen, Y., Huang, G., Tamas, N., and Guo, T. L. (2016). TCDD modulation of gut microbiome correlated with liver and immune toxicity in streptozotocin (STZ)-induced hyperglycemic mice. *Toxicol. Appl. Pharmacol.* 304, 48–58. doi: 10.1016/j.taap.2016.05.016

Lim, J., Lee, D., and Jacobs, D. (2008). Association of brominated flame retardants with diabetes and metabolic syndrome in the US population, 2003-2004. *Diabetes Care* 31, 1802–1807. doi: 10.2337/dc08-0850

Looft, T., Johnson, T. A., Allen, H. K., Bayles, D. O., Alt, D. P., Stedtfeld, R. D., et al. (2012). In-feed antibiotic effects on the swine intestinal microbiome. *Proc. Natl. Acad. Sci. U.S.A.* 109, 1691–1696. doi: 10.1073/pnas.1120238109

Lozupone, C., Faust, K., Raes, J., Faith, J. J., Frank, D. N., Zaneveld, J., et al. (2012). Identifying genomic and metabolic features that can underlie early successional and opportunistic lifestyles of human gut symbionts. *Genome Res.* 22, 1974–1984. doi: 10.1101/gr.138198.112

Marshall, N., and Kerkvliet, N. (2010). Dioxin and immune regulation: emerging role of aryl hydrocarbon receptor in the generation of regulatory T cells. *Ann. N.Y. Acad. Sci.* 1183, 25–37. doi: 10.1111/j.1749-6632.2009.05125.x

Marshall, N. B., Vorachek, W. R., Steppan, L. B., Mourich, D. V., and Kerkvliet, N. I. (2008). Functional characterization and gene expression analysis of CD4+CD25+ regulatory T cells generated in mice treated with 2,3,7,8-tetrachlorodibenzo-p-dioxin. *J. Immunol.* 181, 2382–2391. doi: 10.4049/jimmunol.181.4.2382

Monteleone, I., Pallone, F., and Monteleone, G. (2013). Aryl hydrocarbon receptor and colitis. *Semin. Immunopathol.* 35, 671–675. doi: 10.1007/s00281-013-0396-2

Murray, I., Nichols, R., Zhang, L., Patterson, A., and Perdew, G. (2016). Expression of the aryl hydrocarbon receptor contributes to the establishment of intestinal microbial community structure in mice. *Sci. Rep.* 6:33969. doi: 10.1038/srep33969

Mustafa, A., Holladay, S., Goff, M., Witonsky, S., Kerr, R., Reilly, C., et al. (2008). An enhanced postnatal autoimmune profile in 24 week-old C57BL/6 mice developmentally exposed to TCDD. *Toxicol. Appl. Pharmacol.* 232, 51–59. doi: 10.1016/j.taap.2008.04.015

Nault, R., Colbry, D., Brandenberger, C., Harkema, J., and Zacharewski, T. (2015). Development of a computational high-throughput tool for the quantitative examination of dose-dependent histological features. *Toxicol. Pathol.* 43, 366–375. doi: 10.1177/0192623314544379

Ouchida, R., Mori, H., Hase, K., Takatsu, H., Kurosaki, T., Tokuhisa, T., et al. (2012). Critical role of the IgM Fc receptor in IgM homeostasis, B-cell survival, and humoral immune responses. *Proc. Natl. Acad. Sci. U.S.A.* 109, E2699–E2706. doi: 10.1073/pnas.1210706109

Pamp, S. J., Harrington, E. D., Quake, S. R., Relman, D. A., and Blainey, P. C. (2012). Single-cell sequencing provides clues about the host interactions of segmented filamentous bacteria (SFB). *Genome Res.* 22, 1107–1119. doi: 10.1101/gr.131482.111

Peck, A., and Mellins, E. (2010). Precarious balance: Th17 cells in host defensetle. *Infect. Immun.* 78, 32–38. doi: 10.1128/IAI.00929-09

Qin, J., Li, R., Raes, J., Arumugam, M., Burgdorf, K. S., Manichanh, C., et al. (2010). A human gut microbial gene catalogue established by metagenomic sequencing. *Nature* 464, 59–65. doi: 10.1038/nature08821

Quintana, F., Basso, A., Iglesias, A., Korn, T., Farez, M., Bettelli, E., et al. (2008). Control of T(reg) and T(H)17 cell differentiation by the aryl hydrocarbon receptor. *Nature* 453, 65–71. doi: 10.1038/nature06880

Reis, P. P., Waldron, L., Goswami, R. S., Xu, W., Xuan, Y., Perez-Ordonez, B., et al. (2011). mRNA transcript quantification in archival samples using multiplexed, color-coded probes. *BMC Biotechnol.* 11:46. doi: 10.1186/1472-6750-11-46

Round, J. L., Lee, S. M., Li, J., Tran, G., Jabri, B., Chatila, T. A., et al. (2011). The Toll-like receptor 2 pathway establishes colonization by a commensal of the human microbiota. *Science* 332, 974–977. doi: 10.1126/science.1206095

Round, J. L., and Mazmanian, S. K. (2010). Inducible Foxp3+ regulatory T-cell development by a commensal bacterium of the intestinal microbiota. *Proc. Natl. Acad. Sci. U.S.A.* 107, 12204–12209. doi: 10.1073/pnas.0909122107

Sefik, E., Geva-Zatorsky, N., Oh, S., Konnikova, L., Zemmour, D., McGuire, A., et al. (2015). Individual intestinal symbionts induce a distinct population of RORγ+ regulatory T cells. *Science* 349, 993–997. doi: 10.1126/science.aaa9420

Shukla, R., Ghoshal, U., Dhole, T. N., and Ghoshal, U. C. (2015). Fecal microbiota in patients with irritable bowel syndrome compared with healthy controls using real-time polymerase chain reaction: an evidence of dysbiosis. *Dig. Dis. Sci.* 60, 2953–2962. doi: 10.1007/s10620-015-3607-y

Snedeker, S. M., and Hay, A. G. (2012). Do interactions between gut ecology and environmental chemicals contribute to obesity and diabetes? *Environ. Health Perspect.* 120, 332–339. doi: 10.1289/ehp.1104204

Stedtfeld, R., Sallache, J., Crawford, R., Stedtfeld, T., Williams, M., Waseem, H., et al. (2017a). TCDD administered on activated carbon eliminates bioavailability and subsequent shifts to a key murine gut commensal. *Appl. Microbiol. Biotechnol.* doi: 10.1007/s00253-017-8460-9 [Epub ahead of print].

Stedtfeld, R., Stedtfeld, T., Fader, K., Williams, M., Quensen, J., Zacharewski, T., et al. (2017b). TCDD influences reservoir of antibiotic resistance genes in murine gut microbiome. *FEMS Microbiol. Ecol.* 93:fix058. doi: 10.1093/femsec/fix058

Stedtfeld, R. D., Baushke, S. W., Tourlousse, D. M., Miller, S. M., Stedtfeld, T. M., Gulari, E., et al. (2008). Development and experimental validation of a predictive threshold cycle equation for quantification of virulence and marker genes by high-throughput nanoliter-volume PCR on the OpenArray platform. *Appl. Environ. Microbiol.* 74, 3831–3838. doi: 10.1128/AEM.02743-07

Stedtfeld, R. D., Williams, M. R., Fakher, U., Johnson, T. A., Stedtfeld, T. M., Wang, F., et al. (2016). Antimicrobial resistance dashboard application for mapping environmental occurrence and resistant pathogens. *FEMS Microbiol. Ecol.* 92:fiw020. doi: 10.1093/femsec/fiw020

Suzuki, K., Meek, B., Doi, Y., Muramatsu, M., Chiba, T., Honjo, T., et al. (2004). Aberrant expansion of segmented filamentous bacteria in IgA-deficient gut. *Proc. Natl. Acad. Sci. U.S.A.* 101, 1981–1986. doi: 10.1073/pnas.0307317101

Tan, T., Sefik, E., Geva-Zatorsky, N., Kua, L., Naskar, D., Teng, F., et al. (2016). Identifying species of symbiont bacteria from the human gut that, alone, can induce intestinal Th17 cells in mice. *Proc. Natl. Acad. Sci. U.S.A.* 113, E8141–E8150. doi: 10.1073/pnas.1617460113

Taylor, K. W., Novak, R. F., Anderson, H. A., Birnbaum, L. S., Blystone, C., DeVito, M., et al. (2013). Evaluation of the association between persistent organic pollutants (POPs) and diabetes in epidemiological studies: a national toxicology program workshop review. *Environ. Health Perspect.* 121, 774–783. doi: 10.1289/ehp.1205502

Thigpen, J., Faith, R., McConnell, E., and Moore, J. (1975). Increased susceptibility to bacterial infection as a sequela of exposure to 2,3,7,8-tetrachlorodibenzo-p-dioxin. *Infect. Immun.* 12, 1319–1324.

Troutman, J. M., Sharma, S., Erickson, K. M., and Martinez, C. D. (2014). Functional identification of a galactosyltransferase critical to *Bacteroides fragilis* Capsular Polysaccharide A biosynthesis. *Carbohydr. Res.* 395, 19–28. doi: 10.1016/j.carres.2014.06.003

Troy, E., and Kasper, D. (2010). Beneficial effects of *Bacteroides fragilis* polysaccharides on the immune system. *Front. Biosci.* 15, 25–34. doi: 10.2741/3603

Upadhyay, V., Poroyko, V., Kim, T., Devkota, S., Fu, S., Liu, D., et al. (2012). Lymphotoxin regulates commensal responses to enable diet-induced obesity. *Nat. Immunol.* 13, 947–953. doi: 10.1038/ni.2403

Veldhoen, M., and Duarte, J. (2010). The aryl hydrocarbon receptor: fine-tuning the immune-response. *Curr. Opin. Immunol.* 22, 747–752. doi: 10.1016/j.coi.2010.09.001

Veldhoen, M., Hirota, K., Westendorf, A., Buer, J., Dumoutier, L., Renauld, J., et al. (2008). The aryl hydrocarbon receptor links T(H)17-cell-mediated autoimmunity to environmental toxins. *Nature* 453, 106–109. doi: 10.1038/nature06881

Wang, F.-H., Qiao, M., Su, J.-Q., Chen, Z., Zhou, X., and Zhu, Y.-G. (2014). High throughput profiling of antibiotic resistance genes in urban park soils with reclaimed water irrigation. *Environ. Sci. Technol.* 48, 9079–9085. doi: 10.1021/es502615e

Wiseman, S., Wan, Y., Chang, H., Zhang, X., Hecker, M., Jones, P., et al. (2011). Polybrominated diphenyl ethers and their hydroxylated/methoxylated analogs: environmental sources, metabolic relationships, and relative toxicities. *Mar. Pollut. Bull.* 63, 179–188. doi: 10.1016/j.marpolbul.2011.02.008

Wood, S., Jeong, H., Morris, D., and Holsapple, M. (1993). Direct effects of 2,3,7,8-tetrachlorodibenzo- p-dioxin (TCDD) on human tonsillar lymphocytes. *Toxicology* 81, 131–143. doi: 10.1016/0300-483X(93)90005-D

Yin, Y., Wang, Y., Zhu, L., Liu, W., Liao, N., Jiang, M., et al. (2013). Comparative analysis of the distribution of segmented filamentous bacteria in humans, mice and chickens. *ISME J.* 7, 615–621. doi: 10.1038/ismej.2012.128

Zhang, L., Ma, J., Takeuchi, M., Usui, Y., Hattori, T., Okunuki, Y., et al. (2010). Suppression of experimental autoimmune uveoretinitis by inducing differentiation of regulatory T cells via activation of aryl hydrocarbon receptor. *Invest. Ophthalmol. Vis. Sci.* 51, 2109–2117. doi: 10.1167/iovs.09-3993

Zhang, L., Nichols, R. G., Correll, J., Murray, I. A., Tanaka, N., Smith, P. B., et al. (2015). Persistent organic pollutants modify gut microbiota-host metabolic homeostasis in mice through aryl hydrocarbon receptor activation. *Environ. Health Perspect.* 123, 679–688. doi: 10.1289/ehp.1409055

Zhang, L., Nichols, R. G., and Patterson, A. D. (2017). The aryl hydrocarbon receptor as a moderator of host-microbiota communication. *Curr. Opin. Toxicol.* 2, 30–35. doi: 10.1016/j.cotox.2017.02.001

Zhao, Z., Yu, S., Fitzgerald, D., Elbehi, M., Ciric, B., Rostami, A., et al. (2008). IL-12R beta 2 promotes the development of CD4+CD25+ regulatory T cells. *J. Immunol.* 181, 3870–3876. doi: 10.4049/jimmunol.181.6.3870

15

The Role of Lipoproteins in Mycoplasma-Mediated Immunomodulation

*Alexei Christodoulides, Neha Gupta, Vahe Yacoubian, Neil Maithel, Jordan Parker and Theodoros Kelesidis**

David Geffen School of Medicine, University of California, Los Angeles, Los Angeles, CA, United States

***Correspondence:**
Theodoros Kelesidis
tkelesidis@mednet.ucla.edu

Mycoplasma infections, such as walking pneumonia or pelvic inflammatory diseases, are a major threat to public health. Despite their relatively small physical and genomic size, mycoplasmas are known to elicit strong host immune responses, generally inflammatory, while also being able to evade the immune system. The mycoplasma membrane is composed of approximately two-thirds protein and one-third lipid and contains several lipoproteins that are known to regulate host immune responses. Herein, the immunomodulatory effects of mycoplasma lipoproteins are reviewed. A better understanding of the immunomodulatory effects, both activating and evasive, of Mycoplasma surface lipoproteins will contribute to understanding mechanisms potentially relevant to mycoplasma disease vaccine development and treatment.

Keywords: mycoplasma, lipoproteins, immune system, immune modulation, inflammation

INTRODUCTION

Mycoplasmas cause a wide variety of human disease, such as asthma, bronchiectasis, and pelvic inflammatory diseases (Metaxas et al., 2015). Several species of mycoplasma such as *Mycoplasma pneumoniae* in the respiratory tract, *M. genitalium* in the genitourinary tract cause human disease (Metaxas et al., 2015). Mycoplasma infections can place a big burden on healthcare systems, with more than 100,000 annual hospitalizations arising from *M. pneumoniae* in the US alone (Atkinson et al., 2008). In addition, mycoplasma infections of the respiratory and urogenital tract can be chronic. A better understanding of the pathogenesis of mycoplasma infections will contribute to vaccine development and treatment.

A key characteristic of the pathogenesis of chronic mycoplasma infections is the cross-talk between mycoplasmas and the host immune system (Atkinson et al., 2008). An inflammation response induced by the host's immunity is one of the main characteristics of *M. pneumoniae* infection and contributes to clinical presentations. Elucidating the mycoplasma cellular components will help us understand how the relatively small, and biochemically simple, mycoplasmas are capable of eliciting strong and chronic immune responses (Himmelreich et al., 1996). Mycoplasmas can induce proinflammatory response through secreted toxins, surface antigens and other unclear mechanisms (Yeh et al., 2016). Considering that Mycoplasma lack cell walls, cell wall proteins do not interacting with the host's immune system (Pereyre et al., 2016). Analysis of the mycoplasmal cell membrane demonstrated that several lipoprotein surface antigens elicit strong immune responses (Muhlradt et al., 1997) through a distinct pathway than that seen with lipopolysaccharides (Rawadi and Roman-Roman, 1996). Unlike numerous other bacterial species, a large portion of mycoplasmal genome (6.68%) is dedicated to encoding various lipoproteins (Dandekar et al., 2000; Hallamaa et al., 2006). The functionality of these genes is unknown, but they may drive adhesion and/or the initial stages of mycoplasmal infection since their products are cell surface proteins. Certain mycoplasmal lipoproteins have exonuclease activity that may be involved in the function of the ATP-binding cassette (ABC) transport system to import nucleic acid precursors (Schmidt et al., 2007). Little is known about the transcriptional regulation that occurs within these genes, especially since the mycoplasmal genome lacks many of the transcriptional regulators found in other bacteria (Himmelreich et al., 1996; Dandekar et al., 2000).

The lipoylation mechanism of lipoproteins in mycoplasmas is similar to that of other bacteria (Rottem, 2003). Bacterial lipoproteins play a major role in the cross-talk between bacteria and host immune responses. Bacterial lipoproteins contain a lipoylated amino-terminal cysteinyl residue that is usually *N*-acylated (Braun and Hantke, 1974). However, an *N*-acyltransferase gene has not been found in *M. pneumoniae* or *M. genitalium* genome (Himmelreich et al., 1996) and many mycoplasmal lipoproteins are not *N*-acylated [such as lipoproteins from *M. gallisepticum* (Jan et al., 1996; Muhlradt et al., 1997)]. Triacylation or diacylation of lipoproteins affects their recognition from different Toll like receptors (Jan et al., 1995). Thus, the unique structure of mycoplasmal lipoproteins can determine their immunomodulatory properties. Mycoplasma lipoproteins are all known to induce expression of proinflammatory cytokines including IL-1β, IL-6, and IL-2 (Garcia et al., 1998; Hoek et al., 2005). Several lipoproteins have been identified in mycoplasmas (**Table 1**).

Although Mycoplasma lipoproteins may function as immune-activators within their host, they also regulate mycoplasma colonization and translocation across mucosal membranes and facilitate host immune evasion (Citti et al., 1997; Chambaud et al., 1999). Understanding lipoprotein-induced immunomodulation will aid in developing novel treatments against Mycoplasmas (Martinez de Tejada et al., 2015). Herein, we review the evidence on the effects of mycoplasmal lipoproteins on host immunity (**Figure 1**). Given the complex immunomodulatory effects of mycoplasma lipoproteins we will dissect these effects by specific cell type (epithelial cells, neutrophils, myeloid cells, lymphocytes).

Effects of Mycoplasmal Lipoproteins on Epithelial Cells

Epithelial cells are the main targets of *M. pneumoniae* and secrete cytokines in response to infections (Fahey et al., 2005). Mycoplasmas directly induce *in vitro* production of chemotactic cytokines such as IL-8 by bronchial epithelial cells (Chambaud et al., 1999; Peng et al., 2007; Chen et al., 2016). Mycoplasmal lipoproteins may also have a major role in regulation of the cytokine response in respiratory epithelial cells during *M. pneumoniae* infection (Eckmann et al., 1995; Yang et al., 2002). Similar to the role of respiratory epithelial cells in eliciting a response during *M. pneumoniae* infection, epithelial cells lining the vagina and cervix may induce pro-inflammatory

TABLE 1 | Major lipoproteins in mycoplasma species (isolated in humans).

Lipoprotein/Gene ID	Species of Mycoplasma	Original function	Immunomodulatory effect	References
MPN052, MPN162, MPN415, MPN602, MPN611	*M. pneumoniae*	F_0F_1 ATP Synthase subunit b	NF-kB activation, Pro-inflammatory diacylated lipoprotein	Shimizu et al., 2008, 2014
MPN597	*M. pneumoniae*	F_0F_1 ATP Synthase subunit ε	Induction of inflammation, activation of the autophagy/TLR4-mediated pathway	Shimizu et al., 2014; Shimizu, 2016
MPN611 MPN162 MG-142 MG-149	*M. pneumoniae* *M. pneumoniae* *M. genitalium* *M. genitalium*		Activate NF-κB through TLR pathways	Shimizu et al., 2007
MPN372	*M. pneumoniae*	ADP-ribosylating toxin, CARDS toxin	Induces extensive vacuolization and ultimate cell death of mammalian cells, facilitates adhesion to human surfactant protein A (hSP-A), activation of inflammasome	Kannan et al., 2005; Kannan and Baseman, 2006
MPN333	*M. pneumoniae*	ABC Transporter	Activation of the autophagy/TLR4-mediated pathway	Shimizu, 2016
MPN142, MPN447, MPN453 Lp44	*M. pneumoniae* *M. salivarium*	Cytadherence	Activation of inflammasome	Shibata et al., 2000, p. 2; Waldo and Krause, 2006; Spuesens et al., 2011; Balish, 2014; Widjaja et al., 2015
MPN141	*M. pneumoniae*	Cytadherence, P1 adhesin	Induction of pro-inflammatory cytokine production	Waldo and Krause, 2006; Kannan et al., 2011

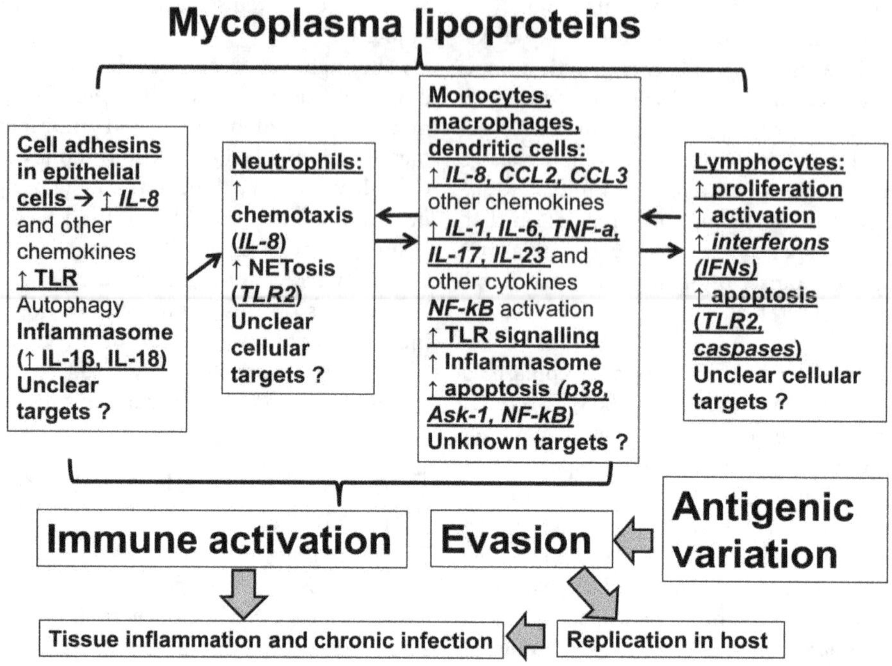

FIGURE 1 | Mechanisms of actions of mycoplasmal lipoproteins: Mycoplasmal lipoproteins lead to inflammatory responses and immune system activation through direct effects on both epithelial and immune cells. Initial adhesion to epithelia of respiratory tract is mediated through adhesins such as P1 (MPN141) as well as other accessory proteins. Epithelial cell activation as well as mycoplasmal lipoproteins induce secretion of chemokines such as IL-8 that promote neutrophilic infiltration and activation of neutrophils (through several mechanisms including NETosis). Neutrophilic activation is followed by activation of myeloid cells (monocytes, macrophages, dendritic cells) that ultimately leads to activation of adaptive immunity (lymphocytes). A key family of receptors that play an important role in recognizing, and inducing responses to Mycoplasmal lipoproteins are the Toll-Like Receptors (TLRs such as TLR2 and TLR6) that are key players in inflammatory responses upon infection. Mycoplasmal lipoproteins can also activate cells through the inflammasome and the pre-cursors of proinflammatory cytokines, such as IL-1β and IL-18, can be cleaved and activated in a caspase-dependent manner prior to their release. Non-TLR or inflammasome dependent mechanisms by which Mycoplasmal lipoproteins can lead to inflammatory responses and immune activation also exist (such as autophagy). TLRs (such as TLR-2 and TLR-6), also play an important role in inducing apoptosis in both monocyte and lymphocyte cell lines through induction of p38 MAPK, the apoptosis signal-regulating kinase (ASK1), caspase and the NF-kB pathways and the release of Nitric Oxide from macrophages. See text for further details. Given poorly understood mechanisms, further studies are needed to elucidate the mechanisms of immunomodulation mediated by mycoplasmal lipoproteins.

cytokines upon exposure to lipoproteins present in *M. genitalium* (McGowin et al., 2009). However, the exact mechanisms that contribute to differential effects of mycoplasma lipoproteins on epithelial compared to immune cells remain unclear. Epithelial cells are also able to have an effect on Mycoplasmas. Upon contact with human epithelial cells *in-vivo, M. pneumoniae* can undergo transcriptional changes in lipoprotein related genes (Hallamaa et al., 2008). Such an alteration in the genetic profile of the Mycoplasma upon coming into contact with epithelial cells represents the two-way dynamic existing between Mycoplasma and the host, where both parties are able to influence each other. Thus, the initial release of proinflammatory cytokines and chemokines by epithelial cells infected by Mycoplasmas can also induce early recruitment of immune cells such as neutrophils.

Effects of Mycoplasmal Lipoproteins on Neutrophils

Mycoplasma respiratory infections lead to the recruitment of polymorphonuclear leukocytes and subsequently monocytes/macrophages (M/M) and lymphocytes (Kruger and Baier, 1997). The attraction of leukocytes to the site of infection is controlled by chemokines, which are chemotactic cytokines. The *M. pneumoniae*/IL-8/neutrophil axis likely plays a vital role in the pathogenesis of MPP and mycoplasmas directly induce *in vitro* production of chemotactic cytokines such as IL-8 by bronchial epithelial cells (Chambaud et al., 1999; Peng et al., 2007; Chen et al., 2016). An *M. fermentans* lipoprotein fraction induces secretion of IL-8 from cultured human M/M (Chambaud et al., 1999; Peng et al., 2007; Chen et al., 2016). The expression of such chemokines allows for the recruitment of leukocytes, such as neutrophils, to the site of infection, and it is this influx of leukocytes that comes to partially contribute to the inflammatory response seen upon mycoplasma infection (Wu et al., 2007).

Except for IL-8 and neutrophil chemotaxis, mycoplasma lipoproteins also induce NETosis. Neutrophil extracellular traps (NETs) are a major component of the first line of defense against invading pathogens and they involve a pathogen facilitated cell death by which neutrophils can extrude chromatin structures loaded with anti-microbial molecules to eliminate pathogens (Gomez-Lopez et al., 2017). Experiments using *M. agalactiae* have shown that mycoplasmas are capable of inducing NETosis upon infection, and mycoplasma lipoproteins are the component primarily responsible for activation of these pathways in neutrophils (Cacciotto et al., 2016). Furthermore, it has also been shown that lipoproteins induce Toll-like Receptor 2 (TLR2) signaling that plays a pivotal role in neutrophil NETosis (Cacciotto et al., 2016; Xu et al., 2017). Notably, NET formation ability decreases with patient age, and this may contribute to the susceptibility of older patients to mycoplasmal pathogens such as *M. pneumoniae* (Xu et al., 2017). More research is needed on the ability of lipoproteins to induce NETosis. Thus, mycoplasmal lipoproteins regulate neutrophilic host immune responses, which are the mainstay of pathogenesis of mycoplasmal infections. These early neutrophilic responses can also contribute to inflammatory responses from myeloid cells.

Effects of Mycoplasmal Lipoproteins on Myeloid Cells

Mycoplasmas induce activation of cytolytic activity of macrophages, and stimulation of cytokines (interleukin [IL]-1, IL-6, tumor necrosis factor-alpha [TNF-α]). Although several mycoplasmal proteins can induce these proinflammatory responses (Chambaud et al., 1999; Peng et al., 2007; Chen et al., 2016), mycoplasmal lipoproteins seem to be a major instigator of production of proinflammatory cytokines by myeloid cells such as M/M and dendritic cells (Cole et al., 2005; He et al., 2009). Non-denaturing detergents enriched with mycoplasmal lipoproteins, have modulatory capacities (Cole et al., 2005; Liu et al., 2012). Synthetic lipopeptides such as the Mycoplasma-derived lipopeptide MALP-2 from *M. fermentans* (Muhlradt et al., 1997), FSL-1 (also known as Pam2C) from *M. salivarium* (Shibata et al., 2000), and MPPL-1 from *M. pneumoniae* (Into et al., 2007) were shown to have immunomodulatory properties. Activation of macrophages by mycoplasmal lipoproteins can occur at pico-molar concentrations of lipoproteins, making them extremely potent activators (Muhlradt et al., 1997).

In vitro and *in vivo* studies demonstrated that the *M. fermentans*-derived membrane component MALP-2 (macrophage-activating lipopeptide 2) is the main active component that induces these proinflammatory responses (Kaufmann et al., 1999). MALP-2 directly induced *in vitro* production of the proinflammatory cytokines TNF-α and IL-6 and the neutrophil-attracting CXC chemokines IL-8 and Growth-regulated Oncogene α (GRO-α) as well as the mononuclear leukocyte-attracting CC chemokines Monocyte chemoattractant protein-1 (MCP-1/CCL2), Macrophage inflammatory protein 1 alpha (MIP-1a/CCL3), and Macrophage inflammatory protein 1 beta (MIP-1b/CCL3) (Garcia et al., 1998; Rawadi et al., 1998). The MALP-2 molecule is a potent activator of human monocytes.

Mycoplasmal lipoproteins in *M. hominis* such as lipoprotein MHO_4720 were recently shown to induce production of Interleukin-23 (IL-23), by dendritic cells through activation of inflammasome (Chen et al., 2017; Goret et al., 2017). Production of proinflammatory cytokines such as IL-23 has been shown to induce the expression of chemokines such as IL-17, allowing for effective containment of the infection (Wu et al., 2007). Additional *in vivo* studies have shown that many of the chemokines induced by mycoplasma infection in humans are conserved across species, such as macrophage inflammatory protein (MIP)-1β (Lam, 2002). Certain mycoplasmal lipoproteins, such as those from *M. hyopneumoniae* also elicit anti-inflammatory cytokines such as Interleukin-10 (Chambaud et al., 1999; Mollazadeh et al., 2017).

Inducing apoptosis of both monocytes and lymphocytes is a key step in allowing Mycoplasma to prolong their survival within their hosts, and has been documented in numerous Mycoplasma, with *M. bovis* being one of the most well-studied (Into et al., 2004; Jimbo et al., 2017). Mycoplasma lipoproteins induce apoptosis in both monocyte (ex. HL-60, THP-1) and lymphocyte cell lines (ex. MOLT-4) (Aliprantis et al., 1999; Into et al., 2002a, 2004) and thus directly contribute to immune evasion.

Thus, mycoplasmal lipoproteins regulate myeloid based host immune responses and inflammatory responses, which are key mediators of pathogenesis of mycoplasmal infections. These innate immune responses may also drive responses from adaptive immunity (such as lymphocytic responses).

Effects of Mycoplasmal Lipoproteins on Lymphocytes

Mycoplasmas induce proliferation of T and B cells (Naot et al., 1979; Cole et al., 1990) through superantigens or unidentified factors. Various mycoplasmas also activate cytotoxic T lymphocytes (CTLs) and natural killer (NK) cells (Wayner and Brooks, 1984) and induce expression of major histocompatibility antigens on B cells (Ross et al., 1992), IL-2 by T cells, interleukin (IL)-1 by macrophages (Muhlradt et al., 1991) and interferons (IFNs) by lymphocytes (Arai et al., 1983). Collectively these mycoplasma-driven immunomodulatory effects contribute to the proliferation and maturation of both T and B lymphocytes as well as the activation of macrophages and NK cells (Arango Duque and Descoteaux, 2014).

During the early phases of infection, mycoplasmas usually induce an inflammatory and a humoral response preferentially directed against their membrane-bound, surface-exposed lipoproteins. Mycoplasmal lipoproteins such as spiralin induce T-cell-independent B-cell blastogenesis and secretion of proinflammatory cytokines (Brenner et al., 1997). Lipoproteins from *M. fermentans* and *M. salivarium* induce TLR2- and caspase-mediated apoptosis in lymphocytes (Into et al., 2004). The effects of mycoplasmal lipoproteins on lymphocytes may not be mediated by effects on TLR signaling on antigen presenting cells such as dendritic cells (Sawahata et al., 2011). Thus, mycoplasmal lipoproteins also regulate adaptive immune and function of both B cells and T cells.

Effects of Mycoplasmal Lipoproteins on Evasion of Host Immunity

Although lipoproteins have a major role as immune system activators, they also facilitate evasion of the host's immune response, leading to chronic mycoplasma infections (Becker and Sander, 2016; Goret et al., 2016). Mycoplasma lipoproteins facilitate immune evasion through several mechanisms such as creation of the mycoplasmal shield, lipoprotein antigenic variation, and protection from growth inhibiting host antibodies (Citti et al., 1997; Chambaud et al., 1999). Understanding the various modes of immune system evasion promises a better approach to treating mycoplasma infections.

Lipoproteins as the Basis for Mycoplasmal Shield Against Host Immune Defense Mechanisms

The ability of mycoplasma to encode numerous forms of lipoproteins that can potentially be expressed on their surface allows mycoplasmas to avoid host immune responses (Simmons et al., 2004). Mycoplasmas are able to create a protective layer around themselves that can sterically hinder access of growth-inhibiting host antibodies and even macrophages (Citti et al., 1997; Simmons et al., 2004). In addition to facilitating Mycoplasmal protection, the lipoprotein shield also plays an important role in hemadsorption and mycoplasmal adherence to surfaces (Bolland and Dybvig, 2012; Xiong et al., 2016). Mycoplasmas that are minimally shielded may be highly adherent while maximally shielded mycoplasmas are less adherent (Bolland and Dybvig, 2012).

Variable Surface Antigen (Vsa) Lipoproteins as Facilitators of Immune Evasion

In addition to the generation of a shield for protecting Mycoplasmas, lipoproteins are also able to protect Mycoplasma by undergoing variation. One major method by which lipoprotein variation in mycoplasmas can contribute to host immune evasion involves altering the length of these variable surface antigens (Vsa) (Xiong et al., 2016). Mycoplasmas use antigenic variation not only to evade immune responses but also to adapt to each host (Bencina et al., 2001). Vsa lipoproteins normally have a 242-amino acid N-terminus with a variable C-terminal domain that can contain up to 60 tandem repeating units which in themselves can range in size from 10 to 19 amino acids (Bencina et al., 2001). Each cell can only transcribe one Vsa gene at a time, with silent Vsa genes missing the sequences necessary to make the conserved N-terminal domain (Shen et al., 2000). To achieve a large variety of Vsa recombination of lipoproteins, mycoplasmas use DNA recombination (Dybvig et al., 1998; Shen et al., 2000). Although a single cell may only transcribe a single Vsa gene, during an infection subpopulations of cells are able to express varying Vsa lipoproteins (Pantoja et al., 2016).

Despite the great importance Vsa size variation plays in facilitating prolonged mycoplasmal survival within hosts, adaptive immunity is still able to decrease mycoplasmal survival, thus necessitating phase variation of the shield as well (Simmons and Dybvig, 2009). Thus, in addition to being able to conduct size variation of surface lipoproteins, mycoplasmas are also able to conduct phase (type) variation of their lipoproteins, hence the name Vsa lipoproteins (Dybvig et al., 1998; Chambaud et al., 1999). Phase variation *in vivo* is only seen upon the onset of an adaptive immune response, with no alterations occurring in Vsa expression if an organism lacks B and T cells (Gumulak-Smith et al., 2001). It is estimated that phase switching occurs at a frequency of around 10^{-3} per CFU per generation (Rosengarten and Wise, 1990). In having the ability to undergo phase variation, mycoplasmas are able to evade host immune responses and indeed lead to chronic infections, similar to how Spirochetes might also use antigenic variation in order to establish a chronic infection (Chambaud et al., 1999; Christodoulides et al., 2017). Thus, Mycoplasmal lipoproteins have pleotropic immunomodulatory effects and their mechanisms of actions need to be elucidated.

MECHANISMS OF ACTION OF MYCOPLASMAL LIPOPROTEINS

A key family of receptors that play an important role in recognizing, and inducing responses to Mycoplasmal lipoproteins are the Toll-Like Receptors (TLRs) that are key players in inflammatory responses upon infection (Akira et al., 2001; Wang et al., 2017). Two of the most well-studied TLRs are TLR2 and TLR6, both of which are pivotal in recognizing Mycoplasmal Macrophage-Activating Lipopeptide-2 (MALP-2), with the absence of either TLR leading to a lack of recognition and macrophage activation (Takeuchi et al., 2002). Mycoplasmal lipoproteins can also activate myeloid cells through the inflammasome (Chen et al., 2017; Goret et al., 2017). Amongst the Mycoplasma capable of activating inflammasome with their lipoproteins are *M. salivarium* and *M. pneumoniae* (Shimizu, 2016; Sugiyama et al., 2016). Through the activation of the inflammasome, the pre-cursors of proinflammatory cytokines, such as IL-1β and IL-18, can be cleaved and activated in a caspase-dependent manner prior to their release (Boyden and Dietrich, 2006).

Non-pathogenic Mycoplasma also express lipoproteins, suggesting that a non-TLR dependent, or inflammasome dependent, mechanism exists by which Mycoplasmal lipoproteins can lead to immune activation (Shimizu, 2016). *M. pneumoniae* was still able to induce a strong inflammatory response in TLR2 KO mice (Shimizu et al., 2014). Introduction of known autophagy inhibitors to the TLR2 KO mice in turn lead to a significant fall in the inflammatory response, suggesting a role of autophagy in also leading to inflammatory responses (Shimizu et al., 2014).

Another mechanism by which Mycoplasmal lipoproteins are able to lead to immune system activation is through their initial adhesion to epithelia such as the respiratory tract in the case of *M. pneumoniae* (Jordan et al., 2001). Such cytadherence is mediated through adhesins such as P1(MPN141) as well as other accessory proteins, and treatment of Mycoplasma with proteases or anti-P1 antibodies was seen to lead to a significant decrease in proinflammatory cytokine release (Yang et al., 2002; Hoek et al., 2005). Cytadherence on behalf of *M. pneumoniae* was seen to generate a proinflammatory response through pathways involving both autophagy/TLR4 as well as inflammasome (Shimizu et al., 2014).

In addition to their roles as inductors of the inflammatory response, TLRs also play an important role in inducing apoptosis in both monocyte cell lines (ex. HL-60, HEK293, THP-1) and lymphocyte cell lines (ex. MOLT-4) upon binding of Mycoplasmal lipoproteins (Aliprantis et al., 1999; Into et al., 2002a; Into et al., 2004). The two main TLRs seen to play a role in this apoptotic pathway are TLR-2 and TLR-6, which through their activation allow induction of NF-kB (Aliprantis et al., 1999; Wu et al., 2008) and the release of Nitric Oxide from macrophages (Muhlradt and Frisch, 1994; Into et al., 2004). Mycoplasmal induced apoptosis seems to be mediated by activation of the p38 MAPK, the apoptosis signal-regulating kinase (ASK1) and the NF-kB pathways (Into and Shibata, 2005). Mycoplasmas such as *M. salivarium* and *M. fermentans* have also been seen to induce apoptosis through the more conventional caspase pathways (Into et al., 2002a,b).

On the other hand, certain mycoplasmal lipoproteins, such as those seen in *M. fermentans*, can inhibit TNF-α mediated apoptosis (Gerlic et al., 2007). Thus, further research is needed to understand the pleotropic effects of mycoplasmal lipoproteins on apoptosis.

A better understanding of mechanisms of immunomodulation mediated by mycoplasmal lipoproteins may lead to therapies to attenuate the detrimental effects of mycoplasma infections.

MYCOPLASMAL LIPOPROTEINS AS THERAPEUTIC TARGETS

One of the most difficult parts of managing a Mycoplasmal infection is the inability to use many antibiotics such as beta-lactams (Bebear and Pereyre, 2005). The development of drugs such as tigecycline that aim to reduce production of chemokines and lipoproteins through targeting of bacterial ribosomes is a growing discipline within the field of Mycoplasma research (Saliba et al., 2009; Salvatore et al., 2009). Studies of tigecycline in a murine model have been able to confirm a significant drop of cytokine and chemokine production following infection with *M. pneumoniae* (Salvatore et al., 2009). Many studies that focus on development of a possible vaccine against Mycoplasma use inactivated Mycoplasma that can then be introduced to patients (Wenzel et al., 1977; David et al., 2010). Atalla et al. (2015) were able to show that inactivation of Mycoplasma using a photoactivatable alkylating agent (INA), with preservation of the surface lipoproteins, might be a possible mechanism by which Mycoplasma can be inactivated for vaccine development (Atalla et al., 2015). Through a better understanding of bacterial lipoproteins and their interaction with the immune system, researchers are now aiming to develop vaccines that rely on the introduction of bacterial lipoproteins into patients to generate antibody responses (Leng et al., 2015). For example, the above has been achieved with the AvgC lipoprotein from *M. agalactiae* and shows promise for a vaccine against *M. agalactiae* infection (Santona et al., 2002). Such an approach to vaccine development is also currently being studied using bacterial lipoproteins, such as the OspA from Spirochetes (Izac et al., 2017; Zhao et al., 2017). An innovative approach for treatment of Mycoplasmal infections would involve direct targeting of lipoproteins; however, such an approach remains to be established given the structure of mycoplasmal lipoproteins and their diverse immunomodulatory mechanisms. Importantly, the polypeptide Aspidasept® which neutralizes endotoxin *in vivo* was previously shown to inhibit cytokines induced by the Mycoplasmal lipoproteins (Martinez de Tejada et al., 2015). Thus, a better understanding of Mycoplasmal lipoprotein epitopes, may promote progress in the field of antibodies, polypeptides or vaccines against Mycoplasma.

CONCLUSION

Further studies are needed to promote understanding of the mechanisms of transcriptional regulation, phase variations and the numerous immunomodulatory effects (both acute and chronic) of Mycoplasmal lipoproteins. Given the decreasing efficacy of antibiotics against mycoplasmas, there is need for novel immunotherapies. Novel strategies such as use of inactivating agents that preserve the mycoplasmal surface lipoproteins, may advance vaccine development (Atalla et al., 2015). Novel approaches such as use of polypeptides that attenuate proinflammatory effects of mycoplasmal lipoproteins need further investigation as novel therapeutic approaches for mycoplasmal infections (Martinez de Tejada et al., 2015). Ultimately, a better understanding of mycoplasmal lipoproteins can set the basis for the development of vaccines or antibodies against mycoplasmal lipoproteins and perhaps shed light on the pathogenesis of other vector based pathogens such as Spirochetes.

AUTHOR CONTRIBUTIONS

AC, NG, VY, JP, NM, and TK wrote and edited the manuscript. TK conceptualized the manuscript.

FUNDING

This work was supported by NIH grants NIH K08AI08272, NIH/NCATS Grant #UL1TR000124.

REFERENCES

Akira, S., Takeda, K., and Kaisho, T. (2001). Toll-like receptors: critical proteins linking innate and acquired immunity. *Nat. Immunol.* 2, 675–680. doi: 10.1038/90609

Aliprantis, A. O., Yang, R. B., Mark, M. R., Suggett, S., Devaux, B., Radolf, J. D., et al. (1999). Cell activation and apoptosis by bacterial lipoproteins through toll-like receptor-2. *Science* 285, 736–739. doi: 10.1126/science.285.5428.736

Arai, S., Munakata, T., and Kuwano, K. (1983). Mycoplasma interaction with lymphocytes and phagocytes: role of hydrogen peroxide released from *M. pneumoniae*. *Yale J. Biol. Med.* 56, 631–638.

Arango Duque, G., and Descoteaux, A. (2014). Macrophage cytokines: involvement in immunity and infectious diseases. *Front. Immunol.* 5:491. doi: 10.3389/fimmu.2014.00491

Atalla, H., Lysnyansky, I., Raviv, Y., and Rottem, S. (2015). *Mycoplasma gallisepticum* inactivated by targeting the hydrophobic domain of the membrane preserves surface lipoproteins and induces a strong immune response. *PLoS One* 10:e0120462. doi: 10.1371/journal.pone.0120462

Atkinson, T. P., Balish, M. F., and Waites, K. B. (2008). Epidemiology, clinical manifestations, pathogenesis and laboratory detection of *Mycoplasma pneumoniae* infections. *FEMS Microbiol. Rev.* 32, 956–973. doi: 10.1111/j.1574-6976.2008.00129.x

Balish, M. F. (2014). *Mycoplasma pneumoniae*, an underutilized model for bacterial cell biology. *J. Bacteriol.* 196, 3675–3682. doi: 10.1128/JB.01865-14

Bebear, C. M., and Pereyre, S. (2005). Mechanisms of drug resistance in *Mycoplasma pneumoniae*. *Curr. Drug Targets Infect. Disord.* 5, 263–271. doi: 10.2174/1568005054880109

Becker, K., and Sander, P. (2016). *Mycobacterium tuberculosis* lipoproteins in virulence and immunity – fighting with a double-edged sword. *FEBS Lett.* 590, 3800–3819. doi: 10.1002/1873-3468.12273

Bencina, D., Drobnic-Valic, M., Horvat, S., Narat, M., Kleven, S. H., and Dovc, P. (2001). Molecular basis of the length variation in the N-terminal part of *Mycoplasma synoviae* hemagglutinin. *FEMS Microbiol. Lett.* 203, 115–123. doi: 10.1111/j.1574-6968.2001.tb10829.x

Bolland, J. R., and Dybvig, K. (2012). *Mycoplasma pulmonis* Vsa proteins and polysaccharide modulate adherence to pulmonary epithelial cells. *FEMS Microbiol. Lett.* 331, 25–30. doi: 10.1111/j.1574-6968.2012.02551.x

Boyden, E. D., and Dietrich, W. F. (2006). *Nalp1b* controls mouse macrophage susceptibility to anthrax lethal toxin. *Nat. Genet.* 38, 240–244. doi: 10.1038/ng1724

Braun, V., and Hantke, K. (1974). Biochemistry of bacterial cell envelopes. *Annu. Rev. Biochem.* 43, 89–121. doi: 10.1146/annurev.bi.43.070174.000513

Brenner, C., Wroblewski, H., Le Henaff, M., Montagnier, L., and Blanchard, A. (1997). Spiralin, a mycoplasmal membrane lipoprotein, induces T-cell-independent B-cell blastogenesis and secretion of proinflammatory cytokines. *Infect. Immun.* 65, 4322–4329.

Cacciotto, C., Cubeddu, T., Addis, M. F., Anfossi, A. G., Tedde, V., Tore, G., et al. (2016). *Mycoplasma* lipoproteins are major determinants of neutrophil extracellular trap formation. *Cell. Microbiol.* 18, 1751–1762. doi: 10.1111/cmi.12613

Chambaud, I., Wroblewski, H., and Blanchard, A. (1999). Interactions between mycoplasma lipoproteins and the host immune system. *Trends Microbiol.* 7, 493–499. doi: 10.1016/S0966-842X(99)01641-8

Chen, Z., Gong, Y., and Shi, Y. (2017). Novel biologic agents targeting interleukin-23 and interleukin-17 for moderate-to-severe psoriasis. *Clin. Drug Investig.* 37, 891–899. doi: 10.1007/s40261-017-0550-z

Chen, Z., Shao, X., Dou, X., Zhang, X., Wang, Y., Zhu, C., et al. (2016). Role of the *Mycoplasma pneumoniae*/interleukin-8/neutrophil axis in the pathogenesis of pneumonia. *PLoS One* 11:e0146377. doi: 10.1371/journal.pone.0146377

Christodoulides, A., Boyadjian, A., and Kelesidis, T. (2017). Spirochetal lipoproteins and immune evasion. *Front. Immunol.* 8:364. doi: 10.3389/fimmu.2017.00364

Citti, C., Kim, M. F., and Wise, K. S. (1997). Elongated versions of Vlp surface lipoproteins protect *Mycoplasma hyorhinis* escape variants from growth-inhibiting host antibodies. *Infect. Immun.* 65, 1773–1785.

Cole, B. C., Kartchner, D. R., and Wells, D. J. (1990). Stimulation of mouse lymphocytes by a mitogen derived from *Mycoplasma arthritidis* (MAM). VIII. Selective activation of T cells expressing distinct V beta T cell receptors from various strains of mice by the "superantigen" MAM. *J. Immunol.* 144, 425–431.

Cole, B. C., Mu, H. H., Pennock, N. D., Hasebe, A., Chan, F. V., Washburn, L. R., et al. (2005). Isolation and partial purification of macrophage- and dendritic cell-activating components from *Mycoplasma arthritidis*: association with organism virulence and involvement with Toll-like receptor 2. *Infect. Immun.* 73, 6039–6047. doi: 10.1128/IAI.73.9.6039-6047.2005

Dandekar, T., Huynen, M., Regula, J. T., Ueberle, B., Zimmermann, C. U., Andrade, M. A., et al. (2000). Re-annotating the *Mycoplasma pneumoniae* genome sequence: adding value, function and reading frames. *Nucleic Acids Res.* 28, 3278–3288. doi: 10.1093/nar/28.17.3278

David, S. A., Volokhov, D. V., Ye, Z., and Chizhikov, V. (2010). Evaluation of *Mycoplasma* inactivation during production of biologics: egg-based viral vaccines as a model. *Appl. Environ. Microbiol.* 76, 2718–2728. doi: 10.1128/AEM.02776-09

Dybvig, K., Sitaraman, R., and French, C. T. (1998). A family of phase-variable restriction enzymes with differing specificities generated by high-frequency gene rearrangements. *Proc. Natl. Acad. Sci. U.S.A.* 95, 13923–13928. doi: 10.1073/pnas.95.23.13923

Eckmann, L., Kagnoff, M. F., and Fierer, J. (1995). Intestinal epithelial cells as watchdogs for the natural immune system. *Trends Microbiol.* 3, 118–120. doi: 10.1016/S0966-842X(00)88894-0

Fahey, J. V., Schaefer, T. M., Channon, J. Y., and Wira, C. R. (2005). Secretion of cytokines and chemokines by polarized human epithelial cells from the female reproductive tract. *Hum. Reprod.* 20, 1439–1446. doi: 10.1093/humrep/deh806

Garcia, J., Lemercier, B., Roman-Roman, S., and Rawadi, G. (1998). A *Mycoplasma fermentans*-derived synthetic lipopeptide induces AP-1 and NF-kappaB activity and cytokine secretion in macrophages via the activation of mitogen-activated protein kinase pathways. *J. Biol. Chem.* 273, 34391–34398. doi: 10.1074/jbc.273.51.34391

Gerlic, M., Horowitz, J., Farkash, S., and Horowitz, S. (2007). The inhibitory effect of *Mycoplasma fermentans* on tumour necrosis factor (TNF)-alpha-induced apoptosis resides in the membrane lipoproteins. *Cell. Microbiol.* 9, 142–153. doi: 10.1111/j.1462-5822.2006.00774.x

Gomez-Lopez, N., Romero, R., Garcia-Flores, V., Xu, Y., Leng, Y., Alhousseini, A., et al. (2017). Amniotic fluid neutrophils can phagocytize bacteria: a mechanism for microbial killing in the amniotic cavity. *Am. J. Reprod. Immunol.* 78:e12723. doi: 10.1111/aji.12723

Goret, J., Beven, L., Faustin, B., Contin-Bordes, C., Le Roy, C., Claverol, S., et al. (2017). Interaction of *Mycoplasma hominis* PG21 with human dendritic cells: interleukin-23-inducing mycoplasmal lipoproteins and inflammasome activation of the cell. *J. Bacteriol.* 199, e213–e217. doi: 10.1128/JB.00213-17

Goret, J., Le Roy, C., Touati, A., Mesureur, J., Renaudin, H., Claverol, S., et al. (2016). Surface lipoproteome of *Mycoplasma hominis* PG21 and differential expression after contact with human dendritic cells. *Future Microbiol.* 11, 179–194. doi: 10.2217/fmb.15.130

Gumulak-Smith, J., Teachman, A., Tu, A. H., Simecka, J. W., Lindsey, J. R., and Dybvig, K. (2001). Variations in the surface proteins and restriction enzyme systems of *Mycoplasma pulmonis* in the respiratory tract of infected rats. *Mol. Microbiol.* 40, 1037–1044. doi: 10.1046/j.1365-2958.2001.02464.x

Hallamaa, K. M., Browning, G. F., and Tang, S. L. (2006). Lipoprotein multigene families in *Mycoplasma pneumoniae*. *J. Bacteriol.* 188, 5393–5399. doi: 10.1128/JB.01819-05

Hallamaa, K. M., Tang, S. L., Ficorilli, N., and Browning, G. F. (2008). Differential expression of lipoprotein genes in *Mycoplasma pneumoniae* after contact with human lung epithelial cells, and under oxidative and acidic stress. *BMC Microbiol.* 8:124. doi: 10.1186/1471-2180-8-124

He, J., You, X., Zeng, Y., Yu, M., Zuo, L., and Wu, Y. (2009). *Mycoplasma genitalium*-derived lipid-associated membrane proteins activate NF-kappaB through toll-like receptors 1, 2, and 6 and CD14 in a MyD88-dependent pathway. *Clin. Vaccine Immunol.* 16, 1750–1757. doi: 10.1128/CVI.00281-09

Himmelreich, R., Hilbert, H., Plagens, H., Pirkl, E., Li, B. C., and Herrmann, R. (1996). Complete sequence analysis of the genome of the bacterium *Mycoplasma pneumoniae*. *Nucleic Acids Res.* 24, 4420–4449. doi: 10.1093/nar/24.22.4420

Hoek, K. L., Duffy, L. B., Cassell, G. H., Dai, Y., and Atkinson, T. P. (2005). A role for the *Mycoplasma pneumoniae* adhesin P1 in interleukin (IL)-4 synthesis and release from rodent mast cells. *Microb. Pathog.* 39, 149–158. doi: 10.1016/j.micpath.2005.07.004

Into, T., Dohkan, J., Inomata, M., Nakashima, M., Shibata, K., and Matsushita, K. (2007). Synthesis and characterization of a dipalmitoylated lipopeptide derived from paralogous lipoproteins of *Mycoplasma pneumoniae*. *Infect. Immun.* 75, 2253–2259. doi: 10.1128/IAI.00141-07

Into, T., Kiura, K., Yasuda, M., Kataoka, H., Inoue, N., Hasebe, A., et al. (2004). Stimulation of human Toll-like receptor (TLR) 2 and TLR6 with membrane lipoproteins of *Mycoplasma fermentans* induces apoptotic cell death after NF-kappa B activation. *Cell. Microbiol.* 6, 187–199. doi: 10.1046/j.1462-5822.2003.00356.x

Into, T., Nodasaka, Y., Hasebe, A., Okuzawa, T., Nakamura, J., Ohata, N., et al. (2002a). Mycoplasmal lipoproteins induce toll-like receptor 2- and caspases-mediated cell death in lymphocytes and monocytes. *Microbiol. Immunol.* 46, 265–276.

Into, T., Okada, K., Inoue, N., Yasuda, M., and Shibata, K. (2002b). Extracellular ATP regulates cell death of lymphocytes and monocytes induced by membrane-bound lipoproteins of *Mycoplasma fermentans* and *Mycoplasma salivarium*. *Microbiol. Immunol.* 46, 667–675.

Into, T., and Shibata, K. (2005). Apoptosis signal-regulating kinase 1-mediated sustained p38 mitogen-activated protein kinase activation regulates mycoplasmal lipoprotein- and staphylococcal peptidoglycan-triggered Toll-like receptor 2 signalling pathways. *Cell. Microbiol.* 7, 1305–1317. doi: 10.1111/j.1462-5822.2005.00558.x

Izac, J. R., Oliver, L. D. Jr., Earnhart, C. G., and Marconi, R. T. (2017). Identification of a defined linear epitope in the OspA protein of the Lyme disease spirochetes that elicits bactericidal antibody responses: implications for vaccine development. *Vaccine* 35, 3178–3185. doi: 10.1016/j.vaccine.2017.04.079

Jan, G., Brenner, C., and Wroblewski, H. (1996). Purification of *Mycoplasma gallisepticum* membrane proteins p52, p67 (pMGA), and p77 by high-performance liquid chromatography. *Protein Expr. Purif.* 7, 160–166. doi: 10.1006/prep.1996.0023

Jan, G., Fontenelle, C., Le Henaff, M., and Wroblewski, H. (1995). Acylation and immunological properties of *Mycoplasma gallisepticum* membrane proteins. *Res. Microbiol.* 146, 739–750. doi: 10.1016/0923-2508(96)81070-9

Jimbo, S., Suleman, M., Maina, T., Prysliak, T., Mulongo, M., and Perez-Casal, J. (2017). Effect of *Mycoplasma bovis* on bovine neutrophils. *Vet. Immunol. Immunopathol.* 188, 27–33. doi: 10.1016/j.vetimm.2017.04.011

Jordan, J. L., Berry, K. M., Balish, M. F., and Krause, D. C. (2001). Stability and subcellular localization of cytadherence-associated protein P65 in *Mycoplasma pneumoniae*. *J. Bacteriol.* 183, 7387–7391. doi: 10.1128/JB.183.24.7387-7891.2001

Kannan, T. R., and Baseman, J. B. (2006). ADP-ribosylating and vacuolating cytotoxin of *Mycoplasma pneumoniae* represents unique virulence determinant among bacterial pathogens. *Proc. Natl. Acad. Sci. U.S.A.* 103, 6724–6729. doi: 10.1073/pnas.0510644103

Kannan, T. R., Coalson, J. J., Cagle, M., Musatovova, O., Hardy, R. D., and Baseman, J. B. (2011). Synthesis and distribution of CARDS toxin during *Mycoplasma pneumoniae* infection in a murine model. *J. Infect. Dis.* 204, 1596–1604. doi: 10.1093/infdis/jir557

Kannan, T. R., Provenzano, D., Wright, J. R., and Baseman, J. B. (2005). Identification and characterization of human surfactant protein a binding protein of *Mycoplasma pneumoniae*. *Infect. Immun.* 73, 2828–2834. doi: 10.1128/IAI.73.5.2828-2834.2005

Kaufmann, A., Muhlradt, P. F., Gemsa, D., and Sprenger, H. (1999). Induction of cytokines and chemokines in human monocytes by *Mycoplasma fermentans*-derived lipoprotein MALP-2. *Infect. Immun.* 67, 6303–6308.

Kruger, T., and Baier, J. (1997). Induction of neutrophil chemoattractant cytokines by *Mycoplasma hominis* in alveolar type II cells. *Infect. Immun.* 65, 5131–5136.

Lam, K. M. (2002). The macrophage inflammatory protein-1beta in the supernatants of *Mycoplasma gallisepticum*-infected chicken leukocytes attracts the migration of chicken heterophils and lymphocytes. *Dev. Comp. Immunol.* 26, 85–93. doi: 10.1016/S0145-305X(01)00053-2

Leng, C. H., Liu, S. J., Chen, H. W., and Chong, P. (2015). Recombinant bacterial lipoproteins as vaccine candidates. *Expert Rev. Vaccines* 14, 1623–1632. doi: 10.1586/14760584.2015.1091732

Liu, Y. C., Lin, I. H., Chung, W. J., Hu, W. S., Ng, W. V., Lu, C. Y., et al. (2012). Proteomics characterization of cytoplasmic and lipid-associated membrane proteins of human pathogen *Mycoplasma fermentans* M64. *PLoS One* 7:e35304. doi: 10.1371/journal.pone.0035304

Martinez de Tejada, G., Heinbockel, L., Ferrer-Espada, R., Heine, H., Alexander, C., Barcena-Varela, S., et al. (2015). Lipoproteins/peptides are sepsis-inducing toxins from bacteria that can be neutralized by synthetic anti-endotoxin peptides. *Sci. Rep.* 5:14292. doi: 10.1038/srep14292

McGowin, C. L., Ma, L., Martin, D. H., and Pyles, R. B. (2009). *Mycoplasma genitalium*-encoded MG309 activates NF-kappaB via Toll-like receptors 2 and 6 to elicit proinflammatory cytokine secretion from human genital epithelial cells. *Infect. Immun.* 77, 1175–1181. doi: 10.1128/IAI.00845-08

Metaxas, E. I., Balis, E., Papaparaskevas, J., Spanakis, N., Tatsis, G., and Tsakris, A. (2015). Bronchiectasis exacerbations: the role of atypical bacteria, respiratory syncytial virus and pulmonary function tests. *Can. Respir. J.* 22, 163–166. doi: 10.1155/2015/783682

Mollazadeh, H., Cicero, A. F. G., Blesso, C. N., Pirro, M., Majeed, M., and Sahebkar, A. (2017). Immune modulation by curcumin: the Role of Interleukin-10. *Crit. Rev. Food Sci. Nutr.* doi: 10.1080/10408398.2017.1358139 [Epub ahead of print].

Muhlradt, P. F., and Frisch, M. (1994). Purification and partial biochemical characterization of a *Mycoplasma fermentans*-derived substance that activates macrophages to release nitric oxide, tumor necrosis factor, and interleukin-6. *Infect. Immun.* 62, 3801–3807.

Muhlradt, P. F., Kiess, M., Meyer, H., Sussmuth, R., and Jung, G. (1997). Isolation, structure elucidation, and synthesis of a macrophage stimulatory lipopeptide from *Mycoplasma fermentans* acting at picomolar concentration. *J. Exp. Med.* 185, 1951–1958. doi: 10.1084/jem.185.11.1951

Muhlradt, P. F., Quentmeier, H., and Schmitt, E. (1991). Involvement of interleukin-1 (IL-1), IL-6, IL-2, and IL-4 in generation of cytolytic T cells from thymocytes stimulated by a *Mycoplasma fermentans*-derived product. *Infect. Immun.* 59, 3962–3968.

Naot, Y., Merchav, S., Ben-David, E., and Ginsburg, H. (1979). Mitogenic activity of Mycoplasma pulmonis. I. stimulation of rat B and T lymphocytes. *Immunology* 36, 399–406.

Pantoja, L. G., Pettit, K., Dos Santos, L. F., Tubbs, R., and Pieters, M. (2016). *Mycoplasma hyopneumoniae* genetic variability within a swine operation. *J. Vet. Diagn. Invest.* 28, 175–179. doi: 10.1177/1040638716630767

Peng, H. H., Liang, S., Henderson, A. J., and Dong, C. (2007). Regulation of interleukin-8 expression in melanoma-stimulated neutrophil inflammatory response. *Exp. Cell Res.* 313, 551–559. doi: 10.1016/j.yexcr.2006.10.030

Pereyre, S., Goret, J., and Bebear, C. (2016). *Mycoplasma pneumoniae*: current knowledge on macrolide resistance and treatment. *Front. Microbiol.* 7:974. doi: 10.3389/fmicb.2016.00974

Rawadi, G., Ramez, V., Lemercier, B., and Roman-Roman, S. (1998). Activation of mitogen-activated protein kinase pathways by *Mycoplasma fermentans* membrane lipoproteins in murine macrophages: involvement in cytokine synthesis. *J. Immunol.* 160, 1330–1339.

Rawadi, G., and Roman-Roman, S. (1996). Mycoplasma membrane lipoproteins induced proinflammatory cytokines by a mechanism distinct from that of lipopolysaccharide. *Infect. Immun.* 64, 637–643.

Rosengarten, R., and Wise, K. S. (1990). Phenotypic switching in mycoplasmas: phase variation of diverse surface lipoproteins. *Science* 247, 315–318. doi: 10.1126/science.1688663

Ross, S. E., Simecka, J. W., Gambill, G. P., Davis, J. K., and Cassell, G. H. (1992). *Mycoplasma pulmonis* possesses a novel chemoattractant for B lymphocytes. *Infect. Immun.* 60, 669–674.

Rottem, S. (2003). Interaction of mycoplasmas with host cells. *Physiol. Rev.* 83, 417–432. doi: 10.1152/physrev.00030.2002

Saliba, R., Paasch, L., and El Solh, A. (2009). Tigecycline attenuates staphylococcal superantigen-induced T-cell proliferation and production of cytokines and chemokines. *Immunopharmacol. Immunotoxicol.* 31, 583–588. doi: 10.3109/08923970902838672

Salvatore, C. M., Techasaensiri, C., Tagliabue, C., Katz, K., Leos, N., Gomez, A. M., et al. (2009). Tigecycline therapy significantly reduces the concentrations of inflammatory pulmonary cytokines and chemokines in a murine model of *Mycoplasma pneumoniae pneumonia*. *Antimicrob. Agents Chemother.* 53, 1546–1551. doi: 10.1128/AAC.00979-08

Santona, A., Carta, F., Fraghi, P., and Turrini, F. (2002). Mapping antigenic sites of an immunodominant surface lipoprotein of *Mycoplasma agalactiae*, AvgC, with the use of synthetic peptides. *Infect. Immun.* 70, 171–176. doi: 10.1128/IAI.70.1.171-176.2002

Sawahata, R., Shime, H., Yamazaki, S., Inoue, N., Akazawa, T., Fujimoto, Y., et al. (2011). Failure of mycoplasma lipoprotein MALP-2 to induce NK cell activation through dendritic cell TLR2. *Microbes Infect.* 13, 350–358. doi: 10.1016/j.micinf.2010.12.003

Schmidt, J. A., Browning, G. F., and Markham, P. F. (2007). *Mycoplasma hyopneumoniae* mhp379 is a Ca2+-dependent, sugar-nonspecific exonuclease exposed on the cell surface. *J. Bacteriol.* 189, 3414–3424. doi: 10.1128/JB.01835-06

Shen, X., Gumulak, J., Yu, H., French, C. T., Zou, N., and Dybvig, K. (2000). Gene rearrangements in the vsa locus of *Mycoplasma pulmonis. J. Bacteriol.* 182, 2900–2908. doi: 10.1128/JB.182.10.2900-2908.2000

Shibata, K., Hasebe, A., Into, T., Yamada, M., and Watanabe, T. (2000). The N-terminal lipopeptide of a 44-kDa membrane-bound lipoprotein of *Mycoplasma salivarium* is responsible for the expression of intercellular adhesion molecule-1 on the cell surface of normal human gingival fibroblasts. *J. Immunol.* 165, 6538–6544. doi: 10.4049/jimmunol.165.11.6538

Shimizu, T. (2016). Inflammation-inducing factors of *Mycoplasma pneumoniae. Front. Microbiol.* 7:414. doi: 10.3389/fmicb.2016.00414

Shimizu, T., Kida, Y., and Kuwano, K. (2007). Triacylated lipoproteins derived from *Mycoplasma pneumoniae* activate nuclear factor-kappaB through toll-like receptors 1 and 2. *Immunology* 121, 473–483. doi: 10.1111/j.1365-2567.2007.02594.x

Shimizu, T., Kida, Y., and Kuwano, K. (2008). *Mycoplasma pneumoniae*-derived lipopeptides induce acute inflammatory responses in the lungs of mice. *Infect. Immun.* 76, 270–277. doi: 10.1128/IAI.00955-07

Shimizu, T., Kimura, Y., Kida, Y., Kuwano, K., Tachibana, M., Hashino, M., et al. (2014). Cytadherence of *Mycoplasma pneumoniae* induces inflammatory responses through autophagy and toll-like receptor 4. *Infect. Immun.* 82, 3076–3086. doi: 10.1128/IAI.01961-14

Simmons, W. L., Denison, A. M., and Dybvig, K. (2004). Resistance of *Mycoplasma pulmonis* to complement lysis is dependent on the number of Vsa tandem repeats: shield hypothesis. *Infect. Immun.* 72, 6846–6851. doi: 10.1128/IAI.72.12.6846-6851.2004

Simmons, W. L., and Dybvig, K. (2009). Mycoplasma biofilms *ex vivo* and *in vivo. FEMS Microbiol. Lett.* 295, 77–81. doi: 10.1111/j.1574-6968.2009.01592.x

Spuesens, E. B., Van De Kreeke, N., Estevao, S., Hoogenboezem, T., Sluijter, M., Hartwig, N. G., et al. (2011). Variation in a surface-exposed region of the *Mycoplasma pneumoniae* P40 protein as a consequence of homologous DNA recombination between RepMP5 elements. *Microbiology* 157, 473–483. doi: 10.1099/mic.0.045591-0

Sugiyama, M., Saeki, A., Hasebe, A., Kamesaki, R., Yoshida, Y., Kitagawa, Y., et al. (2016). Activation of inflammasomes in dendritic cells and macrophages by *Mycoplasma salivarium. Mol. Oral. Microbiol.* 31, 259–269. doi: 10.1111/omi.12117

Takeuchi, O., Sato, S., Horiuchi, T., Hoshino, K., Takeda, K., Dong, Z., et al. (2002). Cutting edge: role of Toll-like receptor 1 in mediating immune response to microbial lipoproteins. *J. Immunol.* 169, 10–14. doi: 10.4049/jimmunol.169.1.10

Waldo, R. H. III, and Krause, D. C. (2006). Synthesis, stability, and function of cytadhesin P1 and accessory protein B/C complex of *Mycoplasma pneumoniae. J. Bacteriol.* 188, 569–575. doi: 10.1128/JB.188.2.569-575.2006

Wang, Y., Wang, Q., Li, Y., Chen, Y., Shao, J., Nick, N., et al. (2017). Mmm-derived lipid-associated membrane proteins activate IL-1beta production through the NF-kappaB pathway via TLR2, MyD88, and IRAK4. *Sci. Rep.* 7:4349. doi: 10.1038/s41598-017-04729-y

Wayner, E. A., and Brooks, C. G. (1984). Induction of NKCF-like activity in mixed lymphocyte-tumor cell culture: direct involvement of mycoplasma infection of tumor cells. *J. Immunol.* 132, 2135–2142.

Wenzel, R. P., Craven, R. B., Davies, J. A., Hendley, J. O., Hamory, B. H., and Gwaltney, J. M. Jr. (1977). Protective efficacy of an inactivated *Mycoplasma pneumoniae* vaccine. *J. Infect. Dis.* 136(Suppl.), S204–S207. doi: 10.1093/infdis/136.Supplement.S204

Widjaja, M., Berry, I. J., Pont, E. J., Padula, M. P., and Djordjevic, S. P. (2015). P40 and P90 from Mpn142 are targets of multiple processing events on the Surface of *Mycoplasma pneumoniae. Proteomes* 3, 512–537. doi: 10.3390/proteomes3040512

Wu, Q., Martin, R. J., Rino, J. G., Breed, R., Torres, R. M., and Chu, H. W. (2007). IL-23-dependent IL-17 production is essential in neutrophil recruitment and activity in mouse lung defense against respiratory *Mycoplasma pneumoniae* infection. *Microbes Infect.* 9, 78–86. doi: 10.1016/j.micinf.2006.10.012

Wu, Y., Qiu, H., Zeng, Y., You, X., Deng, Z., Yu, M., et al. (2008). *Mycoplasma genitalium* lipoproteins induce human monocytic cell expression of proinflammatory cytokines and apoptosis by activating nuclear factor kappaB. *Mediators Inflamm.* 2008:195427. doi: 10.1155/2008/195427

Xiong, Q., Zhang, B., Wang, J., Ni, B., Ji, Y., Wei, Y., et al. (2016). Characterization of the role in adherence of *Mycoplasma hyorhinis* variable lipoproteins containing different repeat unit copy numbers. *Vet. Microbiol.* 197, 39–46. doi: 10.1016/j.vetmic.2016.10.025

Xu, F., Zhang, C., Zou, Z., Fan, E. K. Y., Chen, L., Li, Y., et al. (2017). Aging-related Atg5 defect impairs neutrophil extracellular traps formation. *Immunology* 151, 417–432. doi: 10.1111/imm.12740

Yang, J., Hooper, W. C., Phillips, D. J., and Talkington, D. F. (2002). Regulation of proinflammatory cytokines in human lung epithelial cells infected with *Mycoplasma pneumoniae. Infect. Immun.* 70, 3649–3655. doi: 10.1128/IAI.70.7.3649-3655.2002

Yeh, J. J., Wang, Y. C., Hsu, W. H., and Kao, C. H. (2016). Incident asthma and *Mycoplasma pneumoniae*: a nationwide cohort study. *J. Allergy Clin. Immunol.* 137:1017-1023.e6. doi: 10.1016/j.jaci.2015.09.032

Zhao, H., Bao, F. F., and Liu, A. (2017). Safety, immunogenicity, and efficacy of *Borrelia burgdorferi* outer surface protein a (OspA) vaccine: a meta-analysis. *J. Infect. Dev. Ctries* 11, 1–9. doi: 10.3855/jidc.7999

16

HHV-6A Infection of Endometrial Epithelial Cells Induces Increased Endometrial NK Cell-Mediated Cytotoxicity

*Elisabetta Caselli[1], Daria Bortolotti[1], Roberto Marci[2], Antonella Rotola[1], Valentina Gentili[1], Irene Soffritti[1], Maria D'Accolti[1], Giuseppe Lo Monte[3], Mariangela Sicolo[1], Isabel Barao[4], Dario Di Luca[1] and Roberta Rizzo[1]**

[1] Section of Microbiology and Medical Genetics, Department of Medical Sciences, University of Ferrara, Ferrara, Italy, [2] School of Medicine, University of Geneva, Geneva, Switzerland, [3] Human Reproduction Centre – Brunico Hospital, Brunico, Italy, [4] School of Medicine, University of Nevada, Reno, NV, United States

***Correspondence:**
Roberta Rizzo
rbr@unife.it

Background: We have recently reported the presence of Human herpesvirus-6A (HHV-6A) DNA in the 43% of endometrial epithelial cells from primary idiopathic infertile women, with no positivity in fertile women. To investigate the possible effect of HHV-6A infection in endometrial (e)NK cells functions, we examined activating/inhibitory receptors expressed by eNK cells and the corresponding ligands on endometrial cells during HHV-6A infection.

Methods: Endometrial biopsies and uterine flushing samples during the secretory phase were obtained from 20 idiopathic infertile women and twenty fertile women. HHV-6A infection of endometrial epithelial cells was analyzed by Real-Time PCR, immunofluorescence and flow cytometry. eNKs receptors and endometrial ligands expression were evaluated by immunofluorescence and flow cytometry.

Results: We observed the presence of HHV-6A infection (DNA, protein) of endometrial epithelial cells in the 40% of idiopathic infertile women. The eNK from all the subgroups expressed high levels of NKG2D and NKG2A receptors. Functional studies showed that NKG2D activating receptor and FasL are involved in the acquired cytotoxic function of eNK cells during HHV-6A infection of endometrial epithelial cells. In the presence of HHV-6A infection, eNK cells increased expression of CCR2, CXCR3 and CX3CR1 chemokine receptors ($p = 0.01$) and endometrial epithelial cells up-modulated the corresponding ligands: MCP1 (Monocyte chemotactic protein 1, CCL2), IP-10 (Interferon gamma-induced protein 10, CXCL10) and Eotaxin-3 (CCL26).

Conclusion: Our results, for the first time, showed the implication of eNK cells in controlling HHV-6A endometrial infection and clarify the mechanisms that might be implicated in female idiopathic infertility.

Keywords: endometrium, HHV-6, NK cell, infertility, epithelial cell

INTRODUCTION

Human herpesvirus 6 (HHV-6) is a ubiquitous pathogen of the *Betaherpesvirinae* subfamily, which primarily infects $CD4^+$ T cells (Takahashi et al., 1989). Similarly to other herpesviruses, HHV-6 remains in latency into the host, after an initial productive infection (Sandhoff et al., 1991). HHV-6 is a set of two related viruses known as HHV-6A and HHV-6B (Ablashi et al., 2014). Even if these two viruses present a similar genetical sequence, they differ for biological and pathogenic characteristics. HHV-6B causes exanthema subitum in young children (Yamanishi et al., 1988). HHV-6A seems to be involved in other pathologies, such as multiple sclerosis (Soldan et al., 1997) and encephalitis (McCullers et al., 1995). Moreover, we have recently shown the presence of HHV-6A, but not HHV-6B infection in endometrial epithelial cells of a subgroup of idiopathic infertile women (Marci et al., 2016). HHV-6 infection is implicated in immune-suppressive effects: (i) direct infection and induction of apoptosis of CD4+ T lymphocytes (Lusso et al., 1988; Grivel et al., 2003); (ii) lysis of cytotoxic leukocytes (CD8+ T cells, NK cells) (Lusso et al., 1991; Lusso and Gallo, 1995); (iii) block of dendritic cells and macrophages maturation (Kakimoto et al., 2002; Smith et al., 2005); (iv) inability of macrophages and dendritic cells to produce IL-12p70 after interferon gamma induction (Flamand et al., 1995; Smith et al., 2003, 2005); (v) dysregulation of cytokine networks, with increased secretion of IL-10, RANTES, TNF-alpha and IL-1beta (Flamand et al., 1991); (vi) decreased expression of CD14, CD64 and HLA-DR on the surface of monocytes as a mechanism of immune evasion (Janelle and Flamand, 2006).

Natural killer (NK) cells, positive for the surface marker CD56, are the dominant immune cell type at the uterine mucosa during placentation (Siewiera et al., 2013). They accumulate during implantation, where they support invading placental trophoblast cells and the creation of new vessels, essential for blood supply to the fetus.

The human endometrium contains a substantial population of NK cells (eNK cells) which vary in number and in proportion to the total number of endometrial stromal cells during the menstrual cycle. Although present in proliferative endometrium, eNK cells increase in number substantially in the mid-secretory phase and are the major endometrial lymphocyte population in the late secretory phase and the first trimester of pregnancy. eNK cells are CD56bright CD16+ and also express CD9, which is not expressed by peripheral blood NK cells. In contrast to peripheral blood CD56bright CD16– NK cells, eNK cells have abundant cytoplasmic granules containing perforin and granzyme (Bulmer et al., 1991). There is no consensus about the origin of eNK cells. Mature peripheral blood NK cells or immature precursors may migrate into the endometrium from the blood possibly in response to chemokines produced by cells within the endometrium at specific stages of the menstrual cycle and pregnancy, and be modified by other factors within the endometrium. For example, production of CXCL-12 by extravillous trophoblast (EVT) cells may attract NK cells into the decidua in pregnancy (Wu et al., 2005); interleukin (IL)-15, produced by secretory endometrium and decidua, has a selective chemoattractant effect on peripheral blood CD16– NK cells (Kitaya et al., 2007); and transforming growth factor beta 1 (TGF-1) has been suggested as modifying peripheral blood NK cells to eNK cells (Keskin et al., 2007). An alternative suggestion is that eNK cells are derived from haematopoietic precursor cells within the endometrium (Lynch et al., 2007).

The presence of eNK cells in close proximity to the invading extravillous trophoblast cells suggests that they may play a role in this process. eNK cells produce many different cytokines and growth factors (for example, IL-1, IL-2, IL-4, IL-6, IL-8, IL-10, tumor necrosis factor alpha, granulocyte-macrophage colony stimulating factor, TGF-1, leukemia inhibitory factor and interferon gamma) (Jokhi et al., 1997). eNK cells are also an important source of angiogenic growth factors. Production of angiogenin, angiopoietin (Ang)-1, Ang-2, vascular endothelial growth factor (VEGF)-A, VEGF-C, placental growth factor, keratinocyte growth factor, fibroblast growth factor and platelet-derived growth factor-BB by eNK cells from secretory phase endometrium and early pregnancy decidua has been reported (Li et al., 2001; Lash et al., 2006). eNK cells secrete also matrix metalloproteinases (MMP)-1, MMP-2, MMP-7, MMP-9, MMP-10, tissue inhibitor of metalloproteinases (TIMP)-1, TIMP-2, TIMP-3, urokinase plasminogen activator (uPA) and uPA receptor (Naruse et al., 2009a,b).

The observation of modified percentages of eNK cells in the endometrium of women with reproductive failure (such as infertility, RM and pre-eclampsia) has suggested they may play a role in the pathogenesis. Several studies have shown increased levels of eNK cells in the pre-pregnancy endometrium of women with recurrent miscarriage (Clifford et al., 1999; Tuckerman et al., 2007). There are studies showing an increased number of eNK cells in decidual tissue (Stallmach et al., 1999; Bachmayer et al., 2006) and others showing a reduction in decidual eNK cell numbers in women with pre-eclampsia (Eide et al., 2006; Williams et al., 2009). The presence of a unique type of NK cells in the endometrium is intriguing and the possibility that a microbial infection might affect their functions should be taken into account.

In this article, we provide the first evidence that eNK cells functions are affected by HHV-6A infection of the endometrial epithelial cells and this modification might influence pregnancy outcome.

MATERIALS AND METHODS

Clinical Samples

Endometrial speciments were obtained from patients admitted for tubal patency assessment by Hystero-sono contrast sonography at secretory stage of the menstrual cycle. We selected women with these characteristics: 21–38 years old, regular menstrual cycle (24–35 days), body mass index (BMI) ranging between 18 and 26 Kg/m2, FSH (day 2–3 of the menstrual cycle) <10 mUI/mL, 17-β-Estradiol <50 pg/ml (day 2–3 of the menstrual cycle), normal karyotype. Women that presented endometritis, endometriosis, tubal factor, ovulatory dysfunction, anatomical uterine pathologies and recurrent miscarriage were excluded. Endometrial samples were maintained in HEPES-buffered Dulbecco modified Eagle medium/ Hams F-12 (DMEM/F-12; Invitrogen, Carlsbad, CA, United States) with 1% antibiotic- antimycotic solution (final concentrations: 100 μg/ml penicillin G sodium, 100 μg/ml streptomycin sulfate, 0.25 μg/ml amphotericin B; Invitrogen), and 5% newborn calf serum (NCS; CSL Ltd., Parkville, VIC, Australia), stored at 4°C, and processed within 2 h. Uterine flushing was performed with a 14-gauge Foley three-way balloon catheter (Eschmann) inflating an appropriate (5 mL) amount of sterile physiologic saline solution.

Ethics Statement

This study was approved by the "Ferrara Ethics Committee" and we collected written informed consent from all subjects. All subjects gave written informed consent in accordance with the Declaration of Helsinki.

Preparation of Endometrial Epithelial and Stromal Cells

The endometrium was prepared as previously described (Marci et al., 2016). Cell dissociation was performed in Ca2+ and Mg2+ free phosphate buffered saline (PBS, pH 7.4) additionated with 300 μg/ml collagenase type III (Worthington Biochemical Corporation, Freehold, NJ, United States) and 40 μg/ml deoxyribonuclease type I (Roche Diagnostics, Mannheim, Germany) in a shaking incubator (Bioline 4700; Edwards Instrument Company, Narellan, NSW, Australia) rotating at 150 rpm at 37°C. Every 15 min, the digested tissues were omogenized vigorously and dissociation was checked microscopically. After 45 min, the digests were filtered using a 40-μm sieve (Becton Dickinson Labware, Franklin Lakes, NJ, United States) to obtain a single cells suspension without debris. The digestion process was stopped by the addition of HEPES-buffered DMEM/F-12 containing 5%FCS. We isolated the different endometrial cellular components (mononuclear, stromal and epithelial cells) by centrifugation for 8–10 min at 390 × *g* on Ficoll-Paque (Pharmacia Biotechnology, Uppsala, Sweden). Endometrial cells were collected from the Ficoll-Paque-medium interface using BerEP4-coated magnetic Dynabeads (Dynal Biotech, Oslo, Norway) positive selection system. The sorted epithelial cells were recovered using a magnetic particle collector (Dynal Biotech) and washed in HEPES-buffered DMEM/F-12/1%FCS. The collected cells were finally seeded on culture plates coated with basement membrane extract (BME) (Matrigel®, Collaborative Biomedical Products, Bedford, MA, United States). The fraction containing mononuclear and stromal cells were collected and seeded on 100 mm plastic tissue culture dishes. After 12 h, the supernatant cells were collected from the culture, to recover non-adherent mononuclear cells. Purity of epithelial and stromal components was morphologically evaluated by light microscopy and assessed by cytokeratin-18 (CK18) and vimentin staining for epithelial and stromal cells respectively. Mononuclear cells were $CD45^{pos}$ stained. The purity reached for each cell population was routinely over 98%.

DNA Analysis

DNA extraction and analysis were performed as previously described (Caselli et al., 2012). PCR and real time quantitative (qPCR) specific for the U94 gene were used to determine HHV-6 DNA presence and load. Samples in which 1 μg of cell DNA harbored more than 100 copies of viral DNA, were considered positive. Human RNase P or beta-actin house-keeping genes were used as a control. All clinical samples were randomly and blindly investigated. Furthermore, when enough material to repeat the analysis was present, the analysis was repeated again in a randomized and blinded fashion at a distant time from the first analyses. HHV-6A or B identification was performed as reported previously (Caselli et al., 2012), by restriction enzyme digestion of the U31 nested PCR amplification product and visualization of the digestion products on ethidium bromide stained agarose gel after electrophoresis migration.

RNA Analysis

RNA cell extraction was performed using the RNeasy kit (Qiagen, Hilden, Germany). Extracted RNA did not contain contaminant DNA, as assured by DNase treatment and control β-actin PCR without retrotranscription reverse transcription (Caselli et al., 2012). RNA reverse transcription was performed by the RT2 First strand kit (Qiagen, Hilden, Germany) for analysis of virus transcripts. cDNA aliquots corresponding to 200 ng RNA were used for virus transcription analysis, performed by qPCR detecting the expression of U94 gene, as previously reported (Caselli et al., 2012).

Immunofluorescence Assay for HHV-6 Detection

HHV-6 antigen expression was analyzed by immunofluorescence with a mouse monoclonal antibodies (mAb) that recognized the glycoprotein gp116 (late antigen) of HHV-6 A and B (ABI, Columbia, MD, United States), as previously described (Marci et al., 2016). Epithelial and stromal cells were respectively stained with mouse anti-Cytokeratin-18, a heterotetramer cytoskeleton protein (CK18-FITC) and rabbit anti-vimentin-PE moAbs (Abcam, Cambridge, United Kingdom), respectively. eNK cells were stained for CD56-PE (BD, Milan, Italy). Epithelial cells were stained for IP-10-FITC (Interferon gamma-induced protein 10/CXCL10), Eotaxin-3-PE (CCL26) and MCP-1-PE (Monocyte chemo-attractant protein 1/CCL2) (eBiosciences, Waltham, MA, United States).

NK Cell Purification

Endometrial NK cells were separated from endometrial leukocyte samples using the negative magnetic cell separation (MACS) system (Miltenyi Biotech, Gladbach, Germany) (Marci et al., 2016). The analysis of purified cell fraction by flow cytometry with CD3-PerCp-Cy5.5, CD56-FITC moAbs (e-Bioscience, Frankfurt, DE), demonstrated that the NK cell content was >90% (data not shown). Freshly purified NK cells were cultured for 24 h in presence of suboptimal doses of IL-12 (1 ng/ml).

HHV-6A Cell Infection

Primary endometrial cells and KLE endometrial epithelial cell line (ATCC CRL1622) were cultivated in DMEM F12 medium (ATCC 30-2006) in presence of L-glutamine, 1% penicillin-streptomycine and 10% of FCS at 37°C with the 5% of CO2. The cells were inoculated with HHV-6A (strain U1102) cell-free virus inocula (Marci et al., 2016) and infected with 100 genome equivalents per 1 cell. HHV-6A UV-inactivated viral preparations were used as controls. Infected cells were co-cultured with eNK cells to perform cytotoxicity experiments.

Cytotoxicity Assays

Target cells (1×10^6 cells) were labeled with 7-AAD/CFSE Cell-Mediated Cytotoxicity Assay Kit (Cayman Chemicals, Ann Arbor, MI, United States), that employs CFSE to label target cells within the mixed cell population and 7-AAD to label dead cells. We added eNK effector cells to labeled target cells at various effector:target ratios in replicate in 200 ml DMEM/F12 containing 5% FCS. Microtiter plates were centrifuged at 1200 rpm for 5 min and incubated at 37°C. After 4 or 18 h of culture, the cells were analyzed by flow cytometry.

To block activating receptor engagement or FASL/FAS pathway, CFSE labeled target cells were incubated with soluble NKG2D-Fc IgG1 chimeric protein (0.2 mg/ml) (R&D Systems, Italy) and/or anti-FASL mAb (10 mg/ml; R&D Systems, Italy) or an isotype match control (1.0 mg/ml; mouse IgG1) for 20 min on ice then co-cultured with eNK effector cells. eNK cell cytotoxicity against K562 (ATCC CCL243), classical target cell, was used as control.

ELISA sFASL, sTRAIL, MCP1, IP10, Eotaxin3

Levels of sTRAIL, sFasL, MCP1, IP10 and Eotaxin3 were assessed in duplicates in cell culture supernatants and uterine flushing samples using commercial enzyme-linked immunosorbent assays (ELISAs) (TRAIL, MCP1, IP10, Eotaxin3: R&D Systems, Amersham, United Kingdom; sFasL: Sigma–Aldrich, St. Louis, MO, United States).

Flow Cytometry

Leukocytes were defined as CD45pos, and the different cell subtypes were defined as CD3pos (T cells), CD19pos (B cells) CD14pos (monocytes) and Cd56pos (NK cells). Cell viability was assessed by propidium iodide staining. Anti-isotype controls (Exbio, Praha, CZ) were performed.

1×10^5 eNK cells were labeled with fluorophore-conjugated antibodies: CD3-PE-Cy7, CD16-PE, CD56-APC, NKG2D-PE, NKG2C-PE, NKG2A-PE, NKp30-PE, NKp44-PE, NKp46-PE, KIR2DL2/3-PE, KIR2DL1-PE (BD, Italy), KIR2DL4-PE (R&D Systems, Italy); CXCR1, CXCR2, CXCR3, CX3CR1, CXCR4, CCR1, CCR2, CCR3, CCR5, and CCR7 (R&D Systems, Italy). eNK cells were gated as CD56pos CD3neg. eNK cells activation status was determined by CD107a staining (R&D Systems, Italy), as previously reported (Rizzo et al., 2016).

5×10^5 epithelial cells were stained specific Ab HLA-I (HLA-A,-B,-C)-PE (BD Biosciences, Italy), HLA-E (clone MEM-E/08, Exbio, Praha, CZ) or HLA-DR (BD Biosciences, Italy) and matched isotype controls.

The NKG2D-ligands were detected on epithelial cells by binding of NKG2D-Fc chimera (R&D Systems, Italy) and indirect labeling with the secondary Ab FITC-coupled mouse anti-human IgG1 (Abcam, Cambridge, United Kingdom).

Data were analyzed using FACS CantoII flow cytometer (BD, Milan, Italy) and FlowJo LLC analysis software (Ashland, OR, United States). Ten thousand events were acquired.

Statistical Analysis

Data were analyzed by Student's *t*-test and Fisher exact test [Stat View software (SAS Institute Inc.)]. Statistical significance was assumed for $p < 0.05$ (two tailed).

RESULTS

HHV-6 in Clinical Specimens

We enrolled 20 idiopathic infertile women and 20 fertile women with at least one previous successful pregnancy. As reported in **Table 1**, the two cohorts presented no significant differences.

The endometrial biopsies were analyzed for the presence of HHV-6 infection. As reported in **Table 2**, we found HHV-6B DNA in the peripheral blood mononuclear cells of the 24 and 26% of idiopathic infertile women and control women, respectively ($p = 0.86$; Fisher exact test). These results confirmed the previously reported frequency of the HHV-6B virus in a 25–30% of peripheral blood samples (Caselli and Di Luca, 2007). On the contrary, HHV-6A DNA was not revealed in the peripheral blood of all the subjects. Forty percent (8/20) women with idiopathic infertility were positive for HHV-6 DNA in their endometrial epithelial cells, while fertile women did not present HHV-6A viral DNA in their endometrial epithelial cells ($p = 4.5 \times 10^{-6}$; Fisher exact test). HHV-6B DNA was not

TABLE 1 | Women cohorts: demographical and clinical parameters.

Parameters (median; mean ± SD)	Infertile (20)	Fertile (20)	*p*-value*
Age (years)	34.4 (32.2 ± 2.2)	33.6 (31.5 ± 2.9)	0.95
Duration of infertility (years)	3.2 (3.7 ± 1.9)	–	–
Length of menstrual cycle (days)	3.9 (3.8 ± 1.9)	4.1 (3.7 ± 2.5)	0.54
FSH (mUI/mL) (day 3)	7.9 (8.2 ± 1.7)	7.6 (7.4 ± 2.9)	0.53
LH (mUI/mL) (day 3)	6.8 (6.6 ± 2.5)	7.0 (6.8 ± 2.4)	0.51
Estradiol (pg/mL) (day 3)	71.6 (72.1 ± 63.5)	66.4 (58.2 ± 49.2)	0.052
TSH (uUI/mL)	3.1 (2.8 ± 1.5)	2.8 (2.6 ± 1.4)	0.48
FT4 (pg/mL)	2.4 (2.3 ± 1.2)	2.5 (2.4 ± 1.4)	0.91
Progesterone (pg/mL) (day 21)	15.9 (14.7 ± 6.2)	14.6 (13.9 ± 6.4)	0.72
Smoke habits (%)**	10	9.6	0.92
Day (mestrual cycle) of sample collection	14.1 (13.8 ± 2.6)	14.0 (13.2 ± 2.8)	0.98

*Student's t-test. **Fisher exact test.*

TABLE 2 | HHV-6 DNA results in peripheral blood mononuclear cells (PBMC) and endometrial biopsies.

Samples (*N*)	Infertile (20)	Fertile (20)	*p*-value*
HHV6-A			
Endometrial epithelium	8	0	0,003
Endometrial stroma	0	0	NA
Endometrial leukocytes (CD45pos)	0	0	NA
PBMC	0	0	NA
HHV-6B			
Endometrial epithelium	0	0	NA
Endometrial stroma	0	0	NA
Endometrial leukocytes (CD45pos)	0	0	NA
PBMC	5	6	0,86

**Fisher exact test.*

present in all the endometrial biopsies, as previously reported (Marci et al., 2016).

The average viral load in endometrial epithelial cells (vimentin^{neg} CK18^{pos}; Supplementary Figure S1A) from HHV6-A positive infertile women was 500.000 copies/ug of cellular DNA (range 700.000–240.000 copies/μg DNA), corresponding to about 4 copies of viral DNA per diploid cell (**Figure 1A**). Endometrial epithelial cells were HHV-6A positive as shown by staining for gp116 late viral antigen (**Figure 1B**). Stromal cells (Vimentin^{pos} CK18^{neg}; Supplementary Figure S1B) and leukocytes (CD45^{pos}; Supplementary Figure S1C) were negative for HHV-6 DNA (**Table 2**), confirming a localized HHV-6A infection into endometrial epithelium, as previously reported (Marci et al., 2016).

Endometrial Epithelial Cells Are Permissive to HHV-6A Infection

Primary endometrial epithelial cells, purified from endometrial biopsies from fertile women negative for HHV-6A infection (Vimentin^{neg} and CK18^{pos}, Supplementary Figure S1), and the KLE endometrial epithelial cell line were infected with HHV-6A cell-free inoculum with 100 genome equivalents per cell. Mock infection with UV-inactivated virus was used as control. We evaluated viral replication 1, 3, 7, and 14 days post-infection (d.p.i.) by analyzing virus DNA, transcription and antigen expression. As shown in **Figure 2A**, HHV-6A DNA was present at all times p.i. Virus load, as evaluated by real-time quantitative PCR in primary endometrial epithelial cells and KLE cell line, respectively, corresponded to 7.0×10^4 and 8.1×10^4 genome copies per μg of total cellular DNA at 1 d.p.i., 5.4×10^4 and 6.2×10^4 at 3 d.p.i. and 3.2×10^4 and 4.5×10^4 at 14 d.p.i., when the experiment was discontinued. Virus U94 mRNA, an immediate early gene, was analyzed to establish viral transcription (Pantry and Medveczky, 2017). We observed the persistence of U94 mRNA in all time points (**Figure 2B**). The late HHV-6 gp116 antigen expression confirmed that both primary and KLE endometrial epithelial cells were permissive to HHV-6A replication. gp116 virus antigen expression, indicative of productive infection, peaked at 7 d.p.i., (**Figure 2C**). Control mock-infected endometrial epithelial cells gave no staining (**Figure 2D**).

We previously showed that HHV-6A positive women have an increased cytolytic function of eNK cells toward HHV-6A infected cells (Marci et al., 2016), suggesting an implication of viral infections in the modulation of eNK cell functions. Therefore, to test the ability of eNK cells in controlling HHV-6A infection, we analyzed their cytotoxicity against HHV-6A-infected endometrial epithelial cells, by 7-AAD/CFSE Cell-Mediated Cytotoxicity Assay Kit.

The co-culture of eNK cells with HHV-6A infected endometrial for 4 h did not result in an efficient killing (**Figure 3B**). However, after 18 h of co-culture, eNK cells killed HHV-6A infected endometrial epithelial cells (**Figure 3D**). With eNK cells from HHV-6A positive women at the effector:target ratio of 50 we observed up to 75% of killing, while only 40% of killing was obtained with eNK cells from HHV-6A negative women ($p < 0.001$; Student's t-test). The absence of killing of uninfected endometrial epithelial cells, supports the specificity of the eNK cytotoxic function against HHV-6A infection (**Figures 3A,C**). Taken together, these results suggest that in the presence of HHV-6A infection eNK cells from HHV-6A positive women become more cytotoxic against infected endometrial epithelial cells. To exclude the presence of external factors that could modify the eNK cell cytotoxicity in HHV-6A positive women, we tested the killing of K562 cells, a classical NK cell targets. In agreement with previous studies (Kopcow et al., 2005), we observed a low cytotoxicity of eNK cells in the presence

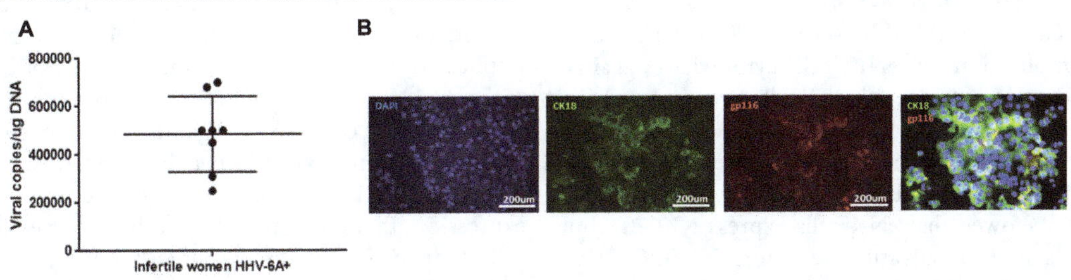

FIGURE 1 | HHV-6A infection of endometrial epithelial cells. **(A)** HHV-6 DNA was searched by real time qPCR specific for U94 gene in endometrial biopsies. Results are expressed in viral copies/ug DNA and represent the mean copy number ± SD referred to duplicates of 2 independent assays. Infertile women: primary idiopathic infertile women; **(B)** Endometrial epithelial cells were characterized by immunofluorescence for cytokeratin18 (CK18, epithelial marker) and gp116 (late viral protein) expression. Images were taken in fluorescence (Nikon Eclipse TE2000S) equipped with a digital camera. Original magnification 20×.

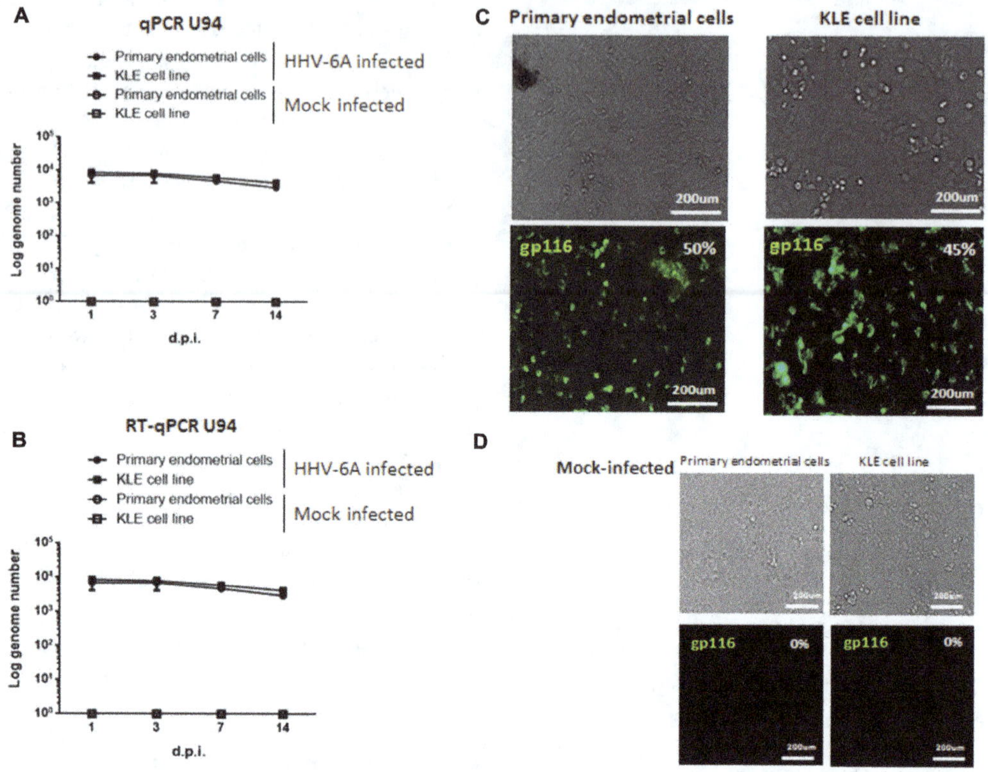

FIGURE 2 | Primary endometrial epithelial cells and KLE cell line (ATCC CRL-1622) were infected with HHV-6A or UV-inactivated (Mock-infected) HHV-6A. The infection was evaluated after 1, 3, 7, and 14 days post infection (d.p.i.). **(A)** DNA and **(B)** RNA expression of viral U94 antigen were evaluated by Real time PCR. Results represent the mean copy number ± SD referred to duplicates of 4 independent assays. **(C,D)** Endometrial epithelial cells were stained for gp116 late viral antigen 7 d.p.i. with HHV-6A **(C)** or mock **(D)**. Images were taken in bright field (*upper panels*) or fluorescence (*lower panels*) (Nikon Eclipse TE2000S) equipped with a digital camera. Original magnification 20×.

of K562 cells in both HHV-6A positive and negative women settings (Supplementary Figures S2A,B). These results suggest a peculiar modification of eNK cells in the presence of HHV-6A-infection, that seems to induce the loss of their tolerance toward endometrial epithelial cells. This condition is enhanced in HHV-6A positive women.

NKG2D Receptor Modulates eNK Cell Responsiveness to HHV-6A-Infected Endometrial Epithelial Cells

NK cells cytotoxicity is controlled by several NKRs. To evaluate their possible implication in eNK cell cytotoxicity against HHV-6A-infected endometrial epithelial cells, we analyzed the expression of activating/inhibitory receptors in eNK cells.

eNK cells, gated as $CD3^{neg}$ and $CD56^{pos}$, were purified from endometrial biopsies from fertile and infertile women. Flow cytometry analysis showed that eNK cells express NKG2D, but express low levels of the activating receptors NKG2C/CD94 and CD16 (**Figure 4A**). Even though the activating receptors NKp44, and NKp30 are expressed in all eNK cells (**Figure 4A**), there is a decreased expression in infertile women positive for HHV-6A infection (**Figures 4A,B**) ($p < 0.001$; Student's t-test). This difference in expression pattern makes eNK cells from infertile women positive for HHV-6A infection quite different from eNK cells commonly present in endometrial tissues (ref J Immunol, **Figure 4**), and from decidual NK cells, which express relatively high levels of NKp30, NKp44, and NKG2D (Hanna et al., 2006).

Expression of inhibitory receptors showed that all eNK cells express high levels of NKG2A/CD94 receptor and low expression of KIRs (Killer immunoglobulin like receptors) (**Figures 4C,D**).

These results demonstrate a possible role of HHV-6A infection in changing in eNK cell receptor repertoire, decreasing NKp30 and NKp44 and maintaining NKG2D and NKG2A expression.

The expression of inhibitory and activating receptors is implicated in the immunoregulation of eNK cells functions to control the uterine environment and embryo implantation. A modification of receptors ligands caused by HHV-6A infection could undermine eNK cells peculiar functions.

We analyzed activation status of eNK cells, measuring CD107a expression, that correlates with both cytokine secretion and NK cell-mediated lysis of target cells (Alter et al., 2004). We observed a slight but not significant increase in the percentage of eNK positive for CD107a expression in HHV-6A positive infertile women ($p = 0.08$; Student's t-test) (**Figure 4E**).

These results suggest that contact of eNK cells with HHV-6A infected cells is detrimental to recognize differences in eNK

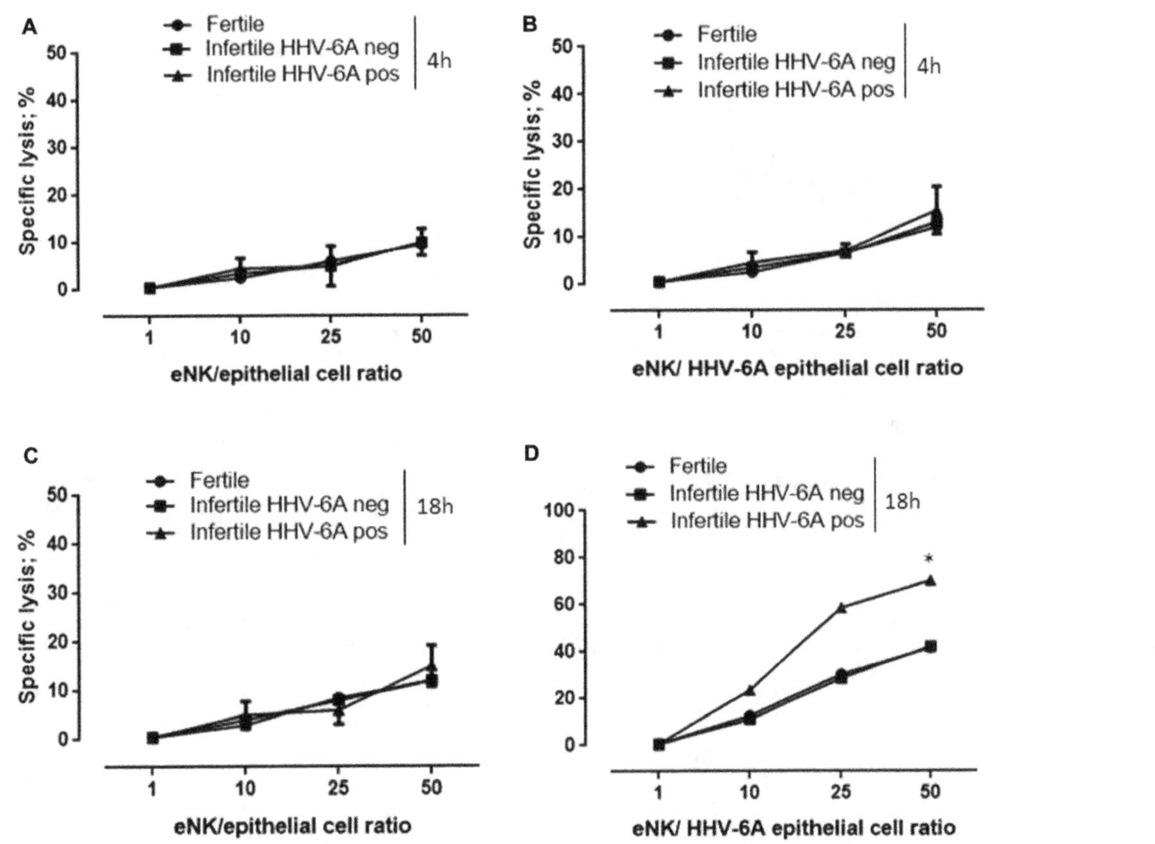

FIGURE 3 | eNK cells are cytotoxic against HHV-6A-infected endometrial epithelial cells. Endometrial epithelial cells were kept **(A,C)** uninfected or **(B,D)** infected for-48 h with HHV-6A. eNK cell cytotoxicity was determined by 7-AAD/CFSE Cell-Mediated Cytotoxicity Assay Kit after **(A,B)** 4 or **(C,D)** 18 h of contact at different E/T ratios. Each data point is calculated as the mean lysis ± SD from at least five independent experiments done in replicate tissue culture wells. *Significant *p*-value; Student's *t*-test.

cells status. For this, we selected to analyze the effect of HHV-6A infection on ligands for the two NK receptors that maintained a high expression in eNK cells: NKG2D and NKG2A.

Because the identities of the cellular ligands of the activating receptor NKG2D is largely unknown, we stained the endometrial epithelial cells with Ig fusion proteins composed of the extracellular portions of NKG2D fused to human IgG1. NKG2D ligands were down-modulated following infection (**Figures 5A,B**). These results suggest the implication of NKG2D activating receptor in the cytotoxic function of eNK cells toward HHV-6A infected endometrial epithelial cells.

We then analyzed the effect of HHV-6A infection and the expression level of HLA-E molecule, the ligand of inhibitory receptor NKG2A. As shown in **Figures 5A,B**, we observed the expression of both the non-classical HLA-E and the classical HLA-A,-B,-C molecules at the surface of endometrial epithelial cells. The infection with HHV-6A reduced HLA-E expression, while no effect was observed for classical HLA-A, -B, -C. This downregulation of HLA-E expression by HHV-6A excluded any effect of NKG2A inhibitory receptor in controlling eNK cell responsiveness to HHV-6A-infected endometrial epithelial cells. HLA-II antigens are not expressed by endometrial epithelial cells, while they are up-modulated during HHV-6A infection, similar to previously reported the effect on thyrocytes (Caselli et al., 2012) (**Figures 5A,B**).

To further confirm that the cytotoxic function of eNK cells is associated to the NKG2D activating receptor, we next investigated lytic capacities of eNK cells from HHV-6A positive women blocking specific receptor/ligand interactions with a Fc-chimeric protein. The addition of NKG2D Fc-chimeric protein decreased eNK cell cytotoxicity resulting in a 20% lysis of infected cells compared to a 60% lysis of HHV-6A-infected cells, that we observed without the block of receptor/ligand interactions (**Figure 5C**) ($p < 0.001$, Student's *t*-test). The reduced eNK cytotoxicity in NKG2D ligation blocking experiments sustains a role for NKG2D receptor in eNK cell cytotoxicity.

When we looked at NKG2D and NKG2A ligands expression by endometrial cells from infertile HHV-6A positive and negative women and fertile women, we observed a slight reduction of HLA-E and a significant decrease in NKG2D ligands expression in HHV-6A positive infertile women (**Figure 5D**) ($p < 0.001$, Student's *t*-test).

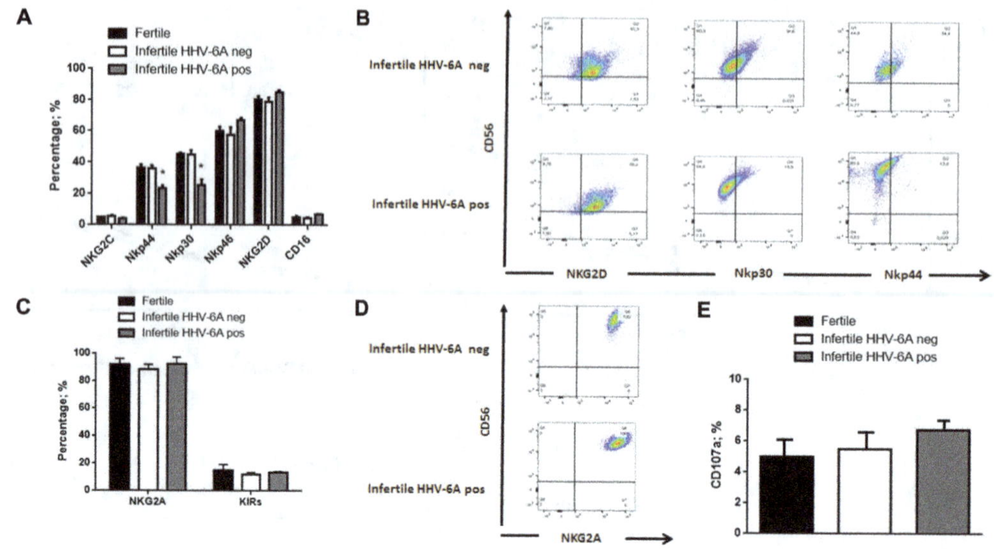

FIGURE 4 | eNK cell receptor repertoire expression. eNK cells purified from endometrial biopsies were stained for surface expression of the indicated **(A)** activating and **(C)** inhibitory receptors and **(E)** CD107a activation marker using fluorochrome-conjugated antibodies and analyzed by flow cytometry. **(B,D)** Representative FACS dot plots gated on CD56pos CD3neg dNK cells are reported. One representative dot plot out of five independent experiments is shown. *Significant *p*-value obtained by Student's *t*-test.

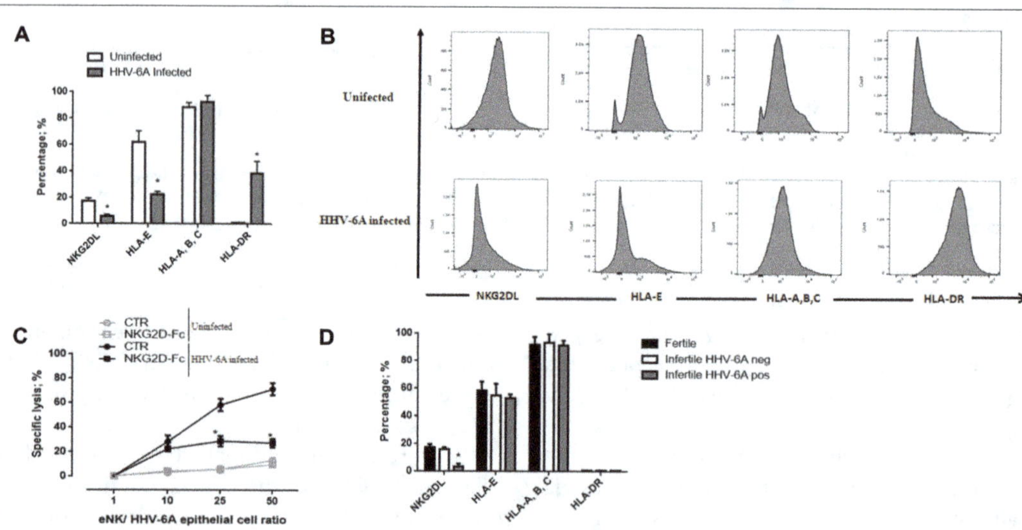

FIGURE 5 | Functional analysis dNK cells specific receptors. **(A,B)** HHV-6A-infection modulates the expression of NKR ligands on endometrial epithelial cells. The binding of human NKG2D-Fc chimera was used to evaluate the cell surface expression of specific receptor ligands. The expression of HLA-E and HLA-A, -B, -C and HLA-DR molecules was evaluated using specific mAb. **(C)** Endometrial epithelial cells uninfected (gray lines) or infected (black lines) were incubated with soluble NKG2D-Fc fusion protein at the concentration of 1 mg/ml and eNK cell cytotoxicity was analyzed by 7-AAD/CFSE Cell- Mediated Cytotoxicity Assay Kit after 18 h of co-culture. **(D)** The expression of NKG2D ligands, NKG2A ligands (HLA-E and HLA-A, -B, -C) and HLA-DR expression on the surface of endometrial epithelial cells from fertile women and HHV-6A positive and negative infertile women. Data sets represent mean lysis ± SD from five independent experiments done in replicate. *Significant *p*-value; Student's *t*-test.

Cytotoxicity of eNK Cells Is Dependent of FasL Killing Pathway

NK cells cytotoxicity is mediated by soluble mediators or by induction of death receptor-ligand pathways such as TRAIL (tumor necrosis factor-related apoptosis-inducing ligand) and Fas ligand (FasL). To evaluate the mechanisms involved in eNK cell killing of HHV-6A-infected endometrial epithelial cells, we analyzed these death receptor-ligand pathways. After 18 h of co-culture, FasL ($p < 0.001$; Student's *t*-test), and not TRAIL, was up-modulated on the surface of eNK cells (**Figures 6A,B**). The blockade of FasL with a neutralizing antibody to FasL reduced eNK cell cytotoxicity against HHV-6A-infected endometrial

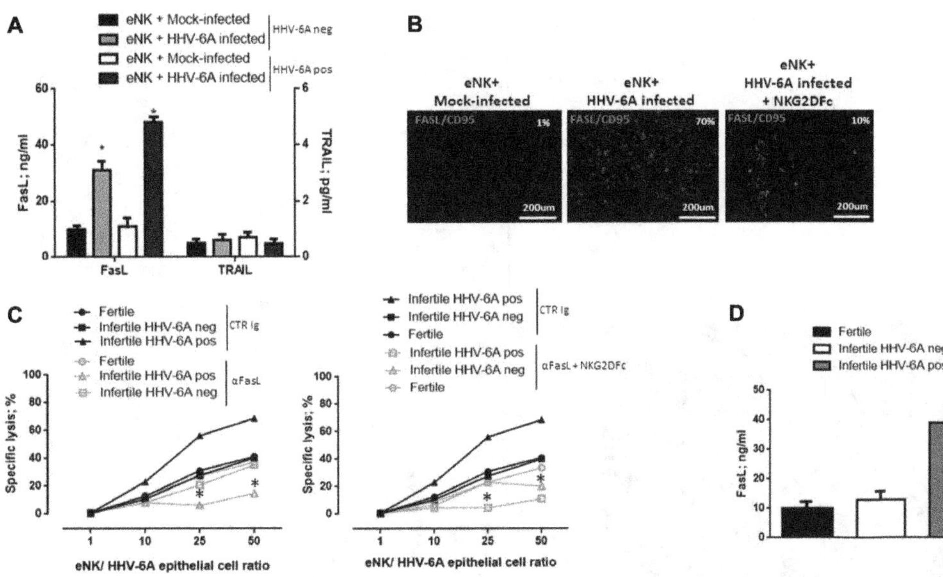

FIGURE 6 | eNK cell cytotoxicity via FasL-Fas pathway. **(A)** Expression of FasL and TRAIL in the culture supernatants of 18 h co-culture of HHV-6A infected endometrial epithelial cells with eNK cells from HHV-6A positive and HHV-6A negative infertile women. **(B)** Expression of FasL in eNK cells after 18 h co-culture with HHV-6A infected endometrial epithelial cells. Images were taken in fluorescence (Nikon Eclipse TE2000S) equipped with a digital camera. Original magnification 20×. **(C)** Functional analysis of FasL. Endometrial epithelial cells were infected for 48 h with HHV-6A. eNK cell cytotoxicity was determined by 7-AAD/CFSE Cell- Mediated Cytotoxicity Assay Kit after 18 h of contact at different E/T ratios, with the addition of a control Ig (CTR Ig; black lines) or of a specific anti FasL Ig (aFasL; gray lines) (left panel) or a specific anti FasL Ig and NKG2DFc (aFasL + NKG2DFc; gray lines). Each data point is calculated as the mean lysis ± SD from at least five independent experiments done in replicate tissue culture wells. **(D)** Expression of FasL in the uterine flushing samples from fertile women and HHV-6A positive and HHV-6A negative infertile women. *Significant *p*-value; Student's *t*-test.

epithelial cells, after 18 h of co-culture (**Figure 6C**). The blockade of NKG2D recognition of its ligands reduced the expression of FasL on eNK cells ($p < 0.03$; Student's *t*-test) and the co-blockade of FasL and NKG2D ligands abolished eNK cells killing of HHV-6A-infected endometrial epithelial cells ($p < 0.02$; Student's *t*-test). These data suggest that NKG2D ligands recognition and mechanisms dependent of the death receptor-ligand Fas/FasL pathway are at the basis of eNK cell killing of HHV-6A infected endometrial epithelial cells.

When we looked at FasL expression by endometrial cells from infertile HHV-6A positive and negative women and fertile women, we observed increased levels of FasL secretion in the uterine flushing samples of infertile HHV-6A positive women (**Figure 6D**) ($p < 0.001$, Student's *t*-test).

HHV-6A Infection Modulates the Repertoire of Chemokine Receptors and Their Ligands

The repertoire of ligand to chemokines receptors plays a critical role in eNK cells homing to infected cells. To evaluate the mechanisms implicated in eNK cell cytotoxicity against HHV-6A infected endometrial epithelial cells, we analyzed the expression of chemokine receptors and ligands on eNK cells in the presence or in the absence of HHV-6A infection.

Flow cytometry analysis showed that eNK cells express very low or undetectable levels of CXCR1, CXCR2, CXCR3, CXCR4, CCR1, CCR2, CCR3, CCR5, CCR7 and CX3CR1 (data not shown). We observed a slight increase CXCR3, CX3CR1 and CCR2 receptors in eNK cells from infertile women positive for HHV-6A infection (**Figures 7A,B**) ($p = 0.02$; $p = 0.012$; $p = 0.01$, respectively; Student's *t*-test).

Meanwhile, we observed an induction of MCP1, IP10 and eotaxin-3 expression on the surface of endometrial epithelial cells 7 d.p.i. (**Figure 7C**). These molecules are the ligands for CCR2, CXCR3 and CX3CR1, respectively, that are upmodulated on eNK cells from HHV-6A positive women (**Figures 7A,B**).

When we analyzed uterine flushing samples for the expression of MCP1, IP10 and eotaxin-3, we observed increased levels in HHV-6A positive infertile women in comparison to HHV-6A negative infertile women and fertile women, with IP10 reaching a significant difference ($p = 0.031$; Student's *t*-test) (**Figure 7D**).

Since eNK cells are in close contact with endometrial epithelial cells, we used an *in vitro* culture model of endometrial epithelial cells to test the ability of eNK cells to get in contact with HHV-6A infected endometrial epithelial cells. Endometrial epithelial cells were infected (72 h) or not and co-cultured with eNK cells from HHV-6A positive infertile women for 2 h. As shown in **Figure 8** eNK cells ($CD56^{pos}$) were able to establish contact with HHV-6A infected endometrial epithelial cells but not with uninfected cells. On the contrary, eNK cells from HHV-6A negative infertile and fertile women were not able to interact with HHV-6A infected endometrial epithelial cells.

Together these results evidence the ability of eNK cells to contact HHV-6A-infected endometrial cells, demonstrating the

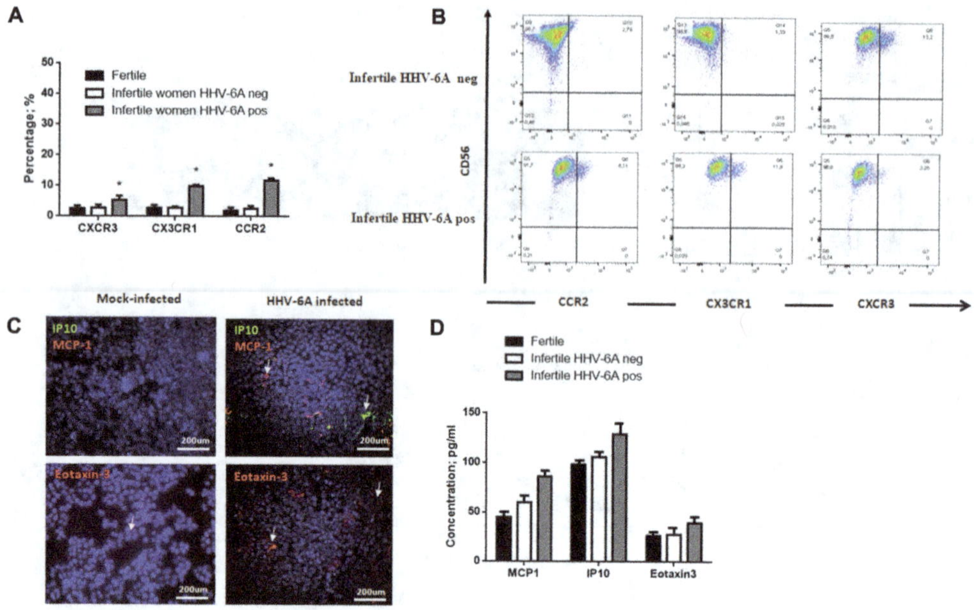

FIGURE 7 | eNK cell receptor repertoire expression. **(A)** eNK cells purified from endometrial biopsies were stained for surface expression of the indicated chemokine receptors using fluorochrome-conjugated antibodies and analyzed by flow cytometry. **(B)** Representative FACS dot plots gated on CD56pos CD3neg dNK cells are reported. One representative dot plot out of five independent experiments is shown. *Significant *p*-value obtained by Student's *t*-test. **(C)** Chemokine receptor ligand expression. MCP1 (Monocyte chemotactic protein 1, CCL2), IP-10 (Interferon gamma-induced protein 10, CXCL10) and Eotaxin-3 (CCL26) expression was evaluated in endometrial epithelial cells 7 d.p.i. White arrows indicate positive staining. Images were taken in fluorescence (Nikon Eclipse TE2000S) equipped with a digital camera. Original magnification 20×. **(D)** Chemokine receptor ligand expression. MCP1 (Monocyte chemotactic protein 1, CCL2), IP-10 (Interferon gamma-induced protein 10, CXCL10) and Eotaxin-3 (CCL26) expression was evaluated in uterine flushing samples from HHV-6A positive and negative infertile women and fertile women. *Significant *p*-value obtained by Student's *t*-test.

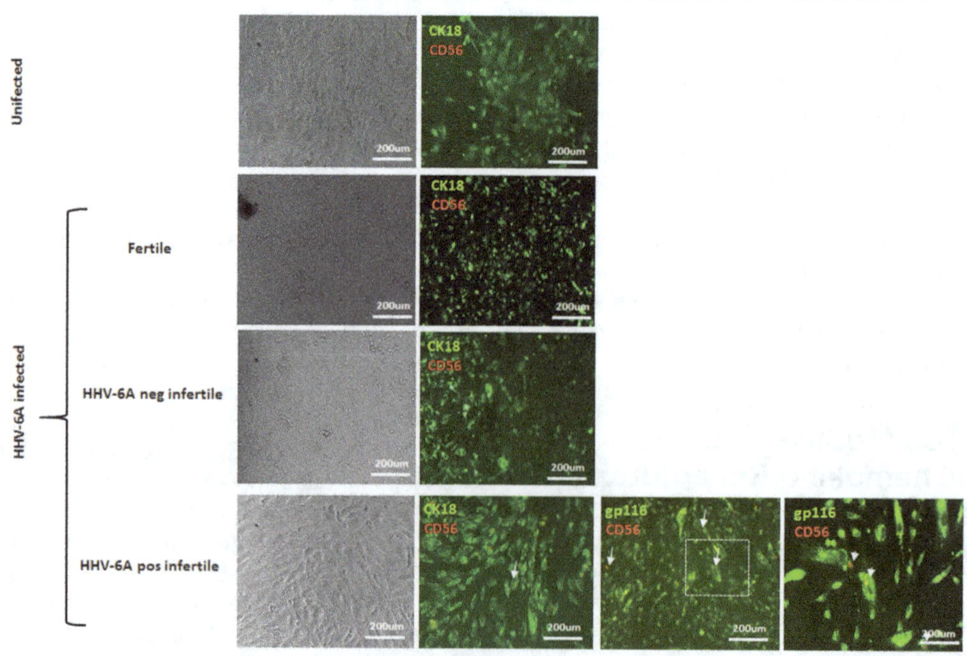

FIGURE 8 | Endometrial epithelial cells were infected for 72 h with HHV-6A. eNK cell were co-cultured for 4 h at a E/T ratio of 10. Endometrial epithelial cells were stained with CK18 (green), eNK cells with CD56 (red) and HHV-6A with gp116 (green). Images were taken in bright field *left panels*) or fluorescence (*right panels*) (Nikon Eclipse TE2000S) equipped with a digital camera. Original magnification 20× and 100×.

role of eNK cells in controlling HHV-6A infection in the endometrial tissue.

DISCUSSION

Our study demonstrates, for the first time, the critical role of eNK cells in counteracting HHV-6A infection in endometrial tissues through cytotoxicity. We showed phenotypic and cellular changes in eNK cells that allow the recognition and killing of HHV-6A-infected cells in a FasL-dependent manner.

We demonstrate that under HHV-6A infectious conditions, a significant fraction of eNK cells rapidly dampened down their Nkp30 and Nkp44 expression level, maintaining NKG2D and NKG2A expression.

We further show that control of HHV-6A infection involves NKG2D receptor and that endometrial epithelial cells decrease NKG2D ligands upon HHV-6A infection. This is true also *in vivo*, where endometrial epithelial cells from HHV-6A positive infertile women decreased the expression of NKG2D ligand. These findings suggest that also HHV-6A, as previously reported for HHV-6B (Schmiedel et al., 2016), modifies the expression of activating NKG2D receptor ligands. It should be noted that we obtained discrepant results with a decrease of NKG2DL expression by endometrial cells and the acquisition of cytotoxic effector functions through NKG2D receptor in eNK cells. We hypothesize a selective decrease in NKG2DL with the maintenance of high affinity ligands. Alternatively, co-engagement of other activating receptors could be enough even if there is less NKG2D ligands. Otherwise, the recruitment of NKG2DL into cholesterol-enriched membrane lipid microdomains may promote their shedding, maintaining their functional activity (Waldhauer et al., 2008; Aguera-Gonzalez et al., 2011). The identification of receptor-ligand interactions sustaining eNK cellular cytotoxicity might help to identify potential therapeutic targets that could limit HHV-6A spreading in endometrial tissues. In fact, it has been previously suggested that NKG2D receptor expressed by a subset of virus-specific lymphocytes might behave as a prototypic costimulatory receptor with a role in the control of viral infection in HLA class II^{pos} $NKG2DL^{pos}$ cells, as we observed in endometrial epithelial cells (Saez-Borderias et al., 2006).

The engagement of NKG2D might trigger cytokine production (i.e., IFN-type 1, IFN-gamma, TNF-alpha) that control cytotoxicity of eNK cells by FasL-Fas pathway (Nguyen et al., 2002). We observed the up-regulation of FasL on the surface of eNK cells and in the uterine flushing samples of HHV-6A positive infertile women, suggesting that eNK cell killing of HHV-6A infected endometrial epithelial cells proceeds through NKG2D engagement and subsequent mechanisms dependent on the death receptor-ligand Fas/FasL pathway. Interestingly, both eNK cells from fertile and infertile HHV-6 negative women presented an increase in specific lysis when co-cultured with HHV-6A infected endometrial cells. However, eNK cells from fertile and infertile HHV-6 negative women present a lower lysis that is similar to that obtained when they are co-cultured with K562 target cells (Supplementary Figure S2). For this, we concluded that the lysis obtained with eNK cells from fertile or infertile HHV-6 negative women is due to the natural cytotoxicity of eNK cells in the presence of target cells. On the contrary, eNK cells from HHV-6A positive infertile women showed a significantly higher lysis of HHV-6A infected endometrial cells, that overcomes the natural cytotoxicity of eNK cells.

Similarly, HLA-E molecules, the ligand of the inhibitory NKG2A receptor, are down-modulated during HHV-6A infection and slightly reduced in endometrial epithelial cells from HHV-6A positive infertile women, thus promoting an activatory profile. On the contrary, classical HLA class I molecules maintain their level of expression during HHV-6A infection. The difference between HLA-E and classical HLA-I molecules might reside in their intrinsic functional differences, where HLA-E has an immune-regulatory function while classical HLA-I antigens are totally involved in antigen presentation (Rizzo et al., 2017). HHV-6A might interfere with HLA-E surface expression impairing protein translocation from endoplasmic reticulum. Endometrial epithelial cells acquired a *de novo* expression of HLA-II DR molecules, as previously reported for thyrocytes (Caselli et al., 2012). This "APC-like" phenotype during HHV-6A infection, might be involved in viral clearance by immune cells. The expression of HLA-II antigens and chemokine receptor ligands could facilitate eNK cells homing to HHV-6A infected endometrial cells, as we demonstrated in *in vitro* culture model of endometrial epithelial cells. Since no evidence of HLA-II up-modulation in endometrial epithelial cells from HHV-6A positive infertile women was observed, further investigations are needed to demonstrate the role of HLA-II molecules expression in HHV-6A antigen presentation.

We demonstrate that during HHV-6A infection, eNK cells seem to become cytotoxic to limit viral infection. We observed phenotipical and functional modifications of both eNK cells and endometrial epithelial cells in HHV-6A positive infertile women samples, suggesting an imprint due to HHV-6A infection on both eNK cell immune-phenotype and receptor repertoire toward a cytotoxic activity. Meanwhile, the down-modulation of NKG2D ligands on endometrial epithelial cells could maintain *in vivo* eNK cells with a low killer profile, allowing the persistence of a subclinical HHV-6A infection. We demonstrate that NKG2D activating and chemokine receptors are implicated in eNK cell cytotoxicity toward HHV-6A-infected endometrial cells. The ability of eNK cells to "recognize" HHV-6A infected endometrial cells *in vitro* support the implication of eNK cells in controlling HHV-6A infection and spreading in endometrial environment. To our knowledge, this is the first time evidence for the involvement of eNK cells in controlling HHV-6A endometrial infection. The persistence of activated eNK and of subclinical HHV-6A infection could alter endometrial environment, as demonstrated by the increase in chemokines, mainly IP10, and FasL in uterine flushing samples from HHV-6A positive infertile women. This perturbation of molecular environment might disadvantage embryo implantation and placentation, which require a correct engagement of eNK cells. The presence of activated eNK cells can potentially have serious adverse side effects, as incorrect or insufficient remodeling of the spiral arteries leading to complications of pregnancy such as pre-eclampsia, fetal growth restriction and stillbirth. Nowadays, there are treatments for the control of NK cells activation, as prednisolone, intravenous Ig (IVIG), intralipid, and TNF-α-blocking agent. Interesting results have been obtained with IVIG treatment in antiphospholipid syndrome with persistent presence of autoantibodies against beta2 glycoprotein 1, where NK cell expansion (Oliver-Minarro et al., 2009) and Th1 shift (Benagiano et al., 2017) seem to be implicated in recurrent miscarriage. It is necessary to underline that during viral infections it is not inhibition of eNK cells that is needed, but rather the right degree of activation that is of importance.

Future studies, with a large cohort of infertile idiopathic women will be necessary to elucidate the possible role of eNK cell cytotoxicity toward HHV-6A endometrial infected cells, endometrial health status and embryo implantation. Understanding mechanisms that regulate eNK cell activation will clarify their involvement in female idiopathic infertility.

AUTHOR CONTRIBUTIONS

EC contributed to the conception of the work and data analysis. DB, AR, VG, IS, MD, MS, and IB contributed to data collection and analysis. RM and GLM contributed to clinical samples collection. DDL contributed to data interpretation and critical revision of the article. RR contributed to the conception of the work, data acquisition and analysis, and writing the article.

FUNDING

This work was supported by HHV-6 Foundation grants (PI: EC and RR), by PRIN grant (PI: EC, cod 2015YZB22C), by Merck grant (PI: RR), and by FISM-Fondazione Italiana Sclerosi Multipla grant (PI: RR, cod 2015/R/20), and Young Scientist Liberati grant (PI: GLM).

ACKNOWLEDGMENTS

The authors thank Iva Pivanti for her excellent technical assistance, and Linda Sartor for revising the English manuscript.

REFERENCES

Ablashi, D., Agut, H., Alvarez-Lafuente, R., Clark, D. A., Dewhurst, S., DiLuca, D., et al. (2014). Classification of HHV-6A and HHV-6B as distinct viruses. *Arch. Virol.* 159, 863–870. doi: 10.1007/s00705-013-1902-5

Aguera-Gonzalez, S., Gross, C. C., Fernandez-Messina, L., Ashiru, O., Esteso, G., Hang, H. C., et al. (2011). Palmitoylation of MICA, a ligand for NKG2D, mediates its recruitment to membrane microdomains and promotes its shedding. *Eur. J. Immunol.* 41, 3667–3676. doi: 10.1002/eji.201141645

Alter, G., Malenfant, J. M., and Altfeld, M. (2004). CD107a as a functional marker for the identification of natural killer cell activity. *J. Immunol. Methods* 294, 15–22. doi: 10.1016/j.jim.2004.08.008

Bachmayer, N., Rafik Hamad, R., Liszka, L., Bremme, K., and Sverremark-Ekstrom, E. (2006). Aberrant uterine natural killer (NK)-cell expression and altered placental and serum levels of the NK-cell promoting cytokine interleukin-12 in pre-eclampsia. *Am. J. Reprod. Immunol.* 56, 292–301. doi: 10.1111/j.1600-0897.2006.00429.x

Benagiano, M., Gerosa, M., Romagnoli, J., Mahler, M., Borghi, M. O., Grassi, A., et al. (2017). β2 glycoprotein I recognition drives Th1 inflammation in atherosclerotic plaques of patients with primary antiphospholipid syndrome. *J. Immunol.* 198, 2640–2648. doi: 10.4049/jimmunol.1600305

Bulmer, J. N., Morrison, L., Longfellow, M., Ritson, A., and Pace, D. (1991). Granulated lymphocytes in human endometrium: histochemical and immunohistochemical studies. *Hum. Reprod.* 6, 791–798. doi: 10.1093/oxfordjournals.humrep.a137430

Caselli, E., and Di Luca, D. (2007). Molecular biology and clinical associations of Roseoloviruses human herpesvirus 6 and human herpesvirus 7. *New Microbiol.* 30, 173–187.

Caselli, E., Zatelli, M. C., Rizzo, R., Benedetti, S., Martorelli, D., Trasforini, G., et al. (2012). Virologic and immunologic evidence supporting an association between HHV-6 and Hashimoto's thyroiditis. *PLOS Pathog.* 8:e1002951. doi: 10.1371/journal.ppat.1002951

Clifford, K., Flanagan, A. M., and Regan, L. (1999). Endometrial CD56+ natural killer cells in women with recurrent miscarriage: a histomorphometric study. *Hum. Reprod.* 14, 2727–2730. doi: 10.1093/humrep/14.11.2727

Eide, I. P., Rolfseng, T., Isaksen, C. V., Mecsei, R., Roald, B., Lydersen, S., et al. (2006). Serious foetal growth restriction is associated with reduced proportions of natural killer cells in decidua basalis. *Virchows Arch.* 448, 269–276. doi: 10.1007/s00428-005-0107-z

Flamand, L., Gosselin, J., D'Addario, M., Hiscott, J., Ablashi, D. V., Gallo, R. C., et al. (1991). Human herpesvirus 6 induces interleukin-1 beta and tumor necrosis factor alpha, but not interleukin-6, in peripheral blood mononuclear cell cultures. *J. Virol.* 65, 5105–5110.

Flamand, L., Gosselin, J., Stefanescu, I., Ablashi, D., and Menezes, J. (1995). Immunosuppressive effect of human herpesvirus 6 on T-cell functions: suppression of interleukin-2 synthesis and cell proliferation. *Blood* 85, 1263–1271.

Grivel, J. C., Santoro, F., Chen, S., Faga, G., Malnati, M. S., Ito, Y., et al. (2003). Pathogenic effects of human herpesvirus 6 in human lymphoid tissue ex vivo. *J. Virol.* 77, 8280–8289. doi: 10.1128/JVI.77.15.8280-8289.2003

Hanna, J., Goldman-Wohl, D., Hamani, Y., Avraham, I., Greenfield, C., Natanson-Yaron, S., et al. (2006). Decidual NK cells regulate key developmental processes at the human fetal-maternal interface. *Nat. Med.* 12, 1065–1074. doi: 10.1038/nm1452

Janelle, M. E., and Flamand, L. (2006). Phenotypic alterations and survival of monocytes following infection by human herpesvirus-6. *Arch. Virol.* 151, 1603–1614. doi: 10.1007/s00705-005-0715-6

Jokhi, P. P., King, A., and Loke, Y. W. (1997). Cytokine production and cytokine receptor expression by cells of the human first trimester placental-uterine interface. *Cytokine* 9, 126–137. doi: 10.1006/cyto.1996.0146

Kakimoto, M., Hasegawa, A., Fujita, S., and Yasukawa, M. (2002). Phenotypic and functional alterations of dendritic cells induced by human herpesvirus 6 infection. *J. Virol.* 76, 10338–10345. doi: 10.1128/JVI.76.20.10338-10345.2002

Keskin, D. B., Allan, D. S., Rybalov, B., Andzelm, M. M., Stern, J. N., Kopcow, H. D., et al. (2007). TGFbeta promotes conversion of $CD16^+$ peripheral blood NK cells into CD16- NK cells with similarities to decidual NK cells. *Proc. Natl. Acad. Sci. U.S.A.* 104, 3378–3383. doi: 10.1073/pnas.0611098104

Kitaya, K., Yamaguchi, T., Yasuo, T., Okubo, T., and Honjo, H. (2007). Post-ovulatory rise of endometrial CD16(-) natural killer cells: *in situ* proliferation of residual cells or selective recruitment from circulating peripheral blood? *J. Reprod. Immunol.* 76, 45–53. doi: 10.1016/j.jri.2007.03.010

Kopcow, H. D., Allan, D. S., Chen, X., Rybalov, B., Andzelm, M. M., Ge, B., et al. (2005). Human decidual NK cells form immature activating synapses and are not cytotoxic. *Proc. Natl. Acad. Sci. U.S.A.* 102, 15563–15568. doi: 10.1073/pnas.0507835102

Lash, G. E., Schiessl, B., Kirkley, M., Innes, B. A., Cooper, A., Searle, R. F., et al. (2006). Expression of angiogenic growth factors by uterine natural killer cells during early pregnancy. *J. Leukoc. Biol.* 80, 572–580. doi: 10.1189/jlb.0406250

Li, X. F., Charnock-Jones, D. S., Zhang, E., Hiby, S., Malik, S., Day, K., et al. (2001). Angiogenic growth factor messenger ribonucleic acids in uterine natural killer cells. *J. Clin. Endocrinol. Metab.* 86, 1823–1834. doi: 10.1210/jcem.86.4.7418

Lusso, P., De Maria, A., Malnati, M., Lori, F., DeRocco, S. E., Baseler, M., et al. (1991). Induction of CD4 and susceptibility to HIV-1 infection in human $CD8^+$ T lymphocytes by human herpesvirus 6. *Nature* 349, 533–535. doi: 10.1038/349533a0

Lusso, P., and Gallo, R. C. (1995). Human herpesvirus 6. *Baillieres Clin. Haematol.* 8, 201–223. doi: 10.1016/S0950-3536(05)80238-0

Lusso, P., Markham, P. D., Tschachler, E., di Marzo Veronese, F., Salahuddin, S. Z., Ablashi, D. V., et al. (1988). In vitro cellular tropism of human B-lymphotropic virus (human herpesvirus-6). *J. Exp. Med.* 167, 1659–1670. doi: 10.1084/jem.167.5.1659

Lynch, L., Golden-Mason, L., Eogan, M., O'Herlihy, C., and O'Farrelly, C. (2007). Cells with haematopoietic stem cell phenotype in adult human endometrium: relevance to infertility? *Hum. Reprod.* 22, 919–926. doi: 10.1093/humrep/del456

Marci, R., Gentili, V., Bortolotti, D., Lo Monte, G., Caselli, E., Bolzani, S., et al. (2016). Presence of HHV-6A in endometrial epithelial cells from women with primary unexplained infertility. *PLOS ONE* 11:e0158304. doi: 10.1371/journal.pone.0158304

McCullers, J. A., Lakeman, F. D., and Whitley, R. J. (1995). Human herpesvirus 6 is associated with focal encephalitis. *Clin. Infect. Dis.* 21, 571–576. doi: 10.1093/clinids/21.3.571

Naruse, K., Lash, G. E., Bulmer, J. N., Innes, B. A., Otun, H. A., Searle, R. F., et al. (2009a). The urokinase plasminogen activator (uPA) system in uterine natural killer cells in the placental bed during early pregnancy. *Placenta* 30, 398–404. doi: 10.1016/j.placenta.2009.02.002

Naruse, K., Lash, G. E., Innes, B. A., Otun, H. A., Searle, R. F., Robson, S. C., et al. (2009b). Localization of matrix metalloproteinase (MMP)-2, MMP-9 and tissue inhibitors for MMPs (TIMPs) in uterine natural killer cells in early human pregnancy. *Hum. Reprod.* 24, 553–561. doi: 10.1093/humrep/den408

Nguyen, K. B., Salazar-Mather, T. P., Dalod, M. Y., Van Deusen, J. B., Wei, X. Q., Liew, F. Y., et al. (2002). Coordinated and distinct roles for IFN-alpha beta, IL-12, and IL-15 regulation of NK cell responses to viral infection. *J. Immunol.* 169, 4279–4287. doi: 10.4049/jimmunol.169.8.4279

Oliver-Minarro, D., Gil, J., Aguaron, A., Rodriguez-Mahou, M., Fernandez-Cruz, E., and Sanchez-Ramon, S. (2009). NK cell expansion in obstetrical antiphospholipid syndrome: guilty by association? *Eur. J. Obstet. Gynecol. Reprod. Biol.* 145:227. doi: 10.1016/j.ejogrb.2009.05.010

Pantry, S. N., and Medveczky, P. G. (2017). Latency, integration, and reactivation of human herpesvirus-6. *Viruses* 9:E194. doi: 10.3390/v9070194

Rizzo, R., Bortolotti, D., Fainardi, E., Gentili, V., Bolzani, S., Baldi, E., et al. (2016). KIR2DL2 inhibitory pathway enhances Th17 cytokine secretion by NK cells in response to herpesvirus infection in multiple sclerosis patients. *J. Neuroimmunol.* 294, 1–5. doi: 10.1016/j.jneuroim.2016.03.007

Rizzo, R., Fainardi, E., Rouas-Freiss, N., and Morandi, F. (2017). The role of HLA-class Ib molecules in immune-related diseases, tumors, and infections 2016. *J. Immunol. Res.* 2017:2309574. doi: 10.1155/2017/2309574

Saez-Borderias, A., Guma, M., Angulo, A., Bellosillo, B., Pende, D., and Lopez-Botet, M. (2006). Expression and function of NKG2D in CD4+ T cells specific for human cytomegalovirus. *Eur. J. Immunol.* 36, 3198–3206. doi: 10.1002/eji.200636682

Sandhoff, T., Kleim, J. P., and Schneweis, K. E. (1991). Latent human herpesvirus-6 DNA is sparsely distributed in peripheral blood lymphocytes of healthy adults and patients with lymphocytic disorders. *Med. Microbiol. Immunol.* 180, 127–134. doi: 10.1007/BF00206116

Schmiedel, D., Tai, J., Levi-Schaffer, F., Dovrat, S., and Mandelboim, O. (2016). Human herpesvirus 6B downregulates expression of activating ligands during lytic infection to escape elimination by natural killer cells. *J. Virol.* 90, 9608–9617. doi: 10.1128/JVI.01164-16

Siewiera, J., El Costa, H., Tabiasco, J., Berrebi, A., Cartron, G., Le Bouteiller, P., et al. (2013). Human cytomegalovirus infection elicits new decidual natural killer cell effector functions. *PLOS Pathog.* 9:e1003257. doi: 10.1371/journal.ppat.1003257

Smith, A., Santoro, F., Di Lullo, G., Dagna, L., Verani, A., and Lusso, P. (2003). Selective suppression of IL-12 production by human herpesvirus 6. *Blood* 102, 2877–2884. doi: 10.1182/blood-2002-10-3152

Smith, A. P., Paolucci, C., Di Lullo, G., Burastero, S. E., Santoro, F., and Lusso, P. (2005). Viral replication-independent blockade of dendritic cell maturation and interleukin-12 production by human herpesvirus 6. *J. Virol.* 79, 2807–2813. doi: 10.1128/JVI.79.5.2807-2813.2005

Soldan, S. S., Berti, R., Salem, N., Secchiero, P., Flamand, L., Calabresi, P. A., et al. (1997). Association of human herpes virus 6 (HHV-6) with multiple sclerosis: increased IgM response to HHV-6 early antigen and detection of serum HHV-6 DNA. *Nat. Med.* 3, 1394–1397. doi: 10.1038/nm1297-1394

Stallmach, T., Hebisch, G., Orban, P., and Lu, X. (1999). Aberrant positioning of trophoblast and lymphocytes in the feto-maternal interface with pre-eclampsia. *Virchows Arch.* 434, 207–211. doi: 10.1007/s004280050329

Takahashi, K., Sonoda, S., Higashi, K., Kondo, T., Takahashi, H., Takahashi, M., et al. (1989). Predominant CD4 T-lymphocyte tropism of human herpesvirus 6-related virus. *J. Virol.* 63, 3161–3163.

Tuckerman, E., Laird, S. M., Prakash, A., and Li, T. C. (2007). Prognostic value of the measurement of uterine natural killer cells in the endometrium of women with recurrent miscarriage. *Hum. Reprod.* 22, 2208–2213. doi: 10.1093/humrep/dem141

Waldhauer, I., Goehlsdorf, D., Gieseke, F., Weinschenk, T., Wittenbrink, M., Ludwig, A., et al. (2008). Tumor-associated MICA is shed by ADAM proteases. *Cancer Res.* 68, 6368–6376. doi: 10.1158/0008-5472.CAN-07-6768

Williams, P. J., Bulmer, J. N., Searle, R. F., Innes, B. A., and Robson, S. C. (2009). Altered decidual leucocyte populations in the placental bed in pre-eclampsia and foetal growth restriction: a comparison with late normal pregnancy. *Reproduction* 138, 177–184. doi: 10.1530/REP-09-0007

Wu, X., Jin, L. P., Yuan, M. M., Zhu, Y., Wang, M. Y., and Li, D. J. (2005). Human first-trimester trophoblast cells recruit CD56brightCD16- NK cells into decidua by way of expressing and secreting of CXCL12/stromal cell-derived factor 1. *J. Immunol.* 175, 61–68. doi: 10.4049/jimmunol.175.1.61

Yamanishi, K., Okuno, T., Shiraki, K., Takahashi, M., Kondo, T., Asano, Y., et al. (1988). Identification of human herpesvirus-6 as a causal agent for exanthem subitum. *Lancet* 1, 1065–1067. doi: 10.1016/S0140-6736(88)91893-4

17

Linking the Gut Microbial Ecosystem with the Environment: Does Gut Health Depend on Where We Live?

Nishat Tasnim, Nijiati Abulizi, Jason Pither, Miranda M. Hart*† and Deanna L. Gibson*†

Department of Biology, The Irving K. Barber School of Arts and Sciences, University of British Columbia, Kelowna, BC, Canada

***Correspondence:**
Miranda M. Hart
miranda.hart@ubc.ca
Deanna L. Gibson
deanna.gibson@ubc.ca
† Co-senior authors.

Global comparisons reveal a decrease in gut microbiota diversity attributed to Western diets, lifestyle practices such as caesarian section, antibiotic use and formula-feeding of infants, and sanitation of the living environment. While gut microbial diversity is decreasing, the prevalence of chronic inflammatory diseases such as inflammatory bowel disease, diabetes, obesity, allergies and asthma is on the rise in Westernized societies. Since the immune system development is influenced by microbial components, early microbial colonization may be a key factor in determining disease susceptibility patterns later in life. Evidence indicates that the gut microbiota is vertically transmitted from the mother and this affects offspring immunity. However, the role of the external environment in gut microbiome and immune development is poorly understood. Studies show that growing up in microbe-rich environments, such as traditional farms, can have protective health effects on children. These health-effects may be ablated due to changes in the human lifestyle, diet, living environment and environmental biodiversity as a result of urbanization. Importantly, if early-life exposure to environmental microbes increases gut microbiota diversity by influencing patterns of gut microbial assembly, then soil biodiversity loss due to land-use changes such as urbanization could be a public health threat. Here, we summarize key questions in environmental health research and discuss some of the challenges that have hindered progress toward a better understanding of the role of the environment on gut microbiome development.

Keywords: gut microbiome, immunity, environment, human health, immune tolerance, microbial colonization, biodiversity, microbe-rich environments

INTRODUCTION

Human health is closely linked to the diverse set of microorganisms in the intestine collectively known as the gut microbiota (Hooper and Gordon, 2001). This population of microorganisms and their genetic potential, or the gut microbiome, has been linked to human metabolism, intestinal homeostasis, immune development (Lynch and Pedersen, 2016), and brain processes and behavior (Mayer et al., 2015). A stable and diverse gut microbiota, optimal for maintaining health, produces metabolites that fuel physiological and metabolic processes. The gut microbiota also tunes local and systemic immune responses to confer protective immunity against pathogens while simultaneously maintaining immune tolerance toward commensals (Cerf-Bensussan and Gaboriau-Routhiau, 2010). Other functions of the gut microbiota include fermentation of indigestible dietary components (Flint et al., 2012), breakdown of environmental pollutants and pharmaceuticals (Claus et al., 2017), and pathogen competitive exclusion (Kamada et al., 2013). Alterations to the gut microbiota, known as dysbiosis, can disrupt these essential health-promoting services and are associated with gastrointestinal, cardiovascular, autoimmune and metabolic diseases (Carding et al., 2015). Therefore, the gut microbiome is a microbial ecosystem that operates much like a microbial organ that functions to promote health and prevent disease.

We are only beginning to understand the ecological processes that lead to the growth and development of a stable and diverse gut microbiome that promotes host-health. The gut microbiota is a diverse ecosystem comprised of bacteria, archaea, fungi and viruses including a diverse bacteriophage community (Manrique et al., 2016). Bacteria dominate the microbiota in abundance and diversity, with commensal members from seven phyla (Firmicutes, Bacteriodetes, Actinobacteria, Fusobacteria, Proteobacteria, Verrucomicrobia, and Cyanobacteria), the majority of which are uncultivated and novel phylotypes (Eckburg et al., 2005). Members of the microbiota can be permanent "residents," transmitted through close contact between individuals, or transient "hitchhikers" from ingested food, water and various components of the environment (Ley et al., 2006; Harmsen and de Goffau, 2016). These transmission routes are important for establishing and maintaining microbial diversity in the gut (Browne et al., 2017). The mechanism of transmission can determine the pattern of colonization which shapes the gut microbial community of the host, but these patterns of transmission are poorly understood. Colonization that leads to the establishment of a stable and diverse adult gut microbiome lays the foundation for a homeostatic host-microbial relationship maintained by balanced immune responses. Colonizing gut microbes provide signals known as microbe-associated molecular patterns (MAMPs) that affect the maturation of the immune system and gut associated lymphoid tissue (GALT) (Wopereis et al., 2014). The development of the GALT is associated with bacterial activation of Toll-like receptors (TLRs) and downstream signaling pathways involved in maintaining host-microbial homeostasis, regulated through cytokines and chemokines (Hooper et al., 2015). Germ free animals have defects in the development of GALT, as well as cellular defects such as decrease in the number of lymphocytes, and molecular immune deficiencies such as reduced antibody production (Round and Mazmanian, 2009; Torrazza and Neu, 2011). Thus, colonization of the gut by microbes is not only important for the development of gut tissue, but also for the establishment of immune tolerance.

Gut bacterial community assembly begins pre-birth (Blaser and Dominguez-Bello, 2016), but rapid colonization takes place at birth and continues for the first 3 years of life (Lozupone et al., 2013). Two key factors that could influence the successful transmission of beneficial gut microbes to the infant are the mother and the external environment. Various studies that have sampled infant fecal microbiota have revealed that early gut microbial settlers that colonize the gut are derived from maternal vaginal, fecal, milk, mouth and skin microbiota during both gestation and birth through vertical transmission, and from the environment through horizontal transmission (Inoue and Ushida, 2003). Therefore, the infant gut microbiome is transmitted from a gut microbial species pool, comprised of gut symbionts from both the mother and the environment (**Figure 1**). The effect of the environment on the diversity and richness of the human gut bacterial species pool and gut microbiota transmission has yet to be explored. If the transmission of gut microbes is primarily parent-child, then environmental factors such as standards of hygiene, contamination of food and water by fecal microbes, delivery mode and hospitalization after birth can alter transmission mechanisms. On the other hand, if colonization patterns and gut microbiota diversity is linked to transmission of microbes from the external environment, then additional factors such as place of birth, geography, urban vs. rural living environment may also alter colonization of the gut microbiota affecting the human health. In this review, we discuss what is known about the role of environmental factors on the gut microbiota composition, diversity and assembly, identify major research challenges for research aiming to elucidate gut microbiota transmission patterns, and make suggestions for future studies that integrate the gut microbiome with environmental health research.

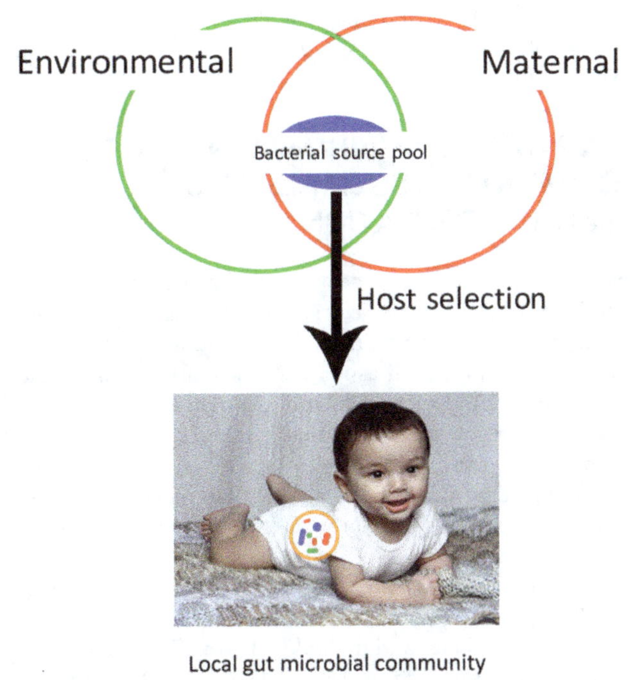

FIGURE 1 | Local microbial community assembly of the infant gut microbiota depends on dispersal from a bacterial source pool. This bacterial source pool is comprised of both maternal microbes, transmitted vertically, and environmental microbes, transmitted horizontally. The development of the local community is shaped primarily by host selection, based on interactions between host and bacterial cells.

INFLUENCE OF ENVIRONMENT ON VARIATIONS IN GUT MICROBIOTA DIVERSITY

The composition and diversity of gut microbiota varies between individuals. Under germ free conditions, gut microbiota transplantation experiments between model organisms such as zebrafish and mice have shown that gut microbiota composition is host-specific (Rawls et al., 2006). In humans, many other factors contribute to variation, such as diet, host genetics and metabolism, familial relationships, culture (Dominguez-Bello and Blaser, 2011), and demographics (Lozupone et al., 2013). According to global surveys of fecal microbiota from healthy populations, variation between individuals in richness of gut microbiota is largely explained by age, ethnicity (Huttenhower et al., 2012), geography (Torrazza and Neu, 2011), medication exposure, blood parameters, bowel, diet, health, anthropometrics and lifestyle (Falony et al., 2016). Of particular interest is the observation that healthy adults from rural societies such as Papua New Guinea (Martínez et al., 2015), Amerindia and Malawi (Clemente et al., 2015), and hunter-gatherers from Tanzania and Amazon (Schnorr et al., 2014) have higher gut bacterial species richness compared to urban populations in Italy and US. Similarly, children (between ages 1 to 5) from rural communities have more diverse gut microbiotas compared to children from Western populations (De Filippo et al., 2010). These host-specific differences in gut microbiota may arise from distinct selective pressures within the host gut habitat including genetics and diet but also may be due, at least in part, to their unique environments.

ROLE OF THE ENVIRONMENT ON GUT COMMUNITY ASSEMBLY AND IMMUNOREGULATION

The role of the environment in the assembly of the gut microbiota has yet to be elucidated, although there is good reason to believe they are linked. Urbanization leads to changes in living conditions such as increased sanitation and antibiotic use (Popkin, 1999), separation from the outdoors (Turner et al., 2004), and poor land management practices that may reduce soil microbial biodiversity (Wall et al., 2015). Accordingly, studies show that infants born via caesarian section have altered colonization patterns and lower total gut microbiota diversity (Biasucci et al., 2010), and individuals who grow up in city environments have a less diverse gut microbiome (Sjögren et al., 2009). Further, urbanites are more prone to inflammatory disorders like diabetes and multiple sclerosis (Kay, 2000) as well as allergic diseases such as asthma (Rook, 2012) during both infancy and adulthood (Garn and Renz, 2007). Although host genetics may in large part determine the composition of the adult gut microbiome, it has been shown that alien microbes from diverse habitats like soil can colonize the germ-free gut (Seedorf et al., 2014). Therefore, horizontal transmission of environmental microbes may be contributing commensal microbes to the gut ecosystem, altering patterns of colonization to increase variation in gut microbiota diversity.

Early-life exposure to microbe-rich environments may be beneficial for human health by increasing the gut bacterial species pool. The "microbial old friends" hypothesis, posits microbe-rich environments are a source of beneficial microbes that promote gut microbiota diversity (Zhou et al., 2015) reducing inflammatory disease risk (Rook et al., 2013). Indeed, growing up in microbe-rich environments, like traditional farms, result in healthier children (Mosca et al., 2016). Therefore, the prevalence of inflammatory disorders may be higher in modern cities because of reduced exposure to beneficial microbes from the environment, such as microbes from house dust or zoonotic microbes from animals. Indeed, exposure to household pets has been shown to alter the infant gut microbiota and reduce allergic disease (Tun et al., 2017). Reduced exposure to pathogenic microorganisms, largely as a result of modern hygienic practices, can also result in defective immunoregulation (Garn and Renz, 2007). The "hygiene hypothesis" makes the argument that infectious stressors are particularly important during early childhood (Wills-karp et al., 2001; Garn and Renz, 2007) and is supported by epidemiological studies showing rural children have reduced asthma (Ege et al., 2011), hay fever (Strachan, 1989) and ectopic eczema (Isolauri et al., 2000). Such allergic diseases are chronic inflammatory disorders caused by a decrease in immune tolerance (Garn and Renz, 2007). Decrease in tolerance is associated with a decrease in Treg cells expressing the transcription factor forkhead box P3 (FOXP3+ Treg cells) (Simon et al., 2015). FOXP3+ Treg cells produce anti-inflammatory cytokines such as interleukin 10 (IL-10) and transforming growth factor-β (TGF-β) which help to suppress exacerbating inflammatory responses and balance CD4+ helper T (Th) Th1 and Th2 cells. In allergic diseases, cytokine stimulation of naïve T cells from IL-4, IL-5 and IL-13 tilt the balance of Th cells toward the Th2 phenotype (Kay, 2000). In infants, there may be a normal Th2 bias observed in both mice (1–3 weeks old) and humans (0–2 years old) (Marchant and Goldman, 2005; Dowling and Levy, 2014). As the infant ages, the Th2 skew is balanced by Th1 responses and induced memory responses through mucosal-associated invariant T cells and interleukin-8 (CXCL8) secreting naïve T cells (Simon et al., 2015). In contrast, allergic infants have a persistent Th2 phenotype, resulting in long term Th2-skewed immunity (Barrios et al., 1996). Therefore, early life exposure to a broad range of immunoregulation-inducing commensal and pathogenic environmental microorganisms can provide a Th1 stimulus, conferring protection against immune disorders.

What is it about urban environments that reduces healthy gut microbiome functioning? Both "old friends" and the "hygiene hypothesis," are contingent on microbial biodiversity. Urban development leading to the loss of local habitats and biodiversity may be detrimental to human health by depleting or otherwise altering the reservoirs of environmental microbes including bacteria, fungi and viruses that may play a role in gut microbiota-mediated immune health. The "biodiversity hypothesis" posits that clinical diseases, caused by poor microbiome, immune dysfunction and inflammation, are linked to biodiversity loss (Anderson et al., 2013). Biodiversity loss due to industrialization is associated with adverse health effects, including inflammatory diseases (Haahtela et al., 2013). Environmental biodiversity and immune function have been linked in epidemiological studies, which show individuals living in built environments have lower diversity of microbiota and higher allergic disposition (Wardle et al., 2004). The World Allergy Organization has proposed that loss of biodiversity is linked to loss of microbial diversity, resulting in microbial deprivation and ultimately, inflammatory disorders (Haahtela et al., 2013). This proposal extends the "old friends" and hygiene hypothesis to include environmental biodiversity as being important in the development of the immune system and gut microbiome (von Hertzen et al., 2011). A biodiverse environment that is microbe-rich may promote the development of healthy gut microbiota and lower disease risk.

Extending the "biodiversity hypothesis" to include soil biodiversity has the potential to provide more insight into the role of the environment and gut mediated immune health. Soils contain a dynamic reservoir of biodiversity (Torsvik and Øvreås, 2002) and this diversity is essential for maintaining biogeochemical processes and ecosystem functioning (Wardle et al., 2004). In this way, soil biodiversity provides benefits to human health indirectly through suppression of soil-borne pathogens, provision of clean air, water and food, and exposure to immunoregulation-inducing soil microorganisms (Wall et al., 2015). Although unknown, we ask if there is a direct link between soil microbial diversity and human health? Certainly, soil microbial diversity varies in taxonomic composition between biomes (Fierer et al., 2012b), physical and chemical gradients (Fierer et al., 2012a; Lauber et al., 2013), and anthropogenic activity (Ramirez et al., 2010). Whether it is species richness that is important, or the composition of key taxa has not been determined. There is some indirect evidence that soil biodiversity and human microbiota are interrelated (Hanski et al., 2012), to provide "natural immunity" (von Hertzen et al., 2011). Further, exposure to soil microbes has been experimentally shown to increase gut microbiota diversity (Zhou et al., 2015). There is also some evidence to suggest that exposure to possible soil pathogens could contribute to immune tolerance (Wall et al., 2015). However, little is known about the impact of soil exposure on gut microbiota transmission and colonization patterns in humans.

EXPLORATION OF THE CONNECTIONS BETWEEN SOIL MICROBIAL COMMUNITIES AND GUT MICROBIAL COMMUNITIES

For soil biodiversity to be relevant to human health requires microbes from local soil to be transmitted horizontally to humans and then established in the gut. If so, then people exposed to similar soil microbial communities should have more similar gut communities. We analyzed soil and gut studies from publicly available datasets on Qiita (http://qiita.microbio.me), to investigate the link between soil and gut microbial diversity, in terms of richness, diversity and species identity. We combined OTU (operational taxonomic unit) tables from 7 gut studies (n= 2,497 human fecal samples) and 4 soil studies (n = 1,123 soil samples) that used 16 s amplicon sequencing to study bacterial communities (**Figures 2A,B**). The human fecal samples were collected from 14 countries, although the vast majority of samples were from USA (n = 1,062), Malawi (n= 1,042) and Venezuela (n = 99). These samples were collected from a range of ages (0–77 years). A small proportion of adult humans were diagnosed with obesity, atherosclerosis (n = 52). Soil studies were from 17 different locations and most samples were from North America (n = 1062). Soil samples ranged from wetland to garden soil from tundra to tropical biomes.

US Studies Dominate

Although our dataset was diverse, we lacked sufficient data to explore global variation in soil-gut microbiota. At the time of analysis, there were 244 studies on Qiita of which we picked four large-scale soil and seven gut studies to pool into a combined dataset (**Figure 2A**). Most studies on soil and human bacterial communities were located in the US. Future efforts should survey populations from different countries and physiographic regions to provide global geographical gut microbial datasets.

There Is Little Overlap between Soil and Gut Microbes at Lower Taxonomic Levels

We performed downstream analysis to compare the relative proportion of bacterial phyla in human gut and soil samples (**Figure 2B**). We visualized the OTUs in human gut and soil samples using taxa summary plots. Samples were grouped and averaged by sample type (gut or soil) and taxonomic composition was summarized on multiple taxonomic levels (e.g., phylum, order, etc.) (Navas-Molina et al., 2013). We found that human fecal samples were dominated by Bacteriodetes and Firmicutes phyla, whereas soil samples were dominated by Proteobacteria and Verrucomicrobia. These differences in taxonomic composition between soil and gut samples were also consistent at lower taxonomic levels (see **Figure 2B** table).

Study Effects Account for Variation

Differences in DNA extraction protocol, primer selection, sequencing platform and sequence analysis pipelines introduce bias to datasets known as study effects. To evaluate the influence of study effects, we pooled all human gut studies from a single investigator (Rob Knight, University of California), and excluded all studies outside the US resulting in four studies. We tested for study effects (n = 935) by considering research group (**Figure 2C**) and primer subfragment (**Figure 2C**). We found that primer target region or research group contributed to strong study-based clustering, similar to clustering patterns found in other meta-analyses of the human microbiota (Lozupone et al., 2013). Our results indicate that soil and gut bacterial communities have few overlapping taxa, but because most gut and soil studies survey North American cohorts, we were not able to determine whether local soil microbial communities influence the composition of gut microbial communities of individuals from different geographical locations.

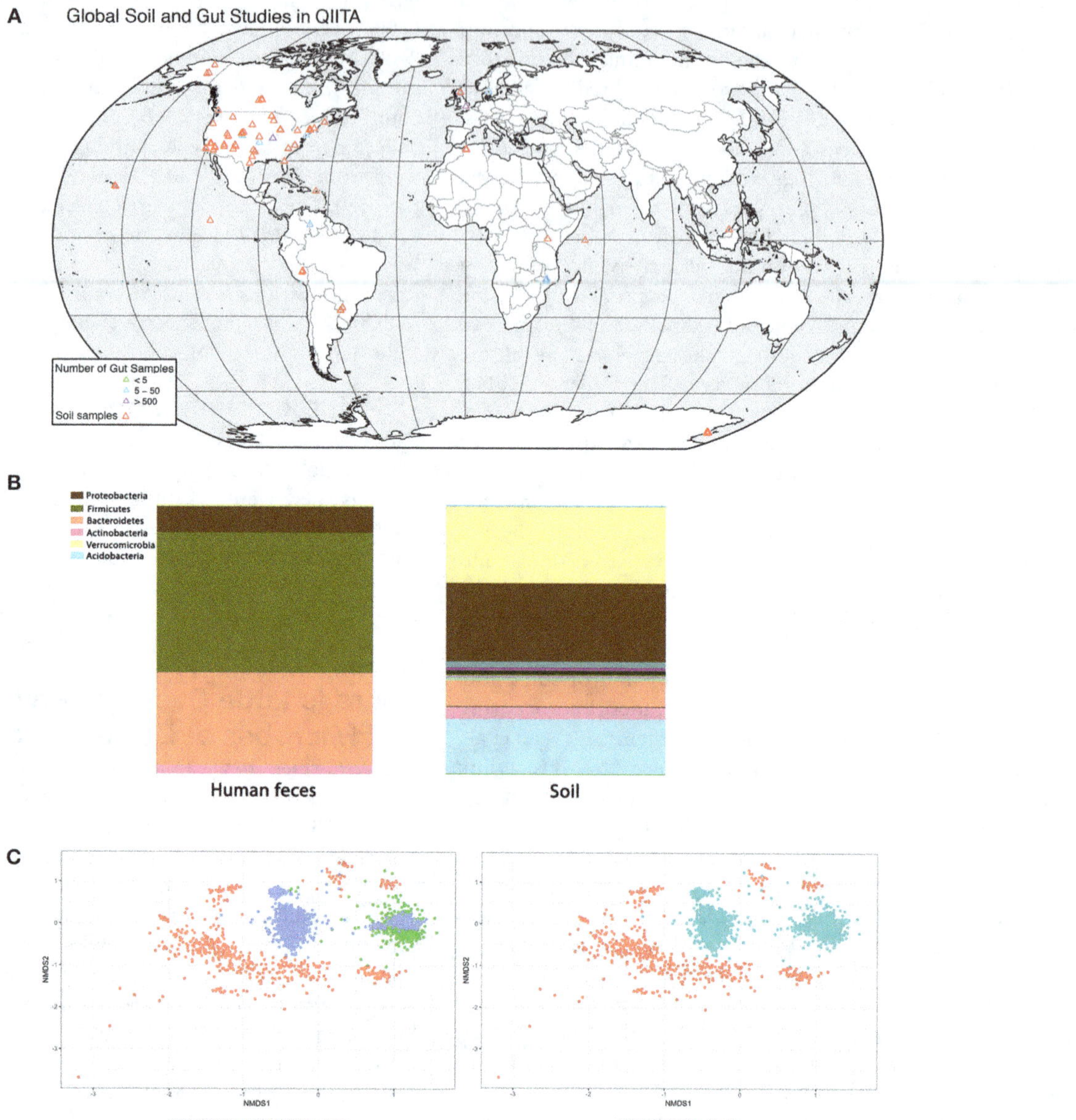

FIGURE 2 | Analysis of concurrence between gut and soil microbiome studies (data deposited in http://qiita.microbio.me) **(A)** Geographical range of soil (red symbols) and gut studies (green, blue, and purple symbols) available on QIITA. Studies are predominantly located in North America and Europe. Human fecal samples were collected from 14 countries, but the vast majority (66%) are from USA, Malawi, and Venezuela. Samples were collected from a range of ages (0–77 years). Soil samples were taken from a variety of habitats, including wetlands, garden soils, tundra, and tropical biomes. **(B)** Relative proportion of bacterial phyla in human feces ($n = 2{,}497$) and soil ($n = 1{,}123$) samples combined from seven gut and four soil studies in QIITA show little overlap of bacterial taxa. **(C)** Non-metric multidimensional scaling (NMDS) ordination plot of Bray-Curtis community dissimilarities on OTUs from 16 s gene sequences from four US gut studies conducted by the same principal investigator (Rob Knight) (2D stress value = 0.16). Samples show clustering according to study center ($n = 935$) (plot on left) as well as primer choice (plot on right) where V2 subfragment ($n = 35$) or V4 subfragment ($n = 900$) is targeted. Symbols represent individual fecal samples.

CHALLENGES FOR STUDYING ENVIRONMENT-GUT MICROBIOTA INTERACTIONS IN HEALTH AND DISEASE

Global surveys on the relationships between environment, gut microbiota and inflammation are yet to be explored, such as how traditional diets consumed in a region may contribute to the gut microbial community or how local soil influences diversity of the gut microbiota of the population through horizontal transmission. The mechanism of horizontal transmission of environmental microbes, whether inhalation, ingestion or cutaneous, also remains to be elucidated. The rate of urbanization and soil degradation may be related to changes in the composition of the gut microbiota, such as an increase abundance of bacterial indicators of dysbiosis such as Proteobacteria (Shin et al., 2015). We cannot begin to understand the link between soil microbial diversity and gut microbial assembly until studies adopt standardized collection, extraction and sample preparation procedures with complete and transparent metadata reporting and appropriate analysis platforms. Some additional challenges for study design and analysis of environment-gut studies are outlined below.

Challenge 1: Quantifying Microbe-Richness and Diversity of the Environment

To link gut microbiota to environmental microbial diversity, it will be important for future studies to develop standardized methods that reliably reflect microbial biodiversity in the environment. In addition to microbial diversity of the direct environment (home, air, soil, water, etc.), biodiversity of the surrounding environment should be estimated by recording information about the landscape, including land use type and predominant vegetation structure, abiotic factors such as climatic factors and information about the biodiversity of resident communities (i.e., plants, animals, etc.; as described by Hanski et al., 2012). Given the logistical challenges associated with such efforts, we recommend choosing sampling locations strategically in relation to desired environmental (Metzger et al., 2013) and other characteristics. This approach will help elucidate associations between microbial exposure, environmental biodiversity, and gut microbiota assembly.

Together, these parameters will help elucidate direct effects of microbial exposure and environmental biodiversity on gut microbiota assembly.

Challenge 2: Collection, Storage and Analysis of Host-Microbiome-Environment Interactions

Developing analysis tools and platforms that are able to store and analyze large datasets will be critical to link gut microbiota assembly to external factors. Currently, limitations in sample collection, processing and storage (Gorzelak et al., 2015), as well as systems of reporting, study design, sample size, variation in demographics and statistical approaches prevent cross study comparisons (Hunter, 2005). The two publicly-available platforms for microbiome-environment studies are Qiita and SourceTracker (Knights et al., 2011), yet these have had little uptake by the community as a whole. To fully understand demographic factors in gut microbial assembly, this will need to be a globally coordinated effort. The utility of the NIH Human Microbiome Project (http://www.hmpdacc.org/) could be enhanced by including protocols and repositories for environmental biodiversity (microbial and otherwise). Applications such as SourceTracker could then be easily used to investigate source-sink dynamics of the microbiota, to investigate microbiome-exposure interactions on the ecology of the microbiome. Once the challenge of data collection, handling and analysis are met, microbiome changes can be used as biomarkers to indicate individual health and disease outcome (Segata et al., 2011).

CONCLUSION

The study of environmental influences on gut microbiota structure and function is especially pertinent because the human living environment is becoming rapidly urbanized. Such drastic changes to the human environment may interrupt the healthy development of the microbiota and increase risk of inflammatory diseases. Moving forward, we must incorporate gut microbiota surveys into a broader framework of environmental exposure, for a thorough understanding of how ecosystem processes contribute to gut microbiota development, and affect the quality of human health.

AUTHOR CONTRIBUTIONS

NT: data collection and analysis; statistical analysis; intellectual design; writing and editing of the manuscript. NA: data collection and analysis; statistical analysis. JP: data analysis; statistical analysis oversight; editing of the manuscript. MH: data analysis; intellectual design; writing and editing of the manuscript; funding support. DG: intellectual design; writing and editing of the manuscript; funding support.

FUNDING

JP and MH are funded through grants from the Natural Sciences and Engineering Research Council. DG is funded through grants from the Natural Sciences and Engineering Research Council and Crohn's and Colitis Canada.

REFERENCES

Anderson, P. M. L., Okereke, C., Rudd, A., and Parnell, S. (2013). *Urbanization, Biodiversity and Ecosystem Services: Challenges and Opportunities.* Dordrecht: Springer.

Barrios, C., Brawand, P., Berney, M., Brandt, C., Lambert, P. H., and Siegrist, C. A. (1996). Neonatal and early life immune responses to various forms of vaccine antigens qualitatively differ from adult responses: predominance of a Th2-biased pattern which persists after adult boosting. *Eur. J. Immunol.* 26, 1489–1496. doi: 10.1002/eji.1830260713

Biasucci, G., Rubini, M., Riboni, S., Morelli, L., Bessi, E., and Retetangos, C. (2010). Mode of delivery affects the bacterial community in the newborn gut. *Early Hum. Dev.* 86 (Suppl. 1), 13–15. doi: 10.1016/j.earlhumdev.2010.01.004

Blaser, M. J., and Dominguez-Bello, M. G. (2016). The human microbiome before birth. *Cell Host Microbe.* 20, 558–560. doi: 10.1016/j.chom.2016.10.014

Browne, H. P., Neville, B. A., Forster, S. C., and Lawley, T. D. (2017). Transmission of the gut microbiota: spreading of health. *Nat. Rev. Micro.* 15, 531–543. doi: 10.1038/nrmicro.2017.50

Carding, S., Verbeke, K., Vipond, D. T., Corfe, B. M., and Owen, L. J. (2015). Dysbiosis of the gut microbiota in disease. *Microb. Ecol. Health Dis.* 26:26191. doi: 10.3402/mehd.v26.26191

Cerf-Bensussan, N., and Gaboriau-Routhiau, V. (2010). The immune system and the gut microbiota: friends or foes? *Nat. Rev. Immunol.* 10, 735–744. doi: 10.1038/nri2850

Claus, S. P., Guillou, H., and Ellero-Simatos, S. (2017). The gut microbiota: a major player in the toxicity of environmental pollutants? *Biofilms Microbiomes* 3:17001. doi:10.1038/npjbiofilms.2017.1

Clemente, J. C., Pehrsson, E. C., Blaser, M. J., Sandhu, K., Gao, Z., Wang, B., et al. (2015). The microbiome of uncontacted Amerindians. *Sci. Adv.* 1:e1500183. doi: 10.1126/sciadv.1500183

De Filippo, C., Cavalieri, D., Di Paola, M., Ramazzotti, M., Poullet, J. B., Massart, S., et al. (2010). Impact of diet in shaping gut microbiota revealed by a comparative study in children from Europe and rural Africa. *Proc. Natl. Acad. Sci. U.S.A.* 107, 14691–14696. doi: 10.1073/pnas.1005963107

Dominguez-Bello, M. G., and Blaser, M. J. (2011). The human microbiota as a marker for migrations of individuals and populations. *Ann. Rev. Anthropol. Anthropol.* 40, 451–474. doi: 10.1146/annurev-anthro-081309-145711

Dowling, D. J., and Levy, O. (2014). Ontogeny of early life immunity. *Trends Immunol.* 35, 299–310. doi: 10.1016/j.it.2014.04.007

Eckburg, P. B., Bik, E. M., Bernstein, C. N., Purdom, E., Dethlefsen, L., Sargent, M., et al. (2005). Diversity of the human intestinal microbial flora. *Science* 308, 1635–1638. doi: 10.1126/science.1110591

Ege, M. J., Mayer, M., Normand, A.-C., Genuneit, J., Cookson, W. O. C. M., Braun-Fahrländer, C., et al. (2011). Exposure to environmental microorganisms and childhood asthma. *New Engl. J. Med.* 364, 701–709. doi: 10.1056/NEJMoa1007302

Falony, G., Joossens, M., Vieira-Silva, S., Wang, J., Darzi, Y., Faust, K., et al. (2016). Population-level analysis of gut microbiome variation. *Science* 352, 560. doi: 10.1126/science.aad3503

Fierer, N., Lauber, C. L., Ramirez, K. S., Zaneveld, J., Bradford, M. A., and Knight, R. (2012a). Comparative metagenomic, phylogenetic and physiological analyses of soil microbial communities across nitrogen gradients. *ISME J.* 6, 1007–1017. doi: 10.1038/ismej.2011.159

Fierer, N., Leff, J. W., Adams, B. J., Nielsen, U. N., Bates, S. T., Lauber, C. L., et al. (2012b). Cross-biome metagenomic analyses of soil microbial communities and their functional attributes. *Proc. Natl. Acad. Sci. U.S.A.* 109, 21390–21395. doi: 10.1073/pnas.1215210110

Flint, H. J., Scott, K. P., Louis, P., and Duncan, S. H. (2012). The role of the gut microbiota in nutrition and health. *Nat. Rev. Gastroenterol. Hepatol.* 9, 577–589. doi: 10.1038/nrgastro.2012.156

Garn, H., and Renz, H. (2007). Epidemiological and immunological evidence for the hygiene hypothesis. *Immunobiology* 212, 441–452. doi: 10.1016/j.imbio.2007.03.006

Gorzelak, M. A., Gill, S. K., Tasnim, N., Ahmadi-Vand, Z., Jay, M., and Gibson, D. L. (2015). Methods for improving human gut microbiome data by reducing variability through sample processing and storage of stool. *PLoS ONE* 10:e0134802. doi: 10.1371/journal.pone.0134802

Haahtela, T., Holgate, S., Pawankar, R., Akdis, C. A., Benjaponpitak, S., Caraballo, L., et al. (2013). The biodiversity hypothesis and allergic disease: world allergy organization position statement. *World Allergy Organ. J.* 6:3. doi: 10.1186/1939-4551-6-3

Hanski, I., von Hertzen, L., Fyhrquist, N., Koskinen, K., Torppa, K., Laatikainen, T., et al. (2012). Environmental biodiversity, human microbiota, and allergy are interrelated. *Proc. Natl. Acad. Sci. U.S.A.* 109, 8334–8339. doi: 10.1073/pnas.1205624109

Harmsen, H. J. M., and de Goffau, M. C. (2016). "The human gut microbiota," in. *Microbiota of the Human Body: Implications in Health and Disease,* ed A. Schwiertz (Cham: Springer International Publishing), 95–108.

Hooper, L. V., and Gordon, J. I. (2001). Commensal host-bacterial relationships in the gut. *Science* 292, 1115–1118. doi: 10.1126/science.1058709

Hooper, L. V., Littman, D. R., Macpherson, A. J., and Program, M. P. (2015). Interactions between the microbiota and the immune system. *Science* 336, 1268–1273. doi: 10.1126/science.1223490

Hunter, D. J. (2005). Gene-environment interactions in human diseases. *Nat. Rev. Genet.* 6, 287–298. doi: 10.1038/nrg1578

Huttenhower, C., Gevers, D., Knight, R., Abubucker, S., Badger, J. H., Chinwalla, A. T., et al. (2012). Structure, function and diversity of the healthy human microbiome. *Nature* 486, 207–214. doi: 10.1038/nature11234

Inoue, R., and Ushida, K. (2003). Vertical and horizontal transmission of intestinal commensal bacteria in the rat model. *FEMS Microbiol. Ecol.* 46, 213–219. doi: 10.1016/S0168-6496(03)00215-0

Isolauri, E., Arvola, T., Sütas, Y., Moilanen, E., and Salminen, S. (2000). Probiotics in the management of atopic eczema. *Clin. Exp. Allergy* 30, 1604–1610. doi: 10.1046/j.1365-2222.2000.00943.x

Kamada, N., Chen, G. Y., Inohara, N., and Nú-ez, G. (2013). control of pathogens and pathobionts by the gut microbiota. *Nat. Rev. Immunol.* 14, 685–690. doi: 10.1038/ni.2608

Kay, A. B. (2000). Overview of 'allergy and allergic diseases: with a view to the future'. *Br. Med. Bull.* 56, 843–864. doi: 10.1258/0007142001903481

Knights, D., Kuczynski, J., Charlson, E. S., Zaneveld, J., Mozer, M. C., Collman, R. G., et al. (2011). Bayesian community-wide culture-independent microbial source tracking. *Nat. Methods* 8, 761–763. doi: 10.1038/nmeth.1650

Lauber, C. L., Ramirez, K. S., Aanderud, Z., Lennon, J., and Fierer, N. (2013). Temporal variability in soil microbial communities across land-use types. *ISME J.* 7, 1641–1650. doi: 10.1038/ismej.2013.50

Ley, R. E., Peterson, D. A., and Gordon, J. I. (2006). Ecological and evolutionary forces shaping microbial diversity in the human intestine. *Cell* 124, 837–848. doi: 10.1016/j.cell.2006.02.017

Lozupone, C., Stombaugh, J., Gonzalez, A., Ackermann, G., Wendel, D., Vázquez-Baeza, Y., et al. (2013). Meta-analyses of studies of the human microbiota. *Genome Res.* 23, 1704–1714. doi: 10.1101/gr.151803.112

Lynch, S. V., and Pedersen, O. (2016). The human intestinal microbiome in health and disease. *New Engl. J. Med.* 375, 2369–2379. doi: 10.1056/NEJMra1600266

Manrique, P., Bolduc, B., Walk, S. T., van der Oost, J., de Vos, W. M., and Young, M. J. (2016). Healthy human gut phageome. *Proc. Natl. Acad. Sci. U.S.A.* 113, 10400–10405. doi: 10.1073/pnas.1601060113

Marchant, A., and Goldman, M. (2005). T cell-mediated immune responses in human newborns: ready to learn? *Clin. Exp. Immunol.* 141, 10–18. doi: 10.1111/j.1365-2249.2005.02799.x

Martínez, I., Stegen James, C., Maldonado-Gómez Maria, X., Eren, A. M., Siba Peter, M., Greenhill Andrew, R., et al. (2015). The gut microbiota of rural papua new guineans: composition, diversity patterns, and ecological processes. *Cell Rep.* 11, 527–538. doi: 10.1016/j.celrep.2015.03.049

Mayer, E. A, Tillisch, K., and Gupta, A. (2015). Gut / brain axis and the microbiota. *J. Clin. Invest.* 125, 926–938. doi: 10.1172/JCI76304

Metzger, M. J., Brus, D. J., Bunce, R. G. H., Carey, P. D., Gonçalves, J., Honrado, J. P., et al. (2013). Environmental stratifications as the basis for national, European and global ecological monitoring. *Ecol. Indic.* 33(Suppl. C), 26–35. doi: 10.1016/j.ecolind.2012.11.009

Mosca, A., Leclerc, M., and Hugot, J. P. (2016). Gut microbiota diversity and human diseases: should we reintroduce key predators in our ecosystem? *Front. Microbiol.* 7:455. doi: 10.3389/fmicb.2016.00455

Navas-Molina, J. A., Peralta-Sánchez, J. M., González, A., McMurdie, P. J., Vázquez-Baeza, Y., Xu, Z., et al. (2013). Advancing our understanding of the human microbiome using QIIME. *Methods Enzymol.* 531, 371–444. doi: 10.1016/B978-0-12-407863-5.00019-8

Popkin, B. M. (1999). Urbanization, lifestyle changes and the nutrition transition. *World Dev.* 27, 1905–1916. doi: 10.1016/S0305-750X(99)00094-7

Ramirez, K. S., Lauber, C. L., Knight, R., Bradford, M. A., and Fierer, N. (2010). Consistent effects of nitrogen fertilization on soil bacterial communities in contrasting systems. *Ecology* 91, 3414–3463. doi: 10.1890/10-0426.1

Rawls, J. F., Mahowald, M. A., Ley, R. E., and Gordon, J. I. (2006). Reciprocal gut microbiota transplants from zebrafish and mice to germ-free recipients reveal host habitat selection. *Cell* 127, 423–433. doi: 10.1016/j.cell.2006.08.043

Rook, G. A. W. (2012). Hygiene hypothesis and autoimmune diseases. *Clin. Rev . Allergy Immunol.* 42, 5–15. doi: 10.1007/s12016-011-8285-8

Rook, G. A. W., Lowry, C. A., and Raison, C. L. (2013). Microbial 'old friends', immunoregulation and stress resilience. *Evol. Med. Public Health.* 2013, 46–64. doi: 10.1093/emph/eot004

Round, J. L., and Mazmanian, S. K. (2009). The gut microbiota shapes intestinal immune responses during health and disease. *Nat. Rev. Immunol.* 9, 313–323. doi: 10.1038/nri2515

Schnorr, S. L., Candela, M., Rampelli, S., Centanni, M., Consolandi, C., Basaglia, G., et al. (2014). Gut microbiome of the Hadza hunter-gatherers. *Nat. Commun.* 5:3654. doi: 10.1038/ncomms4654

Seedorf, H., Griffin, N. W., Ridaura, V. K., Reyes, A., Cheng, J., Rey, F. E., et al. (2014). Bacteria from diverse habitats colonize and compete in the mouse gut. *Cell* 159, 253–266. doi: 10.1016/j.cell.2014.09.008

Segata, N., Izard, J., Waldron, L., Gevers, D., Miropolsky, L., Garrett, W. S., et al. (2011). Metagenomic biomarker discovery and explanation. *Genome Biol.* 12:R60. doi: 10.1186/gb-2011-12-6-r60

Shin, N. R., Whon, T. W., and Bae, J. W. (2015). Proteobacteria: microbial signature of dysbiosis in gut microbiota. *Trends Biotechnol.* 33, 496–503. doi: 10.1016/j.tibtech.2015.06.011

Simon, A. K., Hollander, G. A., and McMichael, A. (2015). Evolution of the immune system in humans from infancy to old age. *Proc. Biol. Sci.* 282:20143085. doi: 10.1098/rspb.2014.3085

Sjögren, Y. M., Jenmalm, M. C., Böttcher, M. F., Björkstén, B., and Sverremark-Ekström, E. (2009). Altered early infant gut microbiota in children developing allergy up to 5 years of age. *Clin. Exp. Allergy* 39, 518–526. doi: 10.1111/j.1365-2222.2008.03156.x

Strachan, D. P. (1989). Hay fever, hygiene, and household size. *BMJ* 299, 1259–1260. doi: 10.1136/bmj.299.6710.1259

Torrazza, R. M., and Neu, J. (2011). The developing intestinal microbiome and its relationship to health and disease in the neonate. *J. Perinatol.* 31, S29–S34. doi: 10.1038/jp.2010.172

Torsvik, V., and Øvreås, L. (2002). Microbial diversity and function in soil: from genes to ecosystems. *Curr. Opin. Microbiol.* 5, 240–245. doi: 10.1016/S1369-5274(02)00324-7

Tun, H. M., Konya, T., Takaro, T. K., Brook, J. R., Chari, R., Field, C. J., et al. (2017). Exposure to household furry pets influences the gut microbiota of infants at 3–4 months following various birth scenarios. *Microbiome* 5, 40. doi: 10.1186/s40168-017-0254-x

Turner, W. R., Nakamura, T., and Dinetti, M. (2004). Global urbanization and the separation of humans from nature. *Bioscience* 54, 585–590. doi: 10.1641/0006-3568(2004)054[0585:GUATSO]2.0.CO;2

von Hertzen, L., Hanski, I., and Haahtela, T. (2011). Natural immunity. Biodiversity loss and inflammatory diseases are two global megatrends that might be related. *EMBO Rep.* 12, 1089–1093. doi: 10.1038/embor.2011.195

Wall, D. H., Nielsen, U. N., and Six, J. (2015). Soil biodiversity and human health. *Nature* 528, 69–76. doi: 10.1038/nature15744

Wardle, D. A., Bardgett, R. D., Klironomos, J. N., Setälä, H., van der Putten, W. H., and Wall, D. H. (2004). Ecological linkages between aboveground and belowground biota. *Science* 304, 1629–1633. doi: 10.1126/science.1094875

Wills-Karp, M., Santeliz, J., and Karp, C. L. (2001). The germless theory of allergic disease: revisiting the hygiene hypothesis. *Nat. Rev. Immunol.* 1, 69–75. doi: 10.1038/35095579

Wopereis, H., Oozeer, R., Knipping, K., Belzer, C., and Knol, J. (2014). The first thousand days - intestinal microbiology of early life: establishing a symbiosis. *Pediatr. Allergy Immunol.* 25, 428–438. doi: 10.1111/pai.12232

Zhou, D., Zhang, H., Bai, Z., Zhang, A., Bai, F., Luo, X., et al. (2015). Exposure to soil, house dust, and decaying plants increases gut microbial diversity and decreases serum IgE levels in BALB/c mice. *Environ. Microbiol.* 18, 1326–1337. doi: 10.1111/1462-2920.12895

18

Dynamics of Viral and Host Immune Cell MicroRNA Expression during Acute Infectious Mononucleosis

Vandana Kaul[1†], Kenneth I. Weinberg[2], Scott D. Boyd[3], Daniel Bernstein[4], Carlos O. Esquivel[1], Olivia M. Martinez[1,5†] and Sheri M. Krams[1,5*†]*

[1] Division of Abdominal Transplantation, Department of Surgery, Stanford University, Stanford, CA, United States, [2] Division of Stem Cell Transplantation, Department of Pediatrics, Stanford University, Stanford, CA, United States, [3] Department of Pathology, Stanford University, Stanford, CA, United States, [4] Division of Cardiology, Department of Pediatrics, Stanford University, Stanford, CA, United States, [5] Stanford Immunology, Stanford University School of Medicine, Stanford, CA, United States

***Correspondence:**
Sheri M. Krams
smkrams@stanford.edu
Olivia M. Martinez
omm@stanford.edu

†Co-senior authors

Epstein–Barr virus (EBV) is the etiological agent of acute infectious mononucleosis (IM). Since acute IM is a self-resolving disease with most patients regaining health in 1–3 weeks there have been few studies examining molecular signatures in early acute stages of the disease. MicroRNAs (miRNAs) have been shown, however, to influence immune cell function and consequently the generation of antibody responses in IM. In this study, we performed a comprehensive analysis of differentially expressed miRNAs in early stage uncomplicated acute IM. miRNAs were profiled from patient peripheral blood obtained at the time of IM diagnosis and at subsequent time points, and pathway analysis performed to identify important immune and cell signaling pathways. We identified 215 differentially regulated miRNAs at the most acute stage of infection when the patients initially sought medical help. The number of differentially expressed miRNAs decreased to 148 and 68 at 1 and 2 months post-primary infection, with no significantly changed miRNAs identified at 7 months post-infection. Interferon signaling, T and B cell signaling and antigen presentation were the top pathways influenced by the miRNAs associated with IM. Thus, a dynamic and regulated expression profile of miRNA accompanies the early acute immune response, and resolution of infection, in IM.

Keywords: RNA, acute infectious mononucleosis, Epstein–Barr virus, immunology

INTRODUCTION

Epstein–Barr virus is a gamma-herpes family virus that infects over 95% of humans globally and is the etiological agent of many acute and chronic infections as well as human malignancies (Khan and Hashim, 2014). While EBV infection is widespread, the outcome of infection can depend upon the age of the host. Pediatric cases are mainly asymptomatic and the infection subsides due to a vigorous host T cell response with the virus subsequently transitioning to latency in a subset

Abbreviations: EBV: Epstein–Barr virus; FDR, false discovery rate; IPA, ingenuity pathway analysis; miRNA, microRNA; PBMC, peripheral blood mononuclear cells.

of memory B cells (Jayasooriya et al., 2015; Gantt et al., 2016). However, in adolescents, primary infection can manifest as glandular fever, lymphadenopathy, and a sore throat, termed infectious mononucleosis (IM) (Balfour et al., 2013). IM is associated with a transient proliferation of EBV-infected B cells followed by a considerable expansion of EBV-specific T cells (Sixbey et al., 1984; Kurth et al., 2000; Chaganti et al., 2009; Hadinoto et al., 2009; Balfour et al., 2013). IM is typically self-limiting and resolves over a period of weeks to months with the virus persisting into a latent phase in infected B cells (Hochberg et al., 2004).

MicroRNAs are small 18–25 nt long single-stranded RNA molecules which regulate gene expression at the post-transcriptional level. miRNA target specific mRNAs by complementary base-pairing, leading to cleavage or repression of translation, and can act as major regulators of key cellular processes. We (Harris et al., 2010) and others (Forte et al., 2012; Mansouri et al., 2014) have shown that EBV infection can alter the expression of host miRNAs and thus modulate various arms of the cellular machinery including cell differentiation and death, proliferation, and the immune response. Along these lines, miR-194 is suppressed by EBV and participates in regulation of IL-10 expression in EBV lymphomas (Harris et al., 2010) while two miRNA families, the let-7 family and the miR-200 family, as well as miR-143-3p, act as tumor-suppressor miRNAs and are significantly downregulated in EBV-infected gastric carcinoma cells (Marquitz et al., 2014). Other studies have found that miR-155 and miR-21 were induced in B cells by EBV infection and potentially play a role in viral tumorigenesis (Linnstaedt et al., 2010; Rosato et al., 2012; Anastasiadou et al., 2015). Furthermore, p53-targeted tumor suppressor, miR-34a, is strongly induced by EBV infection in many EBV and Kaposi's sarcoma-associated herpesvirus-infected lymphoma cell lines and plays a role in B cell transformation (Forte et al., 2012). In addition, miRNAs have been identified that play a critical role in the T cell response to pathogens. For example, miR-155 is essential for the $CD8^{+}$ effector T cell response to mCMV (Dudda et al., 2013).

In addition to host miRNAs, EBV-expressed miRNAs have also been shown to modulate the function of T and B cells during an immune response. In a study by Albanese et al. (2016), EBV-encoded miRNAs were found to inhibit $CD8^{+}$ T cell-mediated viral surveillance at multiple levels. The viral miRNAs downregulate TAP-complex and HLA allotype that present TAP-dependent epitopes, reduce IL-12 secretion by infected B cells to diminish EBV-specific CD8 T cells and repress EBNA1, a viral protein responsible for latency (Albanese et al., 2016). EBV encoded miRNAs miR-BART1, miR-BART2, and miR-BHRF1-2 have also been shown to target the host adaptive immune response by repressing IL-12 secretion resulting in reduced differentiation of $CD4^{+}$ T cells into the Th1 subset and inhibiting lysosomal enzymes involved in MHC class-II peptide processing (Tagawa et al., 2016), while miR-BART16 suppresses Type I IFN signaling (Hooykaas et al., 2017). In the current study, we report the differential expression of host and viral miRNAs in acute IM caused by primary EBV infection. Our findings elucidate the miRNA signature associated with acute IM and demonstrate the dynamic features of this response with the miRNA expression profile reverting to that of healthy individuals within a few months of IM diagnosis in subjects without complications.

MATERIALS AND METHODS

Patient Samples

Peripheral blood samples were obtained from symptomatic patients (aged 18–24 years) who visited Vaden Student Health Center at Stanford University and were diagnosed with clinical IM. Samples were obtained upon diagnosis (time point 0) and then at, 1, 2, and 7 months. Blood samples were processed using Ficoll-Paque PLUS (Amersham Pharmacia Biotech, Piscataway, NJ, United States) then PBMC frozen and maintained in liquid nitrogen until use. PBMCs were isolated from blood derived from healthy age-matched individuals. This study was carried out in accordance with the recommendations of Institutional Review Board at Stanford University with written informed consent from all subjects. All subjects gave written informed consent in accordance with the Declaration of Helsinki.

RNA Isolation and miRNA Microarray

Patient ($n = 16$) and healthy control ($n = 3$) PBMCs were suspended and lysed in TRIzol Reagent (Life Technologies, Foster City, CA, United States) for isolation of total RNA. Glycogen (20 μg) was used for RNA precipitation. Isolated RNA was DNase treated (Qiagen) and clean-up was done on RNeasy spin columns (Qiagen) using a modified protocol which replaced RW1 buffer with RWT buffer for washing. RNA was suspended in RNase free water and stored at −80°C. RNA quantification was done using Nanodrop 2000 Spectrophotometer (Thermo Fisher scientific, Wilmington, DE, United States). Approximately 200 ng RNA was used for microarray analysis using Affymetrix GeneChip miRNA 4.0 arrays (Affymetrix, Santa Clara, CA, United States) through the PAN (Protein and Nucleic acid) facility at Stanford University. Briefly, 130 ng total RNA was assessed for quality using Bioanalyzer 2100 (Agilent), followed by Poly-A tailing and labeling with biotin using a Affymetrix FlashTag Biotin HSR RNA Labeling kit (Affymetrix, Santa Clara, CA, United States) according to the manufacturer's protocol. The labeled targets are hybridized to the GeneChip® miRNA 4.0 arrays per standard miRNA protocol, which includes 16 h (overnight) hybridization at 48°C at 60 RPM in the Affymetrix GeneChip Hybridization oven 645. The arrays were then washed and stained in the Affymetrix GeneChip Fluidics Station 450. The arrays were scanned using the Affymetrix GeneChip Scanner 3000 7G. The GeneChip® miRNA 4.0 arrays contain 30,424 total mature miRNA probe sets including 2578 mature human miRNAs, 2025 pre-miRNA human probes, 1996 Human snoRNA and scaRNA probe sets and miRNAs of 202 other organisms.

Data Analysis

Raw microarray data were statistically analyzed using Partek Genomics Suite software (Partek Inc.). Normalization was done suing Robust Multi-array Average (RMA) and log2 transformation of data was performed, followed by one-way ANOVA statistical testing to identify significantly differentially expressed miRNA between different groups ($P \leq 0.05$). After running ANOVA, the software performs multi-testing correction using Benjamini–Hochberg Step-Up FDR-controlling procedure for all the expressed miRNAs (default FDR Alpha level 0.05). Venn diagram depicting intersection of differentially expressed miRNAs and Unsupervised Hierarchical Clustering analysis was also performed. Raw Fold change and adjusted *p*-value data was exported to dot excel file and data selection and graphic visualization was done using Power BI software (Microsoft Inc.). Differentially expressed EBV miRNAs were also identified using the same miRNA microarray dataset using the miRNA filter as "EBV," mRNA expression data from a publicly available GEO dataset (GSE45924) was used to perform miRNA–mRNA integrated analysis. Briefly, SOFT formatted family file (GSE45924-GPL6883_series_matrix.piv.txt.fmt) were downloaded from the GEO Database and imported into Partek Genomics Suite for mRNA "Gene Expression" workflow. Illumina HumanRef-8 v3.0 expression beadchip annotation files were uploaded to the Partek Software to obtain Fold Change Values for mRNA differential expression between comparison groups of Acute IM subjects (PBMC) and control subjects (PBMC). Pre-normalized data was log2 transformed, followed by one-way ANOVA statistical testing to identify significantly differentially expressed mRNAs and multiple-testing correction using Benjamini–Hochberg Step-Up FDR-controlling procedure (default FDR Alpha level 0.05). Fold increases of >2, and fold decreases of >2 were considered significant. The differentially expressed mRNA data was exported into a text file and converted into a suitable format for upload to IPA for further analysis.

Functional and Pathway Enrichment Analysis of Target Genes Controlled by Differentially Expressed miRNAs

Pathway and molecular function enrichment analysis was performed using IPA software (Qiagen, Redwood city, CA, United States). A list of all twofold differentially expressed miRNAs obtained from Partek Genomics Suite software analysis was uploaded into IPA for analysis. miRNA target enrichment was performed using the "miRNA Target Filter" function, generating a list of 181 miRNAs with available targeting information. An mRNA gene expression dataset (GSE45924) obtained from GEO database was added to the "miRNA Target Filter" setting in IPA and "Expression pairing" was performed. An additional filter applied to this list was "Applied filters: confidence = Experimentally Observed OR High (predicted)." Further "Core Analysis" was performed on the target mRNAs based on different experimental time points to determine the affected networks and canonical pathways. Throughout the analysis, a *p*-value cutoff of 0.05 was applied. The HumanRef-8 v3.0 reference gene list was used to set the population of genes to consider for *p*-value calculations while performing Core Analysis.

RESULTS

Sample QC and Principal Component Analysis

As a means of quality control to determine the biological separation of the groups based on probe intensities, principal component analysis (PCA) was performed using Partek Genomics software. Two separate groups of samples from IM patients at 0 month (at the time of diagnosis) and healthy controls are clearly observed (**Figure 1**). The remaining samples from 1, 2, and 7 months are loosely segregated into groups and fall between these two groups on PC1 with the samples obtained at 7 months grouping closely with those from healthy controls. These findings indicate that the differentially expressed miRNAs are maximal at the time of IM diagnosis and return to the healthy control pattern in subsequent months.

Differentially Expressed miRNAs

The differential expression of miRNAs were compared between patients at the time of IM diagnosis (0 month), and at 1 and 2 months after diagnosis, compared to age-matched healthy controls (**Figure 2A**). We identified 215 differentially regulated miRNAs at the most acute stage of infection (diagnosis, 0 month). The number of differentially expressed miRNAs decreased to 148 and 68 during the course of 1 and 2 months post-primary infection, with no significantly changed miRNAs identified at 7 months post-infection (data not shown). The 27 top differentially expressed miRNAs at diagnosis, and 1 and 2 months after diagnosis, show that most of the differentially expressed miRNAs are increased (25 increased, 2 decreased) (**Figure 2B**).

Unsupervised hierarchical clustering depicted as a heatmap shows the relative intensity for the 215, 148, and 68 differentially expressed miRNAs at diagnosis (**Figure 3**), 1 month (Supplementary Figure S1) and 2 months (Supplementary Figure S2) as compared to healthy controls, respectively. A fold change of two and FDR adjusted *p*-value (Benjamini–Hochberg method for multiple corrections) of 0.05 was considered significant in Partek Genomics Suite Software, with black depicting decreased expression levels and blue depicting upregulation. Furthermore, the differentially expressed miRNAs demonstrate a decreasing absolute fold change over time, with the highest fold change generally observed at the time of diagnosis (**Figure 4**). These 41 miRNAs exhibit a dynamic differential expression pattern that trends toward healthy control levels at 2 months post IM diagnosis. Two miRNAs that are highly upregulated, miR-4417 and miR-4485 (data not shown), exhibit a similar trend of decreasing differential expression from diagnosis to 2 months. A compilation of all statistically significant differentially expressed miRNAs at diagnosis and one, and 2 months versus healthy controls is included in Supplementary Table S1. Supplementary Table S2 provides a list of all differentially expressed miRNAs. A Venn diagram depicts the number of miRNAs in common at IM diagnosis and at 1 and 2 months (**Figure 5**). The intersection shows that 56 miRNAs are differentially expressed at the three time points, thus providing important information regarding possible disease

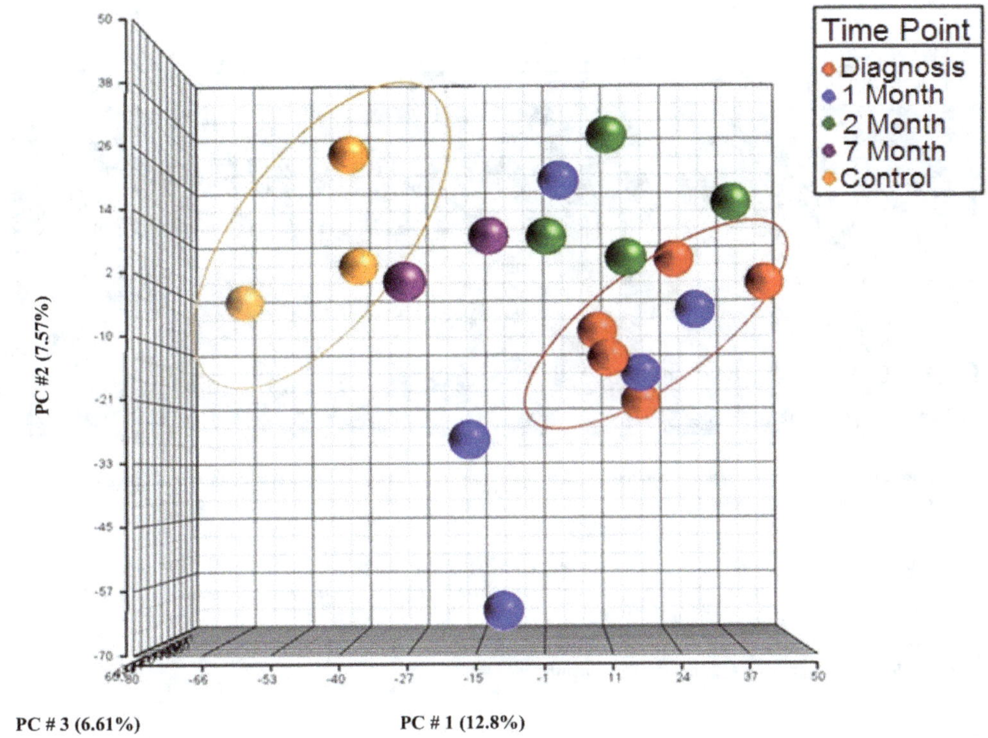

FIGURE 1 | Principal component analysis (PCA) on miRNA expression data from human peripheral blood mononuclear cells (PBMCs) from acute infectious mononucleosis (IM) patients and healthy controls using the first three components. Red, at diagnosis; Blue, 1 month; Green, 2 months; Purple, 7 months; Orange, Healthy control.

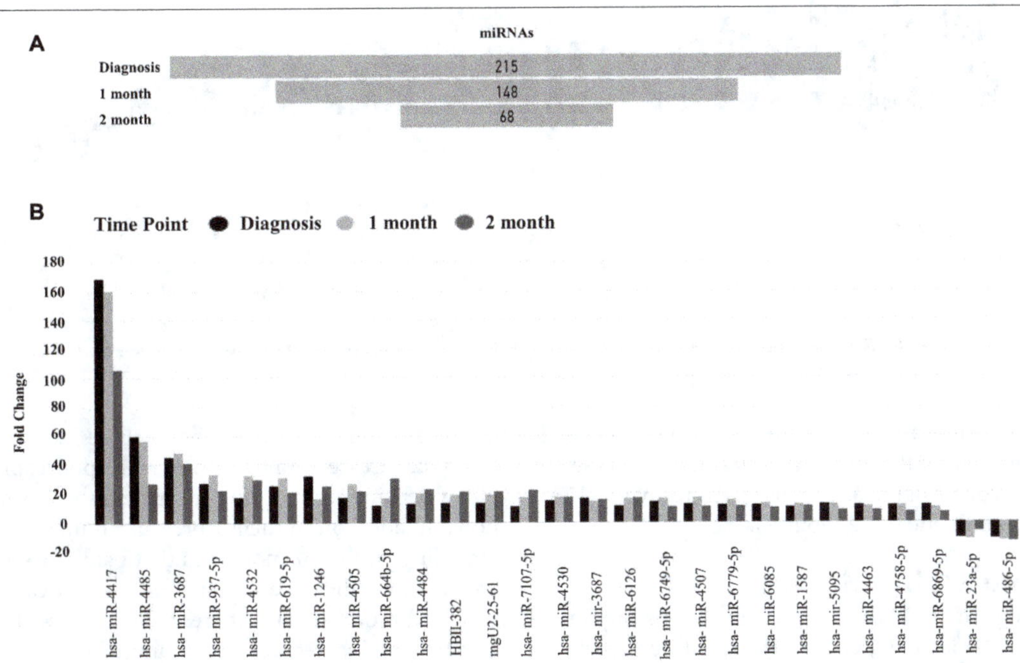

FIGURE 2 | Top differentially expressed microRNAs (miRNAs). **(A)** Differentially expressed miRNAs in IM Patients at Time 0, 1, and 2 months compared to healthy controls, **(B)** Top differentially expressed miRNAs observed at all three time points, at diagnosis, 1, and 2 months vs. healthy controls [false discovery rate (FDR) 0.05, Absolute Fold change > 10].

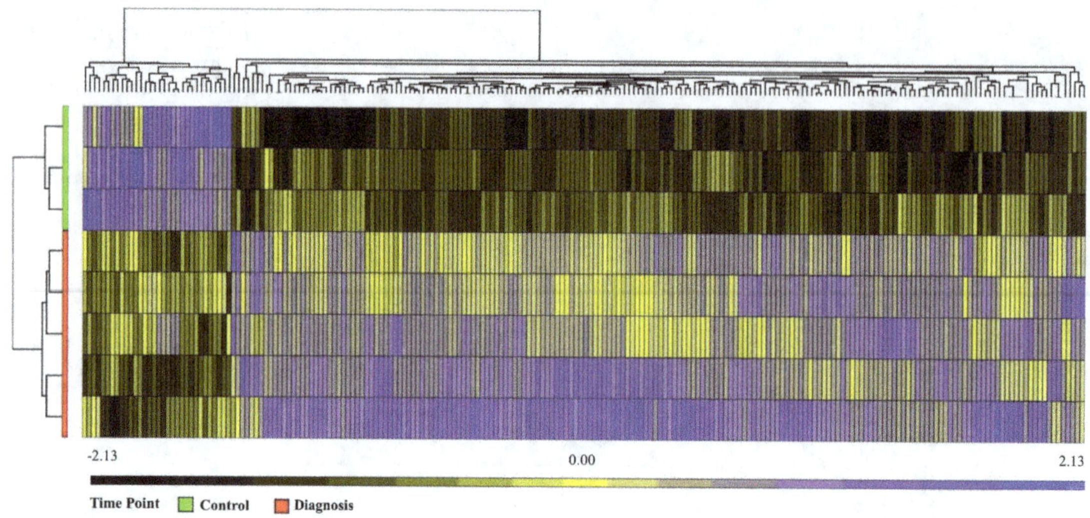

FIGURE 3 | Unsupervised Hierarchical Clustering Heatmap showing relative intensity for 215 miRNAs in Patients at diagnosis versus healthy controls. Analysis using Partek Genomics suite, step up FDR 0.05. Black shows downregulation and blue shows upregulation. Healthy controls (green), IM at diagnosis (red).

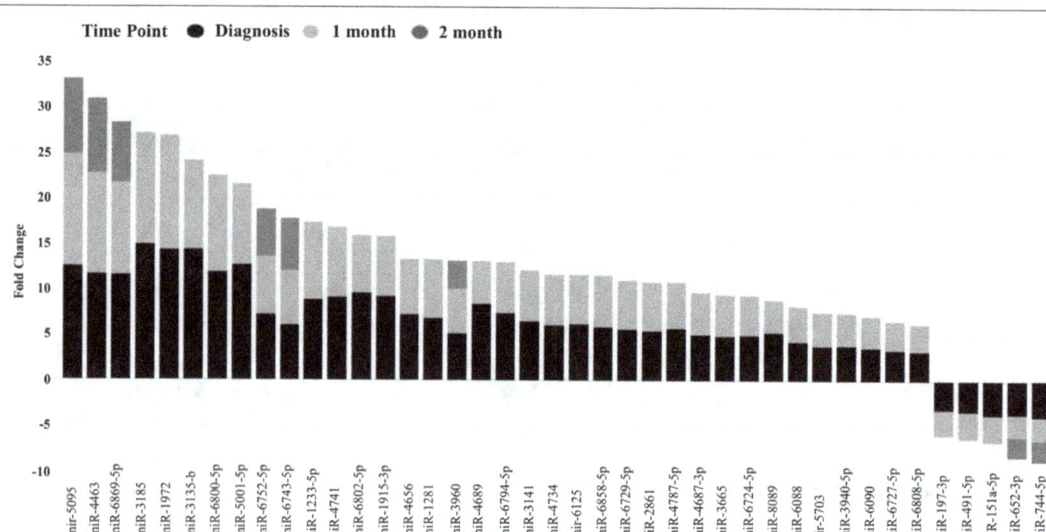

FIGURE 4 | Differentially expressed miRNAs at three time points, at Diagnosis, 1 and 2 months showing a trend toward decreasing absolute fold change (FDR 0.05).

specific signatures. Interestingly, miRNAs uniquely expressed at diagnosis, 1 and 2 months after diagnosis also decrease in number during the course of the infection toward recovery (79 at diagnosis, 15 at 1 month and 9 at 2 months).

Pathways Altered by IM

Expression pairing of miRNA data, from our study and gene expression data from GEO set GSE45924 returned 46 miRNAs targeting 17 mRNAs (**Figure 6A**). Comparative analysis of mRNA targets highlighted the most canonical pathways as well as disease and biological functions (**Figures 6B,C**). Furthermore, functional pathway analysis in IPA using the list of differentially expressed miRNAs at 0 month suggests the most impacted networks include antigen presentation, infectious disease, humoral immune response, protein synthesis, cell cycle, and cell death mechanisms. Networks have been shown in addition to their scores and number of mRNA targets (including particular molecules that pass our set filter criterion) (**Table 1**). Further analysis in IPA for top canonical pathways targeted by our list of differentially expressed miRNAs at IM diagnosis and based on the Illumina HumanRef-8 v3.0 gene superset shows candidates including interferon signaling, altered T and B cell signaling, primary immunodeficiency signaling, antigen presentation and communication between innate and adaptive immune cells as the major affected canonical pathways (Supplementary Figure S3).

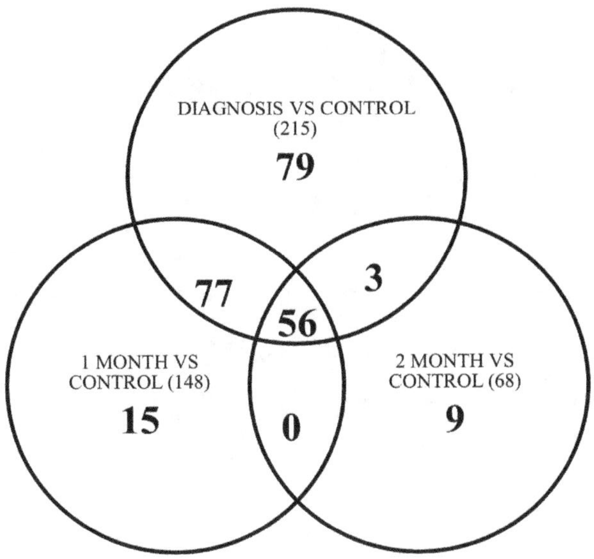

FIGURE 5 | Venn diagram depicting number of miRNAs common between point of diagnosis, 1 and 2 months versus healthy control. Number in brackets () is the total number of differentially expressed miRNAs at that time point vs. control.

Differentially Expressed EBV miRNAs

Interestingly, when the EBV miRNAs are analyzed using specific filtering criteria in Partek, only ebv-miR-BART-16 and ebv-miR-BART5-3p are uniquely upregulated at IM diagnosis and at 1 and 2 months as compared to healthy controls (ANOVA 0.05, unadjusted *p*-value) (**Table 2**). It is notable that no differential expression of any EBV miRNAs is observed at 7 months post-infection, which is expected due to resolution of the symptoms in the acute phase and establishment of EBV latency. Thus, of the more than 40 known EBV miRNAs only two, miR-BART5-3p and miR-BART-16 are expressed during acute IM (Skinner et al., 2017).

DISCUSSION

This study provides the first miRNA expression profile of sequential, peripheral blood samples from college-age patients with acute IM. Our results clearly indicate that primary EBV disease is accompanied by marked expression changes of multiple host and viral miRNA, and that the number of differentially expressed miRNAs decreases substantially after the initial diagnosis. It is noteworthy that there were no differentially expressed miRNAs observed at 7 months as compared to healthy controls, indicating that there is no identifiable miRNA signature that can distinguish between normal college students and those that have resolved IM. Since none of the patients studied had any complications after IM, it remains possible that expression of the differentially expressed host miRNAs would remain dysregulated if IM were not completely resolved.

We determined that 43 of the host miRNAs, including miR-197-3p, miR-491-5p, miR-151a-5p, miR-652-3p, and miR-744-5p, decreased from the levels found at diagnosis over the subsequent 2 months. While the specific function of these miRNA in IM is unknown, other reports have linked these miRNA to disease processes. Recently, miR-197 was found to act synergistically with EBV-BART6-3p to reduce the expression of IL-6R, thereby compromising host immune defense in EBV-positive Burkitt Lymphoma (Zhang et al., 2017). miR-625-3p has been shown to be a potential biomarker for a number of cancerous conditions including malignant pleural mesothelioma (Kirschner et al., 2012). miR-625-3p targets p38

TABLE 1 | List of top five networks with their respective scores obtained from ingenuity pathway analysis (IPA): Data are indicative of networks regulated by mRNA targets of microRNAs (miRNAs) differentially expressed at the time of infectious mononucleosis (IM) diagnosis.

Top diseases and functions	Score	Focus molecules*	Molecules in network
Antigen presentation, protein synthesis, infectious disease	36	13	BCR (complex), ↓**CD79A**, ERK1/2, ↑**FBX06**, ↓**FCRLA**, ↑**GBP2**, ↑**GBP4**, ↑**GBP5,** IFNα, β, IFN type1, Ifnar, Ifnz, IgG, IgM, IL12 (family), ↑**LMNB1**, ↓**LTB**, MHC Class I (complex), NF-κB (complex) Nr1hPirb, ↑**PSMB8**, ↑**RARRES3,** RNA polymerase II, SLFN13, ↑**STAT1**, ↑**TAP1**, TBCB, TCR, ↓**TLR10**, Trbv1
Hematological system development and function, humoral immune response, lymphoid tissue structure and development	3	1	FOXO1, IGHM, KLF3, SOX11, ↓**VPREB3**
Cell morphology, cellular function and maintenance, connective tissue disorders	2	1	APP, HNF4A, HOXD4, LIG4, SAFB2, ZNF24, ZNF396, ZSCAN1, ZSCAN18, ZSCAN20, ↓**ZSCAN32**
Cell cycle cellular assembly and organization, DNA replication, recombination and repair	2	1	BLM, CCND1, CENPS/CENPS-CORT, dihydrotestosterone, ERCC6L, FAAP100, FANCA, FANCM, NOTCH3, RIF3, RMI1, ↑**RMI2**, RPA1, RPA2, RPA3, SPIDR, TOP3A, TOPBP1, TTK
Cell cycle, gene expression, cell death and survival	2	1	All *trans*-retinyl esters, CREBBP, ↓**DHRS3**, ELAVLi, EP300, FSH, GPS2, Lh, N-cor, NADP-retinol dehydrogenase, OSM, PLA2G10, PPARG, RAF1, RDH, RDH10, retinyl ester, SNCA, TNF, TP73, tretinoin

**Focus Molecules (in bold)- molecules that passed the filters and cut-offs that are members of this network.*

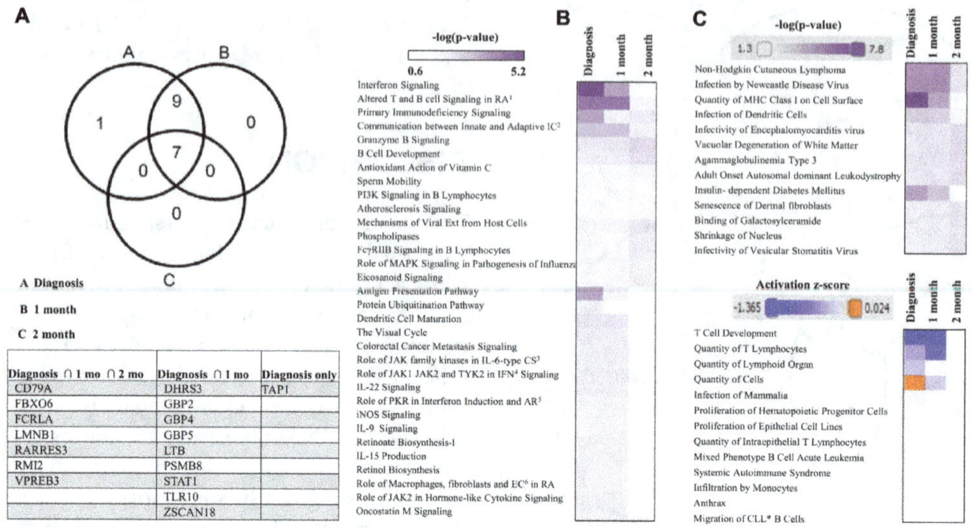

FIGURE 6 | mRNA targets and associated pathways of the differentially expressed miRNAs. **(A)** Venn diagram and table comparison of mRNA targets of differentially expressed miRNAs at Diagnosis, 1 and 2 months. **(B)** Comparison of canonical pathways, **(C)** Comparison of Diseases and Bio Functions; mRNA targets were obtained from miRNA–mRNA expression pairing of differentially expressed miRNAs and GEO dataset GSM1119621–GSM1119636 in ingenuity pathway analysis (IPA).

TABLE 2 | Differentially expressed EBV miRNAs in patients at diagnosis, 1 and 2 months versus healthy controls, ANOVA 0.05, unadjusted *p*-value.

	0 Month (diagnosis)			1 Month			2 Months		
EBV miRNA	**Fold change**	***p*-value**	**↑/↓**	**Fold change**	***p*-value**	**↑/↓**	**Fold change**	***p*-value**	**↑/↓**
ebv-miR-BART16	2.93	0.00	↑	2.75	0.01	↑	2.11	0.04	↑
ebv-miR-BART5-3p	2.44	0.02	↑	2.57	0.01	↑	2.85	0.01	↑

MAPK activator MAP2K6 and induces oxaliplatin resistance by abrogating MAP2K6-p38-regulated apoptosis and cell cycle control networks (Rasmussen et al., 2016). A recent study also shows that miR-625-3p is upregulated in CD8$^+$ T cells during early immune reconstitution following allogeneic stem cell transplantation (Verma et al., 2017). An interesting study with highly virulent H5N2 strain of mouse-adapted avian influenza virus found miR-151a-p as one of the significantly upregulated miRNAs, whose inhibition resulted in a 70% reduction in mortality of inoculated mice (Choi et al., 2014).

The majority of studies to date examining the impact of EBV infection or pathogenesis on miRNA expression have focused on the miRNA profile within the virally infected cell and the implications for tumorigenesis. In contrast, we analyzed the impact of EBV infection on peripheral lymphoid cells that typically participate in the immune response to EBV. A single previous study did examine the cellular miRNAs from pre-adolescent children with IM in China over the first 14 days after primary infection (Gao et al., 2015). They determined the host miRNA expression in B cells and CD8$^+$ T cells and EBV miRNAs in plasma and B cells. Interestingly, some miRNAs such as miR-155 and miR-142 were increased in B cells and decreased in CD8$^+$ T cells, thus, changes would not be reflected in unfractionated PBMC. Our analysis of miRNAs in PBMC demonstrated a different set of host miRNAs as differentially expressed. These distinct patterns are most likely attributed to different methodologies, since our study took an unbiased approach and performed microarray analysis using Affymetrix GeneChip miRNA 4.0 arrays (over 30,000 mature miRNAs) on unfractionated PBMC, whereas the Gao group specifically examined a small subset of 84 miRNAs in sorted B and T cells via PCR. Further, the ages of the subjects were different and there could be other differences including environmental factors and variant strains of EBV. EBV expresses more miRNAs than other characterized human viruses, with at least 44 EBV miRNAs identified to date (Skinner et al., 2017). We determined that ebv-miR-BART16 and ebv-miR-BART5-3p were increased in PBMC as compared to healthy controls. The specific function of these viral miRNA in IM is unknown, but it is interesting that a recent report indicates that BART16 suppresses IFN signaling (Hooykaas et al., 2017). Notably, the EBV miRNA profile we identified in acute IM is distinct from the EBV miRNA profile identified in plasma samples of patients with chronic active EBV infection (Kawano et al., 2013).

In addition to EBV-induced miRNA regulation in infected B cells, others have focused on understanding the EBV pathogenesis and host responses by transcriptomic (mRNA microarray, Illumina) analysis on PBMCs of human subjects in a prospective study of naturally acquired primary EBV infection (Dunmire et al., 2014). The authors found a distinct gene expression profile in acute but not latent EBV infection. Moreover, upon gene expression profiling in sorted $CD8^+$ T cells, NK cells, monocytes, and B cells, it was found that $CD8^+$ T cells and monocytes showed upregulation of key gene groups (Type I interferon regulated genes (IRGs), type II IRGs, and cell cycle/metabolism genes.) during acute infection. This pathway analysis agrees with the pathways predicted to be altered by our miRNA profile during acute IM.

CONCLUSION

We have defined the host immune cell and EBV miRNA profile elicited by primary EBV infection during acute IM. This profile is indicative of a response that is accompanied by complete resolution of disease. Thus, it may be useful in predicting which individuals that present with IM will have an uncomplicated course and ultimately may shed insight into the host immune response to acute EBV infection.

AUTHOR CONTRIBUTIONS

VK designed and performed experiments, analyzed the data, and wrote the manuscript. KW obtained the samples and contributed to development of study design. SB contributed to development of study design and critically revised the manuscript. DB contributed to development of study design. CE contributed to development of study design. OM contributed to study design, provided critical review of the experimental design, wrote, and provided critical review of the manuscript. SK designed the study, analyzed the data, wrote, and critically reviewed the manuscript. All authors reviewed and approved the final manuscript.

FUNDING

VK was supported by fellowship from the Transplant and Tissue Engineering Center of Excellence at Lucile Packard Children's Hospital. Funding was also obtained from the Lucile Packard Children's Hospital Heart Center Research Fund (DB, KW, and SB). OM was partially funded by AI115313, SK was partially funded by AI119686, KW, SB, DB, CE, OM, SK were partially supported by AI104342.

ACKNOWLEDGMENT

The authors would like to acknowledge Natalia V. Kosovilka from Stanford PAN facility for help with microarray experiments.

REFERENCES

Albanese, M., Tagawa, T., Bouvet, M., Maliqi, L., Lutter, D., Hoser, J., et al. (2016). Epstein-Barr virus microRNAs reduce immune surveillance by virus-specific $CD8^+$ T cells. *Proc. Natl. Acad. Sci. U.S.A.* 113, E6467–E6475. doi: 10.1073/pnas.1605884113

Anastasiadou, E., Garg, N., Bigi, R., Yadav, S., Campese, A. F., Lapenta, C., et al. (2015). Epstein-Barr virus infection induces miR-21 in terminally differentiated malignant B cells. *Int. J. Cancer* 137, 1491–1497. doi: 10.1002/ijc.29489

Balfour, H. H., Odumade, O. A., Schmeling, D. O., Mullan, B. D., Ed, J. A., Knight, J. A., et al. (2013). Behavioral, virologic, and immunologic factors associated with acquisition and severity of primary Epstein-Barr virus infection in university students. *J. Infect. Dis.* 207, 80–88. doi: 10.1093/infdis/jis646

Chaganti, S., Heath, E. M., Bergler, W., Kuo, M., Buettner, M., Niedobitek, G., et al. (2009). Epstein-Barr virus colonization of tonsillar and peripheral blood B-cell subsets in primary infection and persistence. *Blood* 113, 6372–6381. doi: 10.1182/blood-2008-08-175828

Choi, E.-J., Kim, H. B., Baek, Y. H., Kim, E.-H., Pascua, P. N. Q., Park, S.-J., et al. (2014). Differential microRNA expression following infection with a mouse-adapted, highly virulent avian H5N2 virus. *BMC Microbiol.* 14:252. doi: 10.1186/s12866-014-0252-0

Dudda, J. C., Salaun, B., Ji, Y., Palmer, D. C., Monnot, G. C., Merck, E., et al. (2013). MicroRNA-155 is required for effector $CD8^+$ T cell responses to virus infection and cancer. *Immunity* 38, 742–753. doi: 10.1016/j.immuni.2012.12.006

Dunmire, S. K., Odumade, O. A., Porter, J. L., Reyes-Genere, J., Schmeling, D. O., Bilgic, H., et al. (2014). Primary EBV infection induces an expression profile distinct from other viruses but similar to hemophagocytic syndromes. *PLOS ONE* 9:e85422. doi: 10.1371/journal.pone.0085422

Forte, E., Salinas, R. E., Chang, C., Zhou, T., Linnstaedt, S. D., Gottwein, E., et al. (2012). The Epstein-Barr virus (EBV)-induced tumor suppressor microRNA MiR-34a is growth promoting in EBV-infected B cells. *J. Virol.* 86, 6889–6898. doi: 10.1128/JVI.07056-11

Gantt, S., Orem, J., Krantz, E. M., Morrow, R. A., Selke, S., Huang, M.-L., et al. (2016). Prospective characterization of the risk factors for transmission and symptoms of primary human herpesvirus infections among ugandan infants. *J. Infect. Dis.* 214, 36–44. doi: 10.1093/infdis/jiw076

Gao, L., Ai, J., Xie, Z., Zhou, C., Liu, C., Zhang, H., et al. (2015). Dynamic expression of viral and cellular microRNAs in infectious mononucleosis caused by primary Epstein-Barr virus infection in children. *Virol. J.* 12:208. doi: 10.1186/s12985-015-0441-y

Hadinoto, V., Shapiro, M., Sun, C. C., and Thorley-Lawson, D. A. (2009). The dynamics of EBV shedding implicate a central role for epithelial cells in amplifying viral output. *PLOS Pathog.* 5:e1000496. doi: 10.1371/journal.ppat.1000496

Harris, A., Krams, S. M., and Martinez, O. M. (2010). MicroRNAs as immune regulators: implications for transplantation. *Am. J. Transplant.* 10, 713–719. doi: 10.1111/j.1600-6143.2010.03032.x

Hochberg, D., Souza, T., Catalina, M., Sullivan, J. L., Luzuriaga, K., and Thorley-Lawson, D. A. (2004). Acute infection with Epstein-Barr virus targets and overwhelms the peripheral memory B-cell compartment with resting, latently infected cells. *J. Virol.* 78, 5194–5204. doi: 10.1128/JVI.78.10.5194-5204.2004

Hooykaas, M. J. G., van Gent, M., Soppe, J. A., Kruse, E., Boer, I. G. J., van Leenen, D., et al. (2017). EBV MicroRNA BART16 suppresses Type I IFN signaling. *J. Immunol.* 198, 4062–4073. doi: 10.4049/jimmunol.1501605

Jayasooriya, S., de Silva, T. I., Njie-jobe, J., Sanyang, C., Leese, A. M., Bell, A. I., et al. (2015). Early virological and immunological events in asymptomatic Epstein-Barr virus infection in African children. *PLOS Pathog.* 11:e1004746. doi: 10.1371/journal.ppat.1004746

Kawano, Y., Iwata, S., Kawada, J.-I., Gotoh, K., Suzuki, M., Torii, Y., et al. (2013). Plasma viral microRNA profiles reveal potential biomarkers for chronic active

Epstein-Barr virus infection. *J. Infect. Dis.* 208, 771–779. doi: 10.1093/infdis/jit222

Khan, G., and Hashim, M. (2014). Global burden of deaths from Epstein-Barr virus attributable malignancies 1990-2010. *Infect. Agent. Cancer* 9:38. doi: 10.1186/1750-9378-9-38

Kirschner, M. B., Cheng, Y. Y., Badrian, B., Kao, S. C., Creaney, J., Edelman, J. J. B., et al. (2012). Increased circulating miR-625-3p: a potential biomarker for patients with malignant pleural mesothelioma. *J. Thorac. Oncol.* 7, 1184–1191. doi: 10.1097/JTO.0b013e3182572e83

Kurth, J., Spieker, T., Wustrow, J., Strickler, G. J., Hansmann, L. M., Rajewsky, K., et al. (2000). EBV-infected B cells in infectious mononucleosis: viral strategies for spreading in the B cell compartment and establishing latency. *Immunity* 13, 485–495. doi: 10.1016/S1074-7613(00)00048-0

Linnstaedt, S. D., Gottwein, E., Skalsky, R. L., Luftig, M. A., and Cullen, B. R. (2010). Virally induced cellular microRNA miR-155 plays a key role in B-cell immortalization by Epstein-Barr virus. *J. Virol.* 84, 11670–11678. doi: 10.1128/JVI.01248-10

Mansouri, S., Pan, Q., Blencowe, B. J., Claycomb, J. M., and Frappier, L. (2014). Epstein-Barr virus EBNA1 protein regulates viral latency through effects on let-7 microRNA and dicer. *J. Virol.* 88, 11166–11177. doi: 10.1128/JVI.01785-14

Marquitz, A. R., Mathur, A., Chugh, P. E., Dittmer, D. P., and Raab-Traub, N. (2014). Expression profile of microRNAs in Epstein-Barr virus-infected AGS gastric carcinoma cells. *J. Virol.* 88, 1389–1393. doi: 10.1128/JVI.02662-13

Rasmussen, M. H., Lyskjær, I., Jersie-Christensen, R. R., Tarpgaard, L. S., Primdal-Bengtson, B., Nielsen, M. M., et al. (2016). miR-625-3p regulates oxaliplatin resistance by targeting MAP2K6-p38 signalling in human colorectal adenocarcinoma cells. *Nat. Commun.* 7:12436. doi: 10.1038/ncomms12436

Rosato, P., Anastasiadou, E., Garg, N., Lenze, D., Boccellato, F., Vincenti, S., et al. (2012). Differential regulation of miR-21 and miR-146a by Epstein–Barr virus-encoded EBNA2. *Leukemia* 26, 2343–2352. doi: 10.1038/leu.2012.108

Sixbey, J. W., Nedrud, J. G., Raab-Traub, N., Hanes, R. A., and Pagano, J. S. (1984). Epstein–Barr virus replication in oropharyngeal epithelial cells. *N. Engl. J. Med.* 310, 1225–1230. doi: 10.1056/NEJM198405103101905

Skinner, C. M., Ivanov, N. S., Barr, S. A., Chen, Y., and Skalsky, R. L. (2017). An Epstein-Barr virus microRNA blocks IL-1 signaling by targeting the interleukin-1 receptor 1. *J. Virol.* 91:e00530-17. doi: 10.1128/JVI.00530-17

Tagawa, T., Albanese, M., Bouvet, M., Moosmann, A., Mautner, J., Heissmeyer, V., et al. (2016). Epstein-Barr viral miRNAs inhibit antiviral $CD4^+$ T cell responses targeting IL-12 and peptide processing. *J. Exp. Med.* 213, 2065–2080. doi: 10.1084/jem.20160248

Verma, K., Jyotsana, N., Buenting, I., Luther, S., Pfanne, A., Thum, T., et al. (2017). miR-625-3p is upregulated in CD8+ T cells during early immune reconstitution after allogeneic stem cell transplantation. *PLOS ONE* 12:e0183828. doi: 10.1371/journal.pone.0183828

Zhang, Y.-M., Yu, Y., and Zhao, H.-P. (2017). EBV-BART-6-3p and cellular microRNA-197 compromise the immune defense of host cells in EBV-positive Burkitt lymphoma. *Mol. Med. Rep.* 15, 1877–1883. doi: 10.3892/mmr.2017.6173

19

Influence of Oral and Gut Microbiota in the Health of Menopausal Women

*Angélica T. Vieira[1], Paula M. Castelo[2,3], Daniel A. Ribeiro[3,4] and Caroline M. Ferreira[2,3]**

[1] Department of Biochemistry and Immunology, Institute of Biological Sciences, Federal University of Minas Gerais, Belo Horizonte, Brazil, [2] Department of Pharmaceutics Sciences, Institute of Environmental, Chemical and Pharmaceutical Sciences, Universidade Federal de São Paulo, Diadema, Brazil, [3] Pathology Graduate Program, Universidade Federal de São Paulo, São Paulo, Brazil, [4] Department of Biosciences, Universidade Federal de São Paulo, Santos, Brazil

***Correspondence:**
Caroline M. Ferreira
caroline.nu.ferreira@gmail.com

Sex differences in gut microbiota are acknowledged, and evidence suggests that gut microbiota may have a role in higher incidence and/or severity of autoimmune diseases in females. Additionally, it has been suggested that oral, vaginal, and gut microbiota composition can be regulated by estrogen levels. The association of vaginal microbiota with vulvovaginal atrophy at menopause is well described in the literature. However, the relevance of oral and gut microbiota modulation in the immune system during estrogen deficiency and its effect on inflammatory diseases is not well explored. Estrogen deficiency is a condition that occurs in menopausal women, and it can last approximately 30 years of a woman's life. The purpose of this mini- review is to highlight the importance of alterations in the oral and gut microbiota during estrogen deficiency and their effect on oral and inflammatory diseases that are associated with menopause. Considering that hormone replacement therapy is not always recommended or sufficient to prevent or treat menopause-related disease, we will also discuss the use of probiotics and prebiotics as an option for the prevention or treatment of these diseases.

Keywords: saliva, oral health, mouth diseases, gut microbiota, estrogen, menopause

INTRODUCTION

We harbor trillions of microorganisms that associate with specific tissues and are termed microbiota. This rich community of microorganisms, mostly bacteria, has co-evolved in a symbiotic relationship with humans in such a way that it is now essential for several physiological functions and controls many aspects of host physiology (Backhed et al., 2005; Backhed, 2012; Grover and Kashyap, 2014).

One of the factors that plays a pivotal role in microbiota modulation, although broadly understudied in current research, is the change in female sexual hormones throughout life. Two phases occur in a woman's life that are characterized by several physiological, metabolic and immunological changes: menarche, or the first menstruation of a woman, which occurs during adolescence between 10 and 15 years of age (Hoffmann et al., 2004), and menopause, which occurs between age 45 and 55 and includes the cessation of menstrual periods and loss of the reproductive function of the ovaries (Brotman et al., 2014). In fact, estrogen and the microbiota of a woman's body tend to be investigated more extensively during the woman's reproductive years than during menopause or the phase of estrogen decline. One exception is the vaginal microbiota, which has been widely investigated during menopause. Here, we consider menopause or the menopausal phase, including perimenopause (before menopause), menopause and postmenopause (after menopause).

Considering that menopause can last for approximately 30 years of a woman's life (Brotman et al., 2014), the purpose of this mini-review is to highlight the importance of alterations in the oral and gut microbiota during estrogen deficiency and determine their relevance in oral infections and inflammatory diseases that are associated with menopause.

THE INTERACTION BETWEEN ORAL MICROBIOTA AND FEMALE SEX HORMONES

The oral cavity (mouth) is composed of several distinct microbial habitats, including the lips, the teeth, the gingival sulcus, the tongue, the cheeks, the palate and the tonsils, which are colonized by hundreds of different bacterial, viral, and fungal species (Dewhirst et al., 2010; Yost et al., 2015). The microbial communities associated with these structures are in symbiosis with the host (Sanz et al., 2017). However, in the presence of stressors that can perturb this homeostasis, several oral infectious diseases may appear, including dental caries and periodontitis (Almstahl et al., 2010; Dewhirst et al., 2010). Many of these disease are recognized to be caused by the consortia of organisms in a biofilm rather than a single pathogen (Jenkinson and Lamont, 2005). In addition, poor oral health and oral diseases may be associated with many systemic diseases (Seymour et al., 2007), such as cardiovascular diseases (Joshipura et al., 1996; Montebugnoli et al., 2004; Belenguer et al., 2006), stroke (Joshipura et al., 2003), preterm birth (Offenbacher et al., 1998), diabetes (Genco et al., 2005), and pneumonia (Awano et al., 2008).

In healthy individuals, the microorganisms found in the mouth with the largest representation include *Streptococcus*, *Actinomyces*, *Veillonella*, *Fusobacterium*, *Porphyromonas*, *Prevotella*, *Treponema*, *Neisseria*, *Haemophilus*, *Eubacteria*, *Lactobacterium*, *Capnocytophaga*, *Eikenella*, *Leptotrichia*, *Peptostreptococcus*, *Staphylococcus*, and *Propionibacterium* (Jenkinson and Lamont, 2005; Liu et al., 2012). The behavior of these organisms can be very dynamic and adapt to a wide range of environments and interactions with other microbial species while aggregated in biofilms over the oral surfaces.

Estrogen receptor-beta has been detected in the oral mucosa and salivary glands (Valimaa et al., 2004), and some evidence shows age-related hormonal changes in the exfoliated normal buccal mucosa of women (Donald et al., 2013). Moreover, the vaginal and buccal epithelia share some microscopic similarities. As observed by Thompson et al. (2001), the patterns of surface keratinization and the distribution and appearance of the lipid lamellae in the intercellular spaces were similar between vaginal and buccal epithelial samples of postmenopausal women. Therefore, given that many menopausal women also suffer from oral discomforts in addition to climacteric symptoms (Meurman et al., 2009), an understanding of the impact of female sex hormones on the characteristics of the oral microbiota may be clinically relevant, especially during menopause. Some of the main complaints from women in menopause include dry mouth and tooth loss, and the existing data have focused on the salivary microbial composition and the microbiota characteristics of the gingival sulcus. Therefore, this review will explore the main findings of the relationship between the oral microbiota and menopause in saliva and periodontal support.

Saliva

Saliva plays an important role in the maintenance of oral health integrity and the protection against dental caries and other oral diseases (Marsh et al., 2016; Wang et al., 2016). The salivary microbiota is highly diverse and complex (Curtis et al., 2011).

Estrogen and menopause-related hormonal imbalances are believed to affect oral health (Cao et al., 2007). According to the literature (Meurman et al., 2009), together with climacteric complaints, various oral discomforts are reported in menopausal women. The main peri- and postmenopausal symptoms include xerostomia (subjective oral dryness) and/or hyposalivation (Mahesh et al., 2014), which may increase the occurrence of mucosal and dental diseases, such as candidiasis. Few studies have investigated the effects of hormone replacement therapy in such patients (Mahesh et al., 2014; Lago et al., 2015), although the existing results show an improvement in symptoms following such treatment (Mahesh et al., 2014; Lago et al., 2015).

The quantitative and qualitative changes in saliva may alter the regular homeostasis of oral health, subsequently leading to specific changes in the salivary bacterial composition (Nasidze et al., 2009, 2011; Belstrøm et al., 2014). However, recent findings have shown that patients with severe hyposalivation do not differ in their bacterial profiles compared with those with normal salivary flow rates (Belstrom et al., 2016), although the corresponding study did not focus on the evaluation of such differences between menopausal and non-menopausal women.

Because the salivary composition may be influenced by the presence of oral diseases, prescribed medications and general health (Belstrom et al., 2016), researchers must pay attention to the sample size and control for confounding factors when revising the existing literature to confirm the external validity of any quantitative and qualitative changes in saliva related to menopause.

Periodontal Support

The periodontium is the specialized tissue that both surrounds and supports the teeth. Periodontal disease, which includes gingivitis and periodontitis, is highly prevalent in adults, and disease severity increases with age. This inflammatory disease develops over time with the accumulation of biofilm (dental plaque), bacterial dysbiosis, the formation of periodontal pockets, gum recession, and tissue destruction (including alveolar bone loss), which can ultimately lead to tooth loss (Michaud et al., 2017).

Fluctuating female sexual hormone levels in menopausal women may represent key factors that respond to changes detected in the oral cavity (Dutt et al., 2013). Menopause is accompanied by decreased bone density, which may have implications for oral health such as the risk of enhanced progression of periodontal infections and tooth loss (Hernandez-Vigueras et al., 2016). According to the literature, sex-related hormonal changes may cause the gums to become more susceptible to plaque and create a much higher risk for gingivitis and advanced periodontitis (Suresh and Radfar, 2004).

Periodontitis is a chronic inflammatory process that occurs in response to an increase in Gram-negative bacteria in the biofilm (Ruby and Barbeau, 2002), affecting the tissues that surround and support the teeth. Specific bacterial species, such as *Porphyromonas gingivalis* and *Tannerella forsythensis*, were found to be important in the etiology of periodontitis in postmenopausal women (Brennan et al., 2007). In addition, changes in periodontal status were found to be associated with variations in sex hormone levels (Mascarenhas et al., 2003), and the occurrence of periodontitis was reported to be greater in postmenopausal women who did not receive hormone replacement than in premenopausal women (Haas et al., 2009). Therefore, from a clinical point of view, the roles of sex hormones and hormone therapy in the prevalence of subgingival bacterial infection in peri- and postmenopausal women are of great interest.

In a cohort study that included 106 women aged 50–58 years, hormone replacement therapy led to a decreased number of positive samples showing the periodontal pathogens *P. gingivalis, Prevotella intermedia,* and *T. forsythia* from the subgingival plaque (Tarkkila et al., 2010). Consistent with this result, a previous study found improved periodontal probing depths and tooth mobility in 190 randomized women who received hormone therapy for 1 year (López-Marcos et al., 2005). Conversely, Pilgram et al. (2002) investigated 135 women in a randomized, controlled trial who received estrogen replacement for 3 years and did not find any changes in clinical parameters such as the attachment of teeth or the bone mineral density of the lumbar spine. In mice, estrogen seems to modulate IL-1 production and participate in the resistance of females to disseminating dentoalveolar infections, leading to the enhanced localization of these infections (Youssef and Stashenko, 2017), which draws attention to the potential role of sex-related hormones in the modulation of oral mucosal infections.

Non-conventional treatment approaches for oral infections, with a particular emphasis on dental biofilm-related diseases, have gained attention in recent years. The use of probiotics and prebiotics to improve gastrointestinal health has now led to an interest in using these treatments to control oral diseases (Allaker and Ian Douglas, 2015). However, few studies have focused on recovery of the oral equilibrium by promoting beneficial microbiota. Despite differences in the composition of the gut and oral microbiota, the community types observed in the gut are predictive of the community observed in the mouth and vice versa (Ding and Schloss, 2014). Among other host factors, the oral microbiota serves as an inoculum for the intestine, and the microorganisms that find adequate conditions in the mouth give rise to distinct types of communities in the intestine. Interestingly, oral inoculation with *P. gingivalis* in experimental models leads to a change in the intestinal microbiota, which is a possible mechanism for the establishment of diseases associated with periodontitis, such as cardiovascular diseases (Arimatsu et al., 2014). In this sense, understanding the role of health-associated microorganisms may have utility in the application of these approaches for the prevention and treatment of disease (Sanz et al., 2017).

THE INTERACTION BETWEEN GUT MICROBIOTA AND FEMALE SEX HORMONES

As mentioned earlier, female sex hormones levels influence the composition of the microbiota in many sites of the body, especially the gut. Due to intimate contact with the larger gut immune system, the gut microbiota has been shown to influence many diseases outside of this organ (**Figure 1**). Accordingly, imbalance of the gut microbiota, called dysbiosis, has been extensively related to metabolic and immunological diseases. Interestingly, the presence or absence of estrogen may be able to alter the gut microbiota equilibrium and corresponding disease pathways. Some autoimmune diseases affect more often women than men, including systemic lupus erythematosus (Jiang et al., 2005), Sjogren's syndrome (Patel and Shahane, 2014) and rheumatoid arthritis (Oliver and Silman, 2009). Gender differences have also been reported for the outcome of microbial infections (Fischer et al., 2015). Interestingly, the onset of autoimmune diseases, asthma (Akinbami et al., 2016) and other diseases occurs after menarche or during the reproductive period of women. Experimental findings in mice have shown that the interactions among the microbiota, female sexual hormones, and immunity are associated with the development of autoimmune diseases (Yurkovetskiy et al., 2013, 2015), including type 1 diabetes (Markle et al., 2013) and rheumatoid arthritis (Wu et al., 2010). The non-obese diabetic (NOD) mouse exhibits spontaneous, immune-mediated pancreatic beta cell destruction causing type 1 diabetes (T1D) with a complex genetic and environmental etiology. The NOD T1D incidence shows a strong 2:1 female to male sex bias (Markle et al., 2013). Interestingly, germ-free NOD female mice lack this gender bias for diabetes. Additionally, after castration, males exhibit a similar microbiota composition and T1D incidence to females (Markle et al., 2013). In general, this study shows that the microbiome is a causal factor and not simply a consequence of autoimmune disease.

The Relevance of the Gut Microbiota in the Health of Menopausal Women

When the interaction between the gut microbiota and estrogen is altered due to a lack of estrogen, this relationship is restructured according to the new circumstances. However, host functional alterations, such as metabolic and immunological changes, also occur.

Obesity affects 65% of postmenopausal women and is associated with the onset of metabolic dysfunction (Leeners et al., 2017). Multiple studies have suggested that postmenopausal women exhibit increased total fat mass and abdominal fat and

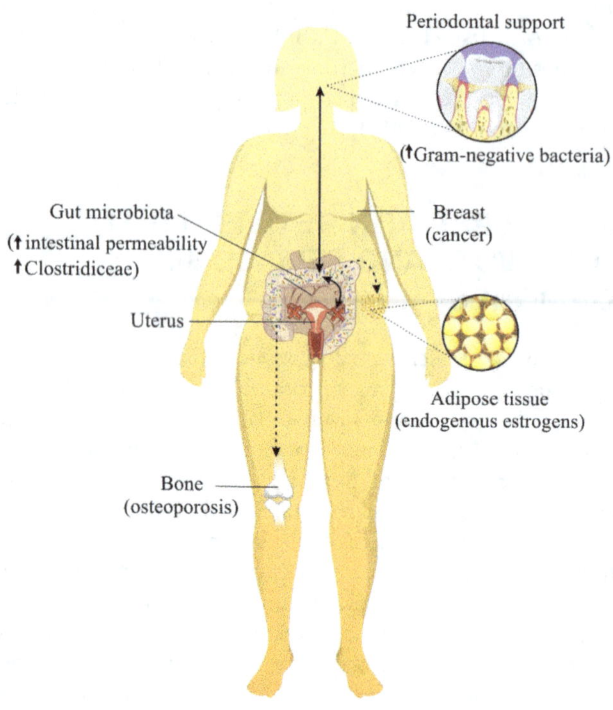

FIGURE 1 | Female sexual hormones levels influence the composition of the microbiota in many sites of the body, especially mouth and gut. The oral and gut microbiota have been shown to influence many diseases, such as osteoporosis, weight gain and lipid deposition, breast cancer and periodontitis.

decreased lean body mass compared with those of premenopausal women, regardless of aging (Aloia et al., 1995; Schreiner et al., 1996; Cordina-Duverger et al., 2016). The accumulation of abdominal fat in postmenopausal women appears to be a critical factor in the development of insulin resistance and type 2 diabetes (Lobo et al., 2014), and the relationship between the gut microbiota and a lack of estrogen is likely responsible for weight gain and lipid deposition during menopause (**Figure 1**). The gut microbiota can metabolize estrogen-like compounds such as isoflavonoids, which are found in soy foods, and promote the growth of some specific bacteria (Frankenfeld et al., 2014; Chen and Madak-Erdogan, 2016; Miller et al., 2017). Indeed, the administration of soy isoflavones to postmenopausal women was shown to increase the concentration of *Bifidobacterium* and suppress Clostridiaceae, which are known to be involved in inflammatory diseases (Frankenfeld et al., 2014; Nakatsu et al., 2014). This suppression of Clostridiaceae, a family of Clostridia associated with obesity (**Figure 1**), likely explains why diets containing phytoestrogens have been shown to improve weight gain in menopausal women.

Few studies have investigated whether prebiotics and probiotics can improve insulin sensitivity in postmenopausal women or body fat in mice. The intake of flaxseed mucilage, a prebiotic, is known to improve insulin sensitivity and alter the gut microbiota in obese postmenopausal women (Brahe et al., 2015). Thus far, the implications of the gut microbiota with low levels or the absence of estrogen hormone in the metabolism of women have not been sufficiently studied and require further clarification.

Another link between the gut microbiome and menopausal health is related to bone. Interesting, the gut microbiota has also been found to influence bone homeostasis. Approximately one in two women over age 50 will break a bone because of osteoporosis. A study that involved twenty postmenopausal women with a mean age of 65 years showed that the group that consumed *Lactobacillus helveticus*-fermented milk had increased serum calcium levels and reduced bone reabsorption compared with those of the control milk consumption group (Narva et al., 2004). Experimental studies have also demonstrated similar results. For instance, *L. reuteri* treatment significantly protected ovariectomized mice from bone loss and increases in bone marrow CD4+ T-lymphocytes, which promote osteoclastogenesis (Britton et al., 2014). Another study that investigated probiotic treatment for cortical bone loss found reduced expression of two inflammatory cytokines, TNF-α and IL-1β, and increased expression of osteoprotegerin, a potent inhibitor of osteoclastogenesis, in the cortical bone of ovariectomized mice (Ohlsson et al., 2014). Additionally, sex steroid deprivation has been reported to promote intestinal permeability (**Figure 1**), and the oral administration of *L. rhamnosus* GG (LGG) or VSL#3 (a combination of tree probiotics) to estrogen-deficient mice significantly reinforced intestinal barrier integrity and completely protected the mice against sex steroid depletion-induced bone loss (Li et al., 2016). Importantly, to confirm the role of the gut microbiota in bone health, another experiment also showed that germ-free mice are protected against the bone loss induced by the absence of sex steroids (Li et al., 2016).

We must mention that the gut microbiota may influence the risk for breast cancer through effects on endogenous estrogens produced by adipose tissue in postmenopausal women (**Figure 1**) (Key et al., 2003). A cross-sectional study on 60 healthy postmenopausal women found that women with a more diverse gut microbiome and an abundance of four Clostridia taxa exhibited an elevated urinary ratio of hydroxylated estrogen metabolites to parent estrogens (Fuhrman et al., 2014), which is related to the etiology of breast cancer (Flores et al., 2012; Kwa et al., 2016). However, another study compared 48 postmenopausal breast cancer patients and 48 control patients and observed that postmenopausal women with breast cancer exhibited an altered composition and estrogen-independent low diversity of their microbiota (Goedert et al., 2015). These different findings on gut microbiota diversity and breast cancer could be explained by the fact that disease outcome or disease stage can also affect the microbiota. In this scenario, the consumption of the soy isoflavone daidzein, which is metabolized by some bacteria of the microbiota to generate equol and O-desmethylangolensin (ODMA), could represent a therapeutic strategy for breast cancer prevention. Some, but not all, studies have shown a lower risk of breast cancer associated with equol production (Hullar et al., 2014). However, only approximately 30–50% of the population can metabolize daidzein (Frankenfeld et al., 2004; Uehara, 2013; Nakatsu et al., 2014) to equol, likely due to the host microbiota. Therefore, an investigation into the administration of the soy isoflavone daidzein together with probiotic bacteria to produce equol is warranted and could offer benefits in the prevention of breast cancer in menopausal women.

CONCLUDING REMARKS

Many chronic diseases can emerge after estrogen levels decline, which will affect a considerable part of a woman's life. Understanding the role of the microbiota in women's health at the menopausal phase could help to improve strategies for microbiota modulation and prevent dysfunction. The oral and gut microbiotas have been extensively studied in women of reproductive age, while the menopausal period has been somewhat overlooked. The use of hormone replacement is not indicated for all menopausal women, and considering that probiotics and prebiotics can affect the dysfunction of bone, adipose tissue, oral and other tissues, such treatments may constitute an important therapeutic strategy. Pro- and prebiotics can also be used in conjunction with menopause hormone therapy and may attenuate the side effects that can arise from hormone replacement. In conclusion, the scientific findings published to date do not definitively demonstrate how non-vaginal microbiota sites influence the health of menopausal women. Thus, many questions remain unanswered and warrant further investigation to improve the quality of life of menopausal women.

AUTHOR CONTRIBUTIONS

AV, PC, DR, and CF drafted and revised the manuscript.

FUNDING

This work was supported by grants awarded by the São Paulo Research Foundation (FAPESP), project number 2012/50410-8 to CF and the National Council for Scientific and Technological Development (CNpq), project number 486037/2012-6.

REFERENCES

Akinbami, L. J., Simon, A. E., and Schoendorf, K. C. (2016). Trends in allergy prevalence among children aged 0–17 years by asthma status, United States, 2001–2013. *J. Asthma* 53, 356–362. doi: 10.3109/02770903.2015.1126848

Allaker, R. P., and Ian Douglas, C. W. (2015). Non-conventional therapeutics for oral infections. *Virulence* 6, 196–207. doi: 10.4161/21505594.2014.983783

Almstahl, A., Carlen, A., Eliasson, L., and Lingstrom, P. (2010). *Lactobacillus* species in supragingival plaque in subjects with hyposalivation. *Arch. Oral. Biol.* 55, 255–259. doi: 10.1016/j.archoralbio.2010.01.007

Aloia, J. F., Vaswani, A., Russo, L., Sheehan, M., and Flaster, E. (1995). The influence of menopause and hormonal replacement therapy on body cell mass and body fat mass. *Am. J. Obstet. Gynecol.* 172, 896–900. doi: 10.1016/0002-9378(95)90018-7

Arimatsu, K., Yamada, H., Miyazawa, H., Minagawa, T., Nakajima, M., Ryder, M. I., et al. (2014). Oral pathobiont induces systemic inflammation and metabolic changes associated with alteration of gut microbiota. *Sci. Rep.* 4:4828. doi: 10.1038/srep04828

Awano, S., Ansai, T., Takata, Y., Soh, I., Akifusa, S., Hamasaki, T., et al. (2008). Oral health and mortality risk from pneumonia in the elderly. *J. Dent. Res.* 87, 334–339. doi: 10.1177/154405910808700418

Backhed, F. (2012). Host responses to the human microbiome. *Nutr. Rev.* 70(Suppl.), S14–S17. doi: 10.1111/j.1753-4887.2012.00496.x

Backhed, F., Ley, R. E., Sonnenburg, J. L., Peterson, D. A., and Gordon, J. I. (2005). Host-bacterial mutualism in the human intestine. *Science* 307, 1915–1920. doi: 10.1126/science.1104816

Belenguer, A., Duncan, S. H., Calder, A. G., Holtrop, G., Louis, P., Lobley, G. E., et al. (2006). Two routes of metabolic cross-feeding between *Bifidobacterium adolescentis* and butyrate-producing anaerobes from the human gut. *Appl. Environ. Microbiol.* 72, 3593–3599. doi: 10.1128/AEM.72.5.3593-3599.2006

Belstrom, D., Holmstrup, P., Fiehn, N. E., Rosing, K., Bardow, A., Paster, B. J., et al. (2016). Bacterial composition in whole saliva from patients with severe hyposalivation–a case-control study. *Oral Dis.* 22, 330–337. doi: 10.1111/odi.12452

Belstrøm, D., Holmstrup, P., Nielsen, C. H., Kirkby, N., Twetman, S., Heitmann, B. L., et al. (2014). Bacterial profiles of saliva in relation to diet, lifestyle factors, and socioeconomic status. *J. Oral Microbiol.* 6. doi: 10.3402/jom.v6.23609

Brahe, L. K., Le Chatelier, E., Prifti, E., Pons, N., Kennedy, S., Blaedel, T., et al. (2015). Dietary modulation of the gut microbiota–a randomised controlled trial in obese postmenopausal women. *Br. J. Nutr.* 114, 406–417. doi: 10.1017/S0007114515001786

Brennan, R. M., Genco, R. J., Hovey, K. M., Trevisan, M., and Wactawski-Wende, J. (2007). Clinical attachment loss, systemic bone density, and subgingival calculus in postmenopausal women. *J. Periodontol.* 78, 2104–2111. doi: 10.1902/jop.2007.070155

Britton, R. A., Irwin, R., Quach, D., Schaefer, L., Zhang, J., Lee, T., et al. (2014). Probiotic *L. reuteri* treatment prevents bone loss in a menopausal ovariectomized mouse model. *J. Cell. Physiol.* 229, 1822–1830. doi: 10.1002/jcp.24636

Brotman, R. M., Shardell, M. D., Gajer, P., Fadrosh, D., Chang, K., Silver, M. I., et al. (2014). Association between the vaginal microbiota, menopause status, and signs of vulvovaginal atrophy. *Menopause* 21, 450–458. doi: 10.1097/GME.0b013e3182a4690b

Cao, M., Shu, L., Li, J., Su, J., Zhang, W., Wang, Q., et al. (2007). The expression of estrogen receptors and the effects of estrogen on human periodontal ligament cells. *Methods Find. Exp. Clin. Pharmacol.* 29, 329–335. doi: 10.1358/mf.2007.29.5.1117560

Chen, K. L., and Madak-Erdogan, Z. (2016). Estrogen and microbiota crosstalk: should we pay attention? *Trends Endocrinol. Metab.* 27, 752–755. doi: 10.1016/j.tem.2016.08.001

Cordina-Duverger, E., Truong, T., Anger, A., Sanchez, M., Arveux, P., Kerbrat, P., et al. (2016). Weight and weight changes throughout life and postmenopausal breast cancer risk: a case-control study in France. *BMC Cancer* 16:761. doi: 10.1186/s12885-016-2793-0

Curtis, M. A., Zenobia, C., and Darveau, R. P. (2011). The relationship of the oral microbiotia to periodontal health and disease. *Cell Host Microbe* 10, 302–306. doi: 10.1016/j.chom.2011.09.008

Dewhirst, F. E., Chen, T., Izard, J., Paster, B. J., Tanner, A. C., Yu, W. H., et al. (2010). The human oral microbiome. *J. Bacteriol.* 192, 5002–5017. doi: 10.1128/JB.00542-10

Ding, T., and Schloss, P. D. (2014). Dynamics and associations of microbial community types across the human body. *Nature* 509, 357–360. doi: 10.1038/nature13178

Donald, P. M., George, R., Sriram, G., Kavitha, B., and Sivapathasundharam, B. (2013). Hormonal changes in exfoliated normal buccal mucosal cells. *J. Cytol.* 30, 252–256. doi: 10.4103/0970-9371.126655

Dutt, P., Chaudhary, S., and Kumar, P. (2013). Oral health and menopause: a comprehensive review on current knowledge and associated dental management. *Ann. Med. Health Sci. Res.* 3, 320–323. doi: 10.4103/2141-9248.117926

Fischer, J., Jung, N., Robinson, N., and Lehmann, C. (2015). Sex differences in immune responses to infectious diseases. *Infection* 43, 399–403. doi: 10.1007/s15010-015-0791-9

Flores, R., Shi, J., Fuhrman, B., Xu, X., Veenstra, T. D., Gail, M. H., et al. (2012). Fecal microbial determinants of fecal and systemic estrogens and estrogen metabolites: a cross-sectional study. *J. Transl. Med.* 10:253. doi: 10.1186/1479-5876-10-253

Frankenfeld, C. L., Atkinson, C., Wahala, K., and Lampe, J. W. (2014). Obesity prevalence in relation to gut microbial environments capable of producing equol or O-desmethylangolensin from the isoflavone daidzein. *Eur. J. Clin. Nutr.* 68, 526–530. doi: 10.1038/ejcn.2014.23

Frankenfeld, C. L., McTiernan, A., Aiello, E. J., Thomas, W. K., LaCroix, K., Schramm, J., et al. (2004). Mammographic density in relation to daidzein-metabolizing phenotypes in overweight, postmenopausal women. *Cancer Epidemiol. Biomarkers Prev.* 13, 1156–1162.

Fuhrman, B. J., Feigelson, H. S., Flores, R., Gail, M. H., Xu, X., Ravel, J., et al. (2014). Associations of the fecal microbiome with urinary estrogens and estrogen metabolites in postmenopausal women. *J. Clin. Endocrinol. Metab.* 99, 4632–4640. doi: 10.1210/jc.2014-2222

Genco, R. J., Grossi, S. G., Ho, A., Nishimura, F., and Murayama, Y. (2005). A proposed model linking inflammation to obesity, diabetes, and periodontal infections. *J. Periodontol.* 76 11(Suppl.), 2075–2084. doi: 10.1902/jop.2005.76.11-S.2075

Goedert, J. J., Jones, G., Hua, X., Xu, X., Yu, G., Flores, R., et al. (2015). Investigation of the association between the fecal microbiota and breast cancer in postmenopausal women: a population-based case-control pilot study. *J. Natl. Cancer Inst.* 107. doi: 10.1093/jnci/djv147

Grover, M., and Kashyap, P. C. (2014). Germ-free mice as a model to study effect of gut microbiota on host physiology. *Neurogastroenterol. Motil.* 26, 745–748. doi: 10.1111/nmo.12366

Haas, A. N., Rosing, C. K., Oppermann, R. V., Albandar, J. M., and Susin, C. (2009). Association among menopause, hormone replacement therapy, and periodontal attachment loss in Southern Brazilian women. *J. Periodontol.* 80, 1380–1387. doi: 10.1902/jop.2009.090082

Hernandez-Vigueras, S., Martinez-Garriga, B., Sanchez, M. C., Sanz, M., Estrugo-Devesa, A., Vinuesa, T., et al. (2016). Oral microbiota, periodontal status, and osteoporosis in postmenopausal females. *J. Periodontol.* 87, 124–133. doi: 10.1902/jop.2015.150365

Hoffmann, J. C., Zeitz, M., Bischoff, S. C., Brambs, H. J., Bruch, H. P., Buhr, H. J., et al. (2004). [Diagnosis and therapy of ulcerative colitis: results of an evidence based consensus conference by the German society of digestive and metabolic diseases and the competence network on inflammatory bowel disease]. *Z. Gastroenterol.* 42, 979–983. doi: 10.1055/s-2004-813510

Hullar, M. A., Burnett-Hartman, A. N., and Lampe, J. W. (2014). Gut microbes, diet, and cancer. *Cancer Treat. Res.* 159, 377–399. doi: 10.1007/978-3-642-38007-5_22

Jenkinson, H. F., and Lamont, R. J. (2005). Oral microbial communities in sickness and in health. *Trends Microbiol.* 13, 589–595. doi: 10.1016/j.tim.2005.09.006

Jiang, J. F., Liu, Y. H., and Zhang, C. X. (2005). [Sex hormones in female patients with systemic lupus erythematosus]. *Zhong Nan Da Xue Xue Bao Yi Xue Ban* 30, 315–317.

Joshipura, K. J., Hung, H. C., Rimm, E. B., Willett, W. C., and Ascherio, A. (2003). Periodontal disease, tooth loss, and incidence of ischemic stroke. *Stroke* 34, 47–52. doi: 10.1161/01.STR.0000052974.79428.0C

Joshipura, K. J., Rimm, E. B., Douglass, C. W., Trichopoulos, D., Ascherio, A., and Willett, W. C. (1996). Poor oral health and coronary heart disease. *J. Dent. Res.* 75, 1631–1636. doi: 10.1177/00220345960750090301

Key, T. J., Appleby, P. N., Reeves, G. K., Roddam, A., Dorgan, J. F., Longcope, C., et al. (2003). Body mass index, serum sex hormones, and breast cancer risk in postmenopausal women. *J. Natl. Cancer Inst.* 95, 1218–1226. doi: 10.1093/jnci/djg022

Kwa, M., Plottel, C. S., Blaser, M. J., and Adams, S. (2016). The Intestinal microbiome and estrogen receptor-positive female breast cancer. *J. Natl. Cancer Inst* 108. doi: 10.1093/jnci/djw029

Lago, M. L., de Oliveira, A. E., Lopes, F. F., Ferreira, E. B., Rodrigues, V. P., and Brito, L. M. (2015). The influence of hormone replacement therapy on the salivary flow of post-menopausal women. *Gynecol. Endocrinol.* 31, 109–112. doi: 10.3109/09513590.2014.959918

Leeners, B., Geary, N., Tobler, P. N., and Asarian, L. (2017). Ovarian hormones and obesity. *Hum. Reprod. Update* 23, 300–321. doi: 10.1093/humupd/dmw045

Li, J. Y., Chassaing, B., Tyagi, A. M., Vaccaro, C., Luo, T., Adams, J., et al. (2016). Sex steroid deficiency-associated bone loss is microbiota dependent and prevented by probiotics. *J. Clin. Invest.* 126, 2049–2063. doi: 10.1172/JCI86062

Liu, B., Faller, L. L., Klitgord, N., Mazumdar, V., Ghodsi, M., Sommer, D. D., et al. (2012). Deep sequencing of the oral microbiome reveals signatures of periodontal disease. *PLOS ONE* 7:e37919. doi: 10.1371/journal.pone.0037919

Lobo, R. A., Davis, S. R., De Villiers, T. J., Gompel, A., Henderson, V. W., Hodis, H. N., et al. (2014). Prevention of diseases after menopause. *Climacteric* 17, 540–556. doi: 10.3109/13697137.2014.933411

López-Marcos, J. F., García-Valle, S., and García-Iglesias, A. A. (2005). Periodontal aspects in menopausal women undergoing hormone replacement therapy. *Med. Oral Patol. Oral Cir. Bucal* 10, 132–141.

Mahesh, D. R., Komali, G., Jayanthi, K., Dinesh, D., Saikavitha, T. V., and Dinesh, P. (2014). Evaluation of Salivary Flow Rate, pH and Buffer in Pre, Post & Post Menopausal Women on HRT. *J. Clin. Diagn. Res.* 8, 233–236. doi: 10.7860/JCDR/2014/8158.4067

Markle, J. G., Frank, D. N., Mortin-Toth, S., Robertson, C. E., Feazel, L. M., Rolle-Kampczyk, U., et al. (2013). Sex differences in the gut microbiome drive hormone-dependent regulation of autoimmunity. *Science* 339, 1084–1088. doi: 10.1126/science.1233521

Marsh, P. D., Do, T., Beighton, D., and Devine, D. A. (2016). Influence of saliva on the oral microbiota. *Periodontol. 2000* 70, 80–92. doi: 10.1111/prd.12098

Mascarenhas, P., Gapski, R., Al-Shammari, K., and Wang, H. L. (2003). Influence of sex hormones on the periodontium. *J. Clin. Periodontol.* 30, 671–681. doi: 10.1034/j.1600-051X.2003.00055.x

Meurman, J. H., Tarkkila, L., and Tiitinen, A. (2009). The menopause and oral health. *Maturitas* 63, 56–62. doi: 10.1016/j.maturitas.2009.02.009

Michaud, D. S., Fu, Z., Shi, J., and Chung, M. (2017). Periodontal disease, tooth loss, and cancer risk. *Epidemiol. Rev.* 39, 49–58. doi: 10.1093/epirev/mxx006

Miller, L. M., Lampe, J. W., Newton, K. M., Gundersen, G., Fuller, S., Reed, S. D., et al. (2017). Being overweight or obese is associated with harboring a gut microbial community not capable of metabolizing the soy isoflavone daidzein to O-desmethylangolensin in peri- and post-menopausal women. *Maturitas* 99, 37–42. doi: 10.1016/j.maturitas.2017.02.006

Montebugnoli, L., Servidio, D., Miaton, R. A., Prati, C., Tricoci, P., and Melloni, C. (2004). Poor oral health is associated with coronary heart disease and elevated systemic inflammatory and haemostatic factors. *J. Clin. Periodontol.* 31, 25–29. doi: 10.1111/j.0303-6979.2004.00432.x

Nakatsu, C. H., Armstrong, A., Clavijo, A. P., Martin, B. R., Barnes, S., and Weaver, C. M. (2014). Fecal bacterial community changes associated with isoflavone metabolites in postmenopausal women after soy bar consumption. *PLOS ONE* 9:e108924. doi: 10.1371/journal.pone.0108924

Narva, M., Nevala, R., Poussa, T., and Korpela, R. (2004). The effect of *Lactobacillus helveticus* fermented milk on acute changes in calcium metabolism in postmenopausal women. *Eur. J. Nutr.* 43, 61–68. doi: 10.1007/s00394-004-0441-y

Nasidze, I., Li, J., Quinque, D., Tang, K., and Stoneking, M. (2009). Global diversity in the human salivary microbiome. *Genome Res.* 19, 636–643. doi: 10.1101/gr.084616.108

Nasidze, I., Li, J., Schroeder, R., Creasey, J. L., Li, M., and Stoneking, M. (2011). High diversity of the saliva microbiome in Batwa Pygmies. *PLOS ONE* 6:e23352. doi: 10.1371/journal.pone.0023352

Offenbacher, S., Jared, H. L., O'Reilly, P. G., Wells, S. R., Salvi, G. E., Lawrence, H. P., et al. (1998). Potential pathogenic mechanisms of periodontitis associated pregnancy complications. *Ann. Periodontol.* 3, 233–250. doi: 10.1902/annals.1998.3.1.233

Ohlsson, C., Engdahl, C., Fak, F., Andersson, A., Windahl, S. H., Farman, H. H., et al. (2014). Probiotics protect mice from ovariectomy-induced cortical bone loss. *PLOS ONE* 9:e92368. doi: 10.1371/journal.pone.0092368

Oliver, J. E., and Silman, A. J. (2009). Why are women predisposed to autoimmune rheumatic diseases? *Arthritis Res. Ther.* 11, 252. doi: 10.1186/ar2825

Patel, R., and Shahane, A. (2014). The epidemiology of Sjogren's syndrome. *Clin. Epidemiol.* 6, 247–255. doi: 10.2147/CLEP.S47399

Pilgram, T. K., Hildebolt, C. F., Dotson, M., Cohen, S. C., Hauser, J. F., Kardaris, E., et al. (2002). Relationships between clinical attachment level and spine and hip bone mineral density: data from healthy postmenopausal women. *J. Periodontol.* 73, 298–301. doi: 10.1902/jop.2002.73.3.298

Ruby, J., and Barbeau, J. (2002). The buccale puzzle: The symbiotic nature of endogenous infections of the oral cavity. *Can. J. Infect. Dis.* 13, 34–41. doi: 10.1155/2002/492656

Sanz, M., Beighton, D., Curtis, M. A., Cury, J. A., Dige, I., Dommisch, H., et al. (2017). Role of microbial biofilms in the maintenance of oral health and in the development of dental caries and periodontal diseases. Consensus report of group 1 of the Joint EFP/ORCA workshop on the boundaries between caries and periodontal disease. *J. Clin. Periodontol.* 44(Suppl. 18), S5–S11. doi: 10.1111/jcpe.12682

Schreiner, P. J., Terry, J. G., Evans, G. W., Hinson, W. H., Crouse, J. R. III, and Heiss, G. (1996). Sex-specific associations of magnetic resonance imaging-derived intra-abdominal and subcutaneous fat areas with conventional anthropometric indices. The Atherosclerosis risk in communities study. *Am. J. Epidemiol.* 144, 335–345. doi: 10.1093/oxfordjournals.aje.xxx a008934

Seymour, G. J., Ford, P. J., Cullinan, M. P., Leishman, S., and Yamazaki, K. (2007). Relationship between periodontal infections and systemic disease. *Clin. Microbiol. Infect.* 13(Suppl. 4), 3–10. doi: 10.1111/j.1469-0691.2007.01798.x

Suresh, L., and Radfar, L. (2004). Pregnancy and lactation. *Oral Surg. Oral Med. Oral Pathol. Oral Radiol. Endod.* 97, 672–682. doi: 10.1016/S1079210404000861

Tarkkila, L., Kari, K., Furuholm, J., Tiitinen, A., and Meurman, J. H. (2010). Periodontal disease-associated micro-organisms in peri-menopausal and post-menopausal women using or not using hormone replacement therapy. A two-year follow-up study. *BMC Oral Health* 10:10. doi: 10.1186/1472-6831-10-10

Thompson, I. O. C., van der Bijl, P., van Wyk, C. W., and van Eyk, A. D. (2001). A comparative light-microscopic, electron-microscopic and chemical study of human vaginal and buccal epithelium. *Arch. Oral Biol.* 46, 1091–1098. doi: 10.1016/S0003-9969(01)00082-6

Uehara, M. (2013). Isoflavone metabolism and bone-sparing effects of daidzein-metabolites. *J. Clin. Biochem. Nutr.* 52, 193–201. doi: 10.3164/jcbn.13-2

Valimaa, H., Savolainen, S., Soukka, T., Silvoniemi, P., Makela, S., Kujari, H., et al. (2004). Estrogen receptor-beta is the predominant estrogen receptor subtype in human oral epithelium and salivary glands. *J. Endocrinol.* 180, 55–62. doi: 10.1677/joe.0.1800055

Wang, A., Wang, C. P., Tu, M., and Wong, D. T. (2016). Oral biofluid biomarker research: current status and emerging frontiers. *Diagnostics* 6:45. doi: 10.3390/diagnostics6040045

Wu, H. J., Ivanov, I. I., Darce, J., Hattori, K., Shima, T., Umesaki, Y., et al. (2010). Gut-residing segmented filamentous bacteria drive autoimmune arthritis via T helper 17 cells. *Immunity* 32, 815–827. doi: 10.1016/j.immuni.2010.06.001

Yost, S., Duran-Pinedo, A. E., Teles, R., Krishnan, K., and Frias-Lopez, J. (2015). Functional signatures of oral dysbiosis during periodontitis progression revealed by microbial metatranscriptome analysis. *Genome Med.* 7, 27. doi: 10.1186/s13073-015-0153-3

Youssef, H., and Stashenko, P. (2017). Interleukin-1 and estrogen protect against disseminating dentoalveolar infections. *Int. J. Oral Sci.* 9, 16–23. doi: 10.1038/ijos.2016.61

Yurkovetskiy, L., Burrows, M., Khan, A. A., Graham, L., Volchkov, P., Becker, L., et al. (2013). Gender bias in autoimmunity is influenced by microbiota. *Immunity* 39, 400–412. doi: 10.1016/j.immuni.2013.08.013

Yurkovetskiy, L. A., Pickard, J. M., and Chervonsky, A. V. (2015). Microbiota and autoimmunity: exploring new avenues. *Cell Host Microbe* 17, 548–552. doi: 10.1016/j.chom.2015.04.010

20

HHV-6A/6B Infection of NK Cells Modulates the Expression of miRNAs and Transcription Factors Potentially Associated to Impaired NK Activity

*Roberta Rizzo, Irene Soffritti, Maria D'Accolti, Daria Bortolotti, Dario Di Luca and Elisabetta Caselli**

Section of Microbiology and Medical Genetics, Department of Medical Sciences, University of Ferrara, Ferrara, Italy

***Correspondence:**
Elisabetta Caselli
csb@unife.it

Natural killer (NK) cells have a critical role in controlling virus infections, and viruses have evolved several mechanisms to escape NK cell functions. In particular, Human herpesvirus 6 (HHV-6) is associated with diseases characterized by immune dysregulation and has been reported to infect NK cells. We recently found that HHV-6 *in vitro* infection of human thyroid follicular epithelial cells and T-lymphocytes modulates several miRNAs associated with alterations in immune response. Since miRNAs are key regulators of many immune pathways, including NK cell functions, we aimed to study the impact of HHV-6A and -6B *in vitro* infection on the intracellular mediators correlated to NK cell function. To this purpose, a human NK cell line (NK-92) was infected *in vitro* with HHV-6A or 6B and analyzed for alterations in the expression of miRNAs and transcription factors. The results showed that both viruses establish lytic replication in NK-92 cells, as shown by the presence of viral DNA, expression of lytic transcripts and antigens, and by the induction of an evident cytopathic effect. Notably, both viruses, although with species-specific differences, induced significant modifications in miRNA expression of miRNAs known for their role in NK cell development, maturation and effector functions (miR-146, miR-155, miR-181, miR-223), and on at least 13 miRNAs with recognized role in inflammation and autoimmunity. Also the expression of transcription factors was significantly modified by HHV-6A/6B infection, with an early increase of ATF3, JUN and FOXA2 by both species, whereas HHV-6A specifically induced a 15-fold decrease of POU2AF1, and HHV-6B an increase of FOXO1 and a decrease of ESR1. Overall, our data show that HHV-6A and -6B infections have a remarkable effect on the expression of miRNAs and transcription factors, which might be important in the induction of NK cell function impairment, virus escape strategies and related pathologies.

Keywords: HHV-6, miRNA, transcription factors, natural killer cells, virus infection

INTRODUCTION

Natural killer (NK) cells belong to the innate immune system and are essential effector cells in the control of virus infections (Cooper et al., 2001). Their activity during antiviral response is crucial to control initial virus replication, by killing virus-infected cells prior to the development of adaptive/specific immunity, but they also act as essential regulators of the adaptive immunity

(Vivier et al., 2008). Their relevance is supported by the observation that individuals with defects in the NK cell component of the innate immunity are more susceptible to virus infection (Orange, 2002), including herpesviruses (Fleisher et al., 1982; Biron et al., 1989), and consequently more prone to develop symptomatic disease following infection. On the other hand, the importance of NK cell activity during virus infections is reflected by the many mechanisms acquired by viruses to evade NK cell-mediated immune responses (Vossen et al., 2002; Arens, 2012). In particular, human herpesvirus 6A and 6B (HHV-6A and 6B), as all viruses belonging to the *Herpesviridae* family, have developed several mechanisms to control and inactivate the immune response in order to establish a lifelong infection in their hosts.

HHV-6A and 6B are members of the *Roseolovirus* group of the β *herpesvirinae* subfamily and, although they share high sequence homology, are classified as distinct species. In fact, they show important differences in biologic properties, epidemiology, and disease association (Ablashi et al., 2014). HHV-6B infects humans in early childhood and is responsible of *Exanthem subitum* (Yamanishi et al., 1988), while primary infection with HHV-6A still has to be clearly identified. Both HHV-6A and -6B establish a latent infection in the host following resolution of primary infection. Reactivations in the adult have been associated to the development of multiple symptomatic diseases often characterized by immune dysregulation (multiple sclerosis, Sjögren's syndrome, autoimmune thyroiditis, and others) (Caselli and Di Luca, 2007). Both viruses are considered lymphotropic, showing an elective tropism for CD4+ T-lymphocytes and being able to infect several different cell types of the immune system, including NK cells (Lusso et al., 1993; Caselli and Di Luca, 2007).

Interestingly, *in vivo* and *in vitro* evidences indicate that HHV-6A/6B interfere with the immune system of the infected host in several ways (Lusso, 2006; Dagna et al., 2013). They can modulate surface antigens important for T-cell activation, such as human leukocyte antigen (HLA) class I molecule expression in dendritic cells (Hirata et al., 2001); they also can affect cytokine and chemokine productions, including selective suppression of IL-12, affecting the generation of effective cellular immune responses (Smith et al., 2003; Dagna et al., 2013). Furthermore, we recently observed that HHV-6A infection induces the expression of the tolerogenic non-classical class I HLA-G molecule in primary human mesothelial cells, leading to impairment of NK cell recognition and killing of infected cells (Caselli et al., 2015). With reference to the NK cell component of the immune response, HHV-6A was reported to establish a productive infection in CD3-negative NK cell clones, leading to the *de novo* expression of CD4 on the NK cell surface (Lusso et al., 1993), and HHV-6B was recently shown to induce down-modulation of the activating NKG2D ligand in infected cells (Schmiedel et al., 2016).

Notably, it has been recently reported that NK cells may be directly involved in the onset and progression of autoimmune diseases, through their potential autoreactivity or through their interaction with the other immune cells (Schleinitz et al., 2010; Poggi and Zocchi, 2014), thus supporting the hypothesis of a correlation between HHV-6A/6B infection, NK cell function and autoimmunity.

On the other hand, miRNAs are known to play an essential role in fine-tuning host immune homeostasis and responses, as miRNA-mediated regulation of gene expression has a profound impact on immune cell development, function, and response to invading pathogens. Interestingly, we recently observed that HHV-6A/6B infection of human thyrocytes and T-lymphocytes profoundly remodulates the expression of cellular miRNAs, inducing specific miRNAs associated to autoimmunity *in vivo* (Caselli et al., 2017), and of transcription factors (unpublished observations).

To study the effects of HHV-6A and -6B on NK cell functions, we analyzed the effect of *in vitro* infection of NK cells on the expression of miRNAs. We also investigated the expression of transcription factors in infected NK cells, in the attempt to further clarify the details of intracellular alterations induced by these viruses with relevance on the immune function.

MATERIALS AND METHODS

Cells and Viruses

The human NK-92 natural killer cell line (ATCC® CRL-2407™) was used for all infection experiments (Gong et al., 1994). Cells were expanded in Alpha Minimum Essential Medium supplemented with 2 mM L-glutamine, 1.5 g/L sodium bicarbonate, 0.1 mM 2-mercaptoethanol, and 20% fetal bovine serum (FBS) (complete medium).

Cell-free virus inocula were obtained as described previously (Caselli et al., 2006; Caruso et al., 2009), and quantified by quantitative real-time PCR (qPCR) (Caselli et al., 2017). All the experiments were performed by using the same virus inoculum, containing 10^{10} genome copies/ml, corresponding to about 10^9 infecting particles/ml, as previously described (Caselli et al., 2015).

All experiments involving virus production and infection were performed under standard BLS-2 biosafety level.

NK Cell Infection

NK-92 cells were seeded at optimal density and after 24 h HHV-6A or 6B were added at a 100:1 multiplicity of infection (MOI, virus genomes:cell ratio). Virus adsorption was carried out in a 2% FBS medium for 3 h, then the excess virus was eliminated by centrifugation and washing in PBS, and cells were finally seeded at 0.5 × 10^6 cells/ml in complete medium with high FBS concentration. Control cells were treated with the same procedure but uninfected. At 1, 2, 3, and 6 days post-infection (d.p.i.) aliquots of cultures were collected and analyzed for virus DNA presence, virus transcription and antigen expression, as well as for expression of miRNAs and transcription factors. Evaluation of cell viability was performed by cell counting after Trypan Blue exclusion test.

qPCR Analyses of Virus DNA Presence

Total DNA was extracted from the infected or uninfected cells by a commercial kit (Exgene Cell SV kit, GeneAll Biotechnology,

Korea), and quantified by spectrophotometric reading at 260 and 280 nm. Virus DNA presence was verified and quantified as previously described by a qPCR detecting the conserved U94 gene of HHV-6A and 6B with equivalent efficiency (Caselli et al., 2017).

Microarray and RT-qPCR Analyses

RNA was extracted from cells by the miRNeasy kit (Qiagen, Hilden, Germany), allowing the extraction of total RNA including miRNA fraction, as previously described (Caselli et al., 2017). Extracted RNA were devoid of contaminant DNA, as assured by DNase treatment and control β-actin PCR without reverse transcription (Caselli et al., 2012). RNA reverse transcription was performed by the RT2 First strand Kit (Qiagen, Hilden, Germany) for analyses of virus transcripts and human transcription factors, whereas for miRNA analyses the miScript RT kit was used (Qiagen, Hilden, Germany). cDNA aliquots corresponding to 200 ng RNA were used for virus transcription analysis, performed by qPCR detecting the expression of U94, U42 and U22 genes, as previously reported (Caselli et al., 2012). The expression of transcription factors was analyzed by the 'Human Transcription Factor' microarray, detecting and quantifying simultaneously 83 different human transcription factors (Qiagen, Hilden, Germany), using 500 ng cDNA as the template.

miRNA analyses were performed on 100 ng of specifically reverse transcribed cDNA, by the 'Human Inflammatory Response & Autoimmunity' Microarray (Qiagen, Hilden, Germany), quantifying simultaneously 84 different miRNAs involved in the immune response, and by 20 individual assays chosen to detect and quantify miRNAs specifically involved in the NK cell functions. Namely, the following individual miRNAs were analyzed: miR155*_1, miR155_2, miR146a_1, miR16-1*_1, miR16_2, miR181a*_1, miR181a_2, miR181b_1, miR181b-3p_1, miR10a*_1, miR10a_2, miR150_1, miR150-3p_1, miR27a_1, miR27a*_1, miR27b*_1, miR27b_2, miR223_1, miR223*_1, miR378*_1; miRTC_1, and SNORD61_11 were used as internal controls (all Qiagen, Hilden, Germany).

All qPCR amplification results obtained by transcription factors microarray, miRNA microarray and individual assays, were analyzed and normalized by a specific Qiagen software, to obtain comparable values between control and infected cells at each time post-infection.

Immunofluorescence Analysis

Immunofluorescence for HHV-6A/6B antigen expression was performed with mouse monoclonal antibodies (mAb) directed against glycoprotein gp116 (late antigen) of HHV-6 A and B (ABI, Columbia, MD, United States), as previously described (Caselli et al., 2006). Briefly, aliquots of infected or uninfected NK-92 cells were collected by centrifugation 10 min at 1000 × *g*, counted, spotted on a glass slide (50,000 cell in 10 μl), dried at room temperature and subsequently stained as described elsewhere (Caselli et al., 2006).

Statistical Analysis

Statistical analysis of collected data was performed using the Stat View software package (SAS Institute, Inc., Cary, NC, United States). Comparative analysis between individual parameters in infected and control groups was performed by Student's *t*-test, and *p*-values ≤ 0.01 were considered significant. For multiple comparisons, the Bonferroni correction was applied, and corrected *p*-values (p_c) ≤ 0.01 were considered significant.

RESULTS

HHV-6A and 6B Infect Productively NK-92 Cells

Both viruses established a productive/lytic infection in NK-92 cells, as shown in **Figure 1**, confirming that human NK cells are permissive to viral infection (Lusso et al., 1993), and showing that the NK-92 cell line could be used for all the subsequent analyses.

In fact, virus DNA was present in infected cells at all time-points post-infection (1 to 6 d.p.i.), as measured by specific U94 qPCR, and the increased genome number, compared to time-point 0, confirmed that virus replication was actually taking place in infected cells. The analysis of virus transcription confirmed the establishment of productive infection in NK cells, as evidenced by the presence of the immediate-early U42 and late U22 transcripts, together with the U94 transcript (which is detected both during lytic and latent HHV-6 infection), at all time-points post-infection (p.i.) (**Figure 1A**). Establishment of lytic infection was confirmed by IFA results, showing abundant expression of the late gp116 envelope glycoprotein at 6 d.p.i. in infected cells (**Figure 1B**).

Infected NK-92 cells appeared damaged and less able to form clusters compared to uninfected controls, with more pronounced effects in the case of HHV-6A, compared to HHV-6B (**Figure 1B**). The virus-induced damages were confirmed by viable cell counts, showing a slight decrease in HHV-6A and 6B infected cells at 1 d.p.i. (−14.5 ± 3.8% compared to control uninfected cells), but a more evident reduction at later time-points, with HHV-6A infection causing a 66.7 ± 9.8% cell loss and HHV-6B a 39.8 ± 6.5% cell loss, at 6 d.p.i., compared to controls.

miRNA Expression Modulation by HHV-6A and 6B Infection

miRNA expression in infected cells was first studied by a microarray assay simultaneously detecting 84 different miRNAs associated to the development of inflammation and autoimmunity. The results, summarized in Supplementary Table S1, show that both HHV-6A and 6B induce evident alterations in the expression of cellular miRNAs. In particular, 23 miRNAs resulted significantly modulated ($p_c \leq 0.01$) compared to controls, in at least one time-point p.i. With the aim to highlight only the most prominent effects caused by virus infection, we focused our attention on those miRNAs showing at least fourfold changes compared to controls, arbitrarily chosen as a cut-off value. Thirteen miRNAs were modulated more than fourfold by virus infections, with clear early and late effects and differences between the two viruses (**Figure 2**). In particular, both HHV-6A and 6B induced an early up-regulation of miR-301a and miR-548e (1 d.p.i.), an increase of miR-101 and a decrease of miR-let-7c

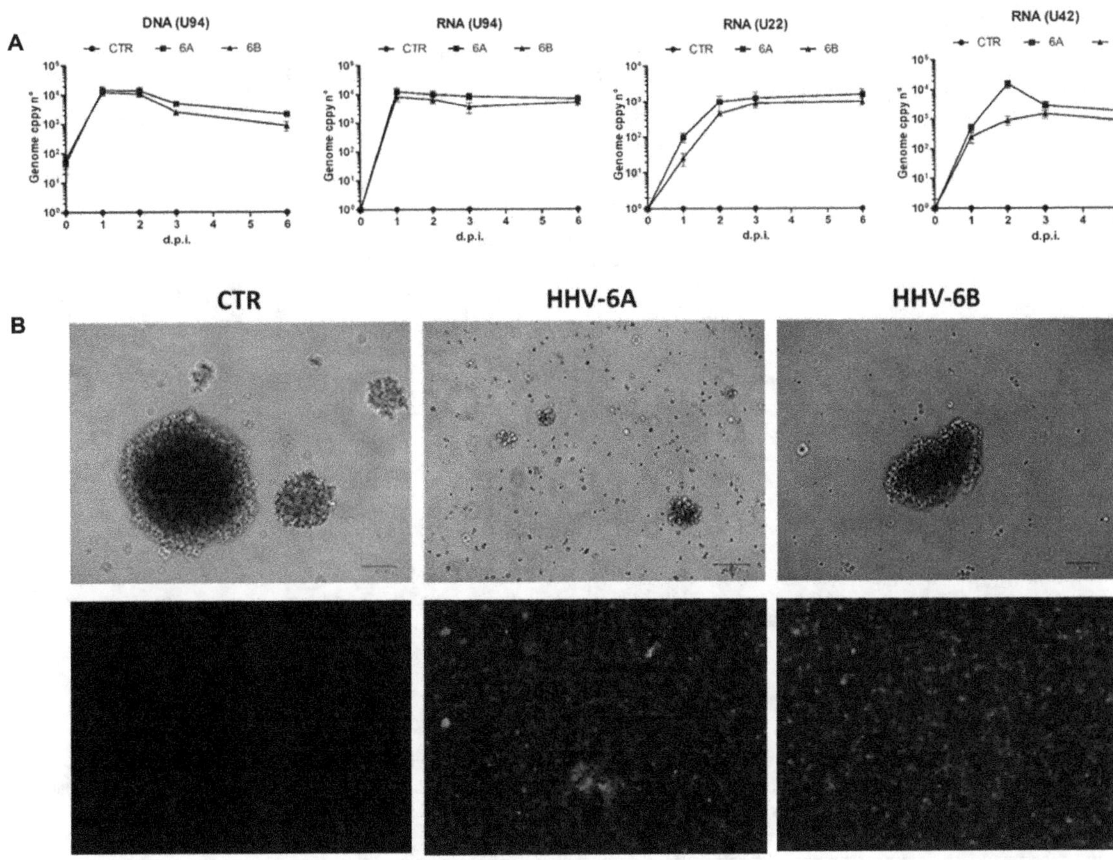

FIGURE 1 | Infection by HHV-6A and 6B in the human NK-92 natural killer cell line. NK-92 cells were infected with HHV-6A or 6B cell-free virus inocula (MOI = 100). **(A)** Virus presence (DNA) and transcription (RNA) were analyzed by qPCR and RT-qPCR for U94, U22, and U42 genes. Results are expressed as genome copy number per 100 ng of DNA or RNA. Results are expressed as mean values ± SD of duplicate samples in three independent experiments. **(B)** *Upper panel*, phase contrast microphotographs of uninfected (CTR) or infected cells at 6 d.p.i., original magnification 40X; *lower panel*, results of IFA assays performed using a mouse mAb recognizing the late gp116 glycoprotein of both virus species. The results shown refer to 6 d.p.i.; original magnification 40X. Size bar = 100 μm.

and miR-340 at 3 d.p.i., and a down-regulation of miR-23 at late time-points p.i. (6 d.p.i.). Other effects were specific for each virus species. Namely, HHV-6A specifically induced an early up-regulation of miR-590 (1 d.p.i.), miR-15a and miR-21 (3 d.p.i.), a sustained up-regulation of miR-29b, miR-101 (3 and 6 d.p.i.), miR-301a and miR-548e (1 and 6 d.p.i.) and a late up-regulation of miR-340 and miR-381 (6 d.p.i.) By contrast, HHV-6B infection specifically up-modulated the expression of miR-301b (2 and 3 d.p.i.) and miR-548e (1 and 3 d.p.i.), whereas it down-regulated miR-590 (2 and 3 d.p.i.) and miR-15a (6 d.p.i.).

Since microarray assays did not include important miRNAs known for their role in NK cell development and function, we analyzed by individual assays the following miRNAs: miR10, miR16, miR27, miR146, miR150, miR155, miR181, miR223, miR378, chosen as they have already been reported to be associated with maturation and activation of NK cells (Liu et al., 2012; Beaulieu et al., 2013; Sullivan et al., 2013).

The results showed that four additional miRNAs were altered by HHV-6A and 6B infection (**Figure 3**), as both viruses, although to a different extent, induced a significant decrease (up to 12-fold compared to controls; $p \leq 0.001$) of miR-155 and miR-181, which are respectively involved in cytotoxicity and maturation of NK cells, and a concomitant significant increase (up to 14-fold; $p \leq 0.001$) in the expression of miR-146 and miR-223, which are associated to NK cell effector functions, including IFNγ and TNFα production.

Transcription Factors Modulation by HHV-6A/6B Infection

We analyzed the impact of HHV-6A and -6B infection on the expression of human transcription factors, with the simultaneous analysis of 83 different transcription factors by microarray.

The results showed that HHV-6 infection strongly modulates the expression of transcription factors (**Figure 4**). In fact, more than 30 transcription factors were significantly up or down-modulated compared to controls, at different time-points p.i ($p_c < 0.01$). In particular, the remodulation of transcription factors was evident at late time-points p.i., whereas at early time-points p.i. viral infection had lower impact, with clear differences between the two species. In fact, while HHV-6A was essentially down-modulating a few transcription factors

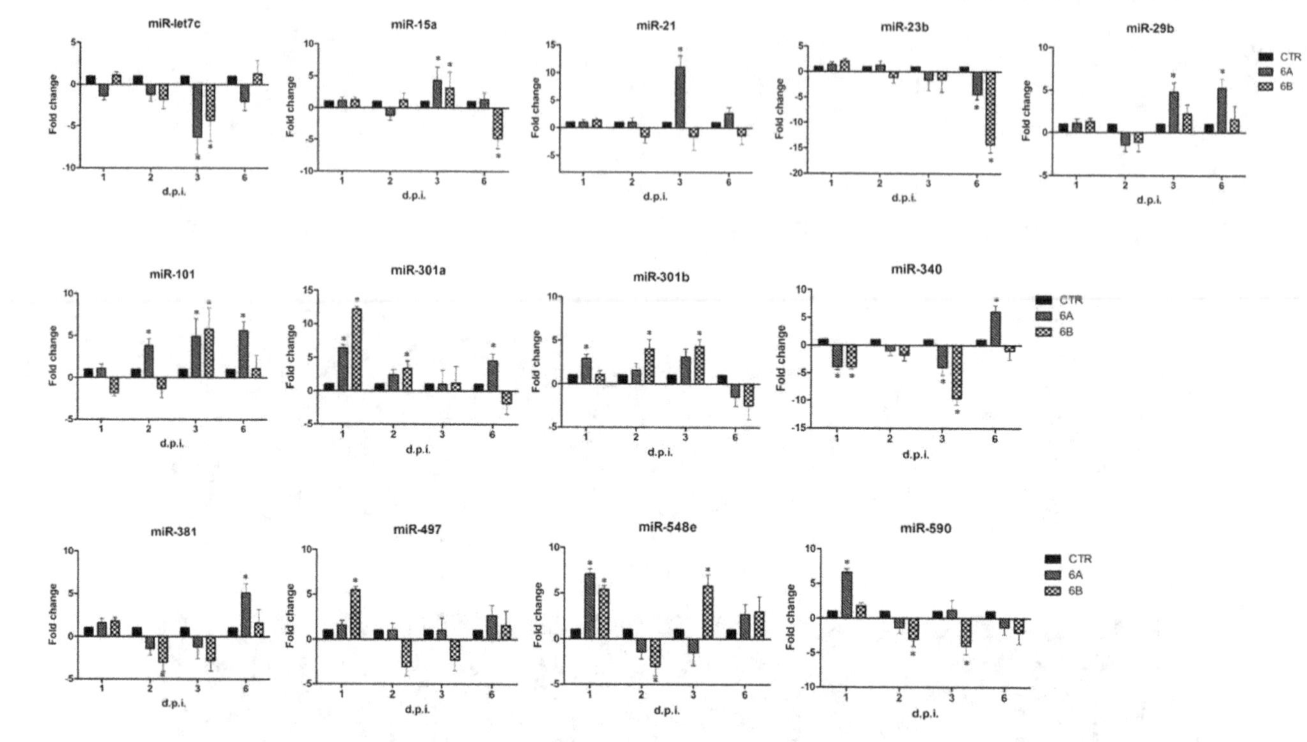

FIGURE 2 | HHV-6A/6B impact on the expression of inflammation and autoimmunity associated miRNAs in NK-92 cells (most affected miRNAs). NK-92 cells were uninfected (control) or infected with HHV-6A or 6B cell-free inocula, then analyzed at 1, 2, 3, and 6 d.p.i. for miRNA expression by a microarray detecting 84 miRNAs. Results represent the fold-changes compared to control values, and are expressed as mean values ± SD (duplicate samples from three independent experiments). Statistically significant alterations, after Bonferroni correction, are marked with asterisks ($p_C \leq 0.01$).

at 1 d.p.i. (DR1, HNF4A, POU2AF1, PPARγ), HHV-6B had an essentially up-regulating effect, increasing the expression of FOXA2, FOXG1, GATA2, HNF1A, and decreasing only the expression of MYOD1. By contrast, at 6 d.p.i. both HHV-6A and HHV-6B infections resulted in the up-modulation of several transcription factors, perhaps related to the evident CPE and cell lysis induced by viruses in the infected NK cells.

Both viruses induced the up-regulation of ATF3, CEBPA, CEBPB, JUN and FOXA2 factors, and the down-modulation of PPARγ factor. However, other factors were modulated by only one virus. For example, EGR1 and FOS were up-regulated only by HHV-6A (at 2, 3, 6 d.p.i.), which also specifically induced the decrease of POU2AF1 expression (at 1, 2 d.p.i.) and NFYB (at 2, 3, 6 d.p.i.). Instead, HHV-6B induced an increase in FOXO1 (2, 3 and 6 d.p.i.) and CREB1 (6 d.p.i.) expression and a down-regulation of ESR1 at 3 d.p.i. Other transcription factors displayed a biphasic modulation, as they were differently regulated by viruses at early and late time-points post-infection: the GATA family, HNF1A and HNF4A.

DISCUSSION

In their continuous interaction with the host immune system, herpesviruses have developed a large array of strategies to escape the host defense mechanisms. In particular, although different for many biological and pathological aspects, both HHV-6A and 6B display a strong tropism toward lymphocytes, causing important modifications and cytopathic effects in infected cells. Both virus species infect preferentially CD4+ T cells, and HHV-6A productively infects also different types of cytotoxic effectors, including CD8+ T cells, γδT cells, and NK cells (Lusso et al., 1993; Caselli and Di Luca, 2007). By contrast, HHV-6B tropism seems to be more restricted compared to HHV-6A, infecting poorly or at all cytotoxic effector cells (Lusso et al., 1991), but it was recently shown to down-modulate the activating NK cell ligands in SupT1 T cells, impairing the recognition of virus-infected cells by NK cells (Schmiedel et al., 2016).

Although the importance of the interplay between immune cells and HHV-6A/6B has been recognized as a key factor in viral immune evasion strategies and in the development of associated pathologies, few mechanisms have been elucidated. Our study shows for the first time that HHV-6A and HHV-6B productively infect NK cells and induce evident modifications in the expression of two sets of intracellular mediators of effector functions: miRNAs and transcription factors. In particular, microarray data showed that HHV-6A and 6B manipulate the expression of cellular miRNAs in NK cells, inducing both common and species-specific effects.

The results show that the two viruses may induce a substantial alteration in NK cell functions, as most of the modulated

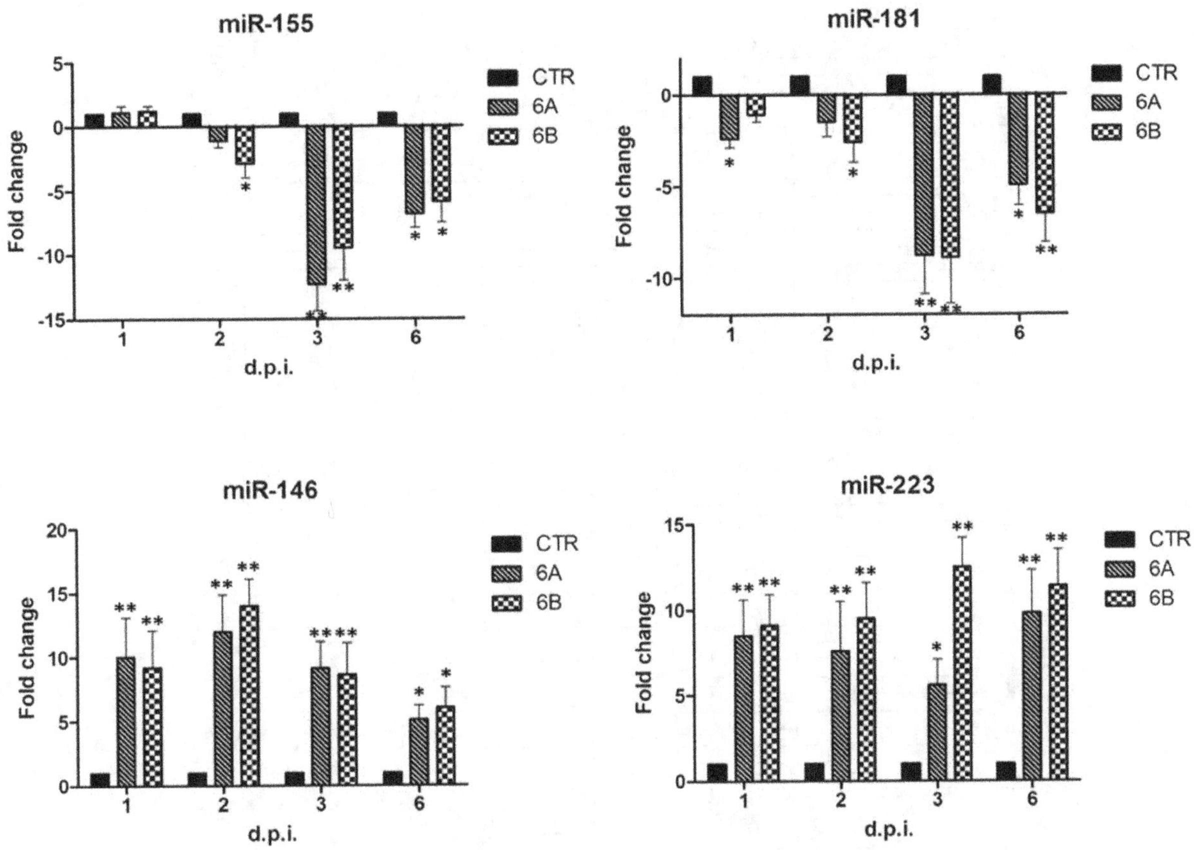

FIGURE 3 | Modulation induced by HHV-6A and 6B infection on specific miRNAs associated to NK cell functions. NK-92 cells were uninfected (control) or infected with HHV-6A or 6B cell-free inocula, then analyzed at 1, 2, 3, and 6 d.p.i. for miRNA expression by individual assays detecting miRNAs already known for their role in NK cell maturation, activation of effector functions. Results are expressed as fold-change ± SD, compared to control values, and represent the mean value of duplicate samples from three independent experiments. Statistically significant values are marked with asterisks (*$p \leq 0.01$; **$p < 0.001$).

miRNAs are involved in important immune functions. In fact, both HHV-6A and 6B down-modulate miR-let-7, which is highly expressed in NK cells, CD4+ and CD8+ T cells. Interestingly, this miRNA was reported to be down-modulated also by murine Cytomegalovirus (Beaulieu et al., 2013) and HIV-1 infection (Swaminathan et al., 2012), where it was associated with an increase of anti-inflammatory IL-10, thus providing viruses with an important immune escape mechanism. Similarly, decrease in miR-340 expression might protect viruses from the immune response, as miR-340 directly targets the Th2 effector proinflammatory cytokine IL-4 (Podshivalova and Salomon, 2013; Kim et al., 2016). Studies have in fact reported that IL-4 can enhance viral virulence in diverse models, including HSV-1 eye disease, possibly by suppressing cytotoxic lymphocyte response (Ghiasi et al., 1999; Jackson et al., 2001; Kerr et al., 2004). On the contrary, the increase of miR-301a (up-regulated by both viruses) has been reported to block the IRF1 innate immune response against Japanese encephalitis virus and might therefore favor HHV-6 pathogenesis by inhibiting IFNβ production (Hazra et al., 2017). Interestingly, miR-301 was also up-regulated in T cells in the central nervous system of animals with experimental autoimmune encephalomyelitis (Mycko et al., 2012), an animal model for the process of autoimmune demyelination occurring during multiple sclerosis, a disease with a possible association with HHV-6 infection (Leibovitch and Jacobson, 2014). The up-regulated miR-101 and miR-381 are involved in the polarization and activation of the cells of the innate immune compartment, regulating the inflammatory response (Zhu et al., 2010; Essandoh et al., 2016; Wen et al., 2016); the increased miR-548 may represent a mechanism facilitating viral pathogenesis as it negatively correlates with IFNγR1 levels (Xing et al., 2014). miR-21 and miR-590, up-regulated by HHV-6A, are involved in differentiation and activation of T cells, particularly during autoimmunity (Sousa et al., 2017), with miR-590 also down-regulating critical genes of signaling pathways similar in cancer and inflammation (Sheikholeslami et al., 2017). miR-29 and miR-15, both increased by HHV-6A infection, have a specific role in regulating the cytotoxic activity of NK cells, inhibiting the production of IFNγ by directly targeting the 3′ UTR of its mRNA (Ma et al., 2011; Leong et al., 2014).

Transcription Factors	1 d.p.i.		2 d.p.i.		3 d.p.i.		6 d.p.i.	
	HHV-6A	HHV-6B	HHV-6A	HHV-6B	HHV-6A	HHV-6B	HHV-6A	HHV-6B
AR	1,38	1,02	1,35	1,34	2,84	-1,47	6,06*	1,92
ARNT	1,09	-1,20	-1,26	-1,13	-1,80	-1,07	-1,09	-1,18
ATF1	-1,12	-1,05	-1,06	1,94	-1,63	1,19	2,35	2,03
ATF2	-1,45	-1,3	1,24	2,03	1,25	-1,07	2,93	1,48
ATF3	-1,16	-1,14	7,61*	8,43*	1,91	6,76*	5,23*	6,69*
ATF4	-1,31	-1,25	1,35	3,90	-1,42	1,57	5,05*	3,42
CEBPA	1,36	2,04	-2,94	1,37	36,01*	-1,47	36,06*	11,84*
CEBPB	-1,05	-1,14	-1,03	1,38	1,16	1,69	7,82*	4,67*
CEBPG	-1,07	-1,19	1,75	3,30	1,13	1,20	3,56	2,51
CREB1	-1,16	-1,03	-1,01	1,91	-1,01	1,64	2,13	47,06*
CREBBP	-1,76	-1,30	1,09	2,64	-4,02*	1,61	2,56	1,80
CTNNB1	1,21	-1,09	1,45	2,65	1,00	4,36*	-2,40	2,23
DR1	-5,76*	-1,18	-1,17	1,46	-1,55	1,30	1,38	1,98
E2F1	1,02	-1,03	-1,17	3,47	-1,41	1,94	4,51*	4,58*
E2F6	-1,33	-1,15	-1,27	1,29	-1,19	1,71	3,42	1,81
EGR1	-1,64	-1,41	16,29*	1,42	8,10*	3,10	5,13*	-1,53
ELK1	-1,44	-1,20	-1,41	1,37	-1,40	1,51	2,11	2,27
ESR1	-3,96	1,77	1,01	-1,01	-1,24	-9,43*	1,79	-3,19
ETS1	-1,02	1,10	1,22	1,51	-1,31	1,31	2,53	1,79
ETS2	-2,19	-2,04	-1,07	2,41	1,14	1,50	2,83	2,76
FOS	-1,91	-1,78	4,06*	1,90	1,43	-1,17	9,45*	1,17
FOXA2	1,36	8,09*	8,82*	1,34	5,82*	-1,26	46,06*	40,23*
FOXG1	-1,12	4,21*	-6,93*	1,23	2,84	-1,47	4,07*	1,92
FOXO1	-1,20	-1,04	1,27	5,61*	-1,53	4,48*	3,28	7,32*
GATA1	1,44	-2,99	-1,82	10,19*	-4,42*	-3,43	9,99*	6,17*
GATA2	1,36	7,33*	-5,44*	1,27	-2,07	1,65	1,25	2,26
GATA3	-2,06	-1,26	-1,24	2,91	-2,22	1,62	5,62*	5,36*
GTF2B	-1,09	-1,08	-1,93	1,29	-2,13	1,61	-1,61	1,39
GTF2F1	-1,28	-1,21	1,03	-1,19	1,51	-1,11	8,98*	1,69
HAND1	1,36	1,02	1,35	3,28	2,84	-1,47	5,58*	1,92
HAND2	1,32	1,04	-2,22	2,91	2,93	-1,47	3,16	1,92
HDAC1	-1,11	-1,09	-2,16	1,44	1,02	1,76	3,31	1,52
HIF1A	-1,15	-1,01	-1,38	2,55	-1,67	2,67	2,04	3,36
HNF1A	1,31	6,43*	9,09*	8,90*	-3,25	-13,56*	6,44*	13,51*
HNF4A	-6,50*	2,69	-17,63*	1,96	5,01*	1,21	42,37*	1,92
HOXA5	-1,05	-1,04	-1,85	-2,54	-2,12	-2,72	2,62	-1,87
HSF1	-1,18	1,06	1,18	1,05	-1,3	1,07	3,28	2,02
ID1	-1,35	1,14	-1,72	1,50	-1,47	1,61	1,76	3,29
IRF1	-1,19	-1,10	-1,54	4,17*	-1,23	2,68	5,02*	5,34*
JUN	-2,05	-1,67	10,69*	9,77*	3,91	6,32*	17,51*	4,01*
JUNB	-1,21	-1,13	1,66	3,52	1,44	3,69	3,66	3,31
JUND	-1,16	-1,07	1,07	2,11	1,09	2,04	3,75	3,26
MAX	-1,37	-1,12	1,06	1,11	1,97	-1,25	3,47	1,71
MEF2A	-1,29	-1,30	-1,06	3,87	-1,49	3,46	3,88	4,50*
MEF2C	-1,37	-1,26	-1,49	4,5*	-1,13	2,32	3,86	3,67
MYB	-1,17	-1,24	-1,11	4,06*	1,09	3,27	3,44	5,87*
MYC	1,08	-1,03	1,51	2,45	1,46	2,10	2,30	3,22
MYF5	-3,33	2,98	-2,44	1,16	2,84	-1,47	2,52	1,92
MYOD1	-3,49	-4,67*	3,66	1,77	2,83	-1,37	7,60*	9,30*
NFAT5	-1,79	-1,29	-1,22	4,12*	1,02	4,25*	3,20	5,88*
NFATC1	-2,38	1,31	1,74	3,07	1,35	-1,57	1,26	-1,24
NFATC2	-1,46	-1,04	1,14	2,24	-2,97	1,25	3,16	2,63
NFATC3	-1,51	-1,33	1,07	1,28	-1,41	-1,28	1,70	1,06
NFATC4	1,36	1,02	1,35	1,34	2,92	-1,47	3,26	1,92
NFKB1	-1,13	-1,13	1,16	1,32	1,01	1,99	2,64	2,04
NFYB	1,15	1,00	-2,11	2,68	-4,82*	2,34	-78,11*	2,65
NR3C1	-1,47	-1,45	1,46	3,77	1,05	1,55	3,81	3,85
PAX6	1,13	-1,10	-4,35*	-1,38	-4,79*	-1,83	3,61	3,59
POU2AF1	-6,48*	1,25	-15,87*	1,19	3,10	-1,47	1,65	1,92
PPARA	-1,06	-1,18	1,56	1,71	-1,04	1,02	3,49	1,98
PPARG	-6,50*	-1,72	-3,33	-1,85	2,99	-11,97*	1,15	-5,77*
RB1	-1,05	-1,02	-1,31	2,17	-2,08	2,31	1,10	2,36
REL	-1,48	-1,28	-1,01	3,14	-1,17	2,99	1,68	3,66
RELA	-1,18	-1,11	1,17	2,35	1,03	1,91	11,63*	3,97
RELB	1,27	1,19	1,58	5,92*	2,26	9,63*	4,90*	4,71*
SMAD1	1,16	-1,14	6,14*	2,21	1,37	2,26	40,26*	1,92
SMAD4	-1,29	-1,15	-1,04	1,77	-1,44	1,07	1,60	2,15
SMAD5	-1,37	-1,22	-1,27	2,02	-1,67	1,54	1,53	2,17
SMAD9	-3,21	-3,93	-4,06*	-1,20	2,66	1,46	3,87	-2,59
SP1	-1,38	-1,48	1,01	2,39	-1,15	1,96	1,45	3,30
SP3	-1,06	1,03	-1,18	1,54	-2,04	1,27	-2,52	1,44
STAT1	-1,20	-1,12	-1,53	2,79	-2,29	1,74	1,03	2,93
STAT2	-1,10	-1,17	-1,34	1,44	-1,87	-2,26	3,72	1,93
STAT3	-1,43	-1,12	1,03	2,13	-1,13	1,57	3,47	2,23
STAT4	1,17	1,09	-1,78	1,29	-2,59	-2,52	1,43	-1,42
STAT5A	-1,06	-1,05	-1,16	1,04	-1,68	-1,47	3,02	1,82
STAT5B	-1,12	-1,03	-1,47	1,26	-2,71	-1,45	1,21	1,82
STAT6	-1,16	-1,02	-1,21	1,01	-1,74	-1,72	2,12	1,31
TBP	-1,48	-1,08	-1,21	1,74	1,05	1,88	3,91	3,62
TCF7L2	-2,92	-1,27	2,36	2,70	2,67	5,73*	3,79	1,78
TFAP2A	-1,30	-1,01	-1,09	1,66	-2,19	1,50	2,84	2,48
TGIF1	-1,36	-1,13	-1,12	3,86	-1,11	2,44	8,51*	9,31*
TP53	-3,51	-1,12	1,16	2,76	-1,18	2,54	8,53*	5,26*
YY1	1,02	1,02	-1,29	1,91	-2,05	2,17	2,53	3,30

FIGURE 4 | Modulation induced by HHV-6A and 6B infection on human transcription factors mRNAs in NK-92 cells. NK-92 cells were uninfected (control) or infected with HHV-6A or 6B cell-free inocula, then analyzed at 1, 2, 3, and 6 d.p.i. for mRNA expression by a microarray detecting 83 transcription factors. Results are expressed as fold-change compared to control values, and represent the mean value of duplicate samples from three independent experiments. Statistically significant differences after Bonferroni correction are marked with asterisks ($p_c \leq 0.01$) and highlighted by colors (yellow ≥ 4-fold up-regulations; blue ≥ 4-fold down-regulations). Exact p_c values of all significant parameters varied from 0.005 to 0.01.

Interestingly, HHV-6B, but not HHV-6A, infection down-modulated miR-590 and miR-15, suggesting that the two species might impact differently on NK cell functions. Notably, however, both species significantly decreased miR-155, important in the effector functions of NK cells as it stimulates IFNγ production in activated NK cells (Trotta et al., 2012), and miR-181, essential for the correct maturation of NK cells (Cichocki et al., 2011). Both viruses induced an increase of miR-146, which negatively regulates NK activity by inhibiting cytotoxicity, IFNγ and TNFα production (Xu et al., 2016), and of miR-223, which inhibits the production of granzyme B by murine NK cells (Fehniger et al., 2010; Leong et al., 2014). Intriguingly, miR-223 has been associated to the pathogenesis of autoimmune thyroiditis, another disease which has been correlated to HHV-6 infection (Caselli et al., 2012). Interestingly, the modifications of miRNA expression induced by HHV-6A and 6B infections in NK cells were not superimposable to those observed in T cells (Caselli et al., 2017), demonstrating that, as well as species-specific, the effects induced by the two viruses are also cell type-specific, as they impact differently on the expression of miRNAs in different immune cell types.

Our analyses showed also that HHV-6A and 6B modulate the expression of several transcription factors in infected NK cells, with effects shared by both viruses, or specifically induced by only one of them, underlining again the different impact of the two viruses on NK cells. In fact, both viruses induced the up-regulation of ATF3, CEBPA, JUN and FOXA2, and down-regulation of PPARγ factor. Whereas HHV-6A induced an increase in EGR1 and FOS expression and a decrease of POU2AF1 expression, HHV-6B induced an increase in FOXO1 and a down-regulation of ESR1 expression. Although many of the modulated factors are not yet associated to specific functions in NK cells biology, some of them have already been described to have a role in this context, or in closely related immune aspects.

Interestingly, ATF3, upregulated by both viruses, was reported to regulate negatively NK cell functions in MCMV infected mice, by modulating IFNγ expression (Rosenberger et al., 2008). On the other hand, although not yet studied in NK cells, several evidences currently associate PPARγ to Th lymphocyte differentiation, B lymphocyte effector functions and cytokine expression (da Rocha Junior et al., 2013). POU2AF1, down-modulated by HHV-6A, was recently reported to induce upregulation of host defense genes, including IL-6, in airway epithelium (Zhou et al., 2016). FOXO1 and ESR1, respectively increased and decreased by HHV-6B, are important regulators of the immune response, being FOXO1 a negative regulator of NK cell maturation and functions (Deng et al., 2015), whereas ESR1 has been associated to regulation of inflammatory pathways of innate immune cells (Kovats, 2015). Other factors, including JUN, FOS, CEBPA, are involved in several biological processes as regulators of cell cycle progression, hematopoietic cell differentiation and apoptosis (Foletta et al., 1998; Wisdom et al., 1999; Ponti et al., 2002; Healy et al., 2013), and might be studied in detail in the NK cell context.

Overall, our data show for the first time that infection by HHV-6A and 6B profoundly impacts the intracellular environment of infected NK cells, likely inducing biological effects helping the viruses to escape the innate immune response. Although the two different HHV-6 species induce many common effects, our data also show species-specific effects on miRNAs and transcription factors expression. The differences might possibly result in a different biological impact of the two viruses, potentially associated to specific pathological conditions.

CONCLUSION

HHV-6A and 6B induce significant alterations on the expression of several miRNAs and transcription factors in infected NK cells. These alterations might lead to important modifications in NK cell ability to control HHV-6 infections, enabling immune evasion and facilitating viral replication cycle, and impacting on NK cell involvement in inflammation and autoimmune reactions.

Functional studies should be conducted to investigate the role of the factors altered by HHV-6 infection, and to evaluate their possible implication in pathological alterations and disease progression.

AUTHOR CONTRIBUTIONS

RR contributed to the conception of the work and data analysis. IS, MD, and DB contributed to data collection and analysis. DDL contributed to data interpretation and critical revision of the article. EC contributed to the conception of the work, data acquisition and analysis, and writing the article.

FUNDING

This work was supported by HHV-6 Foundation grants (PI: EC and RR), by PRIN grant (PI: EC, cod 2015YZB22C), by Merck grant (PI: RR), and by FISM-Fondazione Italiana Sclerosi Multipla grant (PI: RR, cod 2015/R/20).

ACKNOWLEDGMENT

We thank Iva Pivanti for her excellent technical assistance, and Linda Sartor for revising the English manuscript.

REFERENCES

Ablashi, D., Agut, H., Alvarez-Lafuente, R., Clark, D. A., Dewhurst, S., DiLuca, D., et al. (2014). Classification of HHV-6A and HHV-6B as distinct viruses. *Arch. Virol.* 159, 863–870. doi: 10.1007/s00705-013-1902-5

Arens, R. (2012). Rational design of vaccines: learning from immune evasion mechanisms of persistent viruses and tumors. *Adv. Immunol.* 114, 217–243. doi: 10.1016/B978-0-12-396548-6.00009-3

Beaulieu, A. M., Bezman, N. A., Lee, J. E., Matloubian, M., Sun, J. C., and Lanier, L. L. (2013). MicroRNA function in NK-cell biology. *Immunol. Rev.* 253, 40–52. doi: 10.1111/imr.12045

Biron, C. A., Byron, K. S., and Sullivan, J. L. (1989). Severe herpesvirus infections in an adolescent without natural killer cells. *N. Engl. J. Med.* 320, 1731–1735. doi: 10.1056/NEJM198906293202605

Caruso, A., Caselli, E., Fiorentini, S., Rotola, A., Prandini, A., Garrafa, E., et al. (2009). U94 of human herpesvirus 6 inhibits in vitro angiogenesis and lymphangiogenesis. *Proc. Natl. Acad. Sci. U.S.A.* 106, 20446–20451. doi: 10.1073/pnas.0905535106

Caselli, E., Bracci, A., Galvan, M., Boni, M., Rotola, A., Bergamini, C., et al. (2006). Human herpesvirus 6 (HHV-6) U94/REP protein inhibits betaherpesvirus replication. *Virology* 346, 402–414. doi: 10.1016/j.virol.2005.11.018

Caselli, E., Campioni, D., Cavazzini, F., Gentili, V., Bortolotti, D., Cuneo, A., et al. (2015). Acute human herpesvirus-6A infection of human mesothelial cells modulates HLA molecules. *Arch. Virol.* 160, 2141–2149. doi: 10.1007/s00705-015-2490-3

Caselli, E., D'Accolti, M., Soffritti, I., Zatelli, M. C., Rossi, R., Degli Uberti, E., et al. (2017). HHV-6A in vitro infection of thyrocytes and T cells alters the expression of miRNA associated to autoimmune thyroiditis. *Virol. J.* 14:3. doi: 10.1186/s12985-016-0672-6

Caselli, E., and Di Luca, D. (2007). Molecular biology and clinical associations of Roseoloviruses human herpesvirus 6 and human herpesvirus 7. *New Microbiol.* 30, 173–187.

Caselli, E., Zatelli, M. C., Rizzo, R., Benedetti, S., Martorelli, D., Trasforini, G., et al. (2012). Virologic and immunologic evidence supporting an association between HHV-6 and hashimoto's thyroiditis. *PLOS Pathog.* 8:e1002951. doi: 10.1371/journal.ppat.1002951

Cichocki, F., Felices, M., McCullar, V., Presnell, S. R., Al-Attar, A., Lutz, C. T., et al. (2011). Cutting edge: microRNA-181 promotes human NK cell development by regulating Notch signaling. *J. Immunol.* 187, 6171–6175. doi: 10.4049/jimmunol.1100835

Cooper, M. A., Fehniger, T. A., and Caligiuri, M. A. (2001). The biology of human natural killer-cell subsets. *Trends Immunol.* 22, 633–640. doi: 10.1016/S1471-4906(01)02060-9

da Rocha Junior, L. F., Dantas, A. T., Duarte, A. L., de Melo Rego, M. J., Pitta Ida, R., and Pitta, M. G. (2013). PPARgamma agonists in adaptive immunity: what do immune disorders and their models have to tell us? *PPAR Res.* 2013:519724. doi: 10.1155/2013/519724

Dagna, L., Pritchett, J. C., and Lusso, P. (2013). Immunomodulation and immunosuppression by human herpesvirus 6A and 6B. *Future Virol.* 8, 273–287. doi: 10.2217/fvl.13.7

Deng, Y., Kerdiles, Y., Chu, J., Yuan, S., Wang, Y., Chen, X., et al. (2015). Transcription factor Foxo1 is a negative regulator of natural killer cell maturation and function. *Immunity* 42, 457–470. doi: 10.1016/j.immuni.2015.02.006

Essandoh, K., Li, Y., Huo, J., and Fan, G. C. (2016). MiRNA-mediated macrophage polarization and its potential role in the regulation of inflammatory response. *Shock* 46, 122–131. doi: 10.1097/SHK.0000000000000604

Fehniger, T. A., Wylie, T., Germino, E., Leong, J. W., Magrini, V. J., Koul, S., et al. (2010). Next-generation sequencing identifies the natural killer cell microRNA transcriptome. *Genome Res.* 20, 1590–1604. doi: 10.1101/gr.107995.110

Fleisher, G., Starr, S., Koven, N., Kamiya, H., Douglas, S. D., and Henle, W. (1982). A non-x-linked syndrome with susceptibility to severe Epstein-Barr virus infections. *J. Pediatr.* 100, 727–730. doi: 10.1016/S0022-3476(82)80572-6

Foletta, V. C., Segal, D. H., and Cohen, D. R. (1998). Transcriptional regulation in the immune system: all roads lead to AP-1. *J. Leukoc. Biol.* 63, 139–152.

Ghiasi, H., Cai, S., Slanina, S. M., Perng, G. C., Nesburn, A. B., and Wechsler, S. L. (1999). The role of interleukin (IL)-2 and IL-4 in herpes simplex virus type 1 ocular replication and eye disease. *J. Infect. Dis.* 179, 1086–1093. doi: 10.1086/314736

Gong, J. H., Maki, G., and Klingemann, H. G. (1994). Characterization of a human cell line (NK-92) with phenotypical and functional characteristics of activated natural killer cells. *Leukemia* 8, 652–658.

Hazra, B., Kumawat, K. L., and Basu, A. (2017). The host microRNA miR-301a blocks the IRF1-mediated neuronal innate immune response to Japanese encephalitis virus infection. *Sci. Signal.* 10:eaaf5185. doi: 10.1126/scisignal.aaf5185

Healy, S., Khan, P., and Davie, J. R. (2013). Immediate early response genes and cell transformation. *Pharmacol. Ther.* 137, 64–77. doi: 10.1016/j.pharmthera.2012.09.001

Hirata, Y., Kondo, K., and Yamanishi, K. (2001). Human herpesvirus 6 downregulates major histocompatibility complex class I in dendritic cells. *J. Med. Virol.* 65, 576–583. doi: 10.1002/jmv.2075

Jackson, R. J., Ramsay, A. J., Christensen, C. D., Beaton, S., Hall, D. F., and Ramshaw, I. A. (2001). Expression of mouse interleukin-4 by a recombinant ectromelia virus suppresses cytolytic lymphocyte responses and overcomes genetic resistance to mousepox. *J. Virol.* 75, 1205–1210. doi: 10.1128/JVI.75.3.1205-1210.2001

Kerr, P. J., Perkins, H. D., Inglis, B., Stagg, R., McLaughlin, E., Collins, S. V., et al. (2004). Expression of rabbit IL-4 by recombinant myxoma viruses enhances virulence and overcomes genetic resistance to myxomatosis. *Virology* 324, 117–128. doi: 10.1016/j.virol.2004.02.031

Kim, E. S., Choi, Y. E., Hwang, S. J., Han, Y. H., Park, M. J., and Bae, I. H. (2016). IL-4, a direct target of miR-340/429, is involved in radiation-induced aggressive tumor behavior in human carcinoma cells. *Oncotarget* 7, 86836–86856. doi: 10.18632/oncotarget.13561

Kovats, S. (2015). Estrogen receptors regulate innate immune cells and signaling pathways. *Cell Immunol.* 294, 63–69. doi: 10.1016/j.cellimm.2015.01.018

Leibovitch, E. C., and Jacobson, S. (2014). Evidence linking HHV-6 with multiple sclerosis: an update. *Curr. Opin. Virol.* 9, 127–133. doi: 10.1016/j.coviro.2014.09.016

Leong, J. W., Sullivan, R. P., and Fehniger, T. A. (2014). microRNA management of NK-cell developmental and functional programs. *Eur. J. Immunol.* 44, 2862–2868. doi: 10.1002/eji.201444798

Liu, X., Wang, Y., Sun, Q., Yan, J., Huang, J., Zhu, S., et al. (2012). Identification of microRNA transcriptome involved in human natural killer cell activation. *Immunol. Lett.* 143, 208–217. doi: 10.1016/j.imlet.2012.02.014

Lusso, P. (2006). HHV-6 and the immune system: mechanisms of immunomodulation and viral escape. *J. Clin. Virol.* 37(Suppl. 1), S4–S10. doi: 10.1016/S1386-6532(06)70004-X

Lusso, P., De Maria, A., Malnati, M., Lori, F., DeRocco, S. E., Baseler, M., et al. (1991). Induction of CD4 and susceptibility to HIV-1 infection in human CD8+ T lymphocytes by human herpesvirus 6. *Nature* 349, 533–535. doi: 10.1038/349533a0

Lusso, P., Malnati, M. S., Garzino-Demo, A., Crowley, R. W., Long, E. O., and Gallo, R. C. (1993). Infection of natural killer cells by human herpesvirus 6. *Nature* 362, 458–462. doi: 10.1038/362458a0

Ma, F., Xu, S., Liu, X., Zhang, Q., Xu, X., Liu, M., et al. (2011). The microRNA miR-29 controls innate and adaptive immune responses to intracellular bacterial infection by targeting interferon-gamma. *Nat. Immunol.* 12, 861–869. doi: 10.1038/ni.2073

Mycko, M. P., Cichalewska, M., Machlanska, A., Cwiklinska, H., Mariasiewicz, M., and Selmaj, K. W. (2012). MicroRNA-301a regulation of a T-helper 17 immune response controls autoimmune demyelination. *Proc. Natl. Acad. Sci. U.S.A.* 109, E1248–E1257. doi: 10.1073/pnas.1114325109

Orange, J. S. (2002). Human natural killer cell deficiencies and susceptibility to infection. *Microbes Infect.* 4, 1545–1558. doi: 10.1016/S1286-4579(02)00038-2

Podshivalova, K., and Salomon, D. R. (2013). MicroRNA regulation of T-lymphocyte immunity: modulation of molecular networks responsible for T-cell activation, differentiation, and development. *Crit. Rev. Immunol.* 33, 435–476. doi: 10.1615/CritRevImmunol.2013006858

Poggi, A., and Zocchi, M. R. (2014). NK cell autoreactivity and autoimmune diseases. *Front. Immunol.* 5:27. doi: 10.3389/fimmu.2014.00027

Ponti, C., Gibellini, D., Boin, F., Melloni, E., Manzoli, F. A., Cocco, L., et al. (2002). Role of CREB transcription factor in c-fos activation in natural killer cells.

Eur. J. Immunol. 32, 3358–3365. doi: 10.1002/1521-4141(200212)32:12<3358::AID-IMMU3358>3.0.CO;2-Q

Rosenberger, C. M., Clark, A. E., Treuting, P. M., Johnson, C. D., and Aderem, A. (2008). ATF3 regulates MCMV infection in mice by modulating IFN-gamma expression in natural killer cells. *Proc. Natl. Acad. Sci. U.S.A.* 105, 2544–2549. doi: 10.1073/pnas.0712182105

Schleinitz, N., Vely, F., Harle, J. R., and Vivier, E. (2010). Natural killer cells in human autoimmune diseases. *Immunology* 131, 451–458. doi: 10.1111/j.1365-2567.2010.03360.x

Schmiedel, D., Tai, J., Levi-Schaffer, F., Dovrat, S., and Mandelboim, O. (2016). Human herpesvirus 6B downregulates expression of activating ligands during lytic infection to escape elimination by natural killer cells. *J. Virol.* 90, 9608–9617. doi: 10.1128/JVI.01164-16

Sheikholeslami, A., Nabiuni, M., and Arefian, E. (2017). Suppressing the molecular signaling pathways involved in inflammation and cancer in breast cancer cell lines MDA-MB-231 and MCF-7 by miR-590. *Tumour. Biol.* 39:1010428317697570. doi: 10.1177/1010428317697570

Smith, A., Santoro, F., Di Lullo, G., Dagna, L., Verani, A., and Lusso, P. (2003). Selective suppression of IL-12 production by human herpesvirus 6. *Blood* 102, 2877–2884. doi: 10.1182/blood-2002-10-3152

Sousa, I. G., do Almo, M. M., Simi, K. C., Bezerra, M. A., Andrade, R. V., Maranhao, A. Q., et al. (2017). MicroRNA expression profiles in human CD3+ T cells following stimulation with anti-human CD3 antibodies. *BMC Res. Notes* 10:124. doi: 10.1186/s13104-017-2442-y

Sullivan, R. P., Leong, J. W., and Fehniger, T. A. (2013). MicroRNA regulation of natural killer cells. *Front. Immunol.* 4:44. doi: 10.3389/fimmu.2013.00044

Swaminathan, S., Suzuki, K., Seddiki, N., Kaplan, W., Cowley, M. J., Hood, C. L., et al. (2012). Differential regulation of the Let-7 family of microRNAs in CD4+ T cells alters IL-10 expression. *J. Immunol.* 188, 6238–6246. doi: 10.4049/jimmunol.1101196

Trotta, R., Chen, L., Ciarlariello, D., Josyula, S., Mao, C., Costinean, S., et al. (2012). miR-155 regulates IFN-gamma production in natural killer cells. *Blood* 119, 3478–3485. doi: 10.1182/blood-2011-12-398099

Vivier, E., Tomasello, E., Baratin, M., Walzer, T., and Ugolini, S. (2008). Functions of natural killer cells. *Nat. Immunol.* 9, 503–510. doi: 10.1038/ni1582

Vossen, M. T., Westerhout, E. M., Soderberg-Naucler, C., and Wiertz, E. J. (2002). Viral immune evasion: a masterpiece of evolution. *Immunogenetics* 54, 527–542. doi: 10.1007/s00251-002-0493-1

Wen, Q., Zhou, C., Xiong, W., Su, J., He, J., Zhang, S., et al. (2016). MiR-381-3p regulates the antigen-presenting capability of dendritic cells and represses antituberculosis cellular immune responses by targeting CD1c. *J. Immunol.* 197, 580–589. doi: 10.4049/jimmunol.1500481

Wisdom, R., Johnson, R. S., and Moore, C. (1999). c-Jun regulates cell cycle progression and apoptosis by distinct mechanisms. *EMBO J.* 18, 188–197. doi: 10.1093/emboj/18.1.188

Xing, T. J., Xu, H. T., Yu, W. Q., Wang, B., and Zhang, J. (2014). MiRNA-548ah, a potential molecule associated with transition from immune tolerance to immune activation of chronic hepatitis B. *Int. J. Mol. Sci.* 15, 14411–14426. doi: 10.3390/ijms150814411

Xu, D., Han, Q., Hou, Z., Zhang, C., and Zhang, J. (2016). miR-146a negatively regulates NK cell functions via STAT1 signaling. *Cell Mol. Immunol.* 14, 712–720. doi: 10.1038/cmi.2015.113

Yamanishi, K., Okuno, T., Shiraki, K., Takahashi, M., Kondo, T., Asano, Y., et al. (1988). Identification of human herpesvirus-6 as a causal agent for exanthem subitum. *Lancet* 1, 1065–1067. doi: 10.1016/S0140-6736(88)91893-4

Zhou, H., Brekman, A., Zuo, W. L., Ou, X., Shaykhiev, R., Agosto-Perez, F. J., et al. (2016). POU2AF1 functions in the human airway epithelium to regulate expression of host defense genes. *J. Immunol.* 196, 3159–3167. doi: 10.4049/jimmunol.1502400

Zhu, Q. Y., Liu, Q., Chen, J. X., Lan, K., and Ge, B. X. (2010). MicroRNA-101 targets MAPK phosphatase-1 to regulate the activation of MAPKs in macrophages. *J. Immunol.* 185, 7435–7442. doi: 10.4049/jimmunol.1000798

21

Impairment of Intestinal Barrier Function Induced by Early Weaning *via* Autophagy and Apoptosis Associated with Gut Microbiome and Metabolites

*Wenjie Tang, Jingliang Liu, Yanfei Ma, Yusen Wei, Jianxin Liu and Haifeng Wang**

College of Animal Science, Zhejiang University, The Key Laboratory of Molecular Animal Nutrition, Ministry of Education, Hangzhou, China

Correspondence:
Haifeng Wang
haifengwang@zju.edu.cn

Early weaning piglet is frequently accompanied by severe enteric inflammatory responses and microbiota dysbiosis. The links between the gut microbiome and the etiology of gut inflammation are not fully understood. The study is aimed to investigate the potential molecular mechanisms mediating inflammatory reactivity following early weaning, and to find whether these changes are correlated with gut microbiota and metabolite signatures by comparison between suckling piglets (SPs) and weaning piglets (WPs). Histopathology analysis showed a severe inflammatory response and the disruption of epithelial barrier function. Early weaning resulted in reduced autophagy indicated as the suppression of autophagic flux, whereas induced the TLR4/P38MAPK/IL-1β-mediated apoptotic pathway, as well as activation of the IL-1β precursor. The alpha-diversity and microbial composition were changed in WPs, such as the decreased abundances of *Bifidobacterium*, *Bacteroides*, *Bacillus*, *Lactobacillus*, and *Ruminococcus*. Microbial co-concurrence analysis revealed that early weaning significantly decreased network complexity, including network size, degree, average clustering coefficient and number of keystone species, as compared with the SP group. Differentially abundant metabolites were mainly associated with amino acid and purine metabolism. Strong correlations were detected between discrepant microbial taxa and multiple inflammatory parameters. In conclusion, we found that dysregulations of autophagy and apoptosis pathway were involved in colon inflammation during weaned period, which may result from gut microbiota dysbiosis. This study may provide possible intervention modalities for preventing or treating post-weaning infections through maintaining gut microbial ecosystem integrity.

Keywords: weaned piglet, intestinal barrier, apoptosis, autophagy, gut microbiota, metabolome

INTRODUCTION

Early weaning is a widely used strategy for improving sow breeding efficiency in the swine breeding industry. However, early weaning exposes piglets to multiple environmental stresses, such as separation from the sow, a switch in fibrous feed, handling and litter mixing. These experiences result in serious gut health concerns and, eventually, economic losses (1, 2). The circumstances of weaning transition generally induced gastrointestinal infections *via* mucosal surfaces, which attributes to around 17% losses of piglets born in Europe (3). Accumulating evidence has indicated that mammalian offspring are highly susceptible to enteric diseases during the transition of the early weaning (4, 5). Due to the immature gastrointestinal (GI) tract, young animals experience large changes in intestinal morphology, architecture, and physiological functions under weaning stressors (6, 7). The intestinal immune system and barrier function of the pre-weaning piglet have not specialized and expanded completely (3). All these external and internal factors inevitably affect the intestinal development of weaned piglets (WPs) and can lead to inflammation. It is necessary to explore the mechanism how early weaning induces intestinal inflammation.

Autophagy and apoptosis represent distinct adaptive forms of programmed cell death, that are essential for maintaining the complex interplay between the host and gut microbes (8, 9). Excessive apoptosis induced by extracellular stimuli inevitably results in aberrant cell death and inflammation. Autophagy, meanwhile, is a highly conserved mechanism that plays dual roles in routine cell turnover and cellular homeostasis (10). Recent studies have implicated that dysregulated apoptosis and autophagy in intestinal tissues following gut microbiota dysbiosis can lead to bacterial dissemination and an overactive inflammatory response (11, 12). However, it is not clear how these two processes promote specific immunopathological characteristics in the intestinal epithelium of piglets under early weaning stress. Studies have shown that Toll-like receptor 4 (TLR4) is a critical mediator of inflammation and adaptive immunity (13). Mitogen-activated protein kinase (MAPK), a downstream target of TLR4, plays a key role in the progression of mucosal inflammation through the stimulation of an apoptotic cascade (14). These observations imply that the TLR4/P38MAPK signaling pathway may participate in the progression of gut inflammation induced by disturbances in the gut microbiota. However, early weaning-induced regulation of TLR4/P38MAPK or autophagy signaling pathway associated with intestinal homeostasis have not been fully characterized.

The gut microbiota plays a crucial role in the health of the host by producing components and metabolites essential for many biological processes, such as immune regulation, the maintenance of enterocyte function, and the stabilization of the microecosystem (15, 16). The intestinal microbiota of pig comprises a vast and complex community exhibiting dynamic taxonomic richness and diversity that fluctuate over time and along the longitudinal axis of the GI tract (17). Gut microbiota assembly is initiated at birth and develops toward a breastfeeding-oriented microbiome during lactation (18). An abrupt shift from maternal milk to complex solid feed is deemed to result in the remodeling of the gut microbiota structure in piglets. Thus, the examination of the composition of the gut microbiota is important for explaining enteric diseases in WPs. The ecological roles of individual microbial members possess uneven importance within microecosystems (19). The remodeling of the intestinal microbiota structure by weaning transition strongly affects co-occurrence patterns of microorganism. The altered microorganism co-occurrence patterns may further have an impact on the gut health of piglets. Computational-derived co-occurrence network hubs are conducive to determining whether the core ecological modules formed by microorganisms would change within different responsiveness to intervention (20).

The dysbiosis of the intestinal flora frequently alters metabolomic profiles in the GI content, which is thought to be related to modifications in microbe-derived gut metabolites (21). The microbiota-derived metabolites are key intermediates in host-microbiota interactions and influences a wide variety of physiological functions (16, 22). During the weaning transition, solid feed consumed by piglets provides heterogeneous fermentation substrates and prolonged transit time in the GI tract (23). These changes are expected to affect microbial metabolic activity. However, how early weaning influences the gut microbiota and the metabolome of piglets remains incompletely understood. Here, we speculated that the gut metabolome of piglets may undergo profound alterations at the weaning transition period. The exploration of the potential role of the intestinal microbiota and associated metabolomes would help to find the determinants of gut inflammatory disease in piglets.

In this study, the genetic background, age, and feeding environment of the animal were strictly controlled (24). We hypothesized that early weaning induced the colon inflammatory response through dysregulating the autophagy and apoptosis signaling pathways, and alternations of gut microbiota and metabolome are associated with the dysregulation of these two signaling pathways.

MATERIALS AND METHODS

Animal Care and Experimental Design

All procedures involving animals were performed in full compliance with the "Regulation for the Use of Experimental Animals" of Zhejiang Province, China. This research was specifically approved by the Animal Care and Use Committee of Zhejiang University (Ethics Code Permit ZJU20170529). Twelve piglets (Landrace × Yorkshire) were selected from three litters. At age of 21 days, piglets (body weight, 6.95 ± 0.73 kg) from the same litter were randomly allocated to two treatments. The two groups were as follows: suckling piglet group (SP), were continued to be breastfed by sows; and weaning piglet group (WP), were separated from the sows and had *ad libitum* access to water and feed (n = 6/group). At age of 25 days, all piglets were euthanized *via* an intravenous injection of sodium pentobarbital solution (25 mg/kg body weight). Colonic content and tissue were harvested and lyophilized. Tissues adjacent to the colon were stored in 2.5% glutaraldehyde for evaluation by transmission electron microscopy (TEM). Colonic tissue was fixed in 4% buffered formalin for paraffin embedding. Colonic mucosa was collected with a microscope slide and immediately stored at −80°C until use.

Morphology, Histological Score, and TUNEL Labeling

Specimens of the colon were dehydrated with ethanol, cleared with xylene, embedded in paraffin, and cut into 4-µm-thick serial sections. After deparaffinization, the sections were stained with hematoxylin and eosin (H&E) for morphometric analysis. Crypt depth was scored by capturing image of colon tissue in H&E staining slides at 10× using a Bx63-Olympus microscope (Olympus, USA). The images were analyzed using the pen tool form Image J software (ImageJ, NIH, USA). For each sample, at least 20 intact and well-oriented crypts were measured as distance from the apical side to the basal side of crypt. The crypt depth data was shown as mean value. Intestinal acidic and neutral mucin content was examined using periodic acid-Schiff-alcian blue (PAS-AB; Sigma Aldrich) staining. Images were acquired using a scanner (Leica Aperio CS2, San Diego, CA, USA). Morphology was analyzed using the Aperio XT system (San Diego, CA, USA). To assess intestinal inflammation severity, colonic histopathological scoring of H&E-stained sections (100× magnification) were performed. Two blinded histopathological scoring methods were carried out using the following four criteria: 1) the extent of inflammation, 2) bleeding, 3) crypt hyperplasia, and 4) crypt density loss (**Supplementary Table 1**). Each criterion score ranged from 0 to 3 and the sum of the scores for the four criteria were calculated. A TUNEL Apoptosis Assay Kit (Roche, Sweden) was used to visualize the extent of cell apoptosis in paraffin-embedded colonic tissue. Images were captured using an Olympus VS200 digital slide scanner (Japan) to judge the difference in TUNEL-positive cell counts between the two groups. The nuclei of apoptotic cells were identified by the presence of green fluorescence.

Detection of Cytokines in Serum and Colon Mucosa

Venous blood sample was drawn from SPs and WPs into sterile collection tubes. Blood was centrifuged at 3,000 rpm for 10 min at 4°C to collect serum. The colonic mucosa (100 mg) was added to 1 mL of pre-cooled phosphate-buffered saline (PBS) and ground using a tissue grinder (Tissuelyser-24, JingXin, Shanghai, China). The supernatant of the colonic mucosa homogenate was extracted after centrifugation at 3,000 rpm for 12 min at 4°C. The concentrations of IL-1β, IL-6, IL-10, IFN-γ, and TNF-α in the serum and tissue supernatants were detected using porcine ELISA assay kits (R&D Systems, Minneapolis, MN, USA) according to the manufacturer's protocols. To calculate the concentration of each cytokine, the optical density was measured using a standard microplate reader (Phenix Research Products, Hayward, CA).

Immunofluorescence (IF) and Immunohistochemistry (IHC)

Colon sections were kept in neutral formalin buffer for 12 h and then embedded in paraffin and sliced into 4-µm-thick sections. The sections were subsequently dewaxed and rehydrated. For IF staining, the sections were processed with antigen retrieval, permeabilization and blocking. The sections were incubated first with a primary antibody (rabbit anti-MUC2, Biorbyt Ltd, orb372331, 1:400) for 8 h at 4°C. Then, the sections were washed and incubated with a fluorescence-labeled secondary antibody (Alexa Fluor 488-conjugated anti-rabbit IgG, Abcam, #ab150077, 1:600) for 2 h. Nuclei were counterstained with 4′,6-diamidino-2-phenylindole (DAPI) (Cell Signaling Technology, #8961, 150 ng/mL) for 20 min. For IHC, the sections were subjected to antigen retrieval by incubating in AR9 buffer (pH 6.0, PerkinElmer) at 96°C for 20 min. Then, 3% H_2O_2 in methanol was used to quench endogenous peroxidase activity on samples. The sections were followed by incubation with primary antibody (rabbit anti-LC3A/B, Cell Signaling Technology, #12741, 1:450) for 8 h at 4°C. A DAB HRO substrate kit was used for visualization following the manufacturer's instructions. Images were captured using a Bx63-Olympus microscope (Olympus, USA) and analyzed using ImageJ software.

TEM

Small pieces (1.5–2.5 mm^3) of colonic specimens were immersed in a mixture of 2% glutaraldehyde and 0.1 M cacodylate buffer (pH 7.4) until needed. The specimens were washed twice with PBS, incubated with 1% osmium tetroxide in PBS at 4°C for 40 min, and then washed again twice with PBS. The specimens were dehydrated in a series of increasing ethanol concentrations (20%, 40%, 60%, 80%, and 100% *v*/*v*) with 15 min each step. After fixation in pure Spurr resin for 12 h, the specimens were embedded in capsules containing embedding medium and polymerized at 65°C for 4 h. The sections were stained with 0.5% uranyl acetate and alkaline lead citrate (AC20, Leica) for 15 min. Finally, the sections were imaged by TEM using a Model H-7650 microscope.

Immunoblotting

Total protein was extracted from colonic tissue and lysed by lysis buffer (Solarbio, Beijing, China). The protein content of the supernatants or serum was concentrated using StrataClean resin (Agilent, CA, USA). All protein samples were prepared according to the manufacturer's instructions. The protein samples were separated by 12% SDS–PAGE and transferred to PVDF membranes. The membranes were blocked in TBST buffer containing 3% BSA (*w*/*v*) for 60 min at room temperature. Then, the membrane was incubated first with primary antibodies (diluted in TBST buffer containing 1% BSA [*w*/*v*]) targeting primary antibodies overnight at 4°C. They were followed treatment with the appropriate HRP-conjugated secondary antibodies (anti-mouse IgG and anti-rabbit IgG; all 1:4,000) (EMD Millipore, MA, USA) diluted in TBST buffer containing 1% BSA (*w*/*v*) for 1 h at room temperature. Finally, the protein bands were developed using SuperSignal Chemiluminescent Substrate (Thermo Fisher Scientific, MA, USA). Primary antibody details were listed in **Supplementary Table 2**.

16S rRNA Library Construction and Sequencing

Bacterial genomic DNA was extracted from samples of colonic content using the Omega E.Z.N.A. Stool DNA Kit following the manufacturer's protocol. DNA concentration and purity were detected using both a NanoDrop One (Thermo Scientific) spectrophotometer and a Qubit 2.0 Fluorometer (Thermo Scientific). Libraries were constructed and sequenced at the Realbio Genomics Institute (Shanghai, China). Briefly, the V3–V4 region of the 16S rRNA gene was PCR-amplified using the primer pair 341F (5′-CCTACGGGNGGCWGCAG-3′) and 806R (5′-GACTACHVGGGTATCTAATCC-3′). The amplicons were converted to sequencing libraries using the Illumina TruSeq DNA PCR-Free Library Preparation Kit (Illumina, USA). The libraries were sequenced on the MiSeq/HiSeq platform (Illumina, Inc., San Diego, CA, USA) to generate paired-end 500/250 bp reads. Demultiplexed fastq files were generated from the raw data using bcl2fast (v2.20.0.422).

Bioinformatics Analysis of the Sequencing Data

Raw sequencing data from the 16S rRNA V3–V4 hypervariable region were submitted to the following three steps: i) Raw reads were first filtered using Trimmomatic v0.33 and then Cutadapt (version 1.9.1) to remove standard primer sequences to generate high-quality reads; ii) high-quality clean reads were assembled using FLASH v1.2.7; iii) sequences were denoised using dada2 (25) in QIIME2-2020.6 (26) to generate non-chimeric reads. Data quality was estimated based on read length and counts at each stage (**Supplementary Table 2**). An amplicon sequence variant (ASV) table was generated using the standard dada2 workflow. Based on the ASV table, common and unique features between the two groups were visualized using a Venn diagram (27). Taxonomic classification of the ASVs was achieved by Bayesian classifier and BLAST using GreenGene as the reference database. QIIME2 was applied to calculate the abundance of each species and the distribution at each taxonomic level. Alpha diversity was evaluated using species richness and the corresponding significance was determined using the Wilcoxon rank sum test. Beta diversity was estimated using principal coordinate analysis (PCoA) on a matrix of Bray–Curtis distances using QIIME2 software. The statistical significance of the PCoA results was determined using PERMANOVA. According to the NCBI taxonomy database for existing microbial species, MEGAN software was applied to combine species abundance information obtained by sequencing into a taxonomic tree (28). Significant differences in relative abundance between the groups were determined using the Wilcoxon rank sum test and corrected *P*-values (false discovery rate [FDR]). Predictive metabolic functional analysis was performed using the PICRUSt2 plugin for QIIME2 (29). Pathways were assigned based on the KEGG Orthology database while DESeq2 was used for differential abundance testing.

Co-Occurrence Network Diagram

Spearman's rank correlation analysis was used to analyze the differences in the abundance of all species among samples. Data with a correlation coefficient $|\rho\text{-value}| > 0.5$ and a P-value < 0.05 were selected to construct a co-occurrence network. Subnetworks were isolated from the whole network using the following filters: ASVs comprising >0.01% of the total relative abundance and taxa present in >30% of the samples. The network diagram was visualized using a customized Organic layout algorithm in Cytoscape (v3.6.0). For both groups, the five modules were obtained using the vertex and edge betweenness centrality functions in the igraph R package (19). Node-level topological properties were calculated using Gephi (v0.9.2), the properties include degree, clustering coefficient, closeness centrality, betweeness centrality, Zi (within-module connectivity) and Pi (among-module connectivity) (30, 31). Statistically significant differences in node-level attributes were determined by non-parametric Mann–Whitney U tests.

Metabolomics Profiling

A total of 50 ± 1 mg of colonic content was added to 500 µL of a pre-cooled methanol/chloroform extraction mixture in a 3:1 (*v*/*v*) ratio. The samples were mixed with 10 µL of internal standard (Adonitol, 0.5 mg/mL stock). Then, the samples were vortexed and homogenized using a ball mill for 4 min at 50 Hz, and followed by ultrasonication for 5 min in ice-cold water. After centrifugation at 4°C for 15 min at 12,000 rpm, 200 µL of the supernatant was transferred to a fresh tube. To prepare the quality control (QC) sample, 18 µL of each sample were combined. After evaporation in a vacuum concentrator, 80 µL of methoxyamine hydrochloride (20 mg/mL in pyridine) was added followed by incubation at 80°C for 30 min and derivatization by 1 mL of BSTFA regent (1% TMCS, *v*/*v*) at 70°C for 1.5 h. Fatty acid methyl esters (FAMEs; 5 µL in chloroform) were added to the QC sample. Gas chromatography time-of-flight mass spectrometry (GC–TOF–MS) was performed using an Agilent 7890 gas chromatograph coupled with a time-of-flight mass spectrometer (DB-5MS capillary column). A 1 µL aliquot of sample was injected in splitless mode. Helium was used as the carrier gas, the front inlet purge flow was 3 mL/min. The gas flow rate through the column was 1 mL/min. The initial temperature was kept at 50°C for 1 min, raised to 310°C at a rate of 10°C/min, and kept for 8 min at 310°C. The injection, transfer line, and ion source temperatures were set at 250, 280, and 280°C, respectively. The mass spectrometry data were obtained in full-scan mode within the mass range of 50 to 500 *m*/*z* at a rate of 15.5 spectra per second after a solvent delay of 6.25 min.

Metabolomics Data Analysis

Metabolomics data analysis was performed as previously described (32) with some modifications. Briefly, raw data were processed using Chroma TOF4.3x software (32). The LECO-Fiehn Rtx5 database was used for metabolite identification. Finally, peaks detected in less than half of the QC samples or those with a relative standard deviation (RSD) >30% in the QC samples were removed (33). The final dataset was imported into SIMCA15.0.2 (Sartorius Stedim Data Analytics AB, Umea, Sweden) for principal component analysis (PCA) and orthogonal partial least squares discriminant analysis (OPLS-DA). The variable importance in projection (VIP) score of the first principal component in the OPLS-DA was also calculated, which summarizes the importance of each variable to the model. Metabolites with a VIP score >1 and a Student's *t*-test *P*-value <0.05 were determined to display significantly different abundance. The KEGG and MetaboAnalyst (http://www.metaboanalyst.ca) databases were referenced for pathway enrichment analysis. A correlation analysis between genera and metabolites was undertaken using Spearman's correlation in R (Hmisc package, v3.4.3) and visualized using a heatmap.

Statistical Analysis

The statistical significance of differences was assessed using the Student's unpaired *t*-test, the Wilcoxon rank sum test, Mann–Whitney non-parametric tests, or PERMANOVA where appropriate. The results are presented as means ± SEM. Data were analyzed in SPSS (v2.1.0; IBM, USA) or R (for 16S rRNA sequencing data and the metabolomics profile). A *P*-value <0.05 was considered statistically significant and a 0.05 ≤ *P*-value <0.10 was considered a tendency.

RESULTS

Comparison of the Colonic Morphology and Barrier Function Between WPs and SPs

Colonic morphological examination showed that, compared with the SP group, WPs displayed a loosely adherent intestinal epithelial layer structure and less intact surface, as well as erosion and crypt abscesses (**Figure 1A**). The WP group was characterized by a significantly greater crypt depth compared

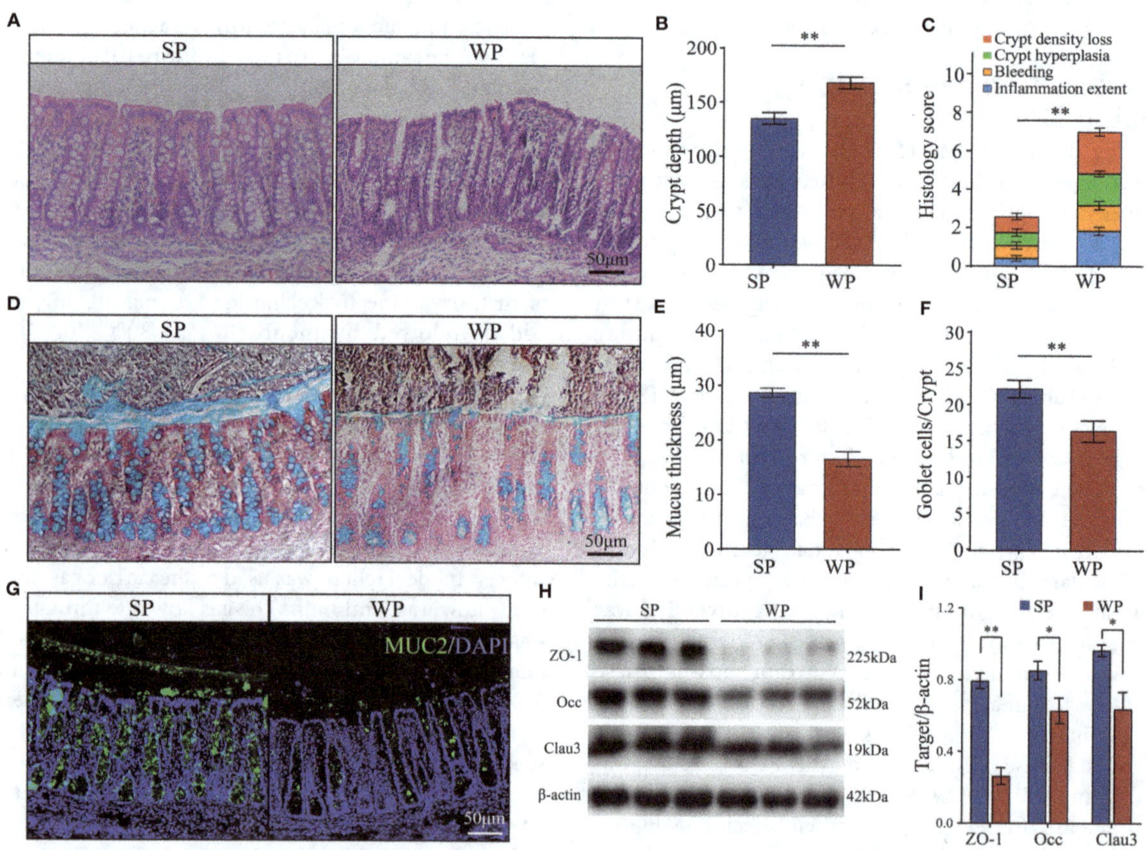

FIGURE 1 | Effects of early weaning on colonic morphology and mucosal barrier function. **(A)** Representative images of hematoxylin and eosin-stained colon sections from SP and WP groups (scale bars, 50 μm). **(B)** Statistical analysis of crypt depth. **(C)** Stacked bar graph showing the total histology scores and individual histological criteria score differences between the two groups. **(D)** Representative images of periodic acid-Schiff-alcian blue (PAS-AB)-stained colonic sections from the SP and WP groups (scale bars, 50 μm). **(E)** Mucin layer width in the colon of SPs and WPs was quantified from images of AB staining. **(F)** Statistical analysis of the numbers of mucus-producing goblet cells. **(G)** Immunofluorescence staining for the goblet cell marker MUC2 (green). Scale bars, 50 μm. **(H, I)** Western blotting results for ZO-1, occludin, and claudin-3 expression in the colon. All data are presented as means ± SEM, Student's *t*-test, *$P < 0.05$, **$P < 0.01$; $n = 6$. SP, suckling piglet; WP, weaning piglets.

with that of the SP group (**Figure 1B**). In addition, histopathological evaluation revealed that the WP group was characterized by significantly greater crypt density loss, degree of bleeding and inflammatory cell infiltration compared with the SP group (**Figure 1C**). PAS-AB staining analysis showed that the thickness of the mucosal layer and the number of secretory goblet cells were significantly decreased in the WP group compared with those in the SP group (**Figures 1D–F**). IF staining for MUC2 further confirmed the reduced abundance of mucin-producing goblet cells in the WP group compared with that in the SP group (**Figure 1G**). The protein expression of zonula occludens-1 (ZO-1), occludin, and claudin 3 were significantly lower in the WP group than in the SP group (**Figures 1H, I** and **Supplementary Figure 1**).

Early Weaning Induced Intestinal Impairment *via* Inhibiting Autophagy and Activating the Apoptotic Signaling Pathway

The TUNEL assay results showed the presence of a significantly greater number of apoptotic cells in the colonic submucosa of WPs compared with that in the SP group (**Figure 2** and **Supplementary Figure 2**). The accumulation of apoptotic cells may be linked with modulating autophagy and apoptotic signal pathway. Therefore, we first examined the expression levels of autophagy-related proteins. The expression levels of beclin-1 and ATG5 were significantly decreased in the WP group compared with those of the SP group, which was in accordance with the reduced expression of microtubule-associated protein light chain 3 (LC3)-I and a decrease trend in expression of LC3-II (**Figures 3A, B** and **Supplementary Figure 3**). Similarly, IHC staining indicated that the number of LC3 puncta was lower in the WP group than in the SP group (**Figure 3C**).

The WP group had significantly higher serum IL-6 and IL-1β concentration, and had significantly higher colonic IL-1β and lower IL-10 content than the SP group (**Figure 4A**). Meanwhile, the colonic TNF-α content had a trend increase in the WPs than the SP group (**Figure 4A**). Ultrastructure analysis showed that a large number of damaged cells were detached and scattered at the bottom of the colon crypts in the WP group, which was accompanied by nuclear fragmentation as a hallmark of cell apoptosis (**Figure 4B** and **Supplementary Figure 4**). Accordingly, we further assessed the status of the TLR4/P38MAPK-mediated apoptotic signaling pathway, which functions upstream of IL-1β. Western blotting results showed that the protein levels of TLR4, pro IL-1β and IL-β were significantly higher in the WP group than in the SP group (**Figures 4C, D** and **Supplementary Figure 5**). Additionally, the ratio of p-P38MAPK to MAPK was significantly increased in the WP group than in the SP group (**Figures 4C, D** and **Supplementary Figure 5**). Moreover, the concentrations of caspase-1 p10, caspase-3, and cleaved (activated) caspase-3 were also significantly higher in the WP group than in the SP group (**Figures 4C, E** and **Supplementary Figure 5**), which indicated the greater rate of IL-1β conversion existed in the WP group than in the SP group.

The Microbial Community Structure and the Co-Existence Pattern Differed Between the WP and SP Groups

The number of denoised clean reads (average of 31,439) was determined for each sample (**Supplementary Table 3**). Rarefaction curves for the ASVs indicated that all the samples achieved a high sampling coverage (>99%) (**Supplementary Figure 6** and **Supplementary Table 3**). These raw data analyses demonstrated that the sequencing depth was sufficient for analyzing the colonic microbiota. Next, we compared the results of 16S rRNA gene sequencing between the SP and WP groups. Common and unique ASV features between the groups were visualized by Venn diagram (**Figure 5A**), from which 235 and 115 unique ASVs were classified in the SP and WP group, respectively. As shown in **Supplementary Table 4**, differences in α-diversity were found between the two groups indicated as common and unique ASV features and the Shannon, Simpson, and Chao1 indices. The WP group had a lower trend inASVs than the SP group (Wilcoxon rank sum test, $P = 0.092$) (**Figure 5B**). The Shannon index was lower in the WP group than in the SP group (Wilcoxon rank sum test, $P = 0.015$) (**Figure 5C**). We found a clear separation between the two groups, which suggests significantly distinct in bacterial community composition between the SP and WP group, respectively (PERMANOVA, $P = 0.045$) (**Figure 5D**).

Relative abundance values were used to calculate the biomass for each species and generate a distribution histogram at each taxonomic level. At the phylum level, bacterial communities in the piglet colon were dominated by *Firmicutes* (61.87%–63.57%), *Bacteroidetes* (22.76%–23.47%), and *Proteobacteria* (4.18%–4.93%) (**Supplementary Figure 7A**). No significant differences were found in read numbers or relative abundance between the SP and the WP groups (**Supplementary Figures 7B, C**). At the genus level, we identified a total of 83 genera from the core bacterial community and combined relative abundance information to taxonomic tree (provided by NCBI) (**Figure 5E**). The results showed a comprehensive framework of the taxonomic branch and differences in the abundance of bacterial members between the two groups. The relative abundance of *Bifidobacterium*, *Bacteroides*, *Bacillus*, *Lactobacillus*, *Faecalibacterium*, and *Ruminococcus* were significantly decreased in the WP group than the SP group (Wilcoxon rank sum test). Conversely, we observed that the genera *Butyrivibrio*, *Coprococcus*, *Roseburia*, and *Succinivibrio* abundances were significantly higher in the WPs than in the SPs (Wilcoxon rank sum test). Moreover, in contrast to the SP group, the WP group was lack of several genera with relatively low proportional abundance, such as *Acinetobacter*, *Campylobacter*, *Enhydrobacter* and *Proteus*.

The SP and WP groups were mainly characterized by two co-occurrence networks with scattered nodes represented by multiple primary genera within distinct phyla. Both ecological networks were obviously parsed into five relatively consistent modules of co-occurring microbial members (**Figure 5F**). The highest degree and clustering coefficient score conceivably pointed out core community members within each ecosystem.

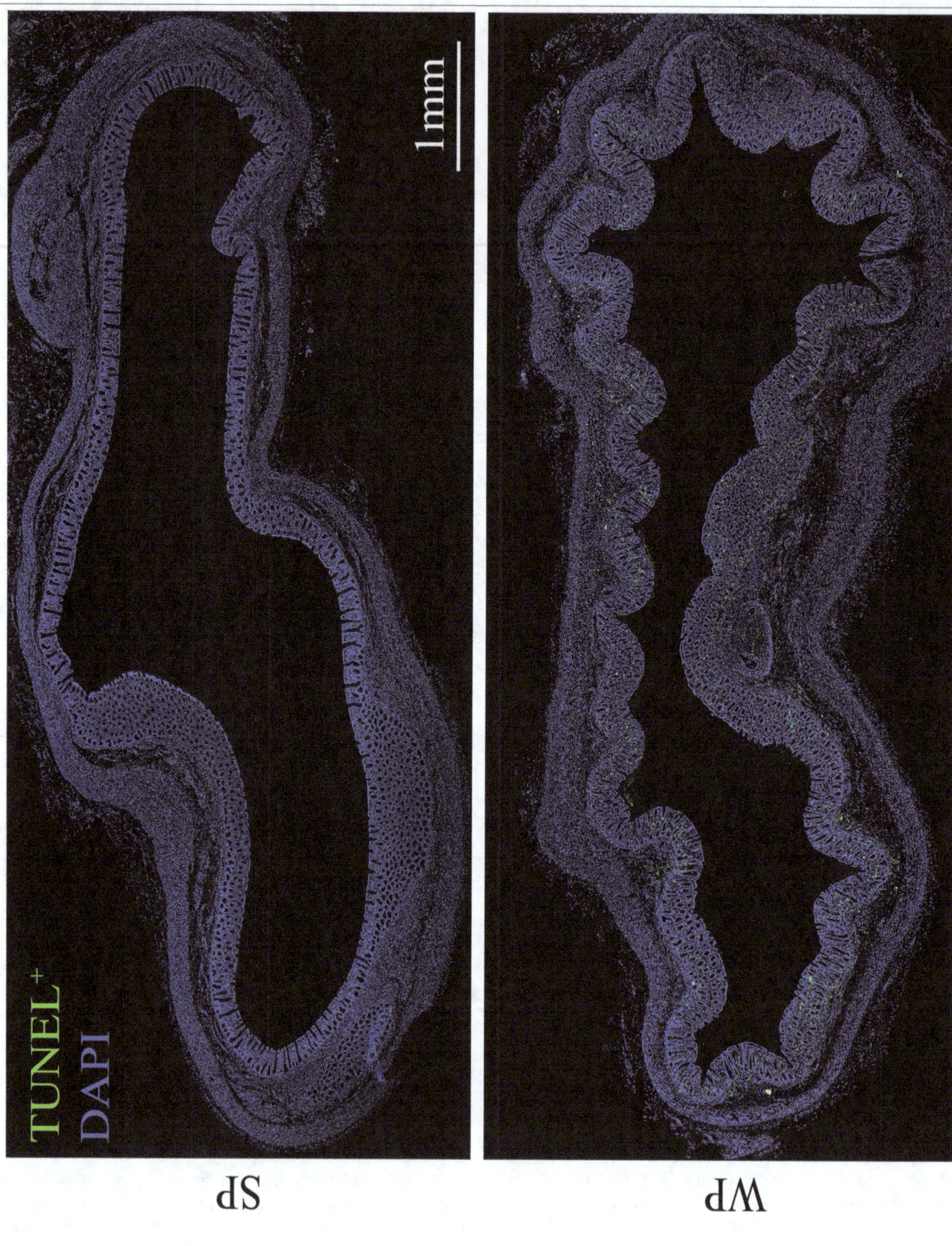

FIGURE 2 | TUNEL staining in colonic sections from SPs and WPs. The nuclei of apoptotic cells are positive for TUNEL staining (green). Scale bars, 1 mm.

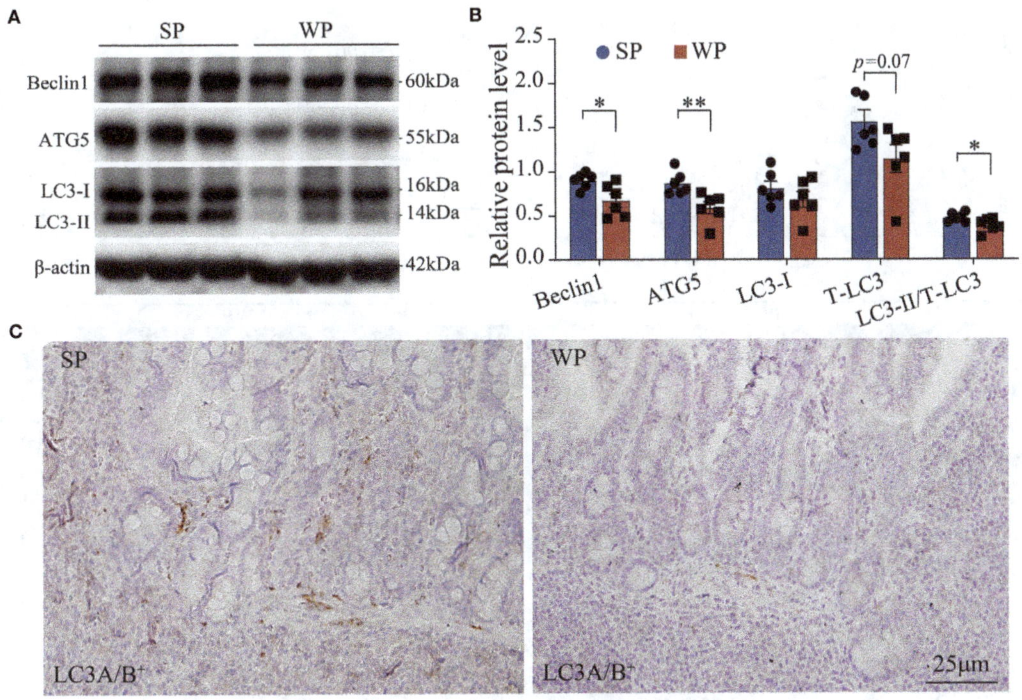

FIGURE 3 | Autophagy-related signaling was suppressed in WPs relative to that in SPs. **(A, B)** The expression of autophagy-related proteins in colonic tissue was determined by immunoblotting. **(C)** Representative images of immunohistochemistry for LC3A/B (n = 6). Scale bars, 25 μm. The data are presented as the means ± SEM, Student's t-test, *$P < 0.05$, **$P < 0.01$; n = 6.

The result showed that *Firmicutes* was the keystone species for determining the network in both the SP and WP groups, while the role of *Bacteroidetes* was minimized in the WP community (**Figure 5F** and **Supplementary Table 5**). We also undertook a detailed statistical analysis of the network characteristics including modularity, diameter, density, average clustering coefficient, and so on. A comparison was carried out for these network property parameters and node-level topological features between the two groups, the result indicated that the overall complexity and composition of the networks for the WP group were clearly reduced compared with those of the SP group (**Figures 5G, H** and **Supplementary Table 6**). Genera with larger degree centrality scores were considered as keystone taxa in the SP group, such as *Peptococcus*, *Ruminococcus*, *Bifidobacterium*, *Lactobacillus*, and *Bacteroides*; however, these genera contributed less to network construction in the WP group, within which *Anaerovibrio*, *Pyramidobacter*, *Butyrivibrio*, and *Collinsella* were more influential.

Metabolomics Analysis Identified Different Metabolic Patterns Between the SP and WP Groups

A total of 215 metabolites were identified (**Supplementary Table 7**). The samples from the SP and WP groups were clearly separated according to the PCA and OPLS-DA ($R2Y = 0.997$, $Q2 = 0.829$, permutation test, **Supplementary Figure 8**), which suggested that the weaning promoted the development of a metabolome composition distinct from that present in breastfeeding (**Figures 6A, B**). We identified the 56 individual metabolites that most contributed to the discrimination between the two groups based on the following criteria: a VIP score >1.0 from OPLS-DA modeling and a $|\log10\ (P\text{-value})| > 1.3$ (Student's t test) (**Figure 6C**). We classified all the metabolites into six major categories. The differences were displayed in overall metabolic clusters between the two groups through a stacked bar graph (**Figure 6D**). We found a higher abundance of organic acids and carbohydrate-associated metabolites in the WP group than in the SP group, whereas lower abundance of amino acids in the WP group. The WP group was largely characterized by a reduction in amino acid (including leucine, isoleucine, lysine, methionine, threonine, valine, and phenylalanine) and purine (including xanthine, inosine, guanosine, and 5-aminoimidazole-4-carboxamide) metabolites (**Figure 6E**). In contrast, the abundance of 9 metabolites associated with carbohydrate and lipid metabolism was significantly increased in the WP group than in the SP group (e.g., cellobiose, octanoate, xylose, monoolein, pelargonic acid, and glycerol) (**Supplementary Table 7**). KEGG pathway analysis of these significantly changed metabolites identified 19 different enrichment pathways between the two groups (**Figure 6F**). The key enrichment pathways identified were aminoacyl-tRNA biosynthesis (enrichment ratio [ER] = 6.24), fatty acid biosynthesis (ER = 5.72), pantothenate and CoA biosynthesis (ER = 5.92), glutathione metabolism (ER = 5.43), and purine metabolism (ER = 7.89).

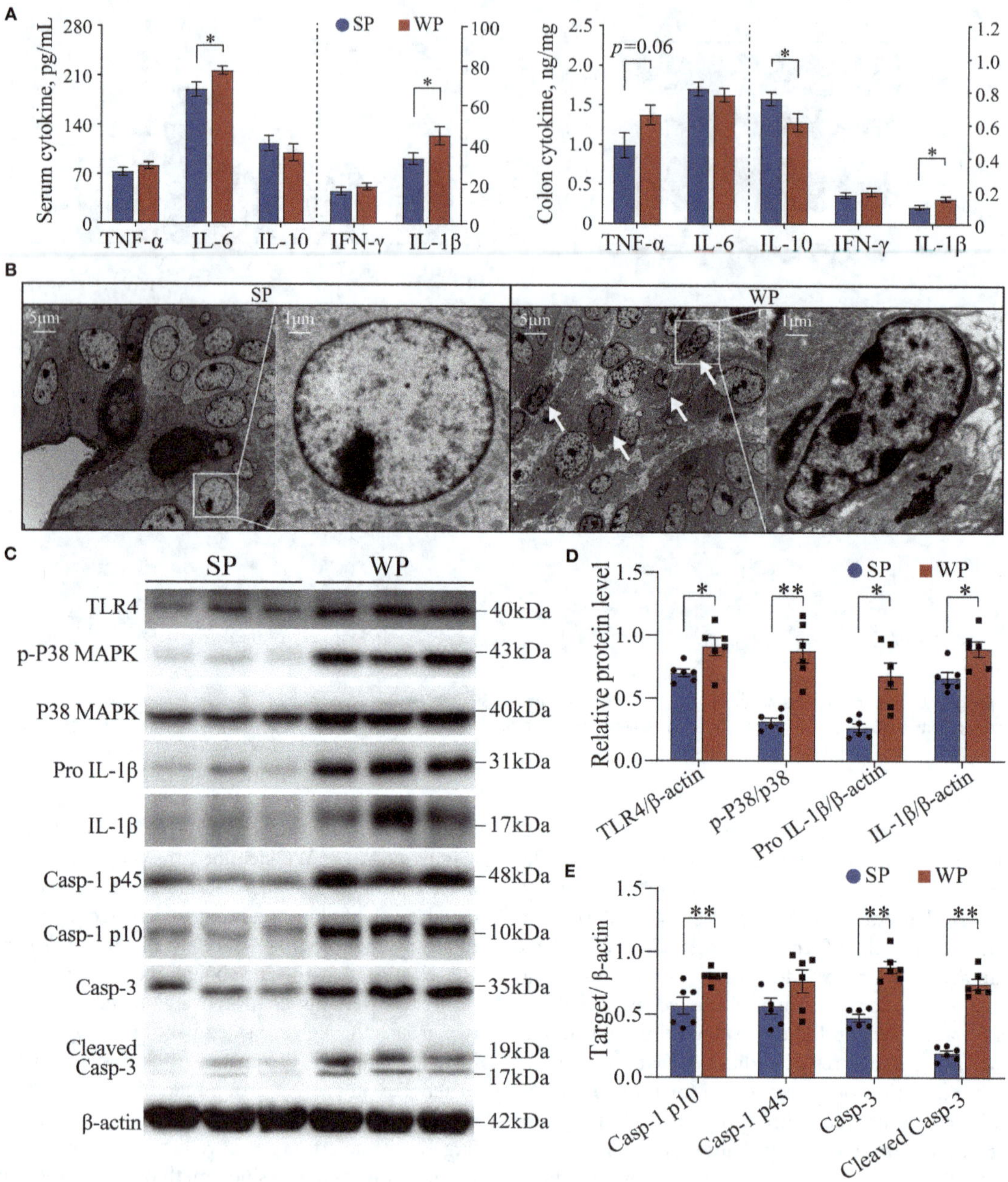

FIGURE 4 | The TLR4/P38MAPK/IL-1β-mediated apoptosis signaling pathway was activated in WPs but not in SPs. **(A)** The levels of various cytokines in serum and colon tissue measured by ELISA. **(B)** Representative transmission electron micrographs of colonic crypts from the SP and WP groups. The low magnification image (scale bar, 5 μm; ×3,000 magnification) demonstrates abundant degeneration and the presence of necrotic cells scattered at the bottom of crypts in the WP group. The higher magnification image (scale bar, 1 μm; ×10,000 magnification) shows a typical apoptosis event characterized by fragmented nuclei and leaking of the nuclear mass (arrow). **(C–E)** The expression of components of the TLR4/P38MAPK/IL-1β signaling pathway and caspase-related proteins in colon tissue were determined by immunoblotting. All data are presented as the means ± SEM, Student's *t*-test, $^{*}P < 0.05$, $^{**}P < 0.01$; $n = 6$.

Correlation Analysis and Functional Prediction of the Microbiome

The results of the 16S rRNA sequencing showed that early weaning disturbed the taxonomic composition of the colonic microbiota. Moreover, a metabolomics analysis indicated that the metabolic profiles of the two groups were different. We further explored the functional correlations between the 26 identified bacterial genomes and the 68 altered colon metabolites. Analysis based on Spearman's correlation coefficient revealed 362 significant associations, many of which involved genera enriched in the SP group. For instance, within the amino acid class, seven metabolites were positively associated

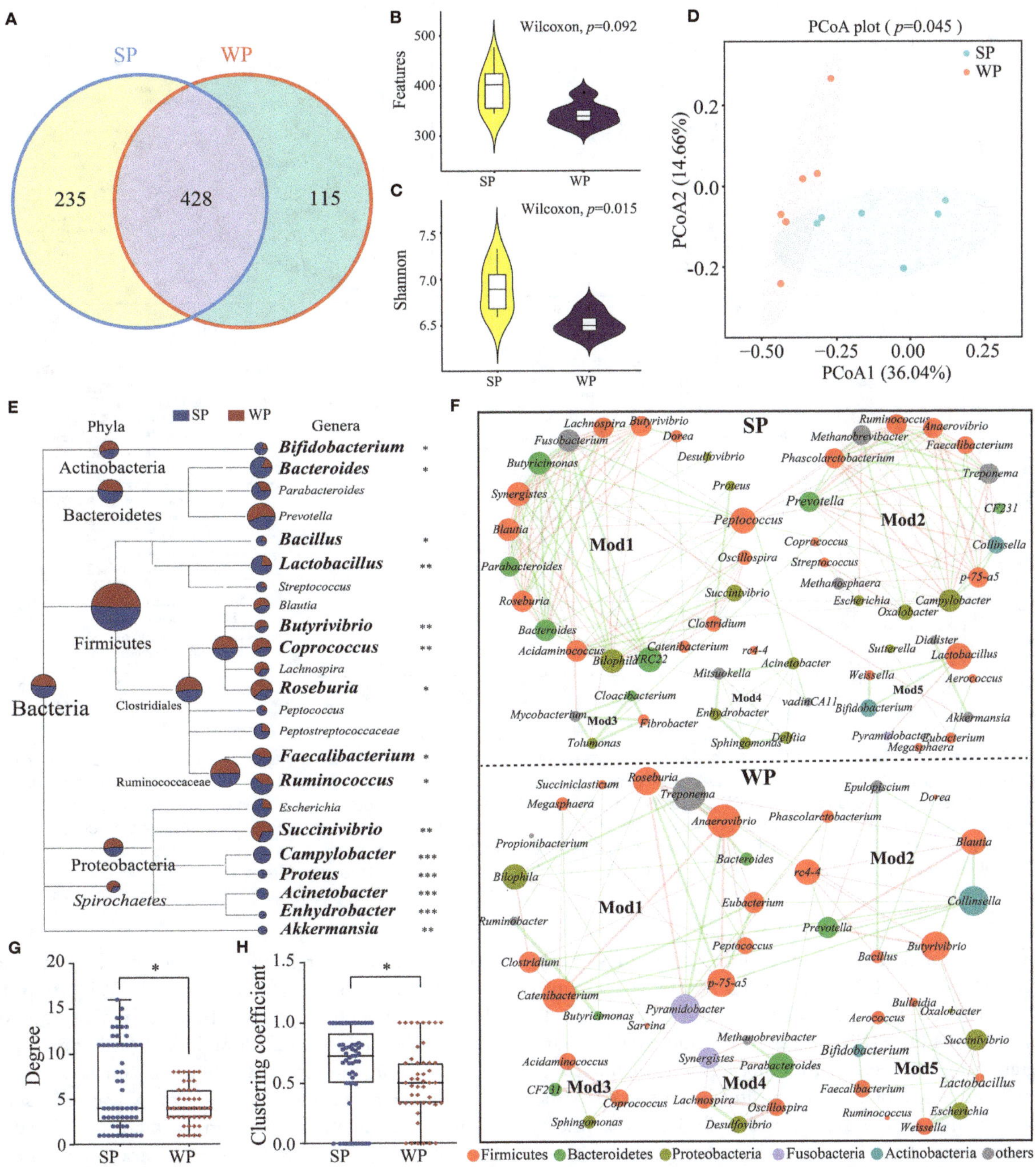

FIGURE 5 | Differences in gut microbiota structure and co-occurrence patterns between the SP and WP groups. **(A)** Venn diagram displaying the numbers of identified amplicon sequence variants (ASVs) in the SP and WP groups. **(B, C)** Differences in alpha diversity in the gut bacteria were assessed based on features and the Shannon index. **(D)** Principal coordinate analysis (PCoA) plots based on the Bray–Curtis distances identified distinct clusters between the SP and WP groups. **(E)** MEGAN taxonomic tree emphasized the evolutionary relationship and differences in abundance of microorganisms in the SP and WP groups. Relative abundance is displayed in a colored pie-chart; the size of the pie-chart indicates relative sequence abundance. **(F)** Microbial co-occurrence patterns in the colon ecosystems of the SP and WP groups were visualized using network diagrams. Co-occurrence relationships with a strong Spearman's correlation coefficient (|ρ value| >0.5 and $P < 0.05$) were selected and formed five modules in both groups; the size of each node is proportional to the degree of correlation. Phylum information for each node is indicated by color. The edges represent the correlation between the two genera, the thickness of the edge represents the strength of the correlation, orange represents a positive correlation, and green a negative correlation. **(G, H)** Topological properties (degree and clustering coefficient) of co-occurrence networks for bacterial communities in the SP and WP groups. All data are presented as means ± SEM. Wilcoxon rank sum test for **(B, C, F)**; PERMANOVA for **(D)**; and the Mann–Whitney non-parametric test for **(G, H)**. *$P < 0.05$, **$P < 0.01$, ***$P < 0.001$; $n = 6$.

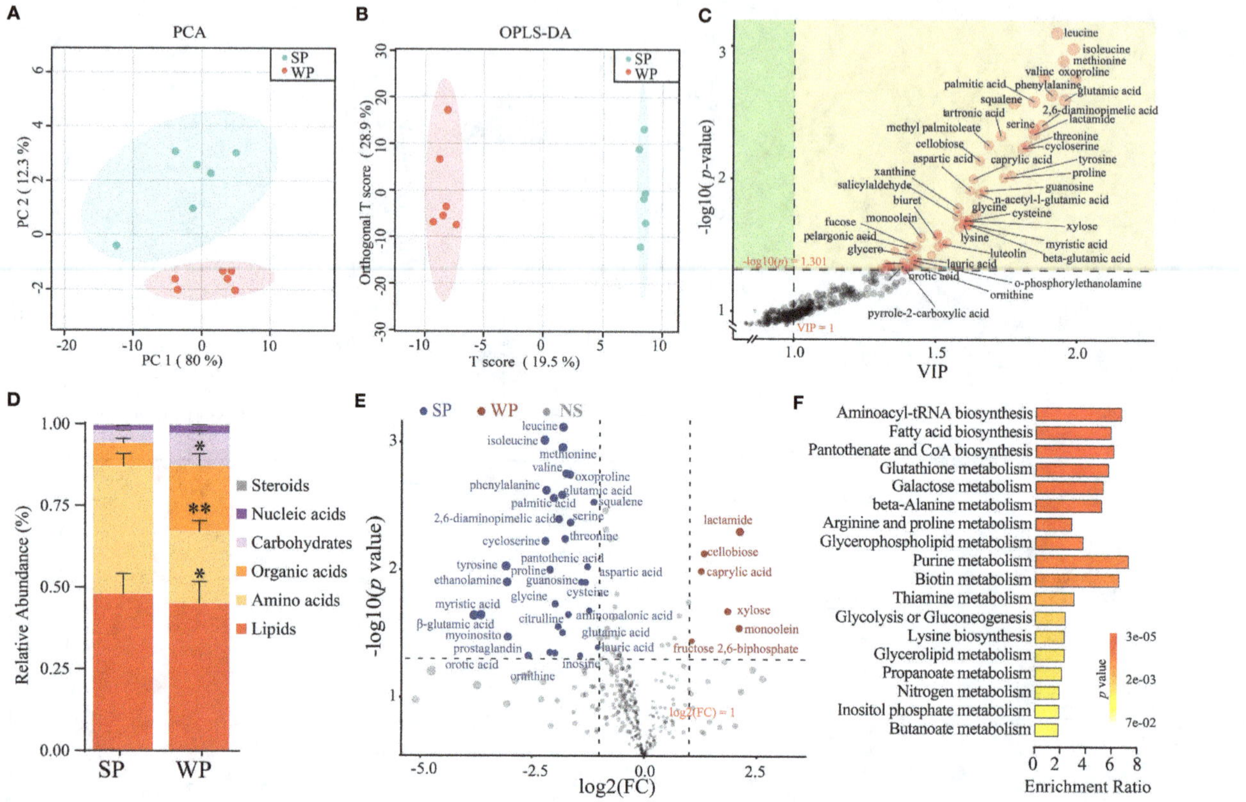

FIGURE 6 | Differences in metabolic patterns between the SP and WP groups. **(A)** The principal coordinate analysis (PCA) plot revealed a separation of the metabolites between the two groups. **(B)** Orthogonal partial least squares discriminant analysis (OPLS-DA) of the metabolomics profiles in the colon. **(C)** Dot diagram determined 56 individual metabolites based on the double criteria of VIP ≥1.0 and $P < 0.05$ (Student's *t*-test). These metabolites strongly contributed to the discrimination of the two groups. **(D)** Stacked bar graph showing the differences in relative abundance of six metabolite categories between the two groups. **(E)** Volcano plots of significantly changed metabolites in the SP and WP groups. **(F)** Metabolic pathway analysis of differentially abundant metabolites between the two groups. The *P*-value for each term is represented by the color intensity. The data are presented as means ± SEM for **(D)**, *$P < 0.05$, **$P < 0.01$, Student's *t*-test; $n = 6$.

with the genera *Lactobacillus*, *Bacillus*, *Bacteroides*, and *Ruminococcus* ($r \geq 0.621$, FDR-corrected *P*-value <0.01) but negatively correlated with *Coprococcus*, *Butytivibrio*, and *Succinivibrio* ($r \geq 0.489$, FDR-corrected *P*-value <0.05). For purine metabolism, the genera *Ruminococcus*, *Acinetobacter*, *Lactobacillus*, and *Bacteroides* were positively correlated with inosine, guanosine, and 5-aminoimidazole-4-carboxamide ($r \geq 0.585$, FDR-corrected *P*-value <0.05). For carbohydrate metabolism, most genera enriched in the SP group were negatively correlated with lactamide, caprylic acid, pelargonic acid, iminodiacetic acid, and fructose 2,6-biphosphate ($r \geq 0.422$, FDR-corrected *P*-value <0.05) (**Figure 7A**). Next, the abundances of the original 16S rRNA sequences were processed with PICRUSt2 to impute the putative biological functional compositions of the microbiomes in the SP and WP groups (**Figure 7B**). In general, symbionts and vigorous fermentation were enriched in the SP group, while pathogens gastroenteritis- and pathogens diarrhea-related genes were more abundant in the WP group. Among these predicted metabolic functions, the abundances of functional genes associated with methanogenesis, starch and sucrose metabolism, and aerobic metabolism significantly increased in the WP group than in the SP group, which suggested that early weaning led to the disturbance of intestinal flora linked with gut inflammation and a shift in metabolic function. In contrast, we found that the gut microbiota of the SP group was characterized by significant enrichment of several metabolism-related pathways. These pathways included nitrogen respiration, nitrate reduction, nitrate respiration, nitrite ammonification, and nucleotide metabolism. Spearman's correlation matrix suggested that the imbalance of the gut microbiota influenced mucosal inflammation and barrier integrity (**Figure 7C**). The relative abundance of *Bifidobacterium*, *Bacteroides*, *Bacillus*, *Lactobacillus*, *Faecalibacterium*, and *Ruminococcus* decreased in the WP group, which was positively correlated with the expression levels of ZO-1, occludin and claudin 3, the number of goblet cells, and mucosal layer thickness. In contrast, the increased relative abundance of *Butyrivibrio*, *Coprococcus*, and *Succinivibrio* in the WP group was positively associated with crypt depth and inflammation scores.

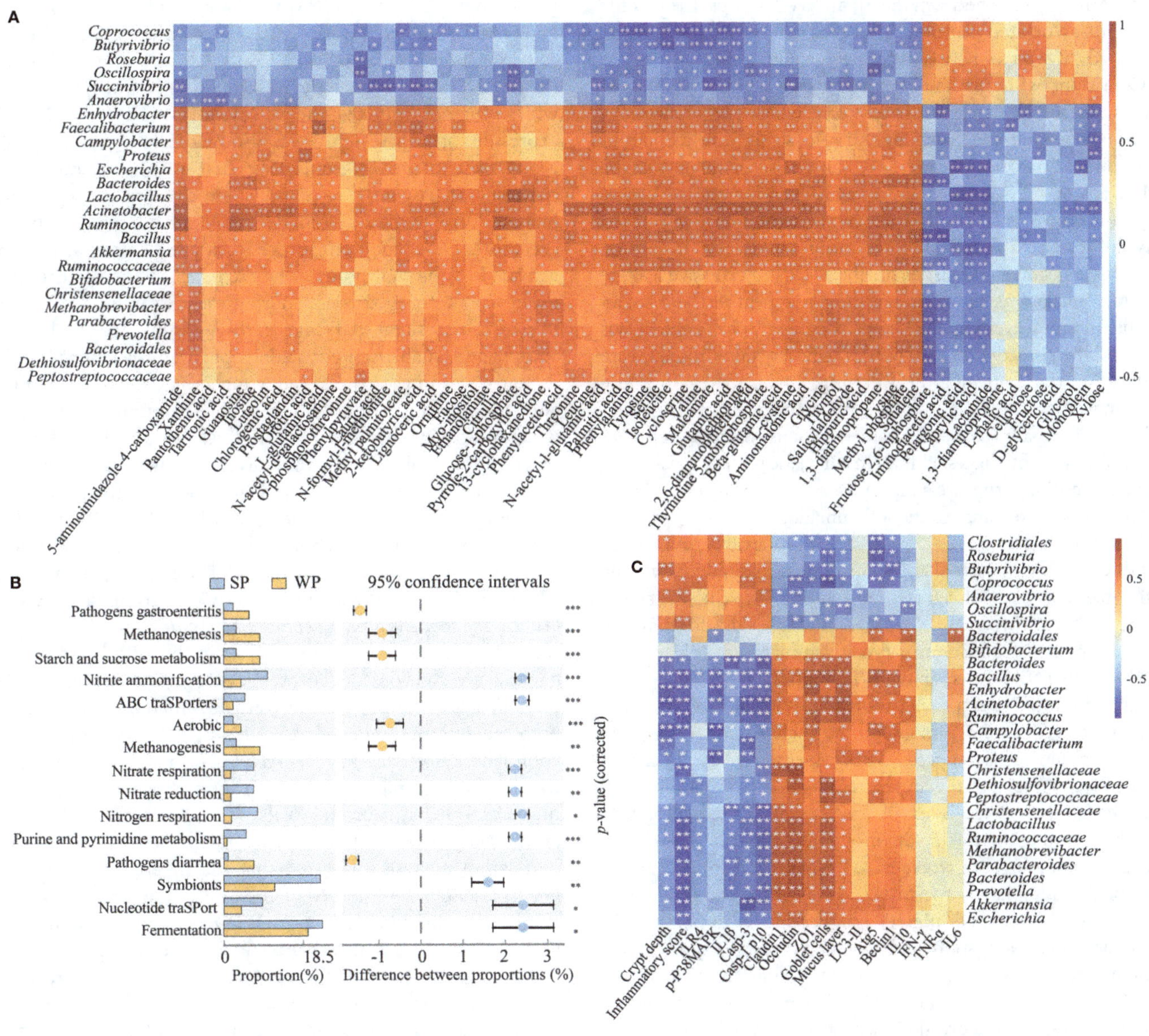

FIGURE 7 | Correlation and pathway analysis of significant differentially abundant metabolites and bacteria. **(A)** Heatmap showing the correlations between gut bacterial genera and individual metabolites. Spearman's rank correlation coefficients and *P*-values for the correlations of genera and their metabolites were calculated. The correlation effect is indicated by a color gradient from red (positive correlation) to blue (negative correlation). **(B)** The enriched pathways of microbial genes between the SP and WP groups. **(C)** Spearman's correlation analysis between the colonic microbiota and gut barrier integrity or inflammation-related signaling parameters. $^{*}P < 0.05$, $^{**}P < 0.01$, $^{***}P < 0.001$.

DISCUSSION

The demand for efficient and healthful pig production has posed challenges for the implementation of early weaning in the modern swine industry (34). Multiple stressors encountered during the early weaning contribute to transient anorexia, gut inflammation, and the disturbance of the intestinal flora of piglets (2). The exploration of cross-interaction between GI inflammation, gut microbiota and metabolomic in weaning piglets is prerequisite of develop strategies to overcome weaning stress and optimize the weaning transition (35). Our integrated analysis revealed that early weaning caused serious colonic inflammation in the piglets, which is linked with impaired mucosal barrier function. We also found that autophagy and apoptosis-related signaling pathways played an important role in promoting the inflammatory process. TLR4 is a major inducer of apoptosis. We observed high levels of TLR4 activation in the WP group, which suggested that the occurrence of intestinal inflammation post-weaning was related with the disturbance of the gut microbiome (13). Although there was a partial overlap in the composition of the gut microbiome and metabolome profiles between the SP and WP groups, the colonic symptom-associated features identified in the current study presented differences between the two groups.

Consistent with previously reported results, weaning stress resulted in severe damage to the colon, which morphologically manifested as high crypt density loss, hyperplasia, and compromised mucosal integrity (36, 37). The intestine of weaning piglets is not fully functionally developed and cannot adapt to sudden dietary transitions and/or environmental changes, which may be the main cause of weaning-associated intestinal inflammation. Impaired barrier function leads to excessive leakage of intraluminal antigens, toxins, and the consequent activation of an intestinal immune response (38). Indeed, the loss of the gut mucus layer and the reduction in the levels of tight junction proteins were evident in the piglets after weaning. Deficiencies in these components indicated that the capacity of the intestinal barrier to defend against pathogens and luminal antigens was impaired (39). These observations suggested that an imbalance in autophagy and apoptosis resulting from weaning stressors could be involved in the etiology of post-weaning enteric inflammation.

In the current study, the TUNEL and TEM analyses confirmed that discontinuous mucosal and transmural inflammation was the noticeable worsening of cell apoptosis seen in the colon tissue of weaned piglets. Meanwhile, ELISA analysis showed that the relatively higher production of pro-inflammatory cytokines (IL-1β, IL-6, and TNF-α) were in the WP group than in the SP group, which indicated that early weaning led to the systemic inflammatory cytokine profiles of the piglets. Conversely, the WP group showed a reduced IL-10, which often exerts critical suppressive effects on the progress of gut inflammation (40). Changes in the release levels of these cytokines can modulate autophagy and apoptosis in response to adverse conditions, such as dysbiosis of the gut microbiota (41). Notably, we found that the level of the autophagosome marker LC3 was reduced in colon tissues of the weaned piglets, suggesting a deficiency in autophagosome elongation and assembly. Beclin-1 and ATG5 proteins are critical for the completion of autophagy involving the LC3-conjugation machinery (42, 43). These autophagy-related molecules were markedly downregulated in WPs, which may account for the decreased autophagic flux seen in the colon of the weaned piglets. Our results supported that a link exists between autophagy and goblet cell function, which is in line with a previous report (44). The emerging evidence has indicated that appropriate levels of autophagy in the intestinal epithelium functions as a deterrent to cytokine-meditated programmed cell apoptosis, thereby promoting intestinal homeostasis and limiting immunopathology (43, 45). In the current study, autophagy deficiency and an abnormal pro-inflammatory cytokine elevation occurred simultaneously in the WP group, which suggested that weaned piglets are susceptible to immunopathology resulting from the activity of proinflammatory cytokines, particularly IL-1β. Accordingly, we further tested the release and activation status of IL-1β. TLR4 modulates the secretion of various cytokines following the sensing of exogenous pathogen-associated molecules, which plays a significant role in mediating gut microbiota disorder-induced enteric infections (46). Similarly, we found that TLR4 and P38MAPK were highly expressed, and P38MAPK phosphorylation was also enhanced in the WP group. Upon microbial invasion, the activation of TLR4/P38MAPK signaling accelerates P38MAPK phosphorylation, which further induces the release of IL-1β (14, 47). The expression of caspase-1 p10 was also markedly higher in the WP group than in the SP group. Caspase-1 p10 is an auto-cleaved fragment of caspase-1 responsible for cleaving pro-IL-1β into mature form to induce cell death (48). Additionally, the key executor of the apoptotic process, caspase-3, was also highly activated in the WP group, which confirmed the occurrence of severe apoptotic progression during early weaning. Collectively, these results suggested that early weaning led to reduced autophagy and aberrant elevated apoptosis in the colon.

Early weaning caused a reduction in gut microbial richness and diversity and shifted the microbial community in piglets, which was in line with previous findings (49, 50). This reduction in gut microbial richness and diversity might be due to the imbalance between symbionts and potentially pathogenic microorganisms by assessment of PICRUSt2 in this study. Differences in sequence abundance in each taxonomic branch were indicative of the existence of taxonomic perturbations, which allowed for distinguishing the WP group from the SP group. *Bifidobacterium*, *Bacillus*, *Bacteroides*, and *Lactobacillus* were abundant in the SP group than in the WP. Most of these bacteria are considered as probiotics for a long history (51, 52). *Faecalibacterium* was found to exert anti-inflammatory effects on both cell and mouse models of colitis (53). The absence of these commensal bacteria may be relative with the gut physiology dysbiosis of the piglets in the WP group. Meanwhile, the gut microbial ecosystem in WPs was characterized by the enrichment of *Butyrivibrio* and *Succinivibrio*. The Spearmen correlation analysis suggested that the differentially abundant gut microbiota community of the WP group was significantly associated with intestinal barrier function and inflammation-related signals. Such disturbances in the intestinal flora and loss of microbial biomass at the early stage of life have previously been reported to be highly associated with GI diseases (54).

Major shifts in microbial composition will lead to an unstable network of microbes, which is often associated with poor host health (55). In this study, co-occurrence analysis was employed to discern the differences in network associations across microbial communities from the SP and WP groups. The bacterial interactions were more intricate and extensive in the SPs than in the WPs. Empirical work has shown that reduced ecological interaction frequencies can disrupt the stability of the microbiome within the mammalian intestine, with detrimental consequences for the health of the host (55). Moreover, based on node properties, we found that the importance of some community members in the network had changed in the weaned piglets. Although five relatively consistent modules of co-occurring gut microbes were detected in both the SP and WP groups. Some species with high 'degree' and 'clustering coefficient' scores contributed equally to the networks of the SP group, which were evenly distributed and dispersed. In contrast, several important species played a dominant role in constructing the network of the WP group, such as *Anaerovibrio*, *Roseburia*, *Pyramidobacter*, *Butyrivibrio*, and *Collinsella*. In addition to changes in diversity, symbiotic relationships tended to be concentrated and monotonous in the WP group, which would be expected to exert a long-term adverse effect on the intestinal health of the piglets (56–58).

The gut metabolites can mediate the interactions between the gut microbiota and the host (16, 21). Multiple-omics analyses yielded unique and differential features of microbiota-metabolic correlations between the SP and WP groups. The abundances of leucine, isoleucine, and lysine were significantly decreased in the WP group than in the SP group. These metabolites were positively correlated with the number of dominant bacteria in the SP group based on correlation analysis. Meanwhile, the prediction of microbial biological function showed that the pattern amino acid metabolites utilization mediated by the intestinal microflora had collapsed in the weaned piglets. The loss of amino acid metabolites may cause an aberrant progression of mucus synthesis (59), because the synthesis of 'mucin domain', a core element of mucins, requires various amino acid residues (60). Furthermore, early weaning resulted in a prominent decrease in the levels of purine metabolites such as xanthine, inosine, and guanosine. We also found that several bacteria, such as *Bacillus*, *Escherichia*, *Akkermansia*, and *Ruminococcus*, may be involved in purine metabolism, which is consistent with previous studies (61, 62). A previous study reported that gut microbial-derived purine metabolites could attenuate intestinal barrier dysfunction (62). These findings may partly explain the inflammatory response present in the colon of the weaned piglets.

In conclusion, early weaning resulted in damage to colonic crypt architecture and a severe inflammatory response, which may be attributable to the dysregulation of autophagy and the TLR4/P38MAPK/IL-1β-mediated apoptotic signaling pathway. Meanwhile, early weaning not only caused the loss of richness and diversity of the microbial community and the dysregulation of the pattern of co-occurrence, but also concomitantly induced metabolic changes in the colonic content. Gut microbiota disturbance caused by early weaning inhibited autophagy and activated the TLR4/P38MAPK/IL-1β apoptosis signaling pathway, ultimately aggravated colon inflammation. These findings provide new knowledge concerning exploiting microbial metabolites to regulate gut barrier integrity and immune responses in weaned piglets. database under accession number PRJNA761570 (https://www.ncbi.nlm.nih.gov/sra/PRJNA761570).

AUTHOR CONTRIBUTIONS

HW and WT conceived the study. HW and WT designed the project and the experiments. WT, JLL, YM, and HW collected the samples, prepared the 16S rRNA library for sequencing, and performed the experiments. WT and YW performed the bioinformatics analysis. JXL, JLL, and YM helped with IF staining. WT wrote the manuscript. HW, JXL, YM, JLL, and YW revised the manuscript. All the authors reviewed and approved the final version of the manuscript.

FUNDING

This study was supported by grants from the Key R & D Projects of Zhejiang Province (2022C04034), the National Natural Sciences Foundation of China (31672430), the Natural Science Foundation of Zhejiang Province (Z19C170001), the Funds of Ten Thousand People Plan of China, and the National Key Research and Development Program of China (2017YFD0500502).

ACKNOWLEDGMENTS

The authors thank the Morphological Platform, Zhejiang University School of Medicine for their technical support. The authors also thank Bio-ultrastructure Analysis Laboratory of the Analysis center of Agrobiology and Environmental Sciences, Zhejiang University for generously sharing their experiment and analysis experiences.

REFERENCES

Ackers J, Clark CG, Diamond LS, Duchêne M, Cantellano ME, Jackson TF, et al. WHO/PAHO/UNESCO report. A consultation with experts on amoebiasis. Mexico City, Mexico 28-29 January, 1997. *Epidemiol Bull* (1997) **18**:13–4.

Pluske JR, Turpin DL, Kim JC. Gastrointestinal Tract (Gut) Health in the Young P ig. *Anim Nutr* (2018) 4(2):187 j.aninu.2017.12.004

Campbell JM, Crenshaw JD, Polo J. The Biological Stress of Early Weaned Piglets. *J Anim Sci Biotechnol* (2013) 4(1):19. doi: 10.1186/2049-1891-4-19

Lallès JP, Bosi P, Smidt H, Stokes CR. Nutritional Management of Gut Health in Pigs Around Weaning. *Proc Nutr Soc* (2007) 66(2):260–8. doi: 10.1017/s0029665107005484

Al Nabhani Z, Dulauroy S, Marques R, Cousu C, Al Bounny S, Déjardin F, et al. A Weaning Reaction to Microbiota is Required for Resistance to Immunopathologies in the Adult. *Immunity* (2019) 50(5):1276–88.e5. doi: 10.1016/j.immuni.2019.02.014

Barroso M, Beth SA, Voortman T, Jaddoe VWV, van Zelm MC, Moll HA, et al. Dietary Patterns After the Weaning and Lactation Period are Associated With Celiac Disease Autoimmunity in Children. *Gastroenterology* (2018) 154 (8):2087–96.e7. doi: 10.1053/j.gastro.2018.02.024

Ren W, Wang P, Yan J, Liu G, Zeng B, Hussain T, et al. Melatonin Alleviates Weanling Stress in Mice: Involvement of Intestinal Microbiota. *J Pineal Res* (2018) 64(2)::e12448. doi: 10.1111/jpi.12448

Ganal-Vonarburg SC, Hornef MW, Macpherson AJ. Microbial-Host Molecular Exchange and its Functional Consequences in Early Mammalian Life. *Science* (2020) 368(6491):604–7. doi: 10.1126/science.aba0478

Maiuri MC, Zalckvar E, Kimchi A, Kroemer G. Self-Eating and Self-Killing: Crosstalk Between Autophagy and Apoptosis. *Nat Rev Mol Cell Biol* (2007) 8 (9):741–52. doi: 10.1038/nrm2239

Haq S, Grondin J, Banskota S, Khan WI. Autophagy: Roles in Intestinal Mucosal Homeostasis and Inflammation. *J BioMed Sci* (2019) 26(1):19. doi: 10.1186/ s12929-019-0512-2

Elshaer D, Begun J. The Role of Barrier Function, Autophagy, and Cytokines in Maintaining Intestinal Homeostasis. *Semin Cell Dev Biol* (2017) 61:51–9. doi: 10.1016/j.semcdb.2016.08.018

Lassen KG, Kuballa P, Conway KL, Patel KK, Becker CE, Peloquin JM, et al. Atg16L1 T300A Variant Decreases Selective Autophagy Resulting in Altered Cytokine Signaling and Decreased Antibacterial Defense. *Proc Natl Acad Sci* (2014) 111(21):7741–6. doi: 10.1073/pnas.1407001111

Campisi L, Barbet G, Ding Y, Esplugues E, Flavell RA, Blander JM. Apoptosis in Response to Microbial Infection Induces Autoreactive TH17 Cells. *Nat Immunol* (2016) 17(9):1084–92. doi: 10.1038/ni.3512

Fitzgerald KA, Kagan JC. Toll-Like Receptors and the Control of Immunity. *Cell* (2020) 180(6):1044–66. doi: 10.1016/j.cell.2020.02.041

Gao L, Yu Q, Zhang H, Wang Z, Zhang T, Xiang J, et al. A Resident Stromal Cell Population Actively Restrains Innate Immune Response in the Propagation Phase of Colitis Pathogenesis in Mice. *Sci Trans Med* (2021) 13 (603):eabb5071. doi: 10.1126/scitranslmed.abb5071

Kamada N, Seo SU, Chen GY, Núñez G. Role of the Gut Microbiota in Immunity and Inflammatory Disease. *Nat Rev Immunol* (2013) 13(5):321–35. doi: 10.1038/nri3430

Fan Y, Pedersen O. Gut Microbiota in Human Metabolic Health and Disease. *Nat Rev Microbiol* (2021) 19(1):55–71. doi: 10.1038/s41579-020-0433-9

Li N, Zuo B, Huang S, Zeng B, Han D, Li T, et al. Spatial Heterogeneity of Bacterial Colonization Across Different Gut Segments Following Inter-Species Microbiota Transplantation. *Microbiome* (2020) 8(1):161. doi: 10.1186/ s40168-020-00917-7

Pannaraj PS, Li F, Cerini C, Bender JM, Yang S, Rollie A, et al. Association Between Breast Milk Bacterial Communities and Establishment and Development of the Infant Gut Microbiome. *JAMA Pediatr* (2017) 171 (7):647–54. doi: 10.1001/jamapediatrics.2017.0378

Yilmaz B, Juillerat P, Øyås O, Ramon C, Bravo FD, Franc Y, et al. Microbial Network Disturbances in Relapsing Refractory Crohn's Disease. *Nat Med* (2019) 25(2):323–36. doi: 10.1038/s41591-018-0308-z

Mainali KP, Bewick S, Thielen P, Mehoke T, Breitwieser FP, Paudel S, et al. Statistical Analysis of Co-Occurrence Patterns in Microbial Presence-Absence Datasets. *PloS One* (20 17) 12 (11) :e0 18713 2. doi : 10 .1 371/ journal.pone.0187132

Lee WJ, Hase K. Gut Microbiota-Generated Metabolites in Animal Health and Disease. *Nat Chem Biol* (2014) 10(6):416–24. doi: 10.1038/nchembio.1535

Koh A, Bäckhed F. From Association to Causality: The Role of the Gut Microbiota and its Functional Products on Host Metabolism. *Mol Cell* (2020) 78(4):584–96. doi: 10.1016/j.molcel.2020.03.005

Roager HM, Hansen LB, Bahl MI, Frandsen HL, Carvalho V, Gøbel RJ, et al. Colonic Transit Time is Related to Bacterial Metabolism and Mucosal Turnover in the Gut. *Nat Microbiol* (2016) 1(9):16093. doi: 10.1038/ nmicrobiol.2016.93

Kurilshikov A, Medina-Gomez C, Bacigalupe R, Radjabzadeh D, Wang J, Demirkan A, et al. Large-Scale Association Analyses Identify Host Factors Influencing Human Gut Microbiome Composition. *Nat Genet* (2021) 53 (2):156–65. doi: 10.1038/s41588-020-00763-1

Callahan BJ, McMurdie PJ, Rosen MJ, Han AW, Johnson AJ, Holmes SP. DADA2: High-Resolution Sample Inference From Illumina Amplicon Data. *Nat Methods* (2016) 13(7):581–3. doi: 10.1038/nmeth.3869

Bolyen E, Rideout JR, Dillon MR, Bokulich NA, Abnet CC, Al-Ghalith GA, et al. Reproducible, Interactive, Scalable and Extensible Microbiome Data Science Using QIIME 2. *Nat Biotechnol* (2019) 37(8):852–7. doi: 10.1038/ s41587-019-0209-9

Chen H, Boutros PC. Venndiagram: A Package for the Generation of Highly-Customizable Venn and Euler Diagrams in R. *BMC Bioinf* (2011) 12:35. doi: 10.1186/1471-2105-12-35

Huson DH, Auch AF, Qi J, Schuster SC. MEGAN Analysis of Metagenomic Data. *Genome Res* (2007) 17(3):377–86. doi: 10.1101/gr.5969107

Douglas GM, Maffei VJ, Zaneveld JR, Yurgel SN, Brown JR, Taylor CM, et al. Picrust2 for Prediction of Metagenome Functions. *Nat Biotechnol* (2020) 38 (6):685–8. doi: 10.1038/s41587-020-0548-6

Deng Y, Jiang YH, Yang Y, He Z, Luo F, Zhou J. Molecular Ecological Network Analyses. *BMC Bioinf* (2012) 13:113. doi: 10.1186/1471-2105-13-113

Zhang L, Delgado-Baquerizo M, Shi Y, Liu X, Yang Y, Chu H. Co-Existing Water and Sediment Bacteria are Driven by Contrasting Environmental Factors Across Glacier-Fed Aquatic Systems. *Water Res* (2021) 198:117139. doi: 10.1016/j.watres.2021.117139

Kind T, Wohlgemuth G, Lee DY, Lu Y, Palazoglu M, Shahbaz S, et al. Fiehnlib: Mass Spectral and Retention Index Libraries for Metabolomics Based on Quadrupole and Time-of-Flight Gas Chromatography/Mass Spectrometry. *Anal Chem* (2009) 81(24):10038–48. doi: 10.1021/ac9019522

Dunn WB, Broadhurst D, Begley P, Zelena E, Francis-McIntyre S, Anderson N, et al. Procedures for Large-Scale Metabolic Profiling of Serum and Plasma Using Gas Chromatography and Liquid Chromatography Coupled to Mass Spectrometry. *Nat Protoc* (2011) 6(7):1060–83. doi: 10.1038/nprot.2011.335

Jayaraman B, Nyachoti CM. Husbandry Practices and Gut Health Outcomes in Weaned Piglets: A Review. *Anim Nutr* (2017) 3(3):205–11. doi: 10.1016/ j.aninu.2017.06.002

Kim HB, Isaacson RE. The Pig Gut Microbial Diversity: Understanding the Pig Gut Microbial Ecology Through the Next Generation High Throughput Sequencing. *Vet Microbiol* (2015) 177(3-4):242–51. doi: 10.1016/ j.vetmic.2015.03.014

Shaoul R, Tiosano D, Hochberg Z. Evo-Devo of Child Growth: The Role of Weaning in the Transition From Infancy to Childhood. *Crit Rev Food Sci Nutr* (2016) 56(6):887–95. doi: 10.1080/10408398.2012.732623

Crispel Y, Shaoul R, Khamaise R, Sabo E, Hochberg Z. Effect of Weaning Age on the Small Intestine Mucosa of Rats. *Appl Physiol Nutr Metab* (2019) 44 (9):985–9. doi: 10.1139/apnm-2018-0454

Bomba L, Minuti A, Moisá SJ, Trevisi E, Eufemi E, Lizier M, et al. Gut Response Induced by Weaning in Piglet Features Marked Changes in Immune and Inflammatory Response. *Funct Integr Genomics* (2014) 14(4):657–71. doi: 10.1007/s10142-014-0396-x

Beaumont M, Paës C, Mussard E, Knudsen C, Cauquil L, Aymard P, et al. Gut Microbiota Derived Metabolites Contribute to Intestinal Barrier Maturation at the Suckling-to-Weaning Transition. *Gut Microbes* (2020) 11(5):1268–86. doi: 10.1080/19490976.2020.1747335

Koelink PJ, Bloemendaal FM, Li B, Westera L, Vogels EWM, van Roest M, et al. Anti-TNF Therapy in IBD Exerts its Therapeutic Effect Through Macrophage IL-10 Signalling. *Gut* (2020) 69(6):1053–63. doi: 10.1136/ gutjnl-2019-318264

Kabat AM, Pott J, Maloy KJ. The Mucosal Immune System and its Regulation by Autophagy. *Front Immunol* (2016) 7:240(240). doi: 10.3389/ fimmu.2016.00240

Sanjuan MA, Dillon CP, Tait SW, Moshiach S, Dorsey F, Connell S, et al. Toll-Like Receptor Signalling in Macrophages Links the Autophagy Pathway to Phagocytosis. *Nature* (2007) 450(7173):1253–7. doi: 10.1038/nature06421

Burger E, Araujo A, López-Yglesias A, Rajala MW, Geng L, Levine B, et al. Loss of Paneth Cell Autophagy Causes Acute Susceptibility to Toxoplasma Gondii-Mediated Inflammation. *Cell Host Microbe* (2018) 23(2):177–90.e4. doi: 10.1016/j.chom.2018.01.001

Wlodarska M, Thaiss CA, Nowarski R, Henao-Mejia J, Zhang JP, Brown EM, et al. NLRP6 Inflammasome Orchestrates the Colonic Host-Microbial Interface by Regulating Goblet Cell Mucus Secretion. *Cell* (2014) 156 (5):1045–59. doi: 10.1016/j.cell.2014.01.026

Pott J, Kabat AM, Maloy KJ. Intestinal Epithelial Cell Autophagy is Required to Protect Against TNF-Induced Apoptosis During Chronic Colitis in Mice. *Cell Host Microbe* (2018) 23(2):191–202.e4. doi: 10.1016/j.chom.2017.12.017

Wang Y, Zhang S, Li H, Wang H, Zhang T, Hutchinson MR, et al. Small-Molecule Modulators of Toll-Like Receptors. *Accounts Chem Res* (2020) 53 (5):1046–55. doi: 10.1021/acs.accounts.9b00631

Saitoh T, Fujita N, Jang MH, Uematsu S, Yang BG, Satoh T, et al. Loss of the Autophagy Protein Atg16L1 Enhances Endotoxin-Induced IL-1beta Production. *Nature* (2008) 456(7219):264–8. doi: 10.1038/nature07383

Vince JE, Silke J. The Intersection of Cell Death and Inflammasome Activation. *Cell Mol Life Sci* (2016) 73(11-12):2349–67. doi: 10.1007/ s00018-016-2205-2

Lu D, Tiezzi F, Schillebeeckx C, McNulty NP, Schwab C, Shull C, et al. Host Contributes to Longitudinal Diversity of Fecal Microbiota in Swine Selected for Lean Growth. *Microbiome* (2018) 6(1):4. doi: 10.1186/s40168- 017-0384-1

Wang W, Hu H, Zijlstra RT, Zheng J, Gänzle MG. Metagenomic Reconstructions of Gut Microbial Metabolism in Weanling Pigs. *Microbiome* (2019) 7(1):48. doi: 10.1186/s40168-019-0662-1

Piewngam P, Zheng Y, Nguyen TH, Dickey SW, Joo HS, Villaruz AE, et al. Pathogen Elimination by Probiotic Bacillus *via* Signalling Interference. *Nature* (2018) 562(7728):532–7. doi: 10.1038/s41586-018-0616-y

Sanders ME, Merenstein DJ, Reid G, Gibson GR, Rastall RA. Probiotics and Prebiotics in Intestinal Health and Disease: From Biology to the Clinic. *Nat Rev Gastroenterol Hepatol* (2019) 16(10):605–16. doi: 10.1038/s41575-019-0173-3

Sokol H, Pigneur B, Watterlot L, Lakhdari O, Bermúdez-Humarán LG, Gratadoux JJ, et al. Faecalibacterium Prausnitzii is an Anti-Inflammatory Commensal Bacterium Identified by Gut Microbiota Analysis of Crohn Disease Patients. *Proc Natl Acad Sci USA* (2008) 105(43):16731– doi: 10.1073/pnas.0804812105

Fouhse JM, Zijlstra RT, Willing BP. The Role of Gut Microbiota in the Health and Disease of Pigs. *Anim Front* (2016) 6(3):30–6. doi: 10.2527/af.2016-0031

Coyte KZ, Schluter J, Foster KR. The Ecology of the Microbiome: Networks, Competition, and Stability. *Science* (2015) 350(6261):663–6. doi: 10.1126/science.aad26026.

Gresse R, Chaucheyras-Durand F, Fleury MA, Van de Wiele T, Forano E, Blanquet-Diot S. Gut Microbiota Dysbiosis in Postweaning Piglets: Understanding the Keys to Health. *Trends Microbiol* (2017) 25(10):851–73. doi: 10.1016/j.tim.2017.05.004

Huang A, Cai R, Wang Q, Shi L, Li C, Yan H. Dynamic Change of Gut Microbiota During Porcine Epidemic Diarrhea Virus Infection in Suckling Piglets. *Front Microbiol* (2019) 10:322. doi: 10.3389/fmicb.2019.00322

Niederwerder MC. Role of the Microbiome in Swine Respiratory Disease. *Vet Microbiol* (2017) 209:97–106. doi: 10.1016/j.vetmic.2017.02.017

Paone P, Cani PD. Mucus Barrier, Mucins and Gut Microbiota: The Expected Slimy Partners? *Gut* (2020) 69(12):2232–43. doi: 10.1136/gutjnl-2020-322260 Johansson MEV, Hansson GC. Immunological Aspects of Intestinal Mucus and Mucins. *Nat Rev Immunol* (2016) 16(10):639–49. doi: 10.1038/nri.2016.88

Sheremet AS, Gronskiy SV, Akhmadyshin RA, Novikova AE, Livshits VA, Shakulov RS, et al. Enhancement of Extracellular Purine Nucleoside Accumulation by Bacillus Strains Through Genetic Modifications of Genes Involved in Nucleoside Export. *J Ind Microbiol Biotechnol* (2011) 38(1):65–70. doi: 10.1007/s10295-010-0829-z

Li D, Feng Y, Tian M, Ji J, Hu X, Chen F. Gut Microbiota-Derived Inosine From Dietary Barley Leaf Supplementation Attenuates Colitis Through PPARg Signaling Activation. *Microbiome* (2021) 9(1):83. doi: 10.1186/ s40168-021-01028-7

Permissions

All chapters in this book were first published by Frontiers; hereby published with permission under the Creative Commons Attribution License or equivalent. Every chapter published in this book has been scrutinized by our experts. Their significance has been extensively debated. The topics covered herein carry significant findings which will fuel the growth of the discipline. They may even be implemented as practical applications or may be referred to as a beginning point for another development.

The contributors of this book come from diverse backgrounds, making this book a truly international effort. This book will bring forth new frontiers with its revolutionizing research information and detailed analysis of the nascent developments around the world.

We would like to thank all the contributing authors for lending their expertise to make the book truly unique. They have played a crucial role in the development of this book. Without their invaluable contributions this book wouldn't have been possible. They have made vital efforts to compile up to date information on the varied aspects of this subject to make this book a valuable addition to the collection of many professionals and students.

This book was conceptualized with the vision of imparting up-to-date information and advanced data in this field. To ensure the same, a matchless editorial board was set up. Every individual on the board went through rigorous rounds of assessment to prove their worth. After which they invested a large part of their time researching and compiling the most relevant data for our readers.

The editorial board has been involved in producing this book since its inception. They have spent rigorous hours researching and exploring the diverse topics which have resulted in the successful publishing of this book. They have passed on their knowledge of decades through this book. To expedite this challenging task, the publisher supported the team at every step. A small team of assistant editors was also appointed to further simplify the editing procedure and attain best results for the readers.

Apart from the editorial board, the designing team has also invested a significant amount of their time in understanding the subject and creating the most relevant covers. They scrutinized every image to scout for the most suitable representation of the subject and create an appropriate cover for the book.

The publishing team has been an ardent support to the editorial, designing and production team. Their endless efforts to recruit the best for this project, has resulted in the accomplishment of this book. They are a veteran in the field of academics and their pool of knowledge is as vast as their experience in printing. Their expertise and guidance has proved useful at every step. Their uncompromising quality standards have made this book an exceptional effort. Their encouragement from time to time has been an inspiration for everyone.

The publisher and the editorial board hope that this book will prove to be a valuable piece of knowledge for researchers, students, practitioners and scholars across the globe.

List of Contributors

Janice K. P. Lam, K. F. Hui, Raymond J. Ning, X. Q. Xu and Alan K. S. Chiang
Department of Paediatrics and Adolescent Medicine, Li Ka Shing Faculty of Medicine, Queen Mary Hospital, The University of Hong Kong, Pokfulam, Hong Kong

K. H. Chan
Department of Microbiology, Li Ka Shing Faculty of Medicine, Queen Mary Hospital, The University of Hong Kong, Pokfulam, Hong Kong

Olga N. Ilinskaya, Vera V. Ulyanova and Dina R. Yarullina
Department of Microbiology, Kazan Federal University, Kazan, Russia

Ilgiz G. Gataullin
Department of Surgery and Oncology, Regional Clinical Cancer Center, Kazan, Russia

Saba Valadkhan
Department of Molecular Biology and Microbiology, Case Western Reserve University School of Medicine, Cleveland, OH, United States

Puri Fortes
Center for Applied Medical Research, Department of Gene Therapy and Hepatology, Navarra Institute for Health Research (IdiSNA), University of Navarra, Pamplona, Spain

Christopher J. Stewart, Daniel P. Smith, Tatiana Y. Fofanova and Joseph F. Petrosino
Alkek Center for Metagenomics and Microbiome Research, Department of Molecular Virology and Microbiology, Baylor College of Medicine, Houston, TX, United States

Nicholas D. Embleton and Janet E. Berrington
Newcastle Neonatal Service, Royal Victoria Infirmary, Newcastle upon Tyne, United Kingdom

Elizabeth Clements, Gillian Taylor, Caroline H. Orr and Stephen P. Cummings
School of Science and Engineering, Teesside University, Middlesbrough, United Kingdom

Pamela N. Luna
Department of Statistics, Rice University, Houston, TX, United States

Andrew Nelson
Faculty of Health and Life Sciences, Northumbria University, Newcastle upon Tyne, United Kingdom

Qinghui Mu, Vincent J. Tavella and Xin M. Luo
Department of Biomedical Sciences and Pathobiology, Virginia-Maryland College of Veterinary Medicine, Virginia Tech, Blacksburg, VA, United States

Nour Sherri, Noor Salloum, Carine Mouawad, Nathaline Haidar-Ahmad, Margret Shirinian and Elias A. Rahal
Department of Experimental Pathology, Microbiology, and Immunology, American University of Beirut, Beirut, Lebanon

Hyoji Kim, Hisashi Iizasa, Yuichi Kanehiro, Sintayehu Fekadu and Hironori Yoshiyama
Department of Microbiology, Faculty of Medicine, Shimane University, Shimane, Japan

Matteo Soverini, Silvia Turroni, Elena Biagi, Sara Quercia, Patrizia Brigidi, Marco Candela and Simone Rampelli
Unit of Microbial Ecology of Health, Department of Pharmacy and Biotechnology, University of Bologna, Bologna, Italy

Marco Toscano and Roberta De Grandi
Laboratory of Clinical Microbiology, Department of Biomedical Sciences for Health, University of Milan, Milan, Italy

Enzo Grossi
Villa Santa Maria Institute, Como, Italy

Lorenzo Drago
Laboratory of Clinical Microbiology, Department of Biomedical Sciences for Health, University of Milan, Milan, Italy
Clinical-Chemistry and Microbiology Lab, IRCCS Galeazzi Orthopedic Institute, University of Milan, Milan, Italy
Lazaros I. Sakkas and Dimitrios P. Bogdanos
Department of Rheumatology and Clinical Immunology, Faculty of Medicine, School of Health Sciences, University of Thessaly, Larissa, Greece

Dimitrios Daoussis and Stamatis-Nick Liossis
Division of Rheumatology, Department of Internal Medicine, Faculty of Medicine, University of Patras, Patras, Greece

Naoko Shibata
Division of Mucosal Immunology, Department of Microbiology and Immunology and International Research and Development Center for Mucosal Vaccines, The Institute of Medical Science, The University of Tokyo, Tokyo, Japan
Department of Mucosal Immunology, School of Medicine, Chiba University, Chiba, Japan
Laboratory of Vaccine Materials and Laboratory of Gut Environmental System, National Institutes of Biomedical Innovation, Health and Nutrition, Osaka, Japan

Jun Kunisawa
Division of Mucosal Immunology, Department of Microbiology and Immunology and International Research and Development Center for Mucosal Vaccines, The Institute of Medical Science, The University of Tokyo, Tokyo, Japan
Laboratory of Vaccine Materials and Laboratory of Gut Environmental System, National Institutes of Biomedical Innovation, Health and Nutrition, Osaka, Japan
Graduate School of Medicine, Graduate School of Pharmaceutical Sciences, Graduate School of Dentistry, Osaka University, Osaka, Japan
Department of Microbiology and Infectious Diseases, Kobe University Graduate School of Medicine, Kobe, Japan

Hiroshi Kiyono
Division of Mucosal Immunology, Department of Microbiology and Immunology and International Research and Development Center for Mucosal Vaccines, The Institute of Medical Science, The University of Tokyo, Tokyo, Japan
Department of Immunology, Graduate School of Medicine, Chiba University, Chiba, Japan

Ira Ekmekciu, Eliane von Klitzing, Stefan Bereswill and Markus M. Heimesaat
Intestinal Microbiology Research Group, Institute of Microbiology, Charité - Universitätsmedizin Berlin, corporate member of Freie Universität Berlin, Humboldt-Universität zu Berlin, and Berlin Institute of Health, Berlin, Germany

Petra Bacher
Department of Cellular Immunology, Clinic for Rheumatology and Clinical Immunology, Charité - Universitätsmedizin Berlin, corporate member of Freie Universität Berlin, Humboldt-Universität zu Berlin, and Berlin Institute of Health, Berlin, Germany

Christian Neumann and Alexander Scheffold
Department of Cellular Immunology, Clinic for Rheumatology and Clinical Immunology, Charité - Universitätsmedizin Berlin, corporate member of Freie Universität Berlin, Humboldt-Universität zu Berlin, and Berlin Institute of Health, Berlin, Germany
German Rheumatism Research Center, Leibniz Association, Berlin, Germany

Lorena Ruiz, Susana Delgado, Patricia Ruas-Madiedo, Borja Sánchez and Abelardo Margolles
Dairy Research Institute, Spanish National Research Council (Instituto de Productos Lácteos de Asturias - CSIC), Villaviciosa, Spain

Robert D. Stedtfeld, Tiffany M. Stedtfeld, Maggie R. Williams and Shao Xiangwen
Department of Civil and Environmental Engineering, East Lansing, MI, United States

Benli Chai, James R. Cole and James M. Tiedje
Center for Microbial Ecology, Michigan State University, East Lansing, MI, United States

Syed A. Hashsham
Department of Civil and Environmental Engineering, East Lansing, MI, United States
Center for Microbial Ecology, Michigan State University, East Lansing, MI, United States

Robert B. Crawford and Norbert E. Kaminski
Institute for Integrative Toxicology, Michigan State University, East Lansing, MI, United States
Department of Pharmacology and Toxicology, Michigan State University, East Lansing, MI, United States

Tomomi Kuwahara
Department of Molecular Bacteriology, Institute of Health Biosciences, University of Tokushima Graduate School, Tokushima, Japan

Alexei Christodoulides, Neha Gupta, Vahe Yacoubian, Neil Maithel, Jordan Parker and Theodoros Kelesidis
David Geffen School of Medicine, University of California, Los Angeles, Los Angeles, CA, United States

Elisabetta Caselli, Daria Bortolotti, Antonella Rotola, Valentina Gentili, Irene Soffritti, Maria D'Accolti, Mariangela Sicolo, Dario Di Luca and Roberta Rizzo
Section of Microbiology and Medical Genetics,
Department of Medical Sciences, University of Ferrara, Ferrara, Italy

Roberto Marci
School of Medicine, University of Geneva, Geneva, Switzerland

Giuseppe Lo Monte
Human Reproduction Centre - Brunico Hospital, Brunico, Italy

Isabel Barao
School of Medicine, University of Nevada, Reno, NV, United States

Nishat Tasnim, Nijiati Abulizi, Jason Pither, Miranda M. Hart and Deanna L. Gibson
Department of Biology, The Irving K. Barber School of Arts and Sciences, University of British Columbia, Kelowna, BC, Canada

Vandana Kaul and Carlos O. Esquivel
Division of Abdominal Transplantation, Department of Surgery, Stanford University, Stanford, CA, United States

Kenneth I. Weinberg
Division of Stem Cell Transplantation, Department of Pediatrics, Stanford University, Stanford, CA, United States

Scott D. Boyd
Department of Pathology, Stanford University, Stanford, CA, United States

Daniel Bernstein
Division of Cardiology, Department of Pediatrics, Stanford University, Stanford, CA, United States

Olivia M. Martinez and Sheri M. Krams
Division of Abdominal Transplantation, Department of Surgery, Stanford University, Stanford, CA, United States
Stanford Immunology, Stanford University School of Medicine, Stanford, CA, United States

Angélica T. Vieira
Department of Biochemistry and Immunology, Institute of Biological Sciences, Federal University of Minas Gerais, Belo Horizonte, Brazil

Paula M. Castelo and Caroline M. Ferreira
Department of Pharmaceutics Sciences, Institute of Environmental, Chemical and Pharmaceutical Sciences, Universidade Federal de São Paulo, Diadema, Brazil
Pathology Graduate Program, Universidade Federal de São Paulo, São Paulo, Brazil

Daniel A. Ribeiro
Pathology Graduate Program, Universidade Federal de São Paulo, São Paulo, Brazil
Department of Biosciences, Universidade Federal de São Paulo, Santos, Brazil

Wenjie Tang, Jingliang Liu, Yanfei Ma, Yusen Wei, Jianxin Liu and Haifeng Wang
College of Animal Science, Zhejiang University, The Key Laboratory of Molecular Animal Nutrition, Ministry of Education, Hangzhou, China

Index

www.ingramcontent.com/pod-product-compliance
Lightning Source LLC
LaVergne TN
LVHW060058220926
848484LV00008BA/2156